Speech, Language, and Hearing Programs in Schools

Speech, Language, and Hearing Programs in Schools

A Guide for Students and Practitioners

◆ ◆ ◆ ◆ ◆ ◆ ◆ ◆ ◆ ◆ ◆ ◆ ◆ ◆ ◆ ◆ ◆

Second Edition

Eileen H. Gravani

Jacqueline Meyer

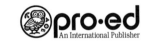
pro·ed
An International Publisher

8700 Shoal Creek Boulevard
Austin, Texas 78757-6897
800/897-3202   Fax 800/397-7633
www.proedinc.com

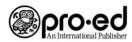

© 2007 by PRO-ED, Inc.
8700 Shoal Creek Boulevard
Austin, Texas 78757-6897
800/897-3202   Fax 800/397-7633
www.proedinc.com

Library of Congress Cataloging-in-Publication Data

Speech, language, and hearing programs in schools : a guide for students and practitioners/[edited by]
Eileen Gravani, Jacqueline Meyer.—2nd ed.
  p. cm.
  Includes bibliographical references (p.) and index
  ISBN-13: 978-1-4164-0071-4
  ISBN-10: 1-4164-0071-0 (softcover : alk. paper)
  1. Speech therapy for children.   2. Language disorders in children—Treatment.   3. Hearing disorders
in children—Treatment.   4. School health services.   I. Gravani, Eileen.   II. Meyer, Jacqueline.
  LB3454.S655 2006
  371.91′4—dc22
                                                                                          2005025071

Art Director: Jason Crosier
Designer: Nancy McKinney-Point
This book is designed in Fairfield Light and MetaPlus.

Printed in the United States of America

1 2 3 4 5 6 7 8 9 10   10 09 08 07 06

Contents

Section I
Overview of the Profession of Speech–Language Pathology in the Schools
1

Chapter 1

Educational History and Legal Landmarks ◆ *3*
Eileen H. Gravani

Chapter 2

The American Speech-Language-Hearing Association ◆ *23*
Regina B. Grantham

Section II
Core Areas of School-Based Speech–Language Pathology
51

Chapter 3

Assessment ◆ *53*
Jacqueline Meyer, with Nanette Clapper

Contributors

Helen Arvidson, PhD
Speech–Language Pathologist
Porter County Education Interlocal
Valparaiso, Indiana

Arlene Balestra-Marko, AuD
Hear 2 Learn
Syracuse, New York

Karen Browning, MEd, OTR/L
Occupational Therapist
Columbia School District
Columbia, Missouri

Li-Rong Lilly Cheng, PhD
Professor
Department of Communication
    Disorders
San Diego State University
San Diego, California

Nanette Clapper, MS, CCC-SLP
Speech–Language Pathologist-2
New York State Office of Mental
    Retardation and Developmental
    Disabilities
Syracuse, New York

Tracy Crouch, MS, CCC-SLP
Speech–Language Pathologist,
    Grades K–5
Bridgeport Elementary School
Chittenango Central School District
Chittenango, New York

Regina B. Grantham, MS
Associate Professor
Department of Speech Pathology
    and Audiology
State University of New York
    College at Cortland
Cortland, New York

Eileen H. Gravani, PhD
Assistant Professor
Department of Speech Pathology
    and Audiology
State University of New York,
    College at Cortland
Cortland, New York

Nancy P. Huffman, MS, CCC-AUD
Consultant
Retired Chair of Speech–Language
    and Audiology Services
Board of Cooperative Educational
    Services #1
Rochester, New York

Donna McGhie-Richmond, PhD
Instructor
Department of Educational
    Psychology
University of Alberta
Edmonton, Alberta, Canada

Jacqueline Meyer, MHS, CCC-SLP
Lecturer Emerita/Supervisor
Department of Speech Pathology
    and Audiology
State University of New York,
    College at Cortland
Cortland, New York

Jill Modafferi, MEd
5th Grade Teacher
Lyncourt Union Free School District
Syracuse, New York

Kim M. Nevins, PhD, LPT
Assistant Professor
Department of Physical Therapy
University of Missouri–Columbia
Columbia, Missouri

Mary Ann O'Brien, MS, CCC-SLP
Retired Director of Support Services
Board of Cooperative Educational
Services #1
Rochester, New York

Luis F. Riquelme, MS, CCC-SLP
Lecturer
Long Island University
Brooklyn, New York

Linda Robinson
Coordinator of Library and
Media Services
Mansfield Public Schools
Mansfield, Connecticut

Ralf W. Schlosser, PhD
Associate Professor
Department of Speech Pathology
and Audiology
Northeastern University
Boston, Massachusetts

Joseph Sheedy, MS, CAS
School Psychologist
Lyncourt Union Free School District
Syracuse, New York

Figures

Tables

Acknowledgments

◆ ◆

A book such as this represents the work of many people. The editors, Eileen H. Gravani and Jacqueline Meyer, thank the contributing authors who produced such valuable work—while working at their day jobs! All of them put forth the thought and effort that demonstrate their committment to their respective fields. Thanks to Regina B. Grantham, Nancy Huffman, Arlene Balestra-Marko, Nanette Clapper, Tracy Crouch, Ralf Schlosser, Donna McGhie-Richmond, Helen Arvidson, Mary Ann O'Brien, Luis Riquelme, Li-Rong Lilly Cheng, Jill Modafferi, Joseph Sheedy, Kim M. Nevins, Karen Browning, and Linda Robinson. We could not have done it without you.

We are grateful for the people behind the scenes, as well: our wonderfully supportive colleagues in the Department of Speech Pathology and Audiology at the State University of New York College at Cortland, particularly our chair, Regina Grantham, who urged us on when spirits were flagging. We thank also Suzannah Campbell, an SLP in a middle school who generously provided us with additional insights; and Marilyn Rogers, Joneen Lowman, and Marcelle Richardson, who reviewed sections of the chapter on IEPs. We thank our PRO-ED editor, Peggy Kipping, for her patience, enthusiasm, and prompt replies to yet another e-mail.

Finally, we thank our families, for their patience, for their support, for their good humor in the face of "Really, just one more hour at the computer...."

Introduction

◆ ◆

This is the second edition of *Speech, Language, and Hearing Programs in Schools: A Guide for Students and Practitioners*. Although it contains updated information, it is not simply a revised version of the first edition. In the introduction to the original text, Pamelia O'Connell, the editor, stated, "Change has been a constant but it cannot completely be captured in writing, which is language made permanent. Remember, as you read, that the guidebook is not the journey" (p. xix). True words, indeed. And prophetic, as well. The single constant in school-based practice remains change, but in the 8 years since the first edition went to press, change has occurred at an exponential rate. Whether we look at increased diagnostic and intervention requirements, expanding roles within school-based practice, newly defined federal and state standards of learning, or the integration of technology, the editors of this edition realize, as did Pamelia O'Connell before us, that we can only outline what appears true at this time. Exactly how the inevitable alterations in our day-to-day professional responsibilities play out in the future will depend on your ability and willingness to apply basic principles to the specific demands you encounter.

Updating the 1997 edition was not a straightforward task. We have remained mindful that we can be only a guide to appropriate services, and as such we were forced to make choices. We recognized, sometimes painfully so, that we cannot provide within our text an additional one exploring school-age language development. That information must be sought elsewhere. Nor can we provide answers to every question you will have when you are faced with a large and diverse caseload of students who need much help in a very limited time. We have attempted, however, to provide sources you can access to expand your own professional knowledge base. Every chapter contains a list of current references, and an appendix at the end of the text features a sampling of Web sites that can serve as a starting point to gain new information.

Some of the alterations we have effected in this edition take place within the confines of the original chapters; others have required that we add new chapters or combine and integrate previously presented information with material that existed in different places within the earlier version. Every chapter was reviewed to be sure that it reflects substantial new findings and requirements and mirrors the schools as they exist now.

We have sought to retain the features of the first edition that readers found particularly useful. As implied above, we continue the practice of multiple authorship, welcoming our authors' different voices and writing styles. Nationally, the training in our field continues to represent a generalist point of view, but clearly no two authors (or editors) possess the expertise needed to discuss every area relevant to school practice. Pam O'Connell's vision was a text for "the novice in our schools, as well as for those who may return to school services after a period of absence" (p. xix). In recent years, significant numbers of speech–language professionals have left the medical setting, some to move to school-based practice. This text provides them with a means to discern the commonalities of practice within the two sites but also affords them specific information to serve as a starting place for the transition. Its chapters not only provide a reasonably detailed portrait of the current scene, they do so within a historical perspective.

This edition replaces the original three-part organizational format of the original with four new sections: "Overview of the Profession of Speech–Language Pathology in the Schools," "Core Areas of School-Based Speech–Language Pathology," "Expanding Roles of Speech–Language Pathology in School-Based Practice," and "The Roles of Related Professionals."

The "Overview" section, Chapters 1 and 2, presents a survey of the speech–language pathologist in school-based practice; the history of that development, including the legal basis of our presence in the schools; and the increasingly important role of ASHA. Two previously separate chapters, "Legal Landmarks" and "History of School Services: Speech, Language, and Hearing" have been combined in the first chapter. The new Chapter 2, "ASHA and the Schools," has been expanded to include that organization's significantly greater focus on school issues since 1997.

"Core Areas of Speech Pathology," Chapters 3–5, constitute the central section of the book, or what Dr. O'Connell dubbed "the heart of the enterprise" (p. xxi). The updated information continues to provide a "unified perspective on the actual operation of school programs for the speech and language disordered student" (p. xxi). It takes the basic roles of the speech pathologist (assess/evaluate, develop goals, provide intervention) and applies them to school-based practice. The first of these chapters introduces a trio of case studies featuring hypothetical but representational students who are followed through Chapters 3, 4, and 5. Chapter 3, "Assessment," includes a section written by a new author who is employed as a school-based speech–language pathologist. Chapter 4, on developing the IEP, reflects the reworkings of IDEA by Congress. Chapter 5, which addresses intervention and different service delivery models, introduces two new authors, both of whom bring to the reader the benefit of their everyday experience as they grapple with the implications of evidence-based practice, new state learning standards, high-stakes testing, and additional demands under the 2004 revision and reauthorization of IDEA. Readers of the previous edition have frequently cited the continuation of the cases through three chapters as a particularly effective way to see how assessment, IEP development, and intervention are connected. This design illustrates that while assessment procedures, specific IEP goals, and intervention approaches change, basic principles remain.

"Expanding Roles," encompassing Chapters 6–10, is devoted to areas that have expanded or changed significantly since the first edition. In Chapter 6, we accept our predecessor's decision not to attempt to describe every condition represented on the caseload of the school-based SLP. The newly revised chapter instead features a brief overview of three disorders that have gained new prominence in schools since 1996: autism spectrum disorders; traumatic brain injury; and medical fragility, including conditions complicated by swallowing problems. It also presents information on the continuing expansion into educational areas once considered to be the exclusive domain of the classroom or special education teacher. Chapter 7, our second entirely new chapter, represents current information on the "hot" topics of literacy and the role of speech–language professionals in reading and writing. Chapter 8, on augmentative communication, reflects three new authors' insights into how that topic applies specifically to the school environment. Chapter 9, "Serving Culturally and Linguistically Diverse Students," reflects updated information by one of the original authors but adds two new authors who address the challenges inherent in serving additional cultural groups. Chapter 10 brings us up to date on the increasingly prevalent but sometimes thorny issues of third-party reimbursement, support personnel, and supervision.

The final section focuses on the roles of related professionals in the schools. New material on the enormous professional changes within the field of audiology, including cochlear implants, is included in Chapter 11. Chapter 12, a new addition, presents information concerning the role of other professionals in the schools whose expertise is closely related to that of the speech–language pathologist: the classroom and special education teachers, the school psychologist, the school librarian, and physical and occupational therapists. The subsections in this chapter were written by the professionals themselves.

It is our hope that the students and instructors who use this text will find it a portal into the exciting, challenging, ever expanding role of the school-based speech–language pathologist. A final word for your journey:

> The Old Man of the Earth stooped over the floor of the cave, raised a huge stone from it, and left it leaning. It disclosed a great hole that went plumb-down.
> "That is the way," he said.
> "But there are no stairs."
> "You must throw yourself in. There is no other way."
> —George MacDonald
> *The Golden Key, Dealings with the Fairies*

REFERENCES

MacDonald, G. (1999). In A. Gash, *What the dormouse said: Lessons for grown-ups from children's books*. Chapel Hill, NC: Algonquin Books of Chapel Hill.

O'Connell, P. (Ed.). (1997). *Speech, language, and hearing programs in schools: A guide for students and practitioners*. Gaithersburg, MD: Aspen.

Overview of the Profession of Speech–Language Pathology in the Schools

This section, consisting of two chapters, provides an overview of the important historical landmarks as well as the major stages of growth in the profession of speech–language pathology. It also includes a description of significant legislation and court opinions that have had an impact on school-based practice in the field. As Pamelia O'Connell stated in her introduction to the first edition of this text,

> An understanding of the past always enriches appreciation of the present and offers hints suggestive of possible futures. The direct antecedents of today's programs in speech and language lie in the early school programs of several large American cities begun in the early decades of the 20th century…. The federal legislation that was initiated in 1975 and the state laws that served as precursors to national standards for the education of children with handicapping conditions are a part of the history of school services [and represent] … an important aspect for the school professional…. [They remain the genesis of] a defining factor in the everyday operations of current school programs. (p. xx)

The history of the field of speech–language pathology also serves as a reminder that legislation enacted today and the professional actions we take during our tenure will have an impact on the practitioners and the children of the future.

REFERENCE

O'Connell, P. (Ed.). (1997). *Speech, language, and hearing programs in schools: A guide for students and practitioners.* Gaithersburg, MD: Aspen.

Chapter 1

Educational History and Legal Landmarks

Eileen H. Gravani

ccording to the *American Heritage Dictionary* (2nd edition), a law is a rule established by authority, society, or custom. In reviewing the legal history of special education, we will discuss several means of establishing the rights of handicapped children. One means is legislation. In our system of government, laws are passed at the federal, state, and local levels. Laws cannot violate the U.S. Constitution. We will be discussing federal law rather than laws of individual states because the purpose of this chapter is to provide you with an overview of the legislative history.

Another means of establishing law that has been important in the rights of handicapped children is case law. Case law involves the judicial system's resolving of disagreements between two parties: for example, between citizens or between a citizen and the government. The courts determine the facts of a disagreement and interpret the meaning of the law in light of those facts.

There are federal, state, and local court systems. The federal court system consists of three levels: trial courts, appellate courts (U.S. appeals courts), and the U.S. Supreme Court. State and local court systems also typically have these three levels. In this chapter, we will discuss some cases that resulted in important decisions in favor of the educational rights of children with special needs.

EDUCATION AND LEGISLATION PRIOR TO THE EDUCATION FOR ALL HANDICAPPED CHILDREN ACT OF 1975

To understand how the present legislation came about, it is important to understand some history. In the 19th century, not all children went to school. Children from poor families, some girls, and children in isolated rural areas often did not attend school or did so only for brief periods. School in the western frontier was typically held for approximately three months per year. There were some special schools for the deaf and blind. Often those schools were residential, not community based. There were no facilities for children with other disabilities, so often those children did not have any type of educational program.

Prior to the early 1800s, some deaf children from wealthy families were sent to Europe to be educated. In 1817, the American Asylum for the Education of the Deaf and Dumb opened in Hartford, Connecticut. It was established by Thomas Hopkins Gallaudet and taught students a system of signs. Gallaudet had studied in France with Abbé Sicard, the successor of Abbé de l'Epée. Later programs were established in New York City, Philadelphia, Kentucky, Ohio, Missouri, and Virginia. Most schools were residential and employed manual (sign) communication. One of these schools, the Columbia Institution for the Deaf and Dumb, later became Gallaudet University, the only liberal arts college for the deaf in the world.

Two Americans, Horace Mann and Samuel Howe, toured schools for the deaf in Germany and returned with an increased interest in the oral approach for deaf education. Soon after, several "oral-only" schools for the deaf were established. Differences in approach led to the "oral versus manual" controversy from 1850 to 1870. The two best-known figures in this controversy were Alexander Graham Bell and Edward Minor Gallaudet, who became the first president of Gallaudet University, named for his father Thomas Hopkins Gallaudet.

There were few educational programs for children with disabilities for several reasons. One was the general political philosophy at that time, which emphasized the rights of the majority rather than the rights of the individual. A second reason was a very narrow or limited interpretation of the definition of education. Education was seen as strictly academic: learning to read and write, do mathematics, and so forth. Other skills, such as daily living or self-help skills, speech and language, preacademics, and vocational skills, were not seen as the responsibility of the schools.

Special education programs, while not typical in the United States, were present in Germany. Following his visit to German institutions, Samuel Howe opened the first school for the severely retarded in Massachusetts in 1848.

A case that illustrates the emphasis on the general welfare is *Beattie v. State Board of Education* in 1919. The case concerned a child with normal intelligence who had cerebral palsy. The boy had attended school in a regular classroom for several years and had been able to complete the academic work. He was described as not having normal use of his overall body. His voice was affected in terms of pitch and prosody. Additionally, he drooled and had uncontrollable facial movements.

The local school board would not allow him to return to school, even though he had made adequate progress. It recommended placement in a school for the deaf because that was the only "special" program available. The parents filed a lawsuit, and the case went before the State of Wisconsin Supreme Court. The ruling favored the school district and stated that it was appropriate to exclude the child because of the depressing effect he had upon the teachers and the other children. The court also indicated that he required more of the teacher's time than most of the students. The minority opinion said that there was no proof that the boy's presence had had a harmful influence upon the rest of the class and there was no legal basis for denying education. It stated that every child has a fundamental right to attend school (*Beattie v. the State Board of Education*).

In the early 1900s, the rigid definition of education began to expand. One reason for this was the child labor laws that were passed first in states such as Massachusetts and then federally. As a result, children from poor families and children with some learning problems entered the schools. To serve these children, school districts began to supply some special services. In 1910, Chicago and Detroit became the first school districts to employ teachers to work with children who demonstrated speech problems. New York City followed in 1911. Soon, services were available in several large cities. But programs varied greatly from state to state, and no programs existed in rural areas. In the 1940s and 1950s, speech programs were available in many more cities and towns. However, services still varied greatly between states and even between different school districts. Services to rural areas were very limited.

Services for children with mental retardation were also scattered. Availability for both residential and community-based programs varied according to geographic location. *Brown v. Board of Education* (BOE) was a historic Supreme Court decision in 1954. That decision essentially stated that segregated education was inherently unequal. Until that decision, schools and other facilities were segregated under a Supreme Court ruling from 1896. In that case, *Plessy v. Ferguson,* the court found that separate facilities were acceptable.

Brown v. BOE actually concerned four cases that were consolidated and heard as one. The case was based on the equal-protection clause in section one of the Fourteenth Amendment, which says that states cannot "deny to any person within its jurisdiction the equal protection of the laws." The Supreme Court's decision indicated that segregated schools violated equal protection and denied minority students the right to an equal educational opportunity.

Brown v. BOE accomplished several things. It illustrated that the Constitution of the United States is the binding law for all government in the United States—federal, state, and local. It also was a major victory for the civil rights movement and provided the basis for school desegregation. In addition to these, it highlighted the *concept* of a right to education. This concept will be important later in decisions on cases concerning children with special needs.

Since *Brown v. BOE,* federal laws have been developed to ensure civil rights. Ten years after that decision, in 1964, the Civil Rights Act was passed. Title VI of that act has two very important components. The first mandated the federal government to withhold federal funds from institutions that excluded benefits to anyone on the basis of race, color, or national origin. The second gave the federal Office of Education the responsibility to determine whether school systems were segregated.

The 1960s have been known as the decade of the civil rights movement. Although the 1970s may be remembered as the decade that emphasized rights for handicapped individuals, there was some federal legislation in the 1960s that provided support for the education of children with disabilities. One of these was Public Law 89-313, an amendment to an education law passed in 1950. This amendment was the beginning of federal support for the education of students with special needs. It provided grant money to state agencies for students with disabilities. The money could be used for education in state-operated or state-supported schools or institutions.

In the following year, 1966, Public Law 89-750 was passed. This provided federal grant money for local school districts to educate students with special needs. This law also established the Bureau of Education for the Handicapped. Some of the purposes of the bureau were to help states to implement and evaluate programs, train teachers to work with students with special needs, and train support staff and parents. The last piece of legislation in the 1960s dealing with special education was Public Law 90-247. This expanded some special education services, established regional resource centers for special education, and established centers to serve children who were deaf or blind.

As indicated, the 1970s may be remembered as the decade that emphasized the rights of individuals with disabilities. This emphasis can be seen in the case laws and legislation that were passed. In 1971, a class-action lawsuit,

Pennsylvania Association for Retarded Children (PARC) *v. Commonwealth of Pennsylvania,* was filed on behalf of 13 children with mental retardation. At that time, Pennsylvania had a policy that children needed to have a mental age of 5 years in order to enter school. As one might predict, this resulted in the exclusion of a large percentage of mentally retarded children. Like *Brown v. BOE,* the PARC case argued from the equal protection clause of the Fourteenth Amendment. PARC also used the due process clause from the Fourteenth Amendment and the Fifth Amendment. Additionally, testimony from legal and educational experts indicated that education was necessary for a child to function in society and that all children can learn from an education. This case was resolved the following year in federal district court by a consent decree, an agreement by all the parties involved and approved by the court. It was agreed that the state and local school districts would identify all children who were excluded from school and provide all mentally retarded children with an appropriate educational program.

While the PARC case was occurring, another class-action suit was being filed in Washington, D.C. This case represented all out-of-school handicapped children who were excluded from school or expelled or suspended. It represented a less specific group than the PARC case. The case, *Mills v. Board of Education* (BOE), took its name from one of the children, Peter Mills. He was a 12-year-old who had been expelled from school as a "behavior problem." Unlike the PARC case, which resulted in an agreement and did not have a judicial ruling, *Mills v. BOE* required a court decision. The court decided against the school board and required that a list of excluded children be developed and that they be provided with a public education. A time limit was put on the BOE so that changes would occur by given dates.

Around this time, there were a variety of similar cases, and states began to pass or revise laws that required the education of all handicapped children. Legislation in Congress used two approaches. Nondiscrimination legislation was passed, as well as federal legislation concerning education. In 1973, the Rehabilitation Act of 1973 (P.L. 93-112) was passed. It dealt with discrimination against people with disabilities and protected their civil rights against discrimination in civil programs. Section 504 of this law states that "no otherwise qualified handicapped individual in the United States shall, solely by reason of his [or her] handicap, be excluded from the participation in, be denied the benefits of, or be subjected to discrimination under any program or activity receiving federal financial assistance." This means that any programs receiving federal funds need to provide equal opportunity to individuals with handicapping conditions. The provision affects school districts, colleges, universities, and employers such as state and local governments and hospitals. This law has been amended several times, and its scope has been broadened. It continues today to protect people with disabilities from discrimination. It also helps to support the Individuals with Disabilities Education Act (IDEA), passed in 1990 (reauthorized in 1997), protecting the rights of students with special needs.

Federal legislation was also passed concerning education. In 1974, Public Law 93-380 was passed. It required that states begin procedures to identify and evaluate all handicapped children, establish a goal of providing full educational opportunities for all handicapped children, and submit to the federal government a plan describing how the state would meet that goal. Other sections of the law included procedural safeguards. These dealt with the evaluation and placement of students and protected families' rights by allowing parents to examine records and, if not satisfied with an educational program, to have a hearing. This procedure is called due process. For the first time, parents and handicapped children were allowed to question a school district's decisions, using systematic procedures and guaranteed rights.

In 1975, Congress held a series of hearings to extend and amend Public Law 93-380. Information was presented by parents, special educators, and professional organizations. American Speech-Hearing Association (ASHA, now American Speech-Language-Hearing Association) involvement was substantial. ASHA members testified in Washington, D.C., and in several regional hearings. They provided input to state departments of education and sent messages to the White House.

The major findings of the hearings indicated that many children ages 3 to 21 years were not receiving appropriate services. Testimony indicated that more than 8 million children and young adults were in this age range. For many of these individuals, special education needs and needs for related services such as speech–language, physical or occupational therapy, audiology, and counseling were not being met. Many of the students who were enrolled in an educational program were not receiving appropriate services. More than 1 million of these children or young adults were excluded from public schools. Although many handicapped children were placed in regular classrooms, their disabilities prevented them from having a successful educational experience. Many families were forced to find services for their children independently. A chart summarizing the laws and key points can be found in Table 1.1.

THE EDUCATION FOR ALL HANDICAPPED CHILDREN ACT OF 1975

In the same year the hearings were held, the Education for All Handicapped Children Act of 1975 was passed. The four major purposes of the act were

1. to ensure that all handicapped children would receive a "free appropriate public education," including special education and related services to meet their needs;
2. to ensure that the rights of handicapped children and their parents would be protected through the due process procedure;
3. to evaluate the effectiveness of federal, state, and local efforts to educate handicapped children; and
4. to provide financial assistance to state and local agencies so that they could provide full educational opportunities to all handicapped children.

Table 1.1 Legislation Concerned with the Education and Rights of Children with Disabilities

Year	Law Number	Title	Primary Intent
1965	P.L. 89-313	The Elementary and Secondary Education Act Amendments of 1965	Provided grant money to state agencies for students with disabilities in state operated or supported institutions.
1966	P.L. 89-750	The Elementary and Secondary Education Act Amendments of 1966	Provided federal grant money to local school districts for the education of students with disabilities.
1968	P.L. 90-247	The Elementary and Secondary Education Act Amendments of 1968	Expanded special education services and established regional resource centers; established centers for deaf and blind students.
1973	P.L. 93-112 (Section 504 often cited)	Rehabilitation Act of 1973	Provided equal opportunity to individuals with handicapping conditions; dealt with discrimination and protected their civil rights in programs receiving federal funds.
1974	P.L. 93-380	Elementary and Secondary Education Act Amendments of 1974 (Part B)	Identified and evaluated all handicapped children; due process rights; procedural safeguards for the evaluation and placement of students.
1975	P.L. 94-142	Education for All Handicapped Children (EHA)	Provided free appropriate public education for all children with handicaps; due process rights; federal money.
1986	P.L. 99-457	Education of the Handicapped Amendments Law	Provided funding for education of preschool children with disabilities; assisted states in program development for infants and toddlers.
1990	P.L. 101-476	Individuals with Disabilities Education Act (renamed EHA as IDEA)	Reauthorized and expanded services for children with disabilities; mandated transition services; added autism and traumatic brain injury to list of categories.
1990	P.L. 101-336	Americans with Disabilities Act (ADA)	Prohibited discrimination against individuals with disabilities for employment, public accommodations and services, telecommunications, etc.
1991	P.L. 102-119	Individuals with Disabilities Education Act Amendments of 1992	Reauthorized services for infants and toddlers.
1997	P.L. 105-17	IDEA Amendments of 1997	Reauthorization of IDEA, encouraged parent involvement; emphasized access to general curriculum.
2004	P.L. 108-446	Individuals with Disabilities Education Improvement Act	Reauthorized and revised IDEA, made changes in IEPs, personnel standards, and other items.

Some basic elements in the act's phrase *free appropriate public education* (FAPE) are extremely important to educational programs. We will discuss them to gain a better understanding of later court cases and the guidelines that school districts follow. The word *free* here means that the service is provided at no cost to the parent. This includes room and board if that is deemed appropriate. Currently, school districts are billing Medicare, HMOs, and private insurance companies for reimbursable services such as audiological evaluations, physical and occupational therapy, speech–language services, and mental health services. (Third-party payments will be discussed in Chapter 10.) Parents are not billed for services.

Another term that needs to be discussed is the word *appropriate*. This means that the special education program and related services provided for handicapped students must meet their needs as adequately as the needs of nonhandicapped students are met. It is clear from this statement that there can be a difference between ideal services and appropriate services. How is it possible to determine what is "appropriate"?

One measure of appropriateness is that the student must be able to benefit from the program and acquire some minimum skills so that the education is considered meaningful. An early case concerned with this issue was *Fialkowski v. Shapp* in 1975. The case involved two brothers who were mentally retarded, with the intellectual level of preschoolers. They were placed in a classroom that emphasized reading and writing. Their lawyer argued that they were not able to find their classroom experience meaningful. We will see this issue of a meaningful education and determining whether a student is demonstrating progress in later cases. To determine what a child's needs are and to document progress, an evaluation must occur. This evaluation needs to consider all areas of suspected disability. Following this evaluation, an educational program with goals is developed. To determine progress, reevaluations need to occur. When hearing officers in due process procedures or courts review information to determine whether placements are appropriate, records documenting evaluations, goals, reevaluations, progress in the general education curriculum, and interactions with nondisabled students are carefully reviewed.

The *least restrictive environment* (LRE) is a key concept relating to the Education for All Handicapped Children Act and to later legislation and cases. According to the law, children with handicapping conditions should be educated with nonhandicapped children to the maximum extent possible. If the nature or the severity of the handicap prevents achievement in a regular classroom, special schools are allowed. The actual wording of the law will be included when we discuss IDEA and its reauthorization.

Because of the immense amount of planning, preparation, and paperwork involved, the Education for All Handicapped Children Act was not implemented until 1978. President Gerald Ford, who signed the legislation, was concerned that it "promised more than the federal government could deliver" (Weiner, 1985, p. 20).

The act resulted in the creation of new programs in special education and the revamping of existing programs. It has continued to have bipartisan support in Congress. In 1982, the Reagan administration proposed a series of revisions that would have weakened the guarantees of the act. Strong negative public response resulted in those proposals being dropped.

The Education of the Handicapped Amendments of 1986 (P.L. 99-457) amended the Education for All Handicapped Children Act of 1975. These amendments had two major purposes. The first was to provide funding for the education of eligible preschool children with disabilities, age 3 to 5 years. The second was to assist states in developing programs for infants and toddlers with disabilities, focusing on early intervention for these children. Public Law 102-119 in 1991 reauthorized these services. We will discuss the procedures used for infants and toddlers (birth to 2 years 11 months) and preschool children (age 3 to 5 years) in Chapter 4.

The Education for All Handicapped Children Act was amended again in 1990. At this time, its name changed to the Individuals with Disabilities Education Act. IDEA has been expanded in several areas. One of these areas is *transition services,* which are now part of Individualized Educational Programs (IEPs). According to IDEA (1990), transition services begin when a student is 15 or 16 years old. Their purpose is to facilitate transition into the community. They will be discussed in more detail in Chapter 4. Because transition services are now mandated, social work and rehabilitation counseling are included under "related services." Another area that IDEA affects is assistive technology. This includes computers and electronic communication boards for augmentative communication. Additionally, changes in the law provide more services and rights to individuals with autism and traumatic brain injury.

Like other legislation that has a time component, IDEA must be periodically reauthorized. Written comments from the public are requested in the *Federal Register*. For the reauthorization in 1997, organizations such as ASHA presented oral and written testimony to Congress. Parents, people with disabilities, and members of ASHA and other organizations maintained pressure on Congress to support IDEA reauthorization. Phone calls, e-mail messages, letters, and telegrams were sent by supporters of IDEA.

REAUTHORIZATION OF IDEA

Following 3 years of debate and information gathering, IDEA was reauthorized as P.L. 105-17 for 5 years when President Clinton signed the 1997 IDEA Amendments into law on June 4, 1997. After that, the U.S. Department of Education worked on regulations to provide interpretation and guidance for the next 2 years. Some of the significant changes include the following:

- increased IEP emphasis on accessing the general education and general education curriculum with appropriate aids and services;
- inclusion of students with special needs in assessments at the state and district levels;
- emphasis on evaluation considering a variety of assessment tools and means to gather relevant information that will assist in identifying the educational needs of the child (IDEA Amendments of 1997);

- increased parent participation in eligibility and placement decisions;
- inclusion in an IEP of an explanation of the amount of time that a child will not be participating in the general education curriculum with nondisabled children; and
- mediation on a voluntary basis for parent–school controversies.

Although some of the implementations have changed, been clarified, or expanded, the basic ideas behind IDEA have not changed. According to the current law, least restrictive environment specifies

1. that to the maximum extent appropriate, children with disabilities, including children in public or private institutions or other care facilities, must be educated with children who are not disabled; and
2. that special classes, separate schooling, or other removal of children with disabilities from the regular educational environment may occur only when the nature or severity of the handicap is such that education in regular classes with the use of supplementary aids and services cannot be achieved satisfactorily. (34 C.F.R. Sec. 300.550)

To educate students with special needs in the least restrictive environment means that districts need to have a *continuum of placements* available, as well as procedures to ensure that these students are educated with students without disabilities to the maximum extent possible.

Implementation of IDEA

The U.S. Office of Special Education and Rehabilitation Services (OSERS) responds to letters from interested parties and gives information and guidance on the implementation of IDEA. An example of this was the response to a congressman in the U.S. House of Representatives from South Carolina, John M. Spratt. He had questioned the policy of inclusion of a student with special needs in general education classes if it was against the parents' wishes. OSERS responded that a regular (or general) education classroom in a local school should be the first option when a placement decision is made for a student with disabilities. The letter noted that placement in a more restrictive setting should be made only on the basis of the educational needs of the child, and that IDEA regulations include parent involvement in the development of the IEP (OSERS, 1994).

IDEA and the Least Restrictive Environment

At times it seems that the benefits of the least restrictive environment need to be compared against a specialized program with possibly more services. Because each child has individual needs and abilities, each case needs to be considered individually. However, some general principles can be followed. The Fifth Circuit Court of Appeals developed a set of criteria or "test" to determine if a school district had fulfilled its obligation to educate students with disabilities in the least restrictive environment. This was done in response to a case that it heard in 1989. The case, *Daniel R.R. v. State Board of Education,* concerned a child with Down syndrome with the classification of mentally retarded. The boy had been in a general education classroom for part of the day. He had not taken part in the classroom activities and had not mastered skills that were part of the classroom program. The school district planned to place him in a special education class. The court held that the special education class was appropriate and that this placement did not violate the least restrictive environment stipulation. The three-judge appeals court developed a two-part test to determine if a school district had attempted to educate students with special needs as much as possible with students without disabilities. The first question is, Can education in the general education classroom be achieved when supplementary aids and services are provided? If it cannot be achieved at a satisfactory level, then the second question is posed: Was the student mainstreamed to the maximum extent possible? In this case, the school district had supplied a continuum of placements and had provided supplementary aids and services, attempting to maintain Daniel in a general education class. The court noted that the school district had provided mainstreaming for Daniel to the maximum extent possible.

The Fifth Circuit Court of Appeals instructed lower courts to consider five factors:

1. the student's ability to comprehend and learn the general classroom curriculum;
2. the type and severity of the disability;
3. the impact that the student's presence would have upon the general education classroom;
4. the student's experiences with mainstream settings; and
5. the extent of contact that the student with special needs would have with students without disabilities.

This two-part test has become a standard in cases involving the LRE. Some of the recent decisions have supported separate settings; others have supported education for some students with special needs within general education (Osborne & Dimatta, 1994).

Oberti v. Board of Education (1993) concerned an 8-year-old boy with Down syndrome. The School District Child Study Team initially recommended a segregated special education class when he was entering the public schools. His parents visited the available classes and rejected them. The school district and the parents then agreed that his IEP for the 1989–1990 school year would include placement in a developmental kindergarten in his neighborhood school for the morning and a special education class in another school district in the afternoon. There were issues with his behavior in the developmental kindergarten class, and the teacher sought input from the Child Study Team and the school psychologist; however, the IEP provided no plan. Similar behavior problems did not occur in the afternoon special education class.

For the 1990–1991 school year, the Child Study Team proposed a segregated special education classroom in a different district. The parents objected and asked that their son be placed in a regular education class in his home school. The district refused, and the parents filed for a due process hearing. Mediation resulted in placement in a special education class for multiply handicapped in another school district. The home school district promised to explore mainstreaming in that district and to consider a placement in a regular kindergarten class in his home district. During the first semester, the child made academic progress, but by December, there were no plans to mainstream him, and he had no meaningful contact with students in regular education. In January 1991, the parents filed a request for another due process hearing. At the first hearing, the hearing officer found that the least restrictive environment was the special education class. The parents filed a civil action in U.S. District Court under IDEA and Section 504 of the Rehabilitation Act of 1973. In 1992, after a 3-day bench trial where new evidence was presented, the district court found that "the School District had failed to establish by a preponderance of the evidence that [the student] could not at that time be educated in a regular classroom with supplementary aids and services" (*Oberti v. Board of Education,* 1993, p. 6). One of the primary issues was the lack of related services and supplementary aids during his placement in the developmental kindergarten. The school district appealed, but the U.S. Court of Appeals, Third Circuit, affirmed the district court's findings and supported the parents. Its decision notes that the hearing officer based the decision on information about the child's behavior problems "without proper consideration of the inadequate level of supplementary aids and services provided by the School District" (*Oberti v. Board of Education,* 1993, p. 18).

One of the court decisions that stressed contact with children without disabilities was *Greer v. Rome City School District* (1990). Christy Greer, a 9-year-old girl with Down syndrome, had been mainstreamed into a kindergarten program for 3 years rather than placed in a separate special education classroom. The court supported the kindergarten placement, noting that the child had made some progress and that she was not disruptive in the classroom. The court did note that although the placement was appropriate at this time, it might not continue to be appropriate in future years. The court also noted that Rome City School District did not consider a range of supplementary aids and services or attempt to modify the classroom curriculum to meet Christy's needs. Additionally, the IEP was developed before the IEP meeting, and a continuum of placement options was not discussed.

Another case, *O'Toole v. Olathe District Schools Unified School District No. 233,* concerned FAPE. The child, M, was diagnosed at age 2½ years with a moderate to severe sensorineural hearing loss in the right ear and a moderate to profound hearing loss in the left ear. In fall 1988, she entered the hearing-impaired program, and an IEP was developed. The case centered on the adequacy of the IEP developed in February 1993 and amended in August 1993. After the IEP meeting in February, the father received a copy of the IEP and agreed to continue the placement. In June 1993, M was evaluated at Central Institute for the Deaf (CID) in Missouri, and learning problems in addition to the hearing impairment were identified. In August, the IEP was changed, with the recommendation for M to remain at the elementary school. The parents disagreed, terminated services, and enrolled their daughter at CID. When the parents' request for tuition reimbursement was denied, they requested a due process hearing. The hearing officer found that the IEP was adequate, that M was making academic progress, and that the degree of progress did not equate with denial of FAPE. The parents appealed, and the reviewing officer affirmed most of the hearing officer's findings. However, the IEP for 1993 was at issue. The parents appealed to the federal district court, which found that M's IEP was adequate (for present levels of performance, annual goals, short-term objectives, and specified related services). The parents appealed based on the claims that M was denied a FAPE and that the IEPs were inadequate. The U.S. Court of Appeals, Tenth Circuit, upheld the district court's decision, stating that the IEP was reasonably designed for M's educational benefit. A previous case was cited in the decision: "As we have said, the 'appropriate' education required by the Act is not one which is guaranteed to maximize the child's potential" (*Johnson v. Independent School District No. 4*).

IDEA and Appropriate Education

IDEA does not employ specific guidelines for defining FAPE. The definition of *appropriate* has been the focus of a variety of cases. The Supreme Court in *Board of Education v. Rowley* (1982) held that although an IEP does not need to maximize a disabled student's potential, it must provide meaningful access to education and confer educational benefit. In *Polk v. Central Susquehana Intermediate Unit 16* (1988), the Third Circuit Court of Appeals noted that IDEA "calls for more than a trivial educational benefit" and requires that IEPs provide "significant learning" with "meaningful benefit." In *Ridgewood Board of Education v. N.E.* (1999), the Third Circuit Court of Appeals cited the above case and noted that the student's intellectual potential must be considered in deciding "significant learning." It also noted that the *Rowley* and *Polk* decisions support a "student-by-student analysis that carefully considers the student's individual abilities" for deciding FAPE (p. 11).

It is clear that these court decisions do not require that all students with special needs be educated in general education classrooms. School districts need to make an effort to provide general education programs using supplemental aids and services for a student with special needs. If the program does not meet the student's needs in terms of academic progress and social interaction, or if the student is disruptive and affects the other students' education negatively, the school district is justified in placing the student in a more restrictive setting (Etscheidt & Bartlett, 1999). The courts have also indicated that school districts may consider cost. An example of this is the four-part test used by the U.S. Court of Appeals for the Ninth Circuit, which said, in considering the LRE, the following need to be considered: (a) the educational benefits related to a student's placement in a regular class when provided with appropriate aids and services compared with benefits of a special education class; (b) the nonacademic benefits of peer interaction with nondisabled students; (c) the effects of the disabled student upon the students in the class and the teacher; and (d) the cost of mainstreaming the child with a disability (*Board of Education v. Rachel H.,* 1994).

The least restrictive environment and the definition of *appropriate* will continue as issues. Another issue that relates to funding is the definition of highest standard requirements for qualified providers. This issue may be dealt with in legislation rather than through litigation. However, the wording for IDEA (2004) concerning highly qualified providers may be a source of litigation. Parental choice over educational placements will continue to be an issue, particularly with private schools. Additionally, the definition of related services for medically fragile students has been an issue (Katsiyannis & Yell, 2000). Finally, schools will need to be in compliance with the Americans with Disabilities Act of 1990.

Litigation Related to Special Education

In reviewing litigation related to special education, researchers noted that the amount of litigation had increased. Typical concerns related to litigation are

- procedural issues,
- liability and negligence actions,
- civil rights violations,
- responsibility for funding of special education,
- least restrictive environment, and
- free appropriate public education (Peters-Johnson, 1995).

A review of 414 published court cases between 1975 and 1995, with 84% of the cases after 1982, indicated that placement was the primary issue in 63% of the cases, with parents favoring a more restrictive setting in approximately 75% of the cases. The appropriateness of the IEP (for issues not related to placement) was an issue in 15% of the cases. Following due process hearings, 60% of the decisions favored the school districts, and 32% favored the parents. Following appeal to state or federal courts (state, federal district courts, and circuit court of appeals), decisions favored the school districts 49% of the time and the parents 41% of the time. For 52.5% of the cases, there was no change from the decisions made at the due process hearings (Newcomer & Zurkel, 1999). Another analysis of due process cases looked at procedural violations. These included lack of adequate notice for IEP meetings, incorrect administration of tests or tests administered by unqualified personnel, IEP goals that were too broad or not meaningful, and failure to provide needed services (Yell & Drasgow, 2000).

IDEA and Reports to Congress

When IDEA was reauthorized in 1997, Congress required the U.S. Department of Education to "undertake a national assessment of activities carried out under the act (Section 674(b))." As a result, there is an annual report to Congress on IDEA implementation and status. In 2002, the findings of the *Twenty-Fourth Annual Report to Congress on the Implementation of the Individuals with Disabilities Act* included the following:

- an increase in the graduation rate for students with disabilities (56.2% in 1999–2000 from 51.9% in 1993–1994);
- a decrease in drop-out rates for students with disabilities as a general group and in most of the categories of disabilities (especially speech–language impairments, specific learning disabilities, orthopedic impairments, hearing impairments, and emotional disturbance);
- inclusion of the majority of students served by IDEA in the categories of specific learning disabilities, speech–language impairment, mental retardation, and emotional disturbance.

The report also notes concerns, such as

- increasing state accountability,
- fostering parental involvement, and
- developing procedures for effective transitions from schools to adult life.

Reauthorization of IDEA

On December 3, 2004, President George W. Bush signed P.L. 108-446, the Individuals with Disabilities Education Improvement Act. Most of the provisions for this law went into effect on July 1, 2005. A few parts were effective immediately. These include changes in the highest qualified special education teacher provisions and the establishment of a National Center for Special Education Research. Some of the changes that became effective in July 2005 include a change in the definition of learning disabilities, more of an emphasis on prevention, and some changes in IEPs. The law also allows the Department of Education to grant waivers of some of the regulatory requirements for 15 states, for a maximum of 4 years. These waivers are an effort to reduce the amount of paperwork and time spent on noninstructional tasks. ASHA has expressed concerns over the wording of the proposed regulations for IDEA (2004). Two of the specific concerns are provision of related services to children with cochlear implants and assessment of children learning English as a second language (ASHA, 2005).

NO CHILD LEFT BEHIND ACT OF 2001

A recent piece of legislation that has had an impact in the schools is the No Child Left Behind Act of 2001 (NCLB), which was signed into law on January 8, 2002. The goal of this act is that each child meet the highest standards possible. The principle components of NCLB are requirements for

- accountability and yearly progress to be reported by states, initially for math and reading/language arts/English, with science to be added later;
- the use of teaching and intervention based upon scientific research;
- parental options for education; and
- increased local control.

NCLB requires that teachers in core academic areas (English/reading/language arts, math, science, history, civics/government, geography, economics, the arts, and foreign language) must be "highly qualified" by the end of the 2005–2006 school year (ASHA, 2004a). Each state can develop a definition of *highly qualified* that is in agreement with NCLB's list of minimum qualifications. In general, a teacher who is highly qualified

- has earned a bachelor's degree,
- has obtained full state certification (not emergency certification) and licensure, and
- demonstrates competency.

The emphasis on highly qualified teachers is based upon studies that link teacher quality to student performance (ASHA, 2004a). The purpose of NCLB is to ensure that students who are members of minority groups or low income "are not taught disproportionately by inexperienced, unqualified or out-of-field teachers" (Radicia & Glimpse, 2004). The overall goal for NCLB is that by 2014, all students must be proficient in core academic areas (Council for Exceptional Children, 2005).

States must set annual performance goals for schools. These goals are based on the percentage of students who have shown proficiency on state assessments. Each school has goals for yearly progress related to student performance. Schools' goals are outlined according to each student subgroup. Subgroups are based upon race or ethnicity, migrant status, limited proficiency in English status, economically disadvantaged status, and special education needs. One of the requirements for testing is that students with limited English proficiency must be tested in English for assessment in language arts/reading/

English if they have attended school for three consecutive years in the U.S. (ASHA, 2004b).

By the 2005–2006 school year, states must assess students (Grades 3–6, 7, & 9) in math and reading/language arts. Students in high school (Grades 10–12) must be assessed once. By the 2007–2008 school year, states must assess students in science at least one time during elementary, middle, and high school. Ninety-five percent of the students in a school district must take the assessments. One percent of the students are allowed to have alternative assessments. Each school district and state must produce an annual report (report card) regarding their progress on the goals.

A great deal of controversy has surrounded NCLB, the mandated assessment and reporting of annual yearly progress. Lawsuits have been filed by several states against the U.S. Department of Education (Council for Exceptional Children, 2005). In response to concerns by states, the U.S. Department of Education indicated that states may apply to the Department of Education to use alternate assessments for an addional 2% of their students. More than 30 states have applied and received permission for the additional 2% option (Council for Exceptional Children, 2005).

Conley and Hinchman (2004) noted that much of the research and policy making related to NCLB is focused upon early literacy. However, there continues to be a crisis in adolescent literacy. They encourage a focus on literacy from preschool through elementary, middle, and high school.

CONCLUSION

Legislation related to serving children with special needs has had a significant impact on their lives, their families, and the professionals who work with them. In the *Twenty-Fourth Annual Report to Congress on the Implementation of the Individuals with Disabilities Education Act,* the Office of Special Education Programs noted that 5,775,722 children (6 to 21 years of age) were being served, and that 95.9% of those children were being educated in regular school buildings (1999–2000 school year). Additionally, in 2000–2001, over 599,678 preschool children (3 to 5 years of age) with disabilities were served.

Recently, No Child Left Behind has had a significant impact upon school and assessment. Clearly, legislation and court decisions will continue to affect services provided to children with special needs in the future. The No Child Left Behind Act is scheduled for reauthorization in 2007. As with IDEA, input from professional organizations, states, school districts, and parents will be important. It is very likely that in your own professional careers, you will see a variety of changes occur.

IDEA was reauthorized in 2004, and the proposed regulations were published in the *Federal Register* (U.S. Department of Education, 2005). Public hearings were held in the summer of 2005 (providing the 75-day comment period required by law) concerning these proposed regulations.

STUDY QUESTIONS

1. How did the U.S. political philosophy and definition of education in the 1800s affect special education services?
2. What provided the basis of civil rights legislation and legislation for special education?
3. What were the four major purposes of Public Law 94-142?
4. What are the two areas in which IDEA (P.L. 101-407) expanded services to special needs students?
5. What is the least restrictive environment? Why is the LRE often the issue in due process hearings and legal cases? Why is the LRE decided on a "case-by-case" basis?
6. What is "appropriate" in FAPE? How can it be determined?
7. What rights and recourses do parents have in the due process procedure?
8. What is the purpose of the No Child Left Behind Act?
9. What is one aspect of IDEA that P.L. 108-446 has changed?

REFERENCES

American Speech-Language-Hearing Association. (2004a). *No Child Left Behind Act: Fact sheet of highly qualified provider.* Retrieved July 20, 2005, from http://www.asha.org/about/legislation-advocacy/federal/nclb/NCLBfactsheetonhighlyqualifiedprovider.htm

American Speech-Language-Hearing Association. (2004b). No Child Left Behind (NCLB). Retrieved on September 5, 2005 from http://www.asha.org/about/legislation-advocay/federal/nclb/exec-summary.htm

American Speech-Language-Hearing Association. (2005). *2005 IDEA Proposed Rules on Part B and Part D.* Retrieved on September 5, 2005 from http://www.asha.org/about/legislation-advocacy/federal/idea/prelim-ideaB-D.htm?print=1

Americans with Disabilities Act of 1990. (1990). Public Law 101-336.

Beattie v. State Board of Education of the City of Antigo, 169 Wis. 231, 172 N.W. 153 (1919).

Board of Education v. Rachel H., 14 F. 3rd 1398 (9th Cir. 1994).

Board of Education v. Rowley, 458 U.S. 176, 203 (1982).

Brown v. Board of Education, 347 U.S. 483 (1954).

Civil Rights Act of 1964. (1964). Public Law 88-352.

Conley, M. W., & Hinchman, K. A. (2004). No child left behind: What it means for U.S. adolescents and what we can do about it. *Journal of Adolescent & Adult Literacy, 48,* 42–50.

Council for Exceptional Children. (2005). *NCLB under siege.* Retrieved on September 5, 2005, from http://www.cec.sped.org/bk/cectoday/summer_2005/NCLB_print.html

Daniel R.R. v. State Board of Education, 874 F.2d 1036, 53 Ed.Law Rep. 824 (5th Cir. 1989).

Education of All Handicapped Children Act. (1975). Public Law 94-142.

Education of the Handicapped Act Amendments of 1986. (1986). Public Law 99-457.

Etscheidt, S. K., & Bartlett, L. (1999). The IDEA amendments: A four-step approach for determining supplementary aide and services. *Exceptional Children, 66,* 163–174.

Fialkowski v. Shapp, 405 F. Supp. 946 (E.D. Pa. 1975).

Greer v. Rome City School District, 762 F. Supp. 936, 67 Ed.Law Rep. 666 (N.D.Ga. 1990); affirmed 905 F.2d 688, 71 Ed. Law Rep. 647 (11th Cir. 1991); withdrawn 956 F.2d 1025, 73 Ed.Law.

IDEA Amendments of 1997. (1998). *National Dissemination Center for Children with Disabilities (NICHCY) News Digest, 26.* Retrieved July 20, 2005, from http://www.nichcy.org

Individuals with Disabilities Education Act Amendments of 1990. (1990). Public Law 102-119.

Individuals with Disabilities Education Act of 1997. (1997). Public Law 101-336.

Individuals with Disabilities Education Improvement Act of 2004. (2004). Public Law 108-446.

Johnson v. Independent School District No. 4, 921 F. 2nd 1022, 1027 (10th Cir. 1990).

Katsiyannis, A., & Yell, M. L. (2000). The Supreme Court and school health services: Cedar Rapids v. Garret F. *Exceptional Children, 67,* 317–326.

Mills v. Board of Education, 348 F. Supp. 866 (D.D.C. 1972).

Newcomer, J. R., & Zurkel, P. A. (1999). An analysis of judicial outcomes of special education cases. *Exceptional Children, 66,* 469–480.

No Child Left Behind Act of 2001. (2001). Public Law 107-110.

Oberti v. Board of Education, 995 F. 2d 1204 (3rd Cir. 1993).

Office of Special Education and Rehabilitation Services. (1994). Letter to Spratt. *Individuals with Disabilities Education Law Report, 20,* 1457–1459.

Osborne, Jr., A. G., & Dimatta, P. (1994). The IDEA's least restrictive environment mandate: Legal implications. *Exceptional Children, 61,* 6–14.

O'Toole v. Olathe District Schools Unified School District No. 233, 97-3125, 1988 WL 251193 (10th Cir. May 19, 1998).

Pennsylvania Association for Retarded Children v. Commonwealth of Pennsylvania, 343 F. Supp. 279 (E.D. Pa. 1972).

Peters-Johnson, C. (1996). Action: School services. *Language, Speech, & Hearing Services in Schools, 27,* 188–189.

Peters-Johnson, C. (1995). Action: School services. *Language, Speech, & Hearing Services in the Schools, 26,* 101.

Plessy v. Ferguson, 163 U.S. 537 (1896).

Polk v. Central Susquehana Intermediate Unit 16, 853 F. 2d. 171, 177 (3rd Cir. 1988).

Radicia, C., & Glimpse, C. (2004). *NICHCY connections . . . to the No Child Left Behind Act.* Retrieved August 15, 2005 from the National Dissemination Center for Children with Disabilities Web site: http://www.nichcy.org/resources/default.asp#az18

Rehabilitation Act of 1973. (1973). Public Law 93-112.

Ridgewood Board of Education v. N.E., 172 F. 3d. 238 (3rd Cir. 1999).

Smith, S. W. (2001). Involving parents in the IEP process. *ERIC Clearinghouse on Disabilities and Gifted Education.* (Eric EC Digest #E611). Retrieved on September 5, 2005 from http://ericec.org/digests/e611.htm

Snyder, N., Diggs, C., Whitmire, K., Karr, S., Clarke, C., & Franklin, R. (2005, January 18). IDEA Reauthorization signed into law. *ASHA Leader, 10,* 1, 22.

Twenty-Fourth Annual Report to Congress on the Implementation of the Individuals with Disabilities Education Act. (2002). Office of Special Education Programs. Retrieved on August 17, 2005 from http://www.ed.gov/about/reports/annual/osep/2002/index.htm

U.S. Department of Education. 34 CFR Parts 300, 301, 304: Assistance to States for the Education of Children with Disabilities: Preschool Grants for Children with Disabilities; and Service Obligations under Special Education—Personnel Development to Improve Services and Results for Children with Disabilities; Proposed Rule. *Federal Register.* Vol. 70, No. 118, June 21, 2005, 35862–35892.

Weiner, R. (1985). *P.L. 94-142: Impact on the schools.* Arlington, VA: Capitol.

Yell, M. L., & Drasgow, E. (2000). Litigating a free appropriate public education: The Lovaas hearings and cases. *The Journal of Special Education, 33,* 205–214.

Chapter 2

◆◆◆◆◆◆◆◆◆◆◆◆◆◆◆◆◆◆◆◆◆◆◆◆◆◆

The American Speech-Language-Hearing Association

Regina B. Grantham

This chapter presents an overview of the American Speech-Language-Hearing Association (ASHA). It discusses the association's history, purpose, governance, membership, standards, code of ethics, guidelines, benefits, and support of school services. Continuing education, special interests divisions, and preferred practices are some of the topics of interest to school-based speech–language pathologists. This information is a valuable resource for practitioners and students in the professions of speech–language pathology and audiology.

ASHA HISTORY

ASHA is a national nonprofit scientific credentialing organization for professionals in the area of speech–language pathology and audiology. It has governing documents such as by-laws, a code of ethics, and parliamentary rules and procedures (ASHA, 2001c, 2001e).

Initially, ASHA was called the American Academy of Speech Correction (AASC). Membership was restricted to members of a related group, the National Association of Teachers of Speech (NATS), who met specific requirements. As the professions grew, the Academy of Speech Correction underwent several name changes. In 1927, it was renamed the American Society for the Study of Speech Disorders (ASSSD), and in 1934, it was renamed the American Speech Correction Association (ASCA). It changed to the American Speech and Hearing Association (ASHA) in 1947. This new name recognized the rapid growth in aural rehabilitation. In 1978, the name was changed again to the American Speech-Language-Hearing Association, but the acronym ASHA was retained. This change recognized the treatment and evaluation of communication disorders in the area of language (Malone, 1999; Paden, 1970). In November of 1995, the association voted to change its name to the American Association of Speech-Language Pathology and Audiology, effective January 1, 1997. This name change acknowledged the profession of audiology. However, because of ASHA's well-established name politically and professionally, this resolution was quickly rescinded. The name of the association remains the American Speech-Language-Hearing Association, with ASHA as its acronym (Malone, 1999).

ASHA PURPOSE

Although ASHA has undergone many name changes, its basic purpose has remained intact: commitment to scientific work in communication disorders. To acknowledge the dynamic nature of the field, the purpose has expanded and now includes stimulating the scientific study of communication, with special reference to speech, language, and hearing; encouraging and promoting appropriate clinical and academic preparation for the professions of speech–language pathology and audiology; maintaining the current knowledge and skills of those within the discipline; promoting the study and prevention of disorders; fostering improvement of services and procedures that address communication disorders; advocating for the rights and interests of people with these disorders; stimulating, distributing, and encouraging the exchange of information; and advancing the interests of the profession and members of the association (ASHA, 1997b, 1997c, 2002b).

The association's mission is to advocate for people with communication disorders and to provide the very highest quality of service for and promote the interests of those in the professions of speech–language pathology, audiology, and speech and hearing science (ASHA, 2001b, 2001e).

ASHA GOVERNANCE

ASHA has a shared governing structure that involves its members in the decision-making process. The Legislative Council (LC) and the Executive Board (EB) share this governance. Both LC and EB are elected by the association membership and therefore serve and are accountable to the membership. LC and EB provide strategic plans and direction as well as developing priorities for annual and multiple years. ASHA committees, boards, and councils make policy recommendations to LC and EB (ASHA, 2002d).

Legislative Council

The role of the Legislative Council is to establish association policies, subject to ratification by the EB. The LC also has the following responsibilities: approve the association's position statements and guidelines; identify member issues and concerns and recommend Focused Initiatives that arise from these issues and concerns; review EB progress reports and inform the membership about the reports; approve the budget; approve any changes in membership categories; approve dues; approve the Code of Ethics and any amendments; approve publications when appropriate; and initiate and approve amendments to the by-laws.

Presently, the LC consists of 150 voting members of the association. They are elected by ASHA members within each state and the District of Columbia, ASHA members who live outside the United States, and representatives from the National Student Speech-Language-Hearing Association (NSSLHA). The speaker of the council is charged with presiding over the business meetings of LC. LC is divided into subgroups called assemblies: the Audiology/Hearing Science Assembly and the Speech–Language Pathology/Speech or Language Science Assembly. LC members (legislative councilors) individually determine the assembly with which they wish to affiliate. The assemblies vote on resolutions and issues that relate to their profession or discipline area. The resolutions passed by each assembly go directly to the EB for ratification. The assemblies provide reports of their actions to the total LC. Resolutions that are not unique to a specific assembly (not discipline-specific issues) are addressed by all members of the LC.

Contacting the legislative councilors in their state and sharing concerns and issues is an ASHA member's way of providing input, making his or her thoughts known to the association. Names of legislative councilors can be found at ASHA's Web site. The legislative councilors are listed by state and by assembly. ASHA members also can present their concerns, questions, issues, and comments by addressing the Membership Forum during ASHA's biannual (spring and fall) meetings. A caucus may be formed. An ASHA member may also address issues of concern in writing, by letter, e-mail, or fax. The expression of ideas and opinions of ASHA members to legislative councilors ensures that the LC appropriately represents and serves its constituents (ASHA, 2000b, 2001e, 2002b, 2002c, 2003h).

ASHA members are encouraged to become legislative councilors. The annual Call for Nominations for Legislative Councilors is noted in the *ASHA Leader* and on the ASHA Web site. ASHA members may nominate themselves. A slate is prepared consisting of the highest-ranked nominees for the available seats from a particular state. Candidates who receive the largest number of votes are designated as duly elected legislative councilors. Legislative councilors represent the association in their state as well as ASHA members of their state. They must be able to receive and integrate information as well as be knowledgeable about ASHA, their state issues, and the will and concerns of ASHA members of their state. During face-to-face meetings in Washington, D.C., legislative councilors also visit senators and representatives of their state to provide information about the professions of speech–language pathology and audiology, as well as speech science. The legislative councilors also lobby for specific legislation that is appropriate for people with communication disorders and the professions that help them. To assist with these responsibilities, the LC provides orientations to help legislative councilors understand the processes and expectations of the position (ASHA, 2002c, 2003h).

Executive Board

The Executive Board directs and supervises the association in collaboration with the LC. It actively pursues the objectives of the association in accordance with programs and policies established by the LC and the ASHA by-laws. EB responsibilities also include providing the ASHA executive director with annual and multiple-year priorities so that implementation strategies, work plans, and budgets can be identified; deciding on Focus Initiatives that have been recommended and prioritized by the LC; monitoring the work of the National Office (NO); approving technical reports; ratifying guidelines and documents approved by the Legislative Council or its assemblies; recommending a budget to the LC; and providing progress reports of its actions to the LC. The Executive Board consists of the president, the president-elect, the past president, the vice president for academic affairs, the vice president for administration and planning (who also serves as treasurer), the vice president for governmental and social policies, the vice president for professional practices in audiology, the vice president for professional practices in speech–language pathology, the vice president for quality of service in audiology, the vice president for quality of service in speech–language pathology, the vice president for research and technology, the executive director of ASHA (a nonvoting member), and the speaker of the legislative council (a nonvoting member) (ASHA, 2005a). To be considered for election to the EB an ASHA member should respond to the Call for Nominations. The call briefly discusses the roles and responsibilities of the various offices. A submission form is included. Again, ASHA members may nominate themselves for the available offices, providing they are eligible (ASHA, 2000c, 2002c, 2003h).

Committees, Boards, Councils, Task Forces, Ad Hoc Committees

The ASHA structure includes numerous committees, boards, councils, task forces, and ad hoc committees such as the Board of Ethics, the Committee on Budget, the Ad Hoc Committee on Caseload Size, and the Multicultural Issues Board (ASHA, 2003g). All of these groups are composed of ASHA members. Each group is responsible to LC or EB and has specific charges and responsibilities, which can be found on ASHA's Web site. There you will find "Who's Who in ASHA Governance," by-laws, committee and board Volunteer Pool forms, Legislative Council members and Executive Board members with their e-mail information so you can contact them, and a section called "How To Get ASHA To Work for You."

ASHA members who are interested in serving on committees, boards, or councils should become familiar with the charges of these groups. It is also helpful to respond to drafts of guidelines, position papers, and peer reviews. Sending in your comments and recommendations helps you become known to the chairs and monitoring vice president. Active involvement in the state association is another way to increase your visibility, as well as develop committee experience. The Volunteer Pool form should also be completed and submitted for a 3-year period (ASHA, 2000c). Appointments will be made from among those who have applied through the volunteer pool, and "high priority will be given to school speech–language pathologists and audiologists, women, and federally designated ethnic minority groups" (ASHA, 1995a, p. 22).

National Office

As the services to members expanded and the officers' responsibilities increased, it became apparent that a National Office was needed to augment the work of ASHA and its governing structure. This office officially opened in 1958 (Paden, 1970) and is currently located in Rockville, Maryland, a suburb of Washington, D.C. Association records, including membership and certification records, are permanently housed in this office (ASHA, 1995g, 1997c, 2002c, 2003h; Malone, 1999).

ASHA MEMBERSHIP

ASHA's membership has increased dramatically, from 25 charter members (Malone, 1999; Paden, 1970) to more than 115,000 professionals and affiliates in 2004 (ASHA, 2003a, 2004e). To accommodate the increased interest in the professions, ASHA offers several categories of membership: (a) membership with certification, (b) membership without certification, and (c) international affiliate. Membership with certification is for those individuals who provide or supervise clinical services. To be eligible for this category, a person must successfully complete the requirements for the Certificate of Clinical Competence (CCC) in speech–language pathology or audiology or both. Qualifications include holding a graduate degree in the field. A person who holds a graduate degree or its equivalent, with a major in speech–language pathology, audiology, or speech–language and hearing science, but is not providing or supervising services qualifies for membership without certification. An individual who holds a graduate degree or its equivalent and demonstrates active research, interest, and performance in the professions but does not provide or supervise clinical services is also eligible for membership without certification. A person who resides abroad and holds a graduate degree or its equivalent may apply for international affiliate membership. There is also a category called certificate holder. This category is reserved for those people who wish to maintain their CCC but not be a member of ASHA. Of course, nonmember certificate holders don't receive ASHA benefits. Applicants for ASHA membership should carefully review all categories to determine the one that best represents their professional status (ASHA, 1997c, 2002b, 2003e).

ASHA BENEFITS AND SERVICES

ASHA offers numerous benefits and services to its members. Services include the development of standards for clinical certification, the development of standards for accreditation of educational programs, the provision of clinical and ethical guidelines for the practice of the professions, lobbying for the professions at various levels of government, the provision for ongoing education opportunities, the provision of occasions to network professionally (a professional connection), the availability of a wide variety of useful resources, easy access to legislative and regulatory data, access to publications, access to employment services for both the job seekers and the employers, availability of professional and personal insurance discounts, access to ASHA's Web site, and toll-free phone access (Action Center Line, 800/498-2071). ASHA members receive the *ASHA Leader* (published 21 times a year) and one scholarly journal of their choice from the following four: *Journal of Speech, Language and Hearing Research; Language, Speech, and Hearing Services in Schools; American Journal of Audiology: A Journal of Clinical Practice; American Journal of Speech–Language Pathology: A Journal of Clinical Practice.* Technical assistance is also available to members via phone, e-mail, and the Web. This assistance covers all professional areas, including policy, practices, health care, schools, industry, and private practice. Assistance can be obtained by calling the Action Center or by e-mailing. Contact information is listed at the end of the chapter.

Membership in ASHA means discounts on convention services such as registration, short courses, institutes, products, and seminars. Discounts are also offered on ASHA's products. ASHA offers numerous self-study products and educational programs to help members obtain their continuing education. This is a very valuable benefit, because as of 2003 for audiologists and 2005 for speech–language pathologists, 30 hours of continuing education (professional development activities) are required every 3 years to maintain ASHA certification (ASHA, 1997c, 2001c, 2003a). Additional information concerning membership benefits is available on the ASHA Web site.

STANDARDS PROGRAM

Standards are a way of making certain that quality services and products are provided to consumers by individuals, agencies, and associations. ASHA certifies individuals and accredits graduate programs to make certain that these quality services are provided to the public.

From 1959 to the present time, ASHA has had boards or councils to ensure quality services for persons with communication disorders. In 1996–1997, a separate body, the Council on Academic Accreditation (CAA) in Audiology and Speech–Language Pathology, assumed the responsibilities of establishing standards as well as applying them in the accreditation of graduate programs, thus replacing another board called the Educational Standards Board (ESB). The council was a response to the rapid growth of the profession, which necessitated change in academic accreditation (ASHA, 1995c, 1995d, 1995e, 1995i, 1997c).

EDUCATIONAL PROGRAM ACCREDITATION

In 1965, ASHA established the master's degree as the minimum level of preparation needed for entry into the professions. To ensure that certain standards are met in obtaining this degree, ASHA accredits graduate programs that train speech–language pathologists and audiologists. These standards for accreditation have moved toward qualitative standards and a focus on outcomes. For example, previously, an educational program had to have a ratio of six students for every faculty member. University programs found this ratio restrictive and often costly. To address this concern, ASHA adopted a more flexible, accommodating approach. The standard was revised to indicate that the educational programs must demonstrate sufficient faculty and staff to support the programs' goals, objectives, and mission (ASHA, 1995a, 1995f, 1997c).

Until 1995, the ESB interpreted and applied the standards for educational programs. As mentioned earlier, CAA assumed those responsibilities. Specifically, the CAA creates and implements the standards for accreditation, evaluates the programs, grants certificates to those programs when they fulfill the accreditation requirements, and maintains a list of accredited programs. When a graduate program applies for accreditation, the institution must meet certain criteria. The institution must have a regional accreditation, offer master's degrees, and conduct a comprehensive self-analysis demonstrating how the program meets the accreditation standards. The standards involve administrative structure and governance, instructional staff, academic and clinical curriculum, the students, and program resources. The program submits its application, and a team of evaluators appointed by ASHA visits the institution. The site visitors are specially trained for this process, and at the site they review such factors as faculty qualifications, academic coursework, clinical supervision, library support, and physical space. After the site visit, the evaluators report to CAA. If the specific criteria are met, including a 3-year probationary period, the department is accredited. To make certain that standards are maintained, a program review cycle occurs with scheduled periodic reviews of the program. Specific standards for accreditation of educational programs can be obtained from ASHA's Web site.

Because of the broad range of diagnostic and remedial services associated with the practice of audiology, the LC voted in 1993 to support the professional doctorate (AuD) as the entry level for audiology. Those who obtain their certification in audiology between January 1, 2007, and January 1, 2012, must have a minimum of 75 semester credit hours of postbaccalaureate education culminating in a doctoral or other recognized degree. After January 1, 2012, applicants for audiology certification must have a doctoral degree (ASHA, 1995e, 1997/1998; 2002c; Lubinski & Frattali, 1994).

The AuD, a bona fide doctoral degree earned at an accredited institution, should not be confused with the "AuD designator." The AuD designator is given by some associations and is received by "earned entitlement" (an award given after review of documentation of time in practice, education, tasks performed, awards received, and publications written). ASHA accepts the AuD that is earned through a regional accredited educational institution (ASHA, 2001i).

PROFESSIONAL SERVICE PROGRAM ACCREDITATION

In the past, ASHA has accredited clinical service delivery programs (clinics, hospital departments, agencies) where treatment and evaluation were provided for people with communication disorders. The Professional Services Board (PSB) of ASHA evaluated the speech–language and hearing services of a clinic or agency that applied for accreditation. Agencies that applied for accreditation received a site visit during which such features as the qualifications of the clinicians, the physical space, the equipment used, and the quality of clinical services provided were reviewed. However, effective December 31, 2001, the accreditation of professional service programs and the Council on Professional Services Accreditation in Audiology and Speech–Language Pathology (CPSA, formerly the Professional Services Board) were eliminated. The majority of eligible programs did not seek this accreditation—even the efforts to encourage programs to participate were not successful. Thus, this accreditation process did not appear necessary (ASHA, 2001j).

CERTIFICATE OF CLINICAL COMPETENCE

ASHA also provides a Certificate of Clinical Competence to individuals who provide services to people with communication disorders. It offers a CCC in audiology and a CCC in speech–language pathology. CPSA had been responsible for developing the standards for clinical certification and for monitoring those standards. In January 2001, the Council for Clinical Certification (CFCC) was established and assumed those functions. A person seeking certification from ASHA in speech–language pathology or audiology must have either a master's or a doctoral degree in the field; must complete a supervised professional clinical experience under the supervision of someone who has a CCC; and must pass the national exam, the Praxis, administered by the Educational Testing Service. The applicant must also abide by ASHA's Code of Ethics (ASHA, 2001f).

Effective January 1, 2005, applicants for certification in speech–language pathology must have a master's or doctorate or other recognized postbaccalaureate degree initiated and completed by an institution accredited by CAA. The applicant must have a minimum of 75 semester credit hours with 400 clock hours of supervised clinical practicum. Of these 400 hours, 25 are in observation, and 375 are in direct patient or client contact, with 325 hours at the graduate level. The applicant must have worked with a client population that was culturally or linguistically diverse and that covered the life span. A Speech Language Pathology Clinical Fellowship (SLPCF, formerly CFY, Clinical Fellowship Year) equivalent to 36 weeks of full-time clinical practice is also required. Again, effective January 1, 2005, demonstration of continued professional development (30 contact hours) is required, with a renewal period of 3 years. This demonstration of continued competence to maintain a CCC became effective January 1, 2003, for members certified in audiology (ASHA, 2001c, 2001k). Starting also in 2005, the Knowledge and Skills Acquisition Summary (KASA) form is used by ASHA-accredited programs and students seeking their CCCs to track the acquisition of the knowledge and skills needed for certification (ASHA, 2002b).

There are and will be numerous changes in certification requirements as our professional knowledge continues to evolve. It would be appropriate for the person seeking certification to call ASHA or visit ASHA's Web site for the most up-to-date information.

ASHA Certification and State Licensure

The ASHA Certificate of Clinical Competence and state licensure are different means of ensuring that speech–language pathologists and audiologists meet set standards related to educational preparation and experience. Licensure requirements vary with each state, but they are often related to ASHA CCC requirements. As of 2004, 44 states had requirements for licensing speech–language pathologists, and 43 states licensed audiologists. Licensure in these states is related to the CCC. In 7 states, the CCC is the only requirement for a state license. In 19 states, possessing the CCC ensures that the individual meets licensing requirements, and in 18 states, the CCC satisfies one or more of the licensing requirements (ASHA, 2004b). Having the CCC makes it easier for speech–language pathologists and audiologists to obtain a state license if they move to a new state (ASHA, 2004b).

Information on the requirements for individual states can be obtained by links from the ASHA Web site. From the Web page for State Education Advocacy Leaders (SEALs), information can be accessed for individual states. This information includes the licensing requirements, contact information, reciprocity agreements, and information regarding the state speech–language and hearing associations.

ASHA CCC and Teacher Certification

As with licensure, requirements for teaching certificates vary from state to state. Some states, like New York, have both an initial teaching certificate and a professional certificate; the latter is received after completion of a variety of requirements including working in the schools for 3 years. Teaching certification is administered by the state education agency in a given state. Speech–language pathologists employed by school districts or educational agencies possess teaching certification. Contact information (addresses) for individual states can be obtained from the ASHA Web site. It is listed with the information on state licensure. Contact information can also be found by using a search engine like Google or Yahoo and typing in the name of the state and the phrase "teacher certification requirements."

Many speech–language pathologists have CCC, a teaching certificate, and a state license. CCC is recognized by federal programs such as Medicaid and other third-party payers. Chapter 10 discusses that information in detail.

POSITION STATEMENTS, GUIDELINES, AND OTHER RELEVANT PAPERS

In addition to setting and implementing standards for certification and accreditation, ASHA develops position statements, guidelines, definitions, bibliographies, reports, tutorial papers, and other relevant documents. The position statements specify ASHA's policy on specific matters such as the delivery of service to individuals with learning disabilities, facilitated communication, augmentative and alternative communication, social dialects, and scope of practice.

Scope of Practice

The document *Scope of Practice, Speech–Language Pathology and Audiology* is of particular interest to students and practitioners. It defines the range of services provided by speech–language pathologists and audiologists. This statement is a list of professional activities that specifies the broad range of services offered within the professions. Not only does it define the scope of practice for speech–language pathologists and audiologists, but it also educates consumers, the general public, and other professionals about the services provided. This statement does not guarantee the skill or proficiency of the professional but merely states the range of activities provided by speech, language, and hearing professionals. Because the professions are continuously developing, the *Scope of Practice* statement will be updated as new clinical practices emerge. To view the statement for speech–language pathology, go to the ASHA Web site (to Desk Reference, volume 3); this can also be used to access *Scope of Practice* for audiology (volume 2). Additional information concerning audiology can also be found in these materials (ASHA, 2001g, 2004f).

Preferred Practice Patterns

To define practices in the professions further, ASHA developed preferred practice patterns (ASHA, 1997d). These practice patterns are not official standards, but they do serve as guidelines for enhancing the quality of professional services to consumers. They represent years of intensive work by the Task Force on Clinical Standards and reflect a consensus of practices based on the most current knowledge available at the time. These practices are universally applicable across work settings. As new procedures and technology develop in the professions, the preferred practice patterns will be updated. Copies of the preferred practice patterns can be obtained from the National Office or by visiting ASHA's Web site.

Many of the preferred practice patterns refer to ASHA's guidelines. The guidelines consist of recommended sets of procedures for specific areas of practice. The procedures are based on research findings and current practice and detail the knowledge and skills necessary to perform the techniques competently. Examples include guidelines for caseload size and speech–language service delivery in schools; suggested competencies for effective clinical supervision; guidelines for identification audiometry; and guidelines for speech–language pathologists serving persons with language, sociocommunicative, or cognitive communicative impairments. A guideline of specific interest to school practitioners is the one on the roles and responsibilities of school-based speech–language pathologists (ASHA, 2000a). That guideline is also available on the ASHA Web site.

Definitions of relevance to the profession (e.g., of communicative disorders and variations, learning disabilities, severely hearing handicapped), along with bibliographies, reports, and other relevant papers, are also published by ASHA for professional reference. These can be found in the *ASHA Desk Reference* (ASHA, 1997a). The *Desk Reference* can be viewed and purchased online at ASHA's Web portal. It can also be purchased by calling ASHA's Product Sales (888/498-6699). A technical report that school speech–language pathologists might like to review in the *Desk Reference* is ASHA's technical report, "Appropriate School Facilities for Students with Speech-Language-Hearing Disorders." It is available at the ASHA Web site. This report can be a reference for professionals in the field. It discusses the minimal requirements for providing optimal learning and assessment environments, including such aspects as the therapy room, equipment, furniture, and confidentiality.

ASHA members and certificate holders are bound by ASHA's Code of Ethics when applying the position statements, practice guidelines, definitions, and other relevant material.

ETHICS

From its inception, ASHA has made a commitment to professional ethics. In 1930, a section headed "Principles of Ethics" was added to ASHA's constitution. It consisted of three parts: "Duties of Members," "Secrecy," and "Unethical Practices" (Malone, 1999; Paden, 1970). In 1951, the "Principles of Ethics" were removed from the by-laws and became a separate document known as the *Code of Ethics*. This document has been revised from time to time to accommodate the changing scope of the professions.

Code of Ethics

The *Code of Ethics* (ASHA, 2002c) provides guidelines for professional practice. It delineates professional boundaries and protects consumers, members, and the professions. The code is divided into two main parts: the preamble, which defines the code; and the four principles of ethics statements, which target specific audiences. Principles 1 and 2 define a member's responsibilities to the persons served. Principle 3 outlines the responsibilities a member has to the public. The responsibilities to the professions of speech–language pathology and audiology are delineated in Principle 4. Specifically, the code incorporates high standards of integrity and is based on the following ethical principles:

1. Individuals shall honor their responsibility to hold paramount the welfare of persons they serve professionally.
2. Individuals shall honor their responsibility to achieve and maintain the highest level of professional competence.
3. Individuals shall honor their responsibility to the public by promoting public understanding of the professions, by supporting the development of services designed to fulfill the unmet needs of the public, and by providing accurate information in all communications involving any aspect of the professions.
4. Individuals shall honor their responsibilities to the professions and their relationships with colleagues, students, and members of allied professions. Individuals shall uphold the dignity and autonomy of the professions, maintain harmonious interprofessional and intraprofessional relationships, and accept the professions' self-imposed standards. (ASHA, 1995h, p. 74)

Each principle includes rules of ethics that state the minimally acceptable professional conduct. The rules include such concepts as providing services in a competent manner; not discriminating against a consumer; not guaranteeing the results of therapy; appropriately representing one's credentials and education; protecting the patient's confidentiality; and not engaging in dishonesty, fraud, or deceit. ASHA members and certificate holders, applicants for membership or certification, and persons in their clinical fellowship year or speech–language pathology clinical fellowship are bound by the Code of Ethics (ASHA, 1995h, 2001d, 2001f, 2003c).

Ethical decision making includes not only decisions of professional ethics (concerns such as fees for service, qualifications, certification, advertising, available resources, and research) but also decisions of clinical ethics (dilemmas involving patient care and management) (Sharp & Genesen, 1996). The numerous challenges such as managed care and IDEA and the expansion of the professions' scope of practice have placed greater demands on the clinical provider, thus posing difficult ethical decisions. The following are a few ethical dilemmas that have arisen in the schools:

- Should the speech–language pathologists in schools evaluate and treat swallowing disorders?
- Should the speech–language pathologists in schools facilitate oral feeding by changing the food texture or the student's posture, especially when the patient is aspirating?
- Should the speech–language pathologists in schools provide evaluation and treatment for children with cognitive communication disorders that have occurred as a result of traumatic brain injury?

- Should the speech–language pathologists or audiologists in schools suction a child in respiratory distress?

To respond to these questions, one must use the *Code of Ethics* as a guideline, consult the *Scope of Practice* and preferred practice patterns, be cognizant of one's skills and training as well as moral values, and use an ethical decision-making process that includes the student's family and related medical and educational professionals. The *Code of Ethics* is a living, breathing document that is revised to meet the needs of the professions. At the time of this writing, the most current version is on ASHA's Web site.

Issues in Ethics

Periodically, additional instruction and analysis about specific ethical issues are necessary to assist ASHA members in the ethical decision-making process. When this occurs, statements that are illustrative of the Code of Ethics are published and entitled "Issues in Ethics Statements." These statements are provided to heighten members' sensitivity and increase awareness about specific features of ethical conduct. Some issues that have been discussed are confidentiality, representation of services for insurance reimbursement or funding, and conflicts of professional interest. These are available in the *Desk Reference* at ASHA's Web site. A complete listing of the "Issues in Ethics Statements" is also available at the ASHA Web site (ASHA, 1994a, 1995h, 2001d, 2003e).

In June 2001 the association and in fact the entire profession was presented with an ethical issue. An article ("Experiment Taught Orphans to Stutter") appeared in the *San Jose Mercury News* alleging that the legendary researcher Wendell Johnson was the faculty advisor for a master's thesis that caused normally speaking children to stutter. There were 22 children in this study, and they were divided into four groups (group 1: children who stuttered were told they did not stutter; group 2: children who stuttered had their stuttering reinforced verbally; group 3: children who were normally fluent were told they stuttered and should avoid stuttering at all costs; and group 4: children who were normally fluent speakers were told they had good speech). In the 4- to 5-month period of the study, the children in group 3 allegedly became people who stuttered (Yairi & Ambrose, 2001). ASHA's response to the article through a letter from its president, Dr. John Bernthal, indicated that that kind of research is now prohibited by the association's Code of Ethics. In addition, Bernthal stated that ASHA members that conduct research involving human subjects must adhere to the ethical considerations in the *Belmont Report: Ethical Principles and Guidelines for the Protection of Human Subjects,* guidelines that protect the rights of all human subjects that participate in research performed in the United States. Yairi and Ambrose (2001) examined the information and data about the Johnson study very carefully. They found that "it is unquestionable that the study was ethically wrong" (p. 17) and the "conclusion that stuttering was/could be induced by labeling is totally unfounded ..."

(p. 17). The true research procedure and results of that study may never be known. We do know now that research that involves human subjects must not be injurious to the subjects.

Ethical Practice

Previously, there were two boards, the Ethical Practices Board (EPB) and the Council on Professional Ethics (COPE), which were responsible for ethics. The EPB had the responsibility of interpreting and enforcing the Code of Ethics. Its charge was to formulate and publish procedures that would be used to process alleged violations of the Code of Ethics (ASHA, 1994c, 1995g). COPE defined and proposed revisions for the Code of Ethics and developed educational materials. EPB and COPE were eventually consolidated into the Board of Ethics (BOE). The BOE has 12 members whose charge is to formulate, publish, and amend the Code of Ethics. The BOE also develops and distributes educational materials and programs on ethics. It formulates and publishes procedures that are used to process alleged violations of the code. If you think a person has violated ASHA's Code of Ethics, send a letter stating your concerns to the chair of the Board of Ethics or the Director of Ethics. Complaints filed by e-mail or fax are not accepted (ASHA, 1993, 1995h, 2004c; Huffman, 2002). For specifics on filing an ethics complaint see the ASHA Web site.

EDUCATION

To keep its membership informed about clinical procedures, scientific research, and professional issues, ASHA provides opportunities for continuing education. The association has established a formal continuing education program. ASHA members earn continuing educational units (CEUs) and are awarded an ACE (Award for Continuing Education) to document and reward their rigorous pursuit of additional and updated information. As mentioned earlier, to renew or maintain a CCC, demonstration of continuing competence is required as of 2003 for audiology and as of 2005 for speech–language pathology. Thirty contact hours of CEUs will fulfill that requirement (ASHA, 2006).

JOURNALS

In its embryonic stages, ASHA mimeographed and sold its convention papers. However, in 1936, the association issued its first publication, the *Journal of Speech Disorders* (Paden, 1970). As mentioned previously, ASHA now has five publications: the *Journal of Speech Language and Hearing Research* (*JSLHR*); *Language, Speech, and Hearing Services in Schools* (*LSHSS*); the *American Journal of Speech–Language Pathology: A Journal of Clinical Practice* (*AJSLP*); the *American Journal of Audiology: A Journal of Clinical Practice* (*AJA*); and the *ASHA*

Leader (ASHA, 1997c; Uffen, 1995). ASHA members automatically receive the *ASHA Leader* and may choose one of ASHA's scholarly publications to receive at no cost. Additional journals are available to members at low rates.

ASHA's research journal is the *Journal of Speech, Language and Hearing Research* (formerly the *Journal of Speech and Hearing Research*). This publication contains studies about the processes and disorders of hearing, language, and speech and about the diagnosis and treatment of these disorders.

The *American Journal of Speech–Language Pathology* is dedicated to clinical issues in speech–language pathology and is published quarterly. Articles in this journal address such topics as screening, assessment, and treatment techniques; professional issues; supervision; and administration. The *American Journal of Audiology* is dedicated to similar issues in the field of audiology. This journal is the first ASHA journal to be available online. Print issues are published in June and December of each year.

Of special interest to school-based clinicians is the *Journal of Language, Speech, and Hearing Services in Schools. LSHSS* is concerned with all aspects of speech, language, and hearing services in the schools. Specifically, it addresses the assessment, nature, and remediation of speech, hearing, and language disorders; program organization; and management and supervision, as well as other issues related to school programming

Asha, which was published four times annually, emphasized the professional and administrative issues of ASHA and of the professions of speech–language pathology and audiology. This publication was discontinued, and the information is now included in the *ASHA Leader.*

The *ASHA Leader* is a four-color newsletter that is published 21 times a year to keep ASHA members abreast of all current news. Its first issue came out in January 1996. The content of the *Leader* is similar to that of the former *Asha.* It provides information on the ever-changing health care system, professional skills, up-to-date treatment techniques and technologies, and employment (ASHA, 2001b). All of these publications keep ASHA members and affiliates informed and involved. You can obtain subscription information, order back issues, or obtain information about authors at ASHA's Web site (ASHA, 2003a).

CONVENTIONS, CONFERENCES, AND OTHER AVENUES OF INFORMATION

ASHA holds annual conferences in various parts of the United States. This allows networking of colleagues and presentation of information through short courses, mini-seminars, professional meetings, and poster and technical sessions. The LC, the EB, and other committees, councils, and boards meet at that time, and the membership has an opportunity to view the various aspects of ASHA governance at work.

ASHA gives teleconferences, regional workshops, and seminars on specific topics of interest. These sessions are usually listed in the *ASHA Leader* or on ASHA's Web site, under Continuing Education.

Brochures and other professional products are available, as well. Upon request, a catalogue of all ASHA products and materials can be acquired from the National Office. ASHA has an annual school conference for the school practitioner, which usually occurs in the month of July. This time is set for the convenience of ASHA school SLP members, as school is usually not in session during July. The program addresses relevant issues for SLPs who work in the schools, such as the role of the SLP in reading disabilities, adolescent reading issues, written language and spelling disabilities, phonological issues, bilingual assessment, assistive technology, research related to school-based practice issues, legislation, and counseling.

ASHA also helps its membership obtain information through the Internet (ASHA, 1996a, 1996b). The Internet offers the opportunity to send and receive electronic mail (e-mail), to join discussion groups and chat lines, to explore databases, and to download programs. In the *Leader,* there is an Internet section that lists Web addresses and list serves related to the professions. The school practitioner might wish to review "Internet Resources in Speech–Language–Hearing" by Judy Kuster, one of her "Internet" columns in the *Leader,* which are listed in the appendix of Web sites at the back of this book.

The ASHA Web site has public information about the professions in general, in addition to professional information. The professional Web site can be accessed from the ASHA Web site by selecting "for ASHA members only." Items listed on ASHA's professional Web site include position statements, state information, other Internet resources, updated information on workshops and conferences, news releases, information for students, specialty recognition, specialty interests divisions, ASHA school settings, advocacy and governmental relations, continuing education, ethics, marketing resources, membership and certification, multicultural information, policy and resource documents, communication disorders prevention strategies, answers to frequently asked questions, and special interest divisions. The site index helps with site navigation.

SPECIAL INTERESTS DIVISIONS

In 1989, Special Interests Divisions were developed. Divisions are groups of ASHA members who wish to meet and share information about specific areas of study. ASHA houses 16 of these divisions, and each one has a designated number:

1. Language Learning and Education promotes activities in the areas of linguistic knowledge and communication interactions of infants, children, and youth from diverse cultures. It looks at how knowledge, interactions,

and culture affect language learning and literacy; how different contexts, like school events, affect children's communication; and the specific diagnostic and therapeutic approaches for people with developmental disabilities or speech–language–hearing disorders.

2. Neurophysiology and Neurogenic Speech and Language Disorders promotes the study of neurophysiologic aspects of speech, language, and cognition and the prevention, assessment, and resolution of communication disorders from central or peripheral nervous systems impairment.

3. Voice and Voice Disorders promotes the study of normal voice production and the nature, presentation, assessment, and treatment of voice disorders.

4. Fluency and Fluency Disorders promotes the study of characteristics and processes of normal fluency of speech and the presentation, assessment, and treatment of fluency disorders. This includes looking at neurophysiologic, cognitive, psychological, social, and cultural factors.

5. Speech Science and Orofacial Disorders focuses on but is not limited to the anatomy and physiology of the speech mechanisms.

6. Hearing and Hearing Disorders: Research and Diagnostics is concerned with both normal and abnormal auditory functions.

7. Aural Rehabilitation and Its Instrumentation focuses on aural rehabilitative methodologies.

8. Hearing Conservation and Occupational Audiology promotes conservation of hearing. It focuses on the prevention of noise exposure and toxic agents, the monitoring and promotion of appropriate regulatory activity and legislation, educating the public and professionals, and support for research in the area.

9. Hearing and Hearing Disorders in Childhood advocates for childhood hearing issues.

10. Issues in Higher Education focuses on strategies and curricula to provide the foundation for the education and skills needed in the professions.

11. Administration and Supervision fosters best practices in administration and supervision through providing resources for the leaders, administrators, directors, and supervisors in our professions.

12. Augmentative and Alternative Communication focuses on training and preparation in this area.

13. Swallowing and Swallowing Disorders (Dysphagia) advocates for education, study, and practice in this area.

14. Communication Disorders and Sciences in Culturally and Linguistically Diverse Populations provides leadership and advocacy for best practices in the area of speech–language pathology and audiology when providing services to a culturally and linguistically diverse clientele.

15. Gerontology is concerned with the communication problems of older individuals.

16. School-Based Issues provides leadership and advocacy for school-based personnel. It is a forum for all school-based issues and promotes the highest-quality services in the schools.

The divisions often bring about immediate action on important issues. They also publish newsletters, sponsor convention short courses, and in some cases sponsor regional conferences (ASHA, 1995a, 1995e, 2003a, 2003f).

SPECIALTY RECOGNITION

Specialty recognition is available for ASHA members in various areas of the professions. Specialty recognition provides opportunities for practitioners to achieve official recognition in a specific practice area and allows consumers to easily identify "specialists" in such areas as neurological disorders, language disorders, pediatric audiology, and geriatric audiology (ASHA, 1995b, 2001h, 2003g). For further information on specialty recognition, see ASHA's Web site.

LOBBYING

ASHA is a strong advocate for the professions of speech, language, and hearing through its governmental affairs division. It uses a proactive strategy and strives to increase awareness of the field at the public, governmental, and legislative levels. It lobbies for more and better funding for research, acts as a consultant to various committees considering laws or legislation that affect the practices of speech–language pathology and audiology, and provides testimony and input on proposed legislation and regulations. It promotes the importance of the services to persons with communication disorders provided by the professions. It lobbies for recognition of these services and for better consumer protection. Recent issues that ASHA has been involved in include the $1,500 cap on Medicare outpatient services, reauthorization of IDEA, infant hearing screening, and federal reading and literacy legislation. ASHA Governmental Relations and Public Policy Updates are available on the ASHA Web site.

An example of ASHA's advocacy for school-based clinicians has been its ongoing involvement with the reauthorization process of IDEA. This involvement has lasted 3 years and two sessions of Congress. Some of ASHA's concerns involved the definitions for speech–language pathology services and audiology services and the description of related services. Other concerns were in the areas of qualification standards, assistive technology, early intervention, and the assessment and eligibility of limited English proficient students (LEP; ASHA 2004a, 2005b).

CONSUMER SERVICES

Consumer protection has been a major thrust for ASHA. To address this area, ASHA established a Consumer Affairs Division in 1988. This division's goals are to advocate on behalf of consumers and to educate them about audiology and speech–language pathology services for persons with communication disorders. The consumer can write to ASHA or call toll free (Action Center, 800/498-2071) to receive information or free educational materials.

Other educational materials for consumers available at ASHA address such topics as hearing loss, adolescent language, bilingualism, pragmatic language tips, brain injury, autism, learning disabilities and dyslexia, deaf culture, and troubleshooting of hearing aids. Members can obtain these materials directly from ASHA and distribute copies to teachers, consumers, libraries, PTAs, day care centers, and referral sources. Resources can also be found on ASHA's Web site.

ASHA makes every attempt to reach out to consumers and consider their needs. One of ASHA's responses to consumer needs has been the creation of a Model Bill of Rights for People Receiving Audiology or Speech–Language Pathology Services (ASHA, 1995i). This model bill was developed by the Task Force on Protection of Client's Rights and is an official statement by ASHA. It provides guidance for individuals who receive services in speech–language pathology and audiology. The technical report "Protection of Rights of People Receiving Audiology or Speech–Language Pathology Services," which includes the Model Bill of Rights, can be found on the Web site.

Another ASHA consumer-sensitive response has been to place consumers on boards and task forces. Also, consumer grants have been awarded to recognize self-help groups who assist people with communication disorders (ASHA, 1995d).

ASHA AND THE PUBLIC SCHOOLS

The public schools have had a major role in the provision of services for children with communication disorders since the early years of the professions of speech–language pathology and audiology. ASHA has been committed to and supportive of practitioners who work in the schools. In fact, one of ASHA's largest memberships consists of professionals who work in the schools; 55% of ASHA-certified speech–language pathologists and 10% of ASHA-certified audiologists work in the schools (Whitmire & Diggs, 2002).

Through the years, the position of associate secretary for school clinic affairs, which supported school-based clinicians, evolved into the School Services Division of ASHA, which was officially established in 1989. This division is dedicated to school issues. Its mission is to "provide leadership, information and support for members employed in public and private school settings on issues related to administration and delivery of service in the schools" (ASHA, 1994b, p. 5). Some of the goals and objectives of this division are providing school-based clinicians with materials and products to enhance service delivery; providing professional consultation to members, consumers, and related organizations; facilitating committee and task force activities and product development related to services in the schools; and developing continuing education programs to increase the members' knowledge base. Now this division has become ASHA's School Services Team. The team staff provides member assistance on topics germane to the practice of speech–language pathology and audiology in the schools, such as caseload issues and guidelines, service delivery models (pullout, collaboration, consultation), public laws and mandates, assessment, education and certification requirements, use of support personnel, entry and exit criteria rating scales, and third-party reimbursement issues. The staff attends professional conferences, gives presentations on school-based issues, serves as an advocate for speech–language pathologists and audiologists, and collaborates with other related professionals. As noted earlier, the School Services Division presents the ASHA Conference for schools.

The School Services Team has professional consultation packets available that contain information relevant to school services. These packets are a compilation of ASHA's position statements, guidelines, technical reports, and other documents that might be school-based. They contain such information as guidelines for caseload, school-based service delivery models, "IDEA and Your Caseload: A Template for Eligibility and Dismissal Criteria for Students Age 3 to 21," and reports on eligibility and dismissal criteria. This information can be obtained from the School Services Team at ASHA's national office. Available Web information is membership protected.

Other ASHA-related resources include "Issues in Determining Eligibility for Language Intervention," "Working for Change: A Guideline for Speech–Language Pathologists and Audiologists Working in the Schools," and "Guidelines for the Roles and Responsibilities of the School-Based Speech–Language Pathologist" (mentioned earlier). They also have a list in the ASHA *Desk Reference* of readings that are related to school services. For information on school services, also see Frequently Asked Questions on the ASHA Web site.

ASHA also established the State Education Advocacy Leaders (SEALs). State speech–language and hearing associations identify a person from their state to participate in this advocacy program. All SEALs network to advocate for school-based issues and to improve and enhance all skills (advocacy, leadership, clinical, management) of school-based ASHA members at the state level. To find out who your SEAL is and obtain more information, check the ASHA Web site.

ASHA has demonstrated a strong interest in the concerns of the ASHA-certified school-based members. The school-based members have informed ASHA that their major concerns are caseload size, implementation of IDEA, and salary supplements. ASHA's first priority in 2000 was school issues. In 2001–2003, there was a focused initiative that addressed caseload size in schools. One of the results of this effort is the ASHA (2002a) Position Statement on workload analysis. Another is the 2004 Schools Survey Caseload Characteristics Report (2004h). ASHA has also demonstrated its commitment to the school practitioners by devoting part or all of the *ASHA Leader* to their issues and concerns. ASHA has also created an e-newsletter called *Access Schools,* which is sent directly to an ASHA member's e-mail. This publication discusses issues and current trends in the schools. Information regarding this newsletter is for members only.

Many ASHA committees, task forces, and ad hoc committees are relevant to school-based services. ASHA members should choose a committee that is relevant to their area of interest. Clinicians working in the schools might want to particularly look at the Ad Hoc Committee on Caseload Size, which is presently revising the ASHA policy document on caseload size. Other areas of interest for the school practitioner are Specialty Interest Divisions 1, Language Learning and Education, and 16, School-Based Issues. These divisions specifically address issues of concern to educational settings. The school practitioner could also serve on a division board.

ASHA's Multicultural Issues Board (MIB), established in 1969, is another area that has much to offer school practitioners. The MIB and Multicultural Resources Teams review, monitor, and recommend to ASHA policies and actions that relate to serving the culturally and linguistically diverse population (ASHA, 2001g). The word *diverse* here includes the underserved and underrepresented population, which may be identified by age, gender, language, religion, race–ethnicity, national origin, physical disabilities, sexual orientation, or socioeconomic status (ASHA, 2001d).

In the early 1990s, ASHA looked at an issue of concern to many school personnel: speech–language pathology assistants (SLPAs). Many schools were using SLPAs, but qualifications and training were not consistent across schools or across the country. SLPAs are support personnel, not speech–language pathologists. They do not diagnose communication disorders, nor do they create a treatment plan on their own. Under the guidance of an SLP, they can carry out therapy activities planned and created by the SLP and other tasks created and engineered by the SLP. In 1995, ASHA established a scope of responsibilities for speech–language pathology assistants. Based on this and the 1999 National Job Analysis of Speech–Language Pathology Assistants conducted by the Educational Testing Service, a curriculum content was designed to provide technical training for SPLAs. In September 2003, there were 27 associate degree programs for SPLAs. For financial reasons, ASHA's Legislative Council voted to discontinue the registration program for SPLAs, as well as the approval process for SPLA training programs. ASHA is considering outsourcing the SPLA program and process. Discussion is ongoing (ASHA, 2004d). If you wish to learn more about SPLAs, visit ASHA's Web site and go to Frequently Asked Questions: Speech–Language Pathology Assistants (ASHA, 2004c).

AMERICAN SPEECH-LANGUAGE-HEARING FOUNDATION

The American Speech-Language-Hearing Foundation, a charitable organization, was established in 1946 by Wendell Johnson. It is dedicated to innovation in communication sciences and disorders. It works to promote a better quality of life for all people who have communication disorders. Specifically, the foundation advances knowledge about the etiology and treatment of communication disorders. It also identifies and facilitates new directions through the promotion of publications and conferences. It supports research and recognizes the clinical excellence of professionals in the field, as well as scholars, through research grants, graduate scholarships, and other awards. School-based practitioners are recognized annually by the foundation with the presentation of the Rolland J. Van Hattum Award at ASHA's national convention (ASHA, 1995d, 2001a). For more information on the foundation, visit the Web site.

NATIONAL STUDENT SPEECH-LANGUAGE-HEARING ASSOCIATION

Founded in 1972, the National Student Speech-Language-Hearing Association (NSSLHA) is for full- and part-time undergraduate and graduate students, including doctoral students, engaged in the study of normal and disordered communication. It is the only official student association recognized by ASHA, and the two organizations work closely together. At this writing, it has approximately 11,000 members with chapters in over 294 colleges and universities. It supports students, promotes the professions, and disseminates information. Although housed at ASHA headquarters, NSSLHA has its own structure and governance. It also has representatives on various ASHA boards and committees. To become a member of NSSLHA, a student must have declared speech–language pathology or audiology as a major and must pay the membership fee. Members receive the annual *Contemporary Issues in Communication Science and Disorders* (*CICSD*), a NSSLHA publication; *News and Notes,* the NSSLHA newsletter; access to the "members only" section of the NSSLHA and ASHA Web sites; the *ASHA Leader* and one of ASHA's scholarly journals; and a reduced fee at ASHA conventions. For students, membership in NSSLHA is an excellent first step toward participation in a professional association (ASHA, 1995d; NSSLHA, 2005). Visit the Web site (www.nsslha.org) to learn more about the organization.

ASHA also offers assistance to students through its online Guide to Graduate Programs. CAA-accredited and candidate programs are listed for each state. ASHA's Web site has a special drop-down menu where students can access information about academic programs, financial aid, job strategies, how to join ASHA, how to obtain a CCC, the Praxis Exam (sample questions are included), and the National Student Speech-Language-Hearing Association. Students can order ASHA's Career Mover CD-ROM and online can find Web links to other information about the communication disorders professions, scholarships, research, academic news, and academic accreditation.

CONCLUSION

ASHA is a national professional organization that promotes the interests of the professions, the consumers, and its members. Members participate in the organization's policy and decision making. Benefits and services accompanying ASHA membership include position statements, guidelines, and reports, along with standards for clinical certification and accreditation for graduate educational programs.

The integrity and ethics of the professions are paramount. The Code of Ethics of ASHA provides the framework and guidelines for maintaining its standards. *Issues in Ethics Statements* are supplied to assist the membership in ethical decision making.

ASHA promotes the continuing education of its members, along with public awareness and representing the professions and the consumers at various governmental levels. It provides forums for debate and networking with other colleagues and professionals.

A large number of ASHA members work in school settings. A special National Office team addresses school-based concerns, an annual professional conference is held specifically for school-based clinicians, and a journal is dedicated to clinical, professional, and academic issues in the schools. Committees, task forces, and other publications also support school practitioners.

CONTACT INFORMATION

ASHA Action Center	800/498-2071 or actioncenter@asha.org
ASHA Audiology	audinfo@asha.org
ASHA Speech–Language Pathology	slpinfo@asha.org
ASHA Health Services	healthservices@asha.org
ASHA School Services	schoolservices@asha.org
ASHA Product Sales	800/498-6699 or http://store.asha.org/shop
American Speech-Language-Hearing Foundation	http://www.ashfoundation.org
National Student Speech-Language-Hearing Association	http://www.nsslha.org

 STUDY QUESTIONS

1. What are the purposes of ASHA?
2. Why should a practitioner in the field of speech–language pathology or audiology become a member of ASHA?
3. If you are a member of ASHA, what should you do to be considered for appointment to a committee, board, or council? What committee would you choose and why?
4. As a member of ASHA, how could you identify and contact your legislative councilor?
5. As a member of ASHA, how could you become a legislative councilor? An ASHA officer?

6. Why is ASHA's Code of Ethics important?
7. What are the four basic principles of ethics in ASHA's Code?
8. What should you do if you feel someone has committed a violation of ASHA's Code of Ethics?
9. How do the *Scope of Practice* and the practice patterns help in the practice of speech–language pathology and audiology?
10. What can you as a student do now to become involved in a professional organization?
11. How does the Schools Services Team work for the school practitioner?
12. What issues concern ASHA with the most recent reauthorization of IDEA?
13. What are CEUs? What is an ACE? Why would they be important for a school practitioner?
14. What is the AuD designator? How does it differ from an AuD from an accredited institution?
15. Identify the following acronyms: LC, EB, ASHA, NO, CAA, CRCC, CCC, AJSLP, LSHSS, JSLHR, MIB, CEU.

REFERENCES

American Speech-Language-Hearing Association. (1993). *Ethics: Resources for professional preparation and practice.* Rockville, MD: Author.

American Speech-Language-Hearing Association. (1994a, March). Issues in ethics. *Asha, 36*(13), 7–27.

American Speech-Language-Hearing Association. (1994b). *School Services Division: 1994 convention highlights, Fall.* Rockville, MD: Author.

American Speech-Language-Hearing Association. (1994c, March). Statement of practices and procedures. *Asha, 36*(13), 3–5.

American Speech-Language-Hearing Association. (1995a). ASHA 1994 annual report. *Asha, 37*(3), 18–26.

American Speech-Language-Hearing Association. (1995b). ASHA reports. *Asha, 37*(2), 12, 17.

American Speech-Language-Hearing Association. (1995c). ASHA reports. *Asha, 37*(4), 23, 29–30, 47.

American Speech-Language-Hearing Association. (1995d). ASHA reports. *Asha, 37*(5), 14–18, 26, 28, 37.

American Speech-Language-Hearing Association. (1995e). ASHA reports. *Asha, 37*(6/7), 18–19, 24–25, 29, 57.

American Speech-Language-Hearing Association. (1995f). At press time. *Asha, 37*(6/7), 7–8.

American Speech-Language-Hearing Association. (1995g). Boards, committees, councils, and task forces. *Asha, 37*(3), 61–73.

American Speech-Language-Hearing Association. (1995h). Code of ethics 1995. *Asha, 37*(3), 74–75.

American Speech-Language-Hearing Association. (1995i). Model bill of rights. *Asha, 37*(3), 37.

American Speech-Language-Hearing Association. (1996a). Contact ASHA over the Internet. *ASHA Leader, 1*(12), 6.

American Speech-Language-Hearing Association. (1996b). New on the website: http://www.asha.org. *ASHA leader, 1*(13), 2.

American Speech-Language-Hearing Association. (1997a). *ASHA desk reference.* Rockville, MD: Author.

American Speech-Language-Hearing Association. (1997b). *Membership and certification handbook, audiology.* Rockville, MD: Author.

American Speech-Language-Hearing Association. (1997c). *Membership and certification handbook, speech–language pathology.* Rockville, MD: Author.

American Speech-Language-Hearing Association. (1997d). *Preferred practice patterns for the profession of speech–language pathology.* Rockville, MD: Author.

American Speech-Language-Hearing Association. (1997–1998). *Council on professional standards in speech–language pathology and audiology: Certification for audiology.* Rockville, MD: Author.

American Speech-Language-Hearing Association. (2000a). *Guidelines for the roles and responsibilities of school-based speech–language pathologists.* Rockville, MD: Author.

American Speech-Language-Hearing Association. (2000b). LC takes action on resolution. *ASHA leader, 5*(24), 8.

American Speech-Language-Hearing Association. (2000c). Nominations. *ASHA Leader, 5*(24), 9.

American Speech-Language-Hearing Association. (2001a). *About the ASH Foundation.* Retrieved August 2, 2005, from http://www.ashfoundation.org/Foundation/about/

American Speech-Language-Hearing Association. (2001b). *An insider's guide to the publication process.* Retrieved August 2, 2005, from http://www.asha.org/about/publications/journal-abstracts/submissions/process.htm

American Speech-Language-Hearing Association. (2001c). *Background information and standards and implementation for the Certificate of Clinical Competence in speech language pathology.* Retrieved August 2, 2005, from http://www.asha.org/about/membership-certification/handbooks/slp/slp_standards_new.htm

American Speech-Language-Hearing Association. (2001d). *Communication development and disorders in multicultural populations: Readings and related materials.* Retrieved August 2, 2005, from http://www.asha.org/about/leadership-projects/multicultural/readings/

American Speech-Language-Hearing Association. (2001e). *Legislative Council handbook.* Rockville, MD: Author.

American Speech-Language-Hearing Association. (2001f). *Membership and certification handbook of the American Speech-Language-Hearing Association.* Retrieved August 2, 2005, from http://www.asha.org/about/membership-certification/handbooks/slp/default.htm

American Speech-Language-Hearing Association. (2001g). *Scope of practice in speech–language pathology.* Rockville, MD: Author.

American Speech-Language-Hearing Association. (2001h). *Specialty recognition: FAQs.* Retrieved August 2, 2005, from http://www.asha.org/about/credentialing/specialty/faq.htm

American Speech-Language-Hearing Association. (2001i). *Statement by the Ethical Practice Board: Use of the AuD designation by members and certificate holders.* Retrieved August 2, 2005, from http://www.asha.org/about/ethics/epb_aud.htm

American Speech-Language-Hearing Association. (2001j). *Three-year phase-out of Professional Services Accreditation Program.* Retrieved August 2, 2005, from http://www.asha.org/about/credentialing/accredited-providers/elimination_accreditation.htm

American Speech-Language-Hearing Association. (2001k). *Using ASHA CEUs for licensure renewal.* Retrieved August 2, 2005, from http://www.asha.org/about/continuing-ed/CEUs/licensure.htm

American Speech-Language-Hearing Association. (2002a). *A workload analysis approach for establishing speech–language caseload standards in the schools: Position statement.* Rockville, MD: Author.

American Speech-Language-Hearing Association. (2002b). *CAA 2002 Update.* Rockville, MD: Author.

American Speech-Language-Hearing Association. (2002c). *Certification and membership handbook: Speech–language pathology.* Rockville, MD: Author.

American Speech-Language-Hearing Association. (2002d). *Legislative council coordinating committee (LCCC): New legislative councilor orientation.* Rockville, MD: Author.

American Speech-Language-Hearing Association. (2003a). *About ASHA.* Retrieved August 2, 2005, from http://www.asha.org/about/

American Speech-Language-Hearing Association. (2003b). *ASHA publications.* Retrieved August 2, 2005, from http://www.asha.org/about/publications/

American Speech-Language-Hearing Association. (2003c). Code of Ethics (revised). *ASHA Supplement, 23,* 13–15.

American Speech-Language-Hearing Association. (2003d). *Issues in Ethics Statements.* Retrieved August 2, 2005, from http://www.asha.org/about/ethics/ethics_issues_index.htm

American Speech-Language-Hearing Association. (2003e). *Membership and certification handbook of the American Speech-Language-Hearing Association for speech–language pathology.* Rockville, MD: Author.

American Speech-Language-Hearing Association. (2003f). *Specialty Interest Division news and events.* Retrieved August 2, 2005, from http://www.asha.org/about/membership-certification/divs/

American Speech-Language-Hearing Association. (2003g). *Committees, boards & councils.* Retrieved August 2, 2005, from http://www.asha.org/about/leadership-projects/committees

American Speech-Language-Hearing Association. (2003h). *2003 orientation manual for new legislative councilors.* Rockville, MD: Author.

American Speech-Language Hearing Association. (2004a). *Analysis of major issues in the IDEA Reauthorization Law.* Retrieved August 23, 2005 from: http://www.asha.org/about/legislation-advocacy/federal/idea/04-law.htm

American Speech-Language-Hearing Association. (2004b). *Benefits of ASHA certification.* Retrieved August 2, 2005, from http://www.asha.org/about/membership-certification/cert_benefits.htm

American Speech-Language-Hearing Association. (2004c). *Frequently asked questions: Speech–language pathology assistants.* Retrieved August 2, 2005, from http://www.asha.org/about/membership-certification/faq_slpasst.htm

American Speech-Language-Hearing Association. (2004d). *Guidelines for the training, use and supervision of speech-language pathology assistants.* Retrieved August 24, 2005 from http://www.asha.org/NR/rdonlyres/2098755B-AC9C-4F81-9011B84000043E59/0/v3GLSupervisionSLPAs.pdf

American Speech-Language-Hearing Association. (2004e). *Highlights and trends: ASHA counts for 2004.* Retrieved August 2, 2005, from http://www.asha.org/about/membership-certification/member-counts.htm

American Speech-Language-Hearing Association. (2004f). *Scope of practice in audiology.* Retrieved August 24, 2005 from http://www.asha.org/NR/rdonlyres/036AC2B1-FB02-4124-870980881C1079A6/0/v1ScopeofPracticeAudiology.pdf

American Speech-Language-Hearing Association. (2004g). *Statement of practices and procedures of the board of ethics.* Retrieved August 24, 2005 from http://www.asha.org/NR/rdonlyres/40C14E5F-C9EB-4580-A79EBD4DD5D41976/0/v1p189ethics.pdf

American Speech-Language-Hearing Association. (2004h). *2004 schools survey-caseload characteristics report.* http://www.asha.org/NR/rdonlyres/22D66325-4CE6-460D-8D61-9E0388219E/0SchoolsSurveycaseloads.pdf

American Speech-Language-Hearing Association. (2005a). *Bylaws and policies associated with the bylaws of the American Speech-Language-Hearing Association.* Retrieved July 22, 2006, from http://www.asha.org/about/Leadership-projects/bylaws.htm

American Speech-Language-Hearing Association. (2005b). *IDEA information center.* Retrieved August 23, 2005 from http://www.asha.org/about//legislation-advocacy/federal/idea/default.htm

American Speech-Language-Hearing Association. (2006). *Maintaining your certification*. Retrieved July 23, 2006, from http://www.asha.org/about/Membership-Certification/certification/

Huffman, N. (2002). ASHA's Board of Ethics—Let's get acquainted. *ASHA Leader, 7*(3), 1, 6–7.

Kuster, J. M., & Kuster, T. A. (1995). Finding treasures on the Internet: Gopher the gold. *Asha, 37*(2), 43–47.

Lubinski, R., & Frattali, C. (Eds.). (1994). *Professional issues in speech–language pathology and audiology: A textbook*. San Diego, CA: Singular.

Malone, R. (1999). *The first 75 years: An oral history of the American Speech-Language-Hearing Association*. Rockville, MD: Author.

National Student Speech-Language-Hearing Association. (2005). *NSSLHA 2005 membership brochure and application*. Retrieved August 24, 2005 from http:www.nsslha.org/NR/rdonlyres/1A351A68-62C7-4D31-BB18-BD02FF7B2EFF/0/05MemAppBrochure.pdf

Paden, E. P. (1970). *A history of the American Speech and Hearing Association, 1925–1958*. Washington, DC: American Speech-Language-Hearing Association.

Sharp, H., & Genesen, L. (1996). Ethical decision-making in dysphagia management. *American Journal of Speech–Language Pathology, 5*, 15–22.

Uffen, E. (1995). Ideas into print: ASHA's scholarly journals. *Asha, 37*(4), 35–38.

Whitmire, K., & Diggs, C. (2002). Making a difference in the schools. *ASHA Leader, 7*(16), 1, 25.

Yairi, E., & Ambrose, N. (2001). The Tudor experiment and Wendell Johnson: Science and ethics reexamined. *ASHA leader, 6*(13), 17.

Note. Access to some documents on the ASHA Web site requires membership.

SECTION II

Core Areas of School-Based Speech–Language Pathology

Regardless of the site in which they practice, all speech–language pathologists are charged with evaluating students, selecting appropriate goals, and providing intervention for the clients they serve. The following three chapters describe how SLPs meet the challenges that these three basic areas of professional competence present within the school environment.

Chapter 3 deals with all aspects of assessment, from tentatively identifying students who may need services to determining the details of individual strengths and weaknesses that will become the basis of educational planning. Three hypothetical students and their presenting problems are described, and the assessment process is followed from observing the student and conducting teacher and parent interviews to selecting appropriate test instruments and other procedures, to scoring and interpreting the results, to eliciting and analyzing language samples, and finally to reporting outcomes.

Chapter 4 details the development of all IEP components and links goals to state standards. The chapter culminates with a complete IEP for each of the three students assessed in Chapter 3.

Chapter 5 provides an overview of intervention considerations for students in kindergarten through high school. Different types of service delivery models are defined, compared, and contrasted. Advantages and disadvantages of each model are described. The three hypothetical students are again encountered, this time with detailed information on how their needs could be addressed through different service models and procedures.

Chapter 3

Assessment

Jacqueline Meyer,
with Nanette Clapper

Even compared with the profound changes that have occurred in school-based speech–language pathology in recent years, assessment and evaluation within that setting is in a particular state of flux. First, as reaffirmed by the reauthorization of the Individuals with Disabilities Education Act of 1997 (IDEA, P.L. 101-336) and its further 2004 reauthorization and revision (P.L. 108-446), school-based assessment involves three different stages, two of which rarely occur in hospital and clinical practice. Stage one consists of "systematically observing and gathering or recording credible information to … [determine] the presence or absence of a disorder" and is common to all sites. Stage two determines whether the disorder "has an adverse effect on educational performance," and during stage three an assessment team decides whether "the student needs special education and related services in order to participate, as appropriate, in the general curriculum" (ASHA, 1999b, p. 14). Clearly, stages two and three apply to school-based practice only.

As part of stages one and two, the reauthorizations of IDEA also mandate that multiple forms of assessment be used to determine if a child is to receive or continue to receive services under the act. Consequently, evaluation has shifted from a primary dependence on standardized instruments to include information acquired through checklists, interviews, observations, and curriculum-based or authentic assessment (IDEA, 1997, Section 300.533). This shift has caused anxiety in many school-based speech–language professionals who have primarily relied on standardized testing. Readers should be aware, however, that the 2004 version of IDEA permits local educational agencies (LEAs) to use some of their local grant funds for early intervening services, the intent of which is to target children "who have not been identified as needing special education or related services but who need additional academic … support to succeed in a general education environment … [including] scientifically based literacy instruction" (Snyder, 2004, p. 27). In other words, SLPs may be evaluating and treating children who do not meet the test of needing special education.

In an attempt to discuss all aspects of evaluation in the schools yet make the amount of information manageable, we have divided the chapter into four major areas. The first describes initial procedures involved in identifying students who may be at risk; the second discusses (for want of a better term) traditional approaches to school-based assessment, including a synopsis of measurement terms and concepts. The third, "New Approaches to Assessment," outlines the history that has led to changes in how we view evaluation and contains a sampling of some exciting new ways to look at measuring language. This section includes an application of Vygotskian developmental theory to the assessment process and descriptions of some of its descendants: authentic, curriculum-based, response to intervention, and dynamic assessment, particularly as it applies to the upper elementary, middle, and high school student. Nanette Clapper reports the why and how of authentic assessment from the point of view of a professional with 18 years in school-based practice. Her work experience reflects her qualifications for discussing new assessment issues: intelligence, disciplined reading skills, a penchant for a careful thought, and an acceptance of the inevitable trial and error associated with any cutting edge endeavor. The last section presents four specific cases that illustrate the general concepts covered in the preceding sections.

Finally, a word about terminology. Routman, among others, makes a distinction between the terms *assessment* and *evaluation,* stating that *assessment* "refers to data collection and the gathering of evidence," and *evaluation* "implies bringing meaning to that data through interpretation, analysis and reflection" (Routman, 1994, p. 302, quoted in ASHA 1999a). For the purposes of this chapter, however, the terms will be used interchangeably, because most speech–language pathologists evaluate as they collect data, deciding how and what to investigate next based on their interpretation of what is happening now as they work with a student. It may help to think of either of the two words as shorthand for a single hyphenated term: assessment–evaluation. The one constant that remains is the function of assessment. Assessment drives intervention, regardless of the type you choose. Discovering a student's strengths as well as the underlying weaknesses that prevent him from succeeding in school allows you to plan and prioritize how to provide services most effectively. Understanding how speech and language deficits affect specific aspects of classroom performance is absolutely key and is required during the second and third stages of the assessment process.

Because this textbook represents many different views, you, as student or instructor, should know where the author of the first part of this chapter (as well as Chapter 5) is coming from. As an SLP who worked in the school environment for many years, and as an instructor of undergraduate and graduate diagnostics, language, and school organization courses, I want this chapter to serve as a practical introduction to school-based assessment and evaluation. At different times, I have served speech pathology students either as their cooperating SLP at my school site or as a college supervisor during their student teaching practicum. These two roles have made me favor lists and examples over an explanation of theory. This is not because theory is unimportant in assessment and intervention. It is important, but whereas theoretical information often answers the why, it usually does not answer the how, particularly when new concepts are being discussed. As befits a text of this type, I hope Chapters 3 and 5 will speak to that ever-present (and nervous) student clinician question, "What should I do tomorrow morning?"

The two chapters are written as if I were talking to you in class or in the speech room—that is, in the first and second person, I and you. I loved Rhea Paul's (2001) description of the first person in the preface to the second edition of *Language Disorders From Infancy Through Adolescence* as "cranky, preachy, and personal" (p. xi). Replacing the third-person point of view serves several purposes. It streamlines sentences, as in "Plan your assessment with great care" versus "Assessment must be planned with great care by the school speech–language professional." It also helps remove infallibility from the statements I make in these two chapters. There is almost never a single correct way to evaluate a student or implement objectives. This inherent flexibility gives us the freedom to try new procedures or disregard or revamp old ones. Theories clash, opinions differ, and personalities dictate different solutions, making ours a vital, intellectually challenging, constantly changing field.

Much of the content of this book deals with services provided to school-age children under the provisions of Public Law No. 94-142 plus later revisions and expansions found in the 1997 and 2004 reauthorizations and revisions of IDEA. Under these laws, plus individual state guidelines, assessment functions as part of the law's charge to "locate, identify and serve all handicapped pupils." So here we have it: One of the major responsibilities of a school speech–language specialist is assessment. And to an inexperienced person, this whole area may be a scary prospect. Most professionals say to themselves, at one time or another, such things as "How do I know what to do? What tests should I choose? What about dynamic assessment? Curriculum-based authentic evaluation? What about language sampling? I've never even *seen* a child with a traumatic brain injury or Fragile X syndrome or swallowing problems. After I finish, how do I know if the child should be labeled? How do I interpret the results and write an Individualized Education Program that will really improve the child's communication skills in school?" First, be assured that these are normal concerns. Every new SLP feels the same way. Second, it is not only those who are relatively new to the field who fret about this; in the course of your career, these questions will recur each time you are faced with a student who represents an area with which you are unfamiliar.

To begin, every competent speech–language professional knows that no one set of tests or procedures can fit every student's needs. With the pressure of a large caseload, limited time for evaluation, and reduced funding, however, it is frequently tempting to make do with the instruments that your district already has or to use the same procedure for every child who is referred for evaluation. Regardless of the temptation, the ethical consideration remains clear: "Individuals shall honor their responsibility to hold paramount the welfare of persons served professionally" (American Speech-Language-Hearing Association [ASHA] *Code of Ethics;* see Chapter 2). That is, you must always ask yourself, when you plan any procedure or assessment, if it is in the best interests of the student. (This is the preachy mode.)

Entire textbooks have been written discussing the theory and ramifications of assessment. Within the past few years, excellent texts specifically addressing general language issues in the school-age population have appeared—for example, those by Paul (2001), Naremore, Densmore, and Harman (2001), Nippold (1998), and Wallach and Butler (1994b). In addition, there has been an explosion of texts designed to help speech–language professionals assess students whose weaknesses are in a specific area (e.g., narrative discourse development or articulation and phonology) or whose deficits appear to stem from a specific disorder (e.g., autism spectrum disorder, Down syndrome, or traumatic brain injury) (Shprintzen, 2000). The entire issue of *Language, Speech, and Hearing Services in Schools* in April 1996 was devoted to one segment of assessment: observing and interpreting behaviors of the school-age child. In October 1995 in the same journal, authors of five articles presented new language norms for this population. ASHA's products catalog lists items that are relevant and topical and meet ASHA's standards for quality instruction and knowledge dissemination (2003). Previously available from ASHA (1997) was a directory that provided information on over 300 instruments that assessed spoken and written language, cognitive communication, fluency, voice, articulation and phonology, swallowing, and oral-motor function, along with test batteries and developmental scales for all ages, including the school-age population. In 2006 ASHA offered this directory online. Titled *Directory of Speech Language Pathology Assessment Instruments,* it is available to members only. Clearly, assessment issues are alive and well in our profession. Yet even with new or refined information, we still struggle to provide appropriate guidelines for when or if a *specific* child should receive (or continue to receive) speech–language services. Consequently, a single chapter like this one can contain only a brief overview of the process involved in choosing and applying procedures to determine whether language deficits exist, whether they are severe enough to warrant intervention, and, if so, how to identify them in enough detail to provide a basis for appropriate intervention. The problem that strikes fear into my author's heart is what to include and what to leave out. (This is the personal mode.)

Therefore, I will start with a disclaimer. This chapter can serve only as a very general guide, rather like a house plan in a magazine that provides an idea of what the house would look like. If you want to build it, however, you will need architectural blueprints. Often the detailed, highly specialized information you need to zero in on the subtle problem of a specific student will be absent from this chapter. The roles and responsibilities of a school-based SLP (ASHA, 1999a) demand that, on a routine basis, you must learn to access the wonderful resources in ASHA school-based publications, journal articles, Web sites, comprehensive texts, and sources of condensed versions of information such as the journal *Word of Mouth,* workshops, conventions, teleconferences, inservice opportunities, and, most important, a network of supportive colleagues. Throughout the four sections of this chapter, I will refer to a number of sources I hope can guide you as you develop your personal professional library.

Finally, be aware that when you develop an Individualized Educational Program (IEP), the Present Level of Performance required as part of the document will reflect assessment information in a specific way. The next chapter will discuss this application of the evaluation process in detail.

Historically, the school speech–language pathologist has investigated suspected deficits in phonology, morphology, syntax, semantics (including discourse), voice, fluency, and pragmatics as separable subdivisions of speech and language (Lund & Duchan, 1993). Within these areas that represent the form, content, and use of language, the SLP has addressed both receptive and expressive skills in oral and, more recently, in written form. In recent years, we have made an additional distinction between language difference and language disorder when we gauge the impact of dialect, English as a second language, or contrasting cultural features on a child's communicative competence (Battle, 1998; Rhyner, Kelly, Brantley, & Drueger, 1999; Roseberry-McKibbin,

1995). As the principle of inclusion has introduced children with more severe handicapping conditions into the general school population, we have also become responsible for decisions concerning augmentative communication (see Chapters 6 and 8). Therefore, because the range of deficits occurring in the school-age population can be so broad and because all linguistic areas are so intertwined with reading and writing, we must plan initial assessment with exquisite care. To recommend that a student should or should not receive our services is an awesome responsibility and not to be taken lightly.

Regardless of the type of evaluation you choose, the process starts with case finding, may proceed to case selection, and ultimately may result in a student being added to your caseload.

CASE FINDING: INITIAL PROCEDURES IN ASSESSMENT

Remember that the Individuals with Disabilities Education Acts of 1997 and 2004, plus their predecessors, require schools to locate, identify, and serve students with any handicapping condition. In our field, case finding involves locating school-age and preschool students who are communicatively impaired or who appear educationally at risk because of suspected language deficits. Different ways for the school district to find preschool students will be discussed in the next chapter, but the most typical means for locating *school-age* children are referral and screening. Because your individual state or district will vary in its specific requirements, you must make every reasonable effort to keep current with its regulations, often referred to as "the regs." The chair of the group within your school or district who deals with issues affecting students with special needs, or your district's director of special education, receives this information on a continuing basis. Regardless of the specifics, your initial contact with one of these students forms the foundation of your professional accountability that continues throughout the intervention process. The spirit of the federal and state guidelines that require you to consider the needs of the student who may have a handicapping condition should be implicit in all decisions as you plan and complete screening, assessment, and intervention procedures.

The following section contains information that deals primarily with periodic rather than ongoing assessment.

Screening

Screening can be defined as a preliminary method of distinguishing individuals with handicaps from the general student population; that is, the means used to identify those in need of further evaluation. Descriptions of different types of screening procedures and general guidelines for choosing each type follow.

Screening Groups of Students

Frequently, the first testing procedure a 4- or 5-year-old encounters is a general preschool or kindergarten screening. Most schools routinely screen all kindergarten and first-grade students; many also screen transfers, regardless of grade, and any student who scores below acceptable levels on certain state-mandated achievement tests, such as a second- or third-grade reading or mathematics examinations. You, as the speech–language professional, will be responsible for part of this process. In fact, screening often serves as an introduction to the concept of team-based evaluation. Many school districts, for example, divide kindergarten screening into stations overseen by the school nurse (medical history, vision and dental screening), the physical education teacher (gross motor ability), the school psychologist (basic cognitive skills, behavioral concerns), the kindergarten teachers (scholastic readiness, including fine motor skills), and the speech–language pathologist (fluency, voice, articulation, and language skills). Hearing screening may be done by an SLP, the school nurse, or, in some large districts, an educational audiologist. (Chapter 11 contains specific information about audiological issues.) Because there is often overlap among these professionals, be careful that the procedures and instruments complement rather than duplicate each other. This is particularly important because children at this age (and their parents) may be very nervous. Testing should not last any longer than necessary.

The portion of a general screening supervised by a speech–language pathologist is not a means to determine whether a child has a speech–language deficit. It serves only to identify those students who appear to be at risk. Therefore, it is neither necessary nor desirable for any one area of language (e.g., phonology, syntax) to be examined in detail. What is important is that screening neither over- nor underidentifies students with potential speech or language problems. Most school clinicians agree, unfortunately, that they have yet to find the "perfect" screening test or procedure. To compound the difficulty, at one time or another, screenings include students from kindergarten through Grade 12.

Let us begin with the easiest. Almost all versions of kindergarten screening include the following, either as part of a standardized screening instrument or through less formal means:

- *Phonology:* usually includes only the most frequently misarticulated sounds (i.e.,/s, /ʃ/, /tʃ/, z, l, r, θ, and f/)
- *Receptive language:* often following two- and three-stage directions (e.g., "Put the ball in the cup and the spoon in your lap")
- *Expressive language:* usually sentence-repetition tasks, story retelling, or talking about an actual incident (e.g., the child's birthday party)
- *Fluency and voice:* evaluated during screening of the previous areas

Several screening instruments, such as the *Speech-Ease Screening Inventory–K–1* (1985), also include a language sample and tasks addressing vocabulary, basic concepts, similarities and differences, sentence repetition, and linguistic relationships. For children in the upper elementary grades, articulation screening can be accomplished by having the student count to 20 or recite the days of the week or the months of the year. This also tells you if these common series have become automatic. Unfortunately, these procedures do not address the underlying receptive, metaphonological, or metalinguistic deficits that can negatively affect reading, spelling, and writing, discussed in Chapter 7.

Some school districts, such as Chappaqua in southern New York State, develop their own instruments. That school district's screening test for Grades 3 through 5 has short sections that address spontaneous verbal expression (e.g., how to play a game or sport), vocabulary (picture identification, analogies, synonyms, multiple meanings, word retrieval), figurative language (riddles, absurdities), verbal comprehension (story questions, memory for sentences, following directions), and syntax (sentence combining and sentence formulation). If the district has not developed such a tool, receptive skills are almost always addressed through a standardized instrument, such as a vocabulary test or one involving classroom spatial and temporal terms. If a standardized screening instrument is not used to address expressive language ability, you can play a game, ask questions about the child's interests, or require the student to explain, for example, how to make a sandwich. Although screening based on less formal procedures may give you a sense of how the child uses language in naturalistic contexts, judging if the student should or should not be assessed further may be more difficult for the inexperienced SLP. Consequently, in this age group, standardized tests are usually employed for at least part of the screening.

Because research has indicated that language deficits can put a child at risk for reading problems (see Chapter 7), children in the kindergarten and first grade in an increasing number of school districts are also being screened for phonological awareness (PA) and other preliteracy skills. The intent of this type of screening, for example, via the PALS–K (a phonological awareness and literacy screening instrument for kindergarten), is to prevent reading problems by determining which children will require additional work in PA and related areas in order to become successful readers (*Phonological Awareness Literacy Screening*, 2004).

For students in high school, screening is usually based on referral—that is, it is almost never of the general variety. It is rare, also, that high school students are referred for the first time unless they have become seriously ill or injured. Almost always, these students have struggled academically at some point in the past and may even have received services but have not been continued on the caseload of an SLP. As the language demands of the school curriculum increase, however, their ability to compensate reaches the breaking point. Owens (1995) stated, "Language impairment may persist across the lifetime of the individual and may vary in symptoms, manifestations, effects, and severity over time and as a consequence of context, content, and learning task" (p. 22). It has been my experience that high school students, if they receive services from a speech–language pathologist at all, do so as a related service, as part of a learning disabilities label, unless they exhibit a severe communication handicap. Consequently, screening is chosen for a specific student and is much more likely to focus on classroom pragmatics or an inability to handle curriculum, often with demonstrated weaknesses in both reading and writing. Therefore, screening procedures that focus on those areas are most useful. Paul (2001) adapted and included in her text two forms to be used with these students, a self-assessment form adapted from Grambau (p. 504), and a checklist adapted from Damico (p. 506). Ehren (2002) argued convincingly that speech–language services to high school students are not as fully implemented as they should be partly because SLPs may assume that students will have been identified as having language disorders before they go to high school. She asserted, "It is common for the language basis of academic problems to go unrecognized in high school students. Therefore it is important … for SLPs to consider identification as an important part of their job" (p. 67).

As noted, school districts vary widely in the instruments they use; a significant number are included in Appendix 3.A. If you are inexperienced and must develop screening procedures, often parts of different instruments can be combined; for young elementary students, you might administer the articulation screening procedure from the *Arizona Articulation Proficiency Scale–3* (Fudala, 2000) or the articulation portion of the *Preschool Language Scale–Fourth Edition* (Zimmerman, Steiner, & Pond, 2002) in addition to a storytelling procedure. For several years, I used an early computerized screening test that included articulation, receptive language, and sentence repetition items combined with the vocabulary plates from the *Joliet 3-Minute Speech and Language Screen* (Kinzler & Johnson, 1993). Because the computerized test contained no normative data, we calculated local norms based on six kindergarten classes over 3 years' time. Be aware that in-depth investigations of likely deficits revealed through screening are planned and take place under quite different circumstances. These will be discussed later under "Case Selection." First, however, let us continue with some additional categories of screening.

Other Types of Screening

Up to this point, articulation and language screening as part of the case-finding process has generally referred to a brief procedure administered to large groups of students, whether or not deficits were suspected. But screening can also help determine if a student who has been referred for a possible handicapping condition should undergo a complete speech–language evaluation, as in the case of the high school screening discussed previously. In this example, you already know that some sort of deficit is interfering with the student's classroom performance. Therefore, you want either to eliminate language as a causative factor or to confirm that a likely connection exists. Other types of screening instruments, usually more lengthy, can be used for this purpose. The *Preschool Language Scale–4* (Zimmerman, Steiner, & Pond, 2002), and the CELF screening instrument (Semel, Wiig, & Secord, 1996) are typical of this type. If a language-based disability appears likely, then you continue and assess deficits in greater depth.

In many screening instruments, there is a "cut-off" point. Depending on the instrument and the child's age, that point determines whether the child has passed or failed that part of the screening. In some school districts, if children have not failed the screening but their scores indicate a weakness, they may be placed in groups for "speech improvement." In essence, this designation refers to children who may benefit from services provided by speech–language or other professionals but do not qualify for a label. Because of a lack of qualified personnel or limited funds, however, many districts have discarded this designation.

Another process that can take place before screening or between a general screening and a formal, complete assessment is *prereferral*. Many districts have created school-based teams that can recommend modifications or other strategies teachers can use to improve a student's ability to function successfully in the classroom. The same team that makes these suggestions usually evaluates their effectiveness. If they have been efficacious, the need for a full evaluation has been avoided, at least for a time. A term newly associated with this procedure is *response to intervention* (RTI). RTI can also refer to the process of providing all children, not just those at risk, with specific assistance—for example, phonological awareness instruction. The entire group is evaluated, and those not responding to the training are given additional help while continuing to be part of the initial group. If the children in this subgroup still do not make appropriate gains, additional evaluation takes place.

Another type of screening addresses a specific deficit area, such as fluency, articulation, or voice. In many cases, you use an instrument specifically devised for this purpose on the basis of a note you have made to yourself, such as "Check for voice problems." Usually, a comment like this one does not suggest a full-scale evaluation but only constitutes a reminder to use an additional screening instrument with a narrower focus. Many screenings take place in the spring and fall when allergies are common; when the pollen disappears, voice quality frequently returns to normal. Voice and fluency screenings are often addressed through checklists, self-inventories, or scales found in any text on assessment in speech–language pathology. Case histories, observation, and interviews are particularly important in these areas and will also be discussed later under "Case Selection." Remember, the whole process may cease at this point. First-grade teachers refer many more students for learning disability (LD) evaluations than are actually diagnosed as LD. Consider a child in the first grade who "sounds funny." Screening may reveal only that this 6-year-old does not pronounce medial or final /r/ correctly or that he uses a dialectical variation (e.g., he is from Houston, Long Island, or Boston).

Guidelines for Screening Choices

What characteristics of screening procedures and instruments should you consider as you make your choices? Different states and districts may vary in their specific rules for general screening, but most of them specify that this type of testing, regardless of the student's age, must

- be fair, unbiased, nondiscriminatory
- be presented in the child's native language

- be normative or criterion referenced
- be completed by a professional or trained paraprofessional
- be valid and reliable
- have clear directions
- be completed within specific time guidelines (e.g., by December 1 of the child's kindergarten year)
- be administered to a group (i.e., not used for an individual student except with the express written consent of the child's parent or guardian)
- test a broad enough span of ages so that it can be given to all children typically in the group or be an alternate test for slightly older or younger students. It is wise to avoid an instrument if the child's age places him or her at the upper or lower limits of the test.
- be easy to administer. Because kindergarten screening is often the first time a child experiences a "school-type" test, you want your attention on the child's responses, not on difficult-to-manipulate materials.
- be easy and quick to score. Some screening tests can be scored by computer, a real time saver. If results do not require interpretation, sometimes scoring can be completed by an aide.

Instruments should also

- screen articulation of age-appropriate phonemes
- screen both receptive and expressive language

If screening features a standardized instrument, check the instruction manual to verify the acceptability of these factors. If you need additional help in interpreting the information, refer to a standard text on measurement; Hutchinson's 1996 article on what to look for and how to interpret the information in the technical manual is also clear and very helpful. Depending on the circumstances, you may choose to emphasize the attributes of one screening procedure or test over another. For example, if you have a huge number of children to screen, you may want to go with one that takes as little time as possible; but if many of your children come from culturally diverse backgrounds, your choice may be quite different. In assessment choices, an enormous "but" seems to lurk perpetually on the horizon; a situation often appears that will dictate a change from an expert's preferred method, or from the last time you completed the procedure, or from the way you expected to do it when you walked through the door. Dealing with whatever arises requires flexibility; remaining open to change is the first prerequisite to keeping current in your profession.

A few last thoughts about screening. First, during the general procedures, you should remain alert to the possibility of a gifted child; this is another reason for choosing an instrument that has a broader age range. Second, the term *screening* can also refer to the procedure of identifying students who fall below a specific reference point on reading or other achievement tests administered to whole grade levels. Although the tests themselves are not screening instruments, you "screen" the results of these tests to identify students who may have undiscovered language deficits (Hill & Haynes, 1992). Last, screenings can refer to annual hearing and vision checks of the entire student body. Although formal screening remains one of the chief ways to locate students who demonstrate communication impairments or are at risk for them—that is, one of the chief methods of case finding—other sources of information are equally important in preliminary assessment or preassessment procedures. They include *referrals, observation, examination of records,* and *language sampling.*

Referrals

Referrals can come from a concerned parent, from almost anyone within the school community, and from outside agencies or individuals, such as a family physician or preschool program. Because they can include both informal and formal requests, they can range from a quick exchange in the teacher's lunchroom ("Please listen to Jonathan") to a written request to the district committee charged with determining if an evaluation is warranted. In New York State this group is called the Committee on Special Education, but different states and districts have adopted different names.

Because referrals constitute an important part of the assessment process (Kelly & Rice, 1986), all school personnel who have contact with a student should be encouraged to share their questions and concerns with the speech–language pathologist. Referrals are the most common form of initial identification of the older student (Larson & McKinley, 1995). They usually specify deficits in classroom performance but may not state specifically how those deficits are linked to language. Appendixes 3.B and 3.C show two different referral forms, one primarily for elementary and young middle school students and the other for older middle school and high school students. These forms do address the language link. Presenting an in-service training session on how to use a referral instrument can be a valuable undertaking for you, as the school's expert on speech and language. The meeting may lead to an avalanche of new referrals at first, but it provides an efficient way to sensitize teachers to the ways that speech–language problems can affect classroom performance and behavior, as well as to acquaint them with what you do. With the new emphasis on standards in many states, teachers are anxious to learn ways they can help their students meet the more sophisticated requirements these standards demand.

Another type of formal referral comes from a preschool committee that deals with children who have special needs. Known by different names, this body is concerned with children prior to their kindergarten year and oversees their educational and developmental needs from birth until the time they enter kindergarten. Here the referral contains much more detailed information, namely results of a full evaluation, the child's present IEP, and a report on the child's progress to date. Usually, although not always, the deficits of these children represent more severe handicapping conditions. Because of space limitations, this chapter will not include typical language profiles of students who represent "special populations," although information in Chapter 6 includes a description of some groups whose type of disorder has become more common since the first edition of this text. In addition, other sources can be helpful if you need information about specific conditions. Owens (1995), for example, described the language implications of traumatic brain injury, mental retardation, language learning disability, specific language impairment, autism, early expressive language delay, and neglect and abuse. Other authors have included severe emotional–social dysfunction, motor disorders (cerebral palsy, spina bifida, degenerative diseases), and visual impairment (McCormick & Schiefelbusch, 1984) and have discussed specific syndromes caused by either chromosomal abnormalities (e.g., Turner, Fragile X, 5p-, Prader-Willi) or metabolic disorders (e.g., PKU, thyroid, Hunter syndrome) (Paul, 2001). Shipley and McAfee (1998) assigned a chapter to assessment of neurologically based communicative disorders, and Richard and Hoge authored two volumes (1999, 2000) that provide information about syndromes with a focus on communication issues.

You can also contact organizations that were created to fund research and provide services for families of children who are included in these special groups; a Web search is often productive. Many times such organizations provide information about attendant speech–language problems. ASHA's new and welcome emphasis on school-based communication has resulted in publications that provide information on various disorders particularly useful to speech–language pathologists. An annual separate conference concerning school issues is now held by ASHA each summer, providing ample opportunity for speech–language professionals to acquire information and discuss concerns with colleagues who work in the same environment. School officials will frequently rely on your expertise and expect you to assume a leadership role regarding the educational and language implications of these disorders (Hux, Morris-Friehe, & Sanger, 1993). In most school districts, however, you will provide language support and intervention on a cross-categorical basis—that is, you will group children by what they need to accomplish to make them more competent language learners and users, not by the cause of their deficits.

Observation

The law (IDEA) makes it clear that students must be observed in the classroom if they have been referred for special education services. Unfortunately, observing a student who is suspected of having language deficits is often relegated to a secondary position in the screening and assessment process because of the perceived time needed. Observation, however, is crucial to gain a clear picture of the student's use and understanding of language within the classroom and other school environments. It is one thing for a student to attend to and reply to an SLP's question in the quiet "speech" room; it is often quite another for the student to perform in the presence of 25 other students in busy, active classrooms six or seven class periods a day. Observing a classroom of "regular" students can also serve as your reality check. It is easy to lose sight of how easily typical students learn, how quick and competent they are. Seeing children with a suspected deficit in the classroom environment where they "live" can be an instructive if painful reminder of how far behind their peers they fall. Observation also assumes a crucial role in authentic assessment procedures, discussed in Nanette Clapper's "Authentic Assessment" section later in this chapter.

Regardless, try to observe the student in as many school locations as possible, particularly if a deficit in pragmatics is suspected. Sites may include "special" classrooms, such as art, music, physical education, or the library, as well as the bus line, the lunchroom, the office, and the hall. Be sensitive to the possibility of culturally based differences if you are observing a child who is not a member of the majority group. Chapter 9 lists a number of cultural factors that can influence a youngster's behavior, such as use of time, individual versus group preference, and organizational style. A typical classroom observation form is included in Appendix 3.D; this can be combined with or replaced by one specifically designed for a student from a different culture. In the case of a preschool referral, it is common that you will be invited to observe the child in his or her preschool setting. At that time, you usually meet with the SLP who is serving the child, as well as the classroom teacher, and you will have an opportunity to ask questions about what you have seen. Observation not only is part of the screening process but is included in assessing deficits as well. When we discuss the four cases at the end of this chapter, we will look at how observation relates directly to evaluation and development of intervention goals.

A final word about observation in the screening process: Try to be alert to information about students wherever it appears. Describe typical or unusual behavior, but resist making a subjective interpretation of the behavior without an adequate foundation. When I was a graduate student, another student SLP and I were evaluating a 3-year-old. While I took data, my partner administered a standardized instrument to our young client, who was moving around in his chair, appeared anxious, and was not following directions very well. A doctoral candidate and several undergraduate students were viewing the procedure from behind a two-way mirror. The PhD candidate explained to the students that they were observing a most certainly hyperactive, perhaps ADD child. When my partner finished—unaware of what had transpired in the observation booth—this experienced mother of little boys knelt down and asked, "Honey, do you have to go potty?" Clutching his front, our small client frantically yelped, "Yeah!" A short trip to the bathroom later, his ADD with hyperactivity had disappeared. Moral: Observe, report, but do not jump to conclusions. At the very least, it can be embarrassing.

School and Other Records

Most schools use a parent information form as part of the kindergarten or first-grade entry process. For the younger student, it usually contains valuable information about language development, medical history, parent educational levels, family members in the household, and so forth. If the student is being seen by a learning disabilities or reading specialist, school psychologist, special education teacher, physical therapist, occupational therapist, social worker, guidance counselor, or other professionals within the school, you should note their perceptions of the student in question. The school nurse usually has current medical information, including developmental information, any prescription drugs the student is taking, and hearing status. The permanent school record can reveal persistent problems in spelling and reading, both of which often have a language base (Butler, 1999; Hill & Haynes, 1992; Temple & Gillet, 1984). Examples of spontaneous (not copied) completed classroom writing assignments should also be analyzed for possible semantic, syntactic, spelling, or organizational weaknesses. Written language is decontextualized; that is, the words alone must convey the message without gestures, intonation, or restatements to help clarify meaning. Consequently, a student's language deficits are often more obvious when they are in written form, particularly in the older student. These procedures are required by IDEA and are essential in authentic assessment.

Language Sampling

Language sampling is not commonly undertaken as part of the screening process in public school settings. Occasionally, however, formal screening instruments will include a brief sample. This topic will be addressed in more detail in the "Case Selection" section later in this chapter.

Once the screening process has identified a student as a possible candidate for services, there is often a meeting of the school-based team to determine whether the assessment process should continue. Depending on the district, this may be a separate committee, or it may be the evaluation committee previously mentioned. This group is also charged with determining if there are supports that can be put in place within the regular classroom that will assist the student in achieving success without undergoing a full evaluation.

If a full evaluation is recommended, there is usually a determination of who will administer what measures. This procedure will be discussed in detail in Chapter 4. During that meeting, the speech–language pathologist typically will outline what areas he or she will focus on during the evaluation and what procedures he or she will follow, including the administration of any standardized instruments. This step cannot proceed without written parental permission. How the speech–language professional decides what to do next will be the subject of the remainder of this chapter.

CASE SELECTION: TRADITIONAL APPROACHES TO ASSESSMENT

The following section contains information that deals primarily with periodic rather than ongoing assessment.

Selection Criteria

As the result of the screening processes, you may have identified 80 or 90 children who appear at risk and could benefit in some way from your services. It is unlikely that all of them have speech–language deficits, so what factors should you consider when deciding whom to recommend for inclusion on your caseload? Most professionals agree that you should reflect on how severe the disorder is in absolute terms, how it specifically affects school performance now and its potential as a causative factor in later problems (its educational significance), the age of the child, the disparity between the child's performance and that of his or her peers, and the length of time the student has exhibited the problem. Federal guidelines in IDEA serve as one source of information, as do your particular state and district standards. Recently, Medicaid funds have been disbursed to pay school districts for services provided to children in families who receive aid. With the money has come an additional list of rules and regulations. Your professional training, including a number of ASHA position statements, has provided you with yet another set of criteria. Predictably, these criteria can be in conflict with one another.

This problem is discussed in "Issues in Determining Eligibility for Language Intervention," an excellent report published in 1989 by ASHA's Committee on Language Disorders. Even though it was published more than a decade ago, its findings are not dated, and the conclusions of the committee remain valid. In brief, the article addresses the "economic, administrative and political factors that affect the determination of eligibility for language intervention [and] that are often beyond the speech–language professional's control" (p. 115). The article questioned the definition or model of language on which decisions are based and spoke to such speech–language professional problems as being required

- to use only district-"approved" standardized tests, discrepancy formulas, or other arbitrary criteria to determine eligibility;
- to exclude certain groups, such as learning-disabled students, if they are being served by other specialists; and
- to maintain an excessively large caseload.

For years, some professionals have expressed concern about these issues—for example, the practice of applying a discrepancy formula (i.e., an arbitrary difference between the student's actual language abilities and his or her anticipated abilities based on either chronological or mental age) to determine eligibility (ASHA, 1999b). Under IDEA P.L. 108-446, the local education authority (LEA) "shall not be required to take into consideration whether a child has a severe discrepancy between achievement and intellectual ability…." The Senate report, in explaining the rationale for this provision, stated that "there is no evidence that the IQ achievement discrepancy formula can be applied in a consistent and educationally reliable and valid manner" (IDEA, 2004). These issues will be discussed further in this chapter under "Standardized Testing" and "New Approaches to Assessment." In its entirety, however, this ASHA report provides a detailed discussion that is particularly useful for new school clinicians. "IDEA and Your Caseload: A Template for Eligibility and Dismissal Criteria for Students Ages 3 to 21" is another source of help for the inexperienced school-based speech–language professional. It is a compilation of material published by ASHA (1999b) and illustrates the excellent information about school-based practice available from your national professional organization.

In addition to the above issues, be aware that personal temptation can rear its ugly head. It can be an appealing idea to include on your caseload John, who has a mild, developmental articulation problem but whose school-board-member parent has been very supportive of programs for children with weaknesses in speech–language; or Jake, a second grader whose teacher is a good friend of yours and has encouraged you to work with him; or Susie, a wonderfully likable child who could use just a *little* help. Conversely, you may feel a strong desire not to include Jimmy, who, behaviorally, has been the bane of every teacher he has ever had; or Alicia, whose deficit represents an absolutely new area for you. Often, you can rationalize your decision or bury it in your unconscious, but how you deal with such temptations will be a test of your professional character. Remember, you are accountable.

Assessing Deficits

Assessing deficits from the traditional perspective is similar to screening in several ways. First, you will gather preassessment information; frequently, you can carry over facts gathered during screening into this new phase. In addition, you will add data collected from a case history, interviews, checklists, additional observations, an oral peripheral examination if indicated, and, of course, formal and informal testing. Although there is no required order in these steps, usually a case history or interviews are accomplished first.

Case History
As mentioned under "Screening," use the information that is already available in the school records, including the parent form completed when the child entered school. If the school district does not administer regular hearing screenings, be sure you check the date of the most recent one on file. If the parent form is very out of date, you may want to either have the parent complete a new form or at least ask during a parent interview about any recent events, such as names and ages of new siblings; a change in occupations; a divorce; any new medical problems, particularly allergies; or any medications that may alter behavior. Although a discussion of the case history is often combined with an interview, send the form home to be completed before talking with the parents or other caregivers. This allows family members time to consult records and each other. Be sure to review the completed form yourself before you talk with the parents either on the telephone or in person. Be aware that not all information

on a case history form is necessarily accurate, particularly if the student in question has a number of siblings. I'm a mother of five, and I can tell you that the amount of available detailed information on my children's development is in inverse proportion to their birth order.

The Oral Peripheral Examination

Appendix 3.E presents an abbreviated form that can be used to screen oral peripheral anatomy (form) and physiology (function). In the school population, these examinations are not usually completed unless the deficit could be caused by a physical problem (e.g., the presence of neurological soft signs, articulation difficulties, hypo- or hypernasality, drooling, eating problems). Remember that you must never conduct an oral peripheral examination without being properly gloved and taking other precautions to prevent the spread of disease.

The Interview

The interview process is as important in school-based practice as it is in other settings. Most texts on diagnosis and evaluation in speech–language pathology devote a chapter or more to the subject, and beginning clinicians can gain valuable general information from them. Any text on assessment has forms or lists of questions that can be adapted to a particular child's case (Owens, 1995; Paul, 2001; Shipley & McAfee, 1998).

Parent or Caregiver's Interview. As a school speech–language pathologist, you may not always conduct a full parent interview prior to assessment. The parents have been informed and have given legal permission for an evaluation, but, rather than an SLP, this contact may have been with the school psychologist, the chair of your school's committee dealing with children who may have special needs, or the vice principal. Often a phone conference suffices, in conjunction with a completed information form. Clinicians who deal primarily with the preschool population are the exception to this. If you are going to meet formally with the parents (or other guardians) before your testing, you must first figure out what you want to ask.

Before discussing questions to ask during an interview, let us look at some general guidelines to help the interaction be as productive as possible. Remember, this is not an inquisition, so do not appear authoritarian or judgmental. Be friendly, open, and noncommittal. Strive for a tone of acceptance and willingness to listen. During an interview, note the way caregivers handle language. Are they glib? Hesitant? Ungrammatical? Critical? Specific? Do they speak in generalities or clichés? Use a dialect? Interacting with parents can be potentially awkward if their educational background is very limited, if you and they represent different cultural groups, or if you do not speak their primary language. Conversely, if one or both parents are MDs, PhDs, or educators, you may feel intimidated. Regardless of the parents' educational background, always explain the purpose of the interview and the use to which you will put the information they give you. Make it clear that you will observe their rights to confidentiality, and expressly state with whom facts they provide may be shared. Remember that by law, your parents have a right to all information in their own language, with some new exceptions noted in the 2004 revision of IDEA. Lund and Duchan (1993) presented an excellent list of questions to ask a cultural informant, as well as other means of working with clients who come from a different background. Garcia (1992) dealt specifically with cultural differences between home and school language, and Damico and Hamayan's *Multicultural Language Intervention* (1992) has a section on ethnographic interviewing and the use of informants. Chapter 11 includes additional information.

Become familiar with the order of questions so you can focus your attention on the caregivers, not on what to ask next. Be prepared for emotional reactions and handle them as tactfully as possible when they occur; parents can be relieved, profane, accusatory, angry, apparently uninterested, or weepy. Caregivers may appear to be primarily interested in not being blamed for the child's problems, or in rationalizing their own or the child's behavior. If this is a first interview, they may be working through their grief at the prospect of losing their "perfect" child. A box of tissues on your desk is as much a part of your professional paraphernalia as your tape recorder. Don't rush! Regardless of your time schedule, try not to appear in a hurry.

Use open-ended questions as much as possible, and avoid leading or "loaded" questions—for example, "You didn't tell him his speech makes him sound like a sissy, did you?" Provide transitions. For example, if you have completed the section on developmental milestones and are moving into medical concerns, make clear the change in topic. Be aware that even the most benign question can be intimidating under some circumstances. Suppose you ask about injuries the child may have suffered. The child's mother may be the only one who knows that when he was 8 months old, he tumbled off her bed onto a hard floor. Her response could be guarded. Be prepared also for questions the parents may have for you. *Don't pretend to have information that you do not have.* The question you will hear again and again is, "Why is my child like this?" If you don't know, and you frequently won't, say so directly.

During the interview, frame direct questions that specifically address any problems in speech–language that the parent has observed in the home. This is equally important whether or not the parent is the referral source. If, for example, a teacher has referred the student, you may be dealing with parents who feel that their child functions just fine at home, thank you. If the parent has referred the child, but the teacher has not expressed concerns, it may be that the child is killing himself to keep up at school and doesn't fall apart until he reaches his front door. The interview may provide insights into parent expectations that do not match the school's, or may reveal a mismatch between home and school language demands. In either case, you have gained information you can use to plan your observations and assessment. If reading or spelling is a problem, be sure to ask if there is a history of either late talking or articulation problems, even if they disappeared over time. Another important factor is the existence of relatives who had problems in school. Research has indicated that there are some language-based reading problems that appear to have a familial base (Tallal, Ross, & Curtiss, 1989; Tomblin, 1991; Wallach & Butler, 1994a).

Don't forget that the family can be a source of strength for both the speech–language professional and the student during the young person's school years. Trivette, Dunst, Deal, Hamer, and Propst (1990) list qualities that characterize the supportive family and suggest that clinicians discover the family's strengths and then encourage the family to use those strengths to assist the child struggling in school. Sometimes we forget to look for and mention what the child, or his family, does well. We will address other aspects of parent counseling in Chapter 5, when we discuss intervention. A final comment: If you forget everything else in these paragraphs of advice, try to remember one thing. Talk less and listen more. Listen hard. Listen for confusion, for contradictions. Listen for concerns. Listen for cues. Listen for what is between the lines.

Teacher Interviews. Because an interview with a teacher is often done "off the cuff," much of the information you could gain from a more structured interview is left to be discovered later as you work with the student. Clearly, this is not the most effective use of your time. Although most college courses in measurement include a form for parent–client interviews, you may not have seen one to use with teachers. One of the most efficient ways to determine a teacher's view of a student's strengths and weaknesses is to use a checklist of communicative skills required in the student's grade—for example, those by Damico (1985, p. 187) and Larson and McKinley (1995). Conversely, you can review a list of typical errors associated with language-based learning disabilities. I have compiled such a list, which appears as Appendix 3.F. Using the referral forms in Appendixes 3.B and 3.C as an outline is another possibility.

School Nurse Interviews. The school nurse represents another source of information about your students that is frequently overlooked. In my experience, if a child is having new problems in the classroom, more frequent trips to the nurse are often the first indication. Stomach aches, headaches, diarrhea, and requests to go home early are common. An increase in absences can also indicate stress. Since school nurses are required to keep a log of student visits, information can be verified. A competent, caring school nurse can be a strong ally, particularly for the inexperienced public school speech–language pathologist.

The Student Interview. Ask even young students specific questions about how they are doing in class. Often children are aware that they are not succeeding, and having someone take their concerns seriously can be wonderfully helpful in establishing rapport. Sometimes students have a very different view from that of their teachers or parents, and this disparity can be clarified in later parent or teacher interviews. As mentioned under "Screening," a student interview is an effective means of gathering information at any age level. It is crucial when dealing with the older student. One of the most direct ways to encourage student communication is to use the pragmatics inventory in Creaghead and Tattershall's work (1985, p. 111). Their questions assess the student's awareness of classroom pragmatic rules, such as "When is it important to be quiet in this class?" and "How important is using correct grammar and spelling when you write for this teacher?" Another list adapted by Paul from Scott and Erwin and presented in her text (Paul, 2001, p. 528) deals with the student's perception of writing demands; some examples include "Did you write anything in school this month that was more than a paragraph long? What was the assignment?" and "What kinds of writing are easiest for you?"

Observations

As was discussed under "Screening," observations are absolutely critical in assessing language-based academic problems. In addition to the reasons stated previously, observation provides you with information that will directly relate to intervention. For example, if you observe a seventh grader during a social studies lesson, and it is obvious that she either cannot or will not take notes, you have identified an area that must be investigated further. Are the teacher's sentences too long or complex for her to follow? Does she have problems seeing any organizational pattern in the material, either narrative or expository? Can she write fast enough to keep up if she knows what to write? Does the teacher provide any overheads? Could the student use a partially completed outline? Does the vocabulary need to be pretaught? Is the classroom too noisy, too visually distracting, too hot, too cold? Can the student see the chalkboard? Can she read well enough for that to help? Regardless of grade level, students function in a variety of educational environments daily, particularly in middle and high school. The more of these in which you can observe the student, the better. If a deficit in pragmatics is likely, completing a checklist such as the Pragmatics Profile of the CELF–4 can be helpful (Semel, Wiig, & Secord, 2003). Setting up and observing how specific intervention techniques affect the student's ability to perform is a vital part of observational assessment, discussed in the second major section of this chapter, "New Approaches to Assessment."

Standardized Testing

The results of any standardized testing procedure are only as good as the tests themselves. A testing corollary of the computer truism "Garbage in, garbage out" is "Put good food into a contaminated container, and it becomes contaminated, too." IDEA P.L. 108-446 states specifically that measures and assessments must be technically sound. Therefore, before you trust the interpretation of standardized test results, you must determine to what extent the instrument in question qualifies as a good measure for your purpose. Part of that process involves understanding what the terms used by the authors of the instrument mean.

I have adapted the most frequently used descriptive terms from a variety of sources; they are listed in Figure 3.1. I am assuming that you have had at least some academic training in testing. If you have completed a recent course on the subject, you may find that you can just scan the table. Otherwise, you should consult a college textbook on measurement to clarify any terms you do

Age equivalent score: the age corresponding to the average or median raw score on a task obtained by students of a particular age. Most authorities caution against using only this score to determine eligibility because it contains no measure of typical variablity.

Anecdotal record: a written report of an incident describing a student's behavior, selected because of its assumed significance. Teachers will often provide reports of behaviors that are "typical" or "surprising"; anecdotal records are an integral part of interpretation-driven assessment.

Basal: the lowest point in testing, from which progress is recorded; all items numerically below this point are assumed to be correct and credit is given for them, even if the student has not completed those items.

Ceiling: the highest item in a sequence of test questions in which a certain number of items have been failed (e.g., 6 out of 8 wrong). It is assumed that all test items numerically beyond this point are incorrect, even if they have not been administered.

Concurrent validity: a measure of criterion-related validity that compares subjects' performance on the test to those on a similar test administered at about the same time.

Content sampling reliability: the internal consistency of a test; a measure of the interrelationship of test items.

Content validity: the extent to which a particular domain of content, e.g., expressive single-word vocabulary, represents a balanced and adequate sampling of what the test purports to measure (e.g., overall semantic ability).

Contrasted groups validity: a measure of criterion-related validity that compares the extent to which a test significantly discriminates between normal subjects and subjects known to possess disabilities for the skills being assessed. This is particularly important in screening.

Criterion-referenced test: establishes the criteria for acceptable responses; measures skills in terms of absolute levels of mastery (e.g., a multiplication test). Usually, criterion-referenced tests cover relatively small units of content. They tell what a student can or can't do, rather than assessing his performance in relation to other students. See McCauley (1996) for an application to speech and language.

Criterion-related validity: the extent to which scores on a test are related to some true measure of the behavior being assessed; this is often a question in language tests: Do they really measure language?

Derived scores: scores computed from raw scores that allow comparison of a student's performance with the performances of the normative sample (e.g., a percentile rank, standard score).

Face validity: a reference to the apparent content validity of a test when it is examined superficially or by an untrained individual.

Grade equivalent: a score that states the student's achievement in terms of the average expectations for a grade level. A common score in end-of-the-year tests in reading, math, etc. Like age equivalents, these scores contain no measure of variability.

Inter-examiner reliability: a measure of the validity with which different examiners administer or score a test.

Mean: the average score of a subject age group on a task. It is computed by dividing the sum of scores by the number of scores: the statistical average.

Mental age: a measure of a child's level of mental development, based on her performance on a test of mental ability and determined by the level of difficulty of the test items passed. If a child, regardless of age, can pass only those items passed by an average 6-year-old, the child will be assigned a mental-age (MA) score of 6 years; see Francis et al. (1996) for a discussion of this topic as it applies to language assessment.

Normative study: the procedure by which the final version of a test is administered to a large sample of subjects. The performances are then statistically analyzed and reported as test norms and derived scores.

Figure 3.1. Common testing terminology.

Norm-referenced test: a test that compares a student's performance to the performances of a representative sample of peers. It identifies where the child's performance on a particular instrument falls compared to others.

Percentile rank: the ranking that indicates the percentage of raw scores within a particular age or grade group that were lower than the raw score in question. If your raw score places you at the 35th percentile, then 34% of your peers scored lower, and 65% scored higher than you did. Caution: Parents often confuse this term with a percentage.

Practice effect: the change in scores on a test, usually a gain, resulting from previous practice with the test. This is one of the reasons that you should not repeat the same standardized test too soon, usually 6 months to a year before readministering it to the same student. Alternate forms of a test can circumvent this effect.

Predictive validity: a measure of criterion-related validity that estimates the extent to which test performances can be expected to relate to future performances on a criterion measure.

Raw score: the number earned when correct test items are computed (e.g., if there are 16 correct answers and each is worth 2 points, the raw score is 32). The raw score is usually converted into another type of score.

Reliability: in general, the consistency with which a test measures a given attribute or behavior: the stability, precision, and accuracy of scores. These can include test–retest, content sampling, split-half, and inter-examiner reliability.

Split-half reliability: a measure of a task's reliability by comparing scores obtained on one half of the task with scores obtained on the other half of the test.

Standardization: the process of administering a test in a systematic and consistent way to a large sample of subjects.

Standardized test: a test composed of selected materials with definite directions for use, predetermined norms, and data on reliability and validity.

Standard score: transforms raw scores into a set of scores having the same mean and standard deviation.

Test norms: the statistical summary of the raw scores received by the normative sample, usually represented in a table.

Test–retest reliability: the stability of test scores over time, measured by repeat testing of a group of students within a relatively short time.

Validity: the extent to which a test actually assesses the skills that it was designed to assess. It can include content, face, criterion-related, concurrent, predictive, and contracted groups validity.

Figure 3.1. *Continued.*

not understand or review other aspects of formal assessment not discussed in the following paragraphs. It is a valuable exercise to restate the definitions in your own words. Often you will have to explain these terms to parents, many of whom may have a limited educational background. Casually using the terms in a meeting with a parent who does not understand them can defeat the reason for the conference.

Lund and Duchan (1993) warned that reliability can be adversely affected by factors other than the test items themselves, such as unclear or complicated directions or individual test administrators' interpreting the questions differently. They also pointed out that the model of language on which the test is developed is an important factor in judging whether the questions on the instrument actually measure language—that is, their basic validity. If you frequently deal with dialectical differences or pragmatics—for example, if you wish to discover in which environments different kinds of language are or are not appropriate—you may conclude that the "mismatch" language model is most germane. At other times, you may be more interested in the etiology of a language problem, such as autism, mental retardation, or cerebral palsy. Other commonly used models are those that involve information processing, a neuropsychological basis, auditory processing, or descriptive developmental aspects. Rather than being identified as models per se, this information is sometimes described as a series of approaches and is covered during a historical review of diagnosis in speech–language pathology. The relationship of either to assessment lies in the fact that changing views about what language *is* lead to new tests and procedures. At some point, you must evaluate them and decide whether to use them in your practice or disregard them. Sabers (1996) cautioned that "by deciding to use one test over another, the clinician adopts the operational definition of the test's authors" (p. 103). Lest you consider this an esoteric issue, during legal hearings attorneys commonly question specialists like speech–language pathologists on the validity of their assessment procedures. A single chapter like this one obviously cannot include any real discussion of these issues, but most texts on language development go into the subject thoroughly, and a review of them can be very helpful as you analyze tests or procedures. I refer you to them. Hutchinson's (1996) article on how to use a technical manual is very helpful for inexperienced clinicians who must choose tests for their districts.

A frequently overlooked avenue of information about a specific test is the publisher of the instrument. If you have specific questions about the normative group or about whether, for example, you can repeat an instruction to a student, you should ask the publisher, preferably in writing. This serves not only to clear up your confusion but also to alert the publisher that you, as a user and potential buyer of future tests and "new, improved" versions of the instrument in question, require more detailed or more clearly written information. In other words, if the test directions or lack of them drives you crazy, complain. If you do not understand, ask. If the instrument does not include in the normative group members of the body to which your student belongs, do not use the test, and tell the publisher why. (We have reached the cranky mode.)

In addition to the technical considerations, all of us, teachers and students alike, should check tests for possible cultural bias. The issue of multicultural sensitivity addressed in Chapter 11 is particularly important in assessment because of the danger of overidentification—that is, of increasing "false positives" and consequent overrepresentation of minority students in special education programs. Federal law states that assessment must be racially or culturally nondiscriminatory. As a beginning, make sure that the normative data reflect the plurality of our population, and specifically include the group to which your student belongs. Some commonly administered instruments, such as the *Peabody Picture Vocabulary Test–Revised* (PPVT–R; Dunn & Dunn, 1981) and the *Goldman–Fristoe Test of Articulation* (Goldman & Fristoe, 1986), have been investigated for cultural and gender bias (Washington & Craig, 1992; Willabrand & Iwata-Reuyl, 1994). As a result of concerns, revised editions of both of these heavily used tests are now available: *Goldman–Fristoe Test of Articulation–2* (Goldman & Fristoe, 2000) and the *Peabody Picture Vocabulary Test–III* (Dunn & Dunn, 1997). McFadden's (1996) article on what constitutes "normal" in normative sampling raises some crucial issues regarding overidentification in general. It remains difficult, however, to determine whether a test is fair, unbiased, and nondiscriminatory for every child to whom you administer it. As you pursue your professional life, adopt the habit of sharing with colleagues your experiences using new tests and procedures; this is how the body of information on which we all rely grows.

In judging a test, we should also routinely investigate how easy or complicated it is to learn, administer, and score it. Note the time actually required to administer it completely and then score it. I remember with a shudder the first time I tried to score the then "new" *Clinical Evaluation of Language Fundamentals–Revised* (CELF–R; Semel, Wiig, & Secord, 1987). I was familiar with the original CELF (Semel & Wiig, 1980) and assumed I would have no problem scoring the newest version because I had just administered it with no difficulty. Several hours later, I was still flipping pages in the instructor's manual trying to figure out the confidence intervals. I can now score this instrument in minutes, even without computer assistance, but I feel obligated to warn students in my classes that the CELF–3 (Semel, Wiig, & Secord, 1995) is not an instrument to score "cold" the night before they have to present results in a formal meeting. The CELF–4 (Semel, Wiig, & Secord, 2003) has simplified the scoring process, leading me to believe that users informed the publisher that changes were in order. Other tests, such as the *Token Test for Children* (DiSimoni, 1978), the *Test of Word Finding–Second Edition* (German, 2000), and the *Lindamood Auditory Conceptualization Test–Third Edition* (Lindamood & Lindamood, 2004), require significant practice to administer smoothly and correctly. As overwhelming as the "alphabet soup" of test names may seem, be sure also that you can pronounce and spell them accurately: It is the *CELF*, not the SELF; the *TACL*, not the TACKLE; and, my favorite student "goof," the *Lindamood Test*, not Linda's Mood Test.

Apart from these issues, the single most important fact is whether the test addresses the specific suspected deficits of the student for whom the evaluation is planned. In the final section of this chapter, "Case Studies," we will plan initial assessment procedures for four different profiles of student deficits; part of that process will be choosing appropriate standardized instruments. Some of what you will need to absorb in this section of the chapter has been discussed earlier (e.g., testing terminology, multicultural concerns in testing), and you may want to review those areas before continuing.

Generally, assessing deficits can be divided into two main components: standardized testing and other procedures. In recent years the use of standardized instruments has come under increasing fire (Duchan, 1982; Muma, Lubinski, & Pierce, 1982; Siegel & Broen, 1976). Peterson and Marquardt (1990) stated, "No test is ever completely valid, and tests are only valid to the extent that they serve their function" (p. 11). Lund and Duchan (1993) contended that "one cannot judge the adequacy of a child's syntax or semantics without considering what the child is attempting to do" (p. 54); that is, one should not artificially separate form from the overall communicative contexts in which it occurs. They stated, "Part of the unnaturalness of tests comes from the removal of contextual clues in order to assure [that] the child 'knows' the answer only from the language forms given.... The language is often characteristically different from language in everyday communicative exchanges" (p. 324). Other concerns have been expressed because, as noted previously, the results of norm-referenced instruments can be misinterpreted or applied incorrectly, particularly to a population not adequately considered in the normative group. Particular concerns have been expressed by members of the African American, Hispanic, Native American, and Asian communities (Westby, 1994).

Another issue in using standardized tests to determine eligibility is that of assigning a number to a skill as incredibly complex as language comprehension and use. Kamhi (1993), applying the term *reification* to language assessment, defined it as "the process by which something abstract is turned into a material and concrete entity" (p. 111). Once we have done this, he asserts, our human tendency takes over "to rank complex variation into a gradual ascending scale" (p. 111). A quarter of a century ago, Muma (1978) warned that because behavior (and by extension, language) is "relative, conditional, complex and dynamic, [it follows that] clinical assessment must be relative, contextual, process-oriented and dynamic, ... not ... categorical, quantitative or normative.... [It] should be about an individual as he functions in natural contexts or deals with systems and processes directly relevant to natural behavior" (p. 211). According to Kamhi, inappropriate quantification and ranking can create and perpetuate potentially damaging misconceptions about competence and skill. We need to develop and use assessment procedures that better reflect the behaviors we are trying to change in treatment; for example, to reflect the underlying language skills that, when improved, will allow a student to reach his intellectual potential and be as successful as possible in the school environment.

Remember also that standardized tests can include both norm-referenced and criterion-referenced tests, used for different purposes. McCauley's (1996) article on the latter clarifies the differences. Norm-referenced tests rank individuals, their items are chosen to distinguish among individuals, they address broad content, and they summarize performances into percentile or standard scores. Criterion-referenced instruments distinguish specific levels of performance in a clearly specified domain and are summarized meaningfully using raw scores. Both types have their uses.

Although you should be keenly aware of why IDEA states that case selection cannot be based solely on the scores of standardized instruments, such instruments will undoubtedly remain part of the initial evaluation in the school environment. First, state or district guidelines often require that a child's scores on two standardized measures must fall 1.5 (or in some cases 2.0) standard deviations below the mean before a label indicating the presence of a disorder can be assigned. Standardized tests are also less subjective than informal means, and in many cases are less time consuming to administer, as well. This is an important consideration because you cannot afford to waste evaluation time on unnecessary or inefficient procedures. In addition, good standardized measures have been specifically designed to be administered and scored and the results interpreted using clearly stated procedures. Finally, issues of validity, reliability, correlation to other tests, and the presence of a normative group for comparison purposes (for norm-referenced measures) have been considered in their construction.

Caution, caution: Just because a test says it is standardized, it does not automatically follow that all these issues have been addressed properly. When Plante and Vance (1994) investigated 21 tests of language skills that included norms for children aged 4 and 5, only 38% met half or more of the following 10 psychometric criteria (see definitions in Figure 3.1). Each criterion is important in ensuring diagnostic accuracy.

- description of normative sample
- sample size
- item analysis
- means and standard deviations
- concurrent validity
- predictive validity
- interexaminer reliability
- description of test procedures
- description of tester qualifications

Plante and Vance also cautioned against comparing the results of two instruments if the standard deviations for the tests are markedly different.

All standardized tests have specific ways to be administered that must be followed if the accuracy of the scores is not to be compromised. It is part of your professional responsibility to review the directions carefully and practice as necessary before actually administering any instrument. The instructions may address some or all of the following: the permissible age range for the student; where the examiner and the student should sit in relation to each other and the test materials; how much training the examiner must have; whether test questions can be repeated; what prompts, if any, can be given; where to begin and end the testing procedure; the form the answers must be in (standards for the response); how the scoring is to be computed; time limits of the test; how long an examiner can wait for a question to be answered; training questions; and permissible reinforcers. A word of encouragement: You will be astonished at how quickly you become proficient once you gain some experience.

Types of Standardized Tests. As discussed previously, the two main categories of standardized tests are (a) norm-referenced and (b) criterion-referenced measures.

NORM-REFERENCED TESTS. These instruments are designed to determine relative ranking based on a comparison with members of the student's peer group. They are usually administered to answer the general question "Does this child have a problem?" Typical examples of this type of test in our field include the CELF–4 (Semel, Wiig, & Secord, 2003), the PPVT–III (Dunn

& Dunn, 1997), and the *Language Processing Test–Revised* (Richard & Hanner, 1995). As stated, one use of this type of test is to verify that the student's performance is inferior to that of his or her peers. If the instrument has a number of subtests, as in the case of the CELF–4, which has 10, it can also help identify specific areas within language that are deficient, such as receptive semantics or expressive syntax. The TOLD tests and the CELF–4 also use a composite of subtests to identify underlying skills and behaviors—for example, language content and memory.

CRITERION-REFERENCED TESTS. Tests of this type measure a child's performance in terms of mastery. They answer the question "Does this student exhibit these specific skills?" or conversely, "What is it this child can't do?" *Evaluating Communicative Competence–Revised* (Simon, 1994) and the *Test of Problem Solving–Adolescent* (Bowers, Barrett, Huisingh, Orman, & LoGiudice, 1991) are typical of this type; others include language sample analyses, pure-tone threshold screening, and percentage of intelligible words (Weiss, 1980). Almost all classroom examinations, ranging from weekly spelling tests to end-of-the-year examinations in chemistry and earth science, are also criterion referenced.

Reporting Scores Using Standard Deviations. After you have chosen and administered a standardized test, you must often report the scores orally and as part of a written report. Two examples of a speech–language diagnostic report are presented in Appendixes 3.G and 3.H. Standardized results often include terms such as *percentile rank, stanine, NCE score, deviation quotient, z or T score,* or *standard score* based on a mean of 100, 50, or 10. A score with a mean of 10 is sometimes called a *scaled score*. When you share numerical results of standard scores with other professionals, such terms as *stanine* or *z score* usually pose no problem. To expect parents to interpret what they mean, however, is expecting too much, particularly if the information is presented in the emotionally stressful atmosphere of an initial meeting to discuss whether their child has a disability.

One way to make results more understandable is to translate each score into a score based on the approximate standard deviation, as follows. Scores that fall between –1 and +1 *SD* are considered within normal limits. As mentioned before, most school districts do not consider that a child has a handicapping condition unless scores fall at least 1.5 or, in some districts, 2.0 standard deviations below the mean. The example below shows test scores and their translations into approximate standard deviations:

Test	Test Score	Standard Deviation
PPVT–III	Percentile rank 12	−1.0 to −1.5
CELF–4 Formulated Sentences	Standard score 6	−1.0 to −1.5
CELF–3 Expressive Language	Standard score 71	−1.5 to −2.0
Language Processing Test	Standard score 42	−0.5 to −1.0
Year-end reading score	Stanine 3	−1.0

There are precise numerical tables available to translate values exactly, but you can use the bell-shaped curve chart in Figure 3.2 to make the quick approximations given in the preceding table. Caution: Some standard scores, called *linear standard scores,* are computed from the mean and standard deviation of the sample; others, called *normalized standard scores,* are based on percentile ranks and their relationship to the z score in a normal distribution. To make the comparisons in the preceding table, the tests must be using the same unit of measurement.

Interpreting Scores Using Other Means. Other common ways to determine eligibility used by schools are based on discrepancy, age delay, and descriptive approaches. *Discrepancy* is usually defined in terms of a "significant language delay." Either the child's chronological age (CA) or "mental" age (MA) serves as the comparison. If you choose the former, be aware that all cognitively challenged children will likely be labeled as speech–language impaired, even if their language is on a par with or superior to their intellectual level. Choosing MA as the comparison, however, also presents problems, because using MA could eliminate students with mental retardation, even if they clearly need help in applying language skills to school situations.

Using MA to determine eligibility is called "cognitive profiling" and is in violation of ASHA and IDEA guidelines because it violates both the requirement that students not be denied (or granted) services on the basis of their disability category, and the requirement that all consideration of services must be on an individual basis. In addition, recent research has indicated that "language may surpass cognition ... [and] language intervention has been shown to benefit children whose cognitive levels were commensurate with their language levels, as well as children whose cognitive levels exceeded their language levels" (Cole, quoted in ASHA, 1999b, p. 17).

There are additional problems with using MA as the basis of comparison. First, the means used to calculate mental age can be affected by environmental factors, achievement history, motivation, ethnicity, and the problems inherent in any kind of standardized testing, such as validity or reliability issues. Often an IQ score is used as a measure of MA, and critics have stated for years that that measure may be contaminated because language skills themselves are used to determine the number. Not sure what this means? Think of it this way: Suppose you need to know if Medicine X lowers blood pressure. Before you can say that it does, you have to determine what "normal" blood pressure is. So you take readings, but only from people who are already on a medication. Clearly, you have contaminated your results. Francis et al. (1996) discuss this issue in detail. It is necessary to understand how IQ is measured before you can discuss comparisons with the school psychologist or in a meeting in which you have to justify services based on discrepancy. Chapter 12 contains a description of intelligence testing authored by a school psychologist. It contains important information for the SLP because of the similarities and differences to language testing.

Other colleagues in our field criticize discrepancy scores (and, by extension, standardized testing in general) because they are often based on a single

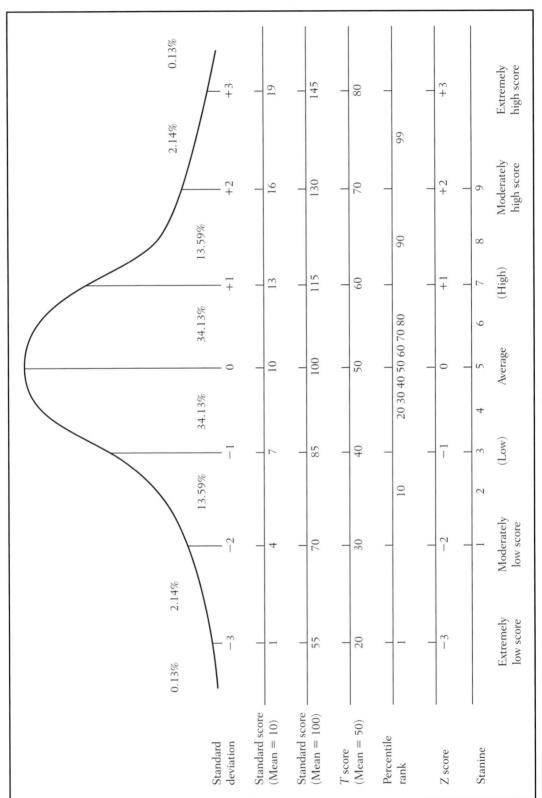

Figure 3.2. Bell-shaped curve used to convert test scores to approximate standard deviation.

area of language, such as phonology or syntax, and ignore others, such as pragmatics, expository and narrative discourse, or the relationship of language to reading or writing. Indeed, little generally accepted specific normative data for the latter three areas exist. Consequently, although a child may be judged as having weaknesses in syntax, the discrepancy in that specific area may not be considered large enough to warrant labeling the student—even though the youngster's overall communicative skills are too weak to allow success in the school environment. Closely linked to this criticism is the fact that deficits in some areas of language are potentially more serious than others in terms of their effect on school performance at advanced grade levels. These underlying problems with discrepancy formulas are the likely reason that the 2004 revision of IDEA states that when a specific learning disability is suspected, the school shall not be required to consider whether a discrepancy exists between achievement and intellectual ability.

An *age delay*, the second means of comparison, varies across grades and stages of development. Clearly, a child who is "one year behind," whether the comparison is to CA or MA, has a potentially higher degree of deficit if he is a 6-year-old first grader than if he is a 15-year-old in the 10th grade. Charts have been developed that present a sliding scale, but they are more often used with preschool than with school-age students. Age delays are also often based on *age equivalent* (AE) scores that, unlike standardized scores, do not consider normal variability. Take this example: A student who is 11 years 8 months old achieves a raw score of 120 on the *Peabody Picture Vocabulary Test–IIIA*. This score translates into an AE of 9 years 2 months, which seems to indicate a deficit. What the AE alone does not tell you, however, is that this raw score of 120 also represents a standard score of 87, which in turn indicates a standard deviation of –1, that is, a score that falls roughly within normal limits.

Descriptive approaches are almost always used as an addition to normative data. You employ them to indicate how the child applies (or does not apply) language during a specific school situation—for example, describing how a lack of organizational skills or memory deficits can be devastating to a high school student, regardless of subject area.

A severity rating can also be considered as an example of a descriptive approach if it is based on a subjective decision of the SLP—for example, if you evaluate a student's voice as having severe hypernasality, or his articulation as moderately deficient if it is intelligible with careful listening. A fluency disorder can also be described as mild, moderate, or severe. Other severity ratings, however, are linked to percentiles or standard scores. Customarily, a mild to moderate level is equated with a score between 1.0 and 1.5 standard deviations below the mean, a moderate level with a score between 1.5 and 2.0 standard deviations below the mean, and a severe level with a score 2.0 or more standard deviations below the mean. The value of descriptive approaches is that they often make more sense to parents and teachers.

Although we have concluded the topic many of you thought was synonymous with evaluation, standardized testing, keep in mind that the second section of this chapter, "New Approaches to Assessment," will acquaint you with other valuable ways to measure a student's competence.

Language Sampling

Like almost every aspect of assessment, language sampling has its advantages and disadvantages. Some of the advantages are obvious. A language sample not only allows you to say with absolute surety that a child can produce a structure or word spontaneously, but it can also provide more specific information concerning intervention goals, because, as Blau, Lahey, and Oleksiuk-Velez (1984) stated, it includes both the content and the context of language. Owens (1995) added, "If the goal of language intervention is generalization to the language used by the child in everyday situations, it is essential that the speech–language professional collect a language sample that is a good reflection of that language in actual use" (p. 120). In addition, spontaneous language sampling allows you to make an informal judgment concerning any possible voice, fluency, or articulation problems in connected speech. So if language sampling is such a good idea, why isn't it used routinely by all speech–language specialists?

Typical of relatively inexperienced clinicians, many of my speech–pathology students are scared to death of language samples or language sampling procedures in general, let alone the prospect of eliciting one from a school-age child. First, they worry that the child will not talk. Second, they fear that even if they do manage to collect a decent sample, their background in grammar and discourse analysis may be insufficient to evaluate the child's language correctly. Next, unlike standardized instruments, no script exists to tell them exactly what to say. Finally, clinicians often do not know the child well and may not know the child at all. Perhaps this common early experience is the reason that I have always compared language sampling in the schools to regular strenuous exercise. Every school-based speech–language professional understands how important taking a language sample is to the diagnostic procedure and knows how to do it, but many tend to avoid it as much as possible.

Another obstacle to language sampling among school-based speech–language professionals, in addition to general reluctance, is the obvious time constraints when you are dealing with caseloads of 40 to 60 students; this is particularly crucial when intervention time must be sacrificed because you are evaluating another student. Some school clinicians also cite the lack of accepted norms and procedures for the older school-age population. Few can dispute that, historically, this age group, compared with preschoolers, has been treated with benign neglect by those involved in basic language research. Fortunately, in the last decade there has been new interest in this area. The October 1995 issue of *Language, Speech, and Hearing Services in Schools* featured five articles that provided new normative data for school-age children, and Gummersall and Strong (1999) discuss complex sentence structure in a narrative context; the textbooks referred to earlier also include new useful data.

Even with new data, however, the problem of obtaining a truly representative sample remains. Hux et al. (1993) warned that school speech–language pathologists who create their own abbreviated procedures may "forfeit the benefits offered by standardized procedures with respect to reliability and validity" (p. 90). This quote appears at the end of an interesting survey conducted by the three authors, who reported on the analysis and collection procedures of 239 school-based speech–language pathologists in California, as well as their attitudes toward formal language sampling. Although the survey respondents recognized the importance of language sampling and reported using a variety of published standardized and nonstandardized guidelines to analyze the samples, most of them employed self-designed procedures. Usually, those procedures measured mean length of utterance (MLU) and the overall pragmatic, syntactic, morphological, and semantic aspects of language. The most popular elicitation technique was conversation, distantly followed by descriptions, story retelling, explanations, question-answer formats, and story-generation activities. The majority of respondents, however, employed language sampling only with younger or more severely involved students, not with older or mildly impaired ones.

If you decide to take a language sample as part of an assessment, here is a five-step procedure to consider: First, collect information to determine the best time and location for the sample. Next, decide what linguistic area or areas you wish to tap. Third, determine the means to elicit those areas. Following elicitation, interpret the sample. Finally, report the results.

Determining Time and Location. The questions of where and when will depend on the underlying purpose of your sample. Wallach and Butler (1994a, 1994b), Paul (1995, 2001), Owens (1995), Brinton and Fujiki (1992), and Simon (1985) have all spoken to this issue. Other authors have indicated that the most representative samples occur when children's language is evaluated in seminaturalistic and naturalistic situations (Lund & Duchan, 1993; Nelson, 1990). However, within those situations, what is your purpose? Are you interested primarily in the student's pragmatic behavior in a typical school setting? Or, because the student's written grammar is so poor, is your main focus the complexity (or lack of it) in his oral language? Do you feel, as Nelson (1994) suggested, that you should identify "the curricular contexts where language-related problems are evident" (p. 106)? Van Kleeck (1994) suggested taking a sample while the student pushes the limits of his competence as he uses language to work through problems. Indeed, many experts suggest that clinicians take several samples in different environments because a child's production will obviously undergo changes as he switches from the school setting to a casual setting outside the classroom when he converses with friends. Taking samples in different environments can also serve to indicate if the child can "switch code" as he moves from one setting to another. Even if you are primarily interested in expressive language, remember that, as Nelson (1985) stated, "it is often observed that children who have difficulty comprehending connected discourse or text also have difficulty expressing their own thoughts in a connected fashion" (p. 84). In other words, do not treat comprehension as a separate issue.

If you are not sure where or how to proceed, first review pertinent records, or complete your teacher or student interviews and your student observations.

If this is the student's initial evaluation, other school personnel will be investigating her academic achievement, learning characteristics, social and physical development, and management needs as required by federal and state statute. Often these assessments contain valuable information concerning language, such as the pragmatic implications of social development, the possible language basis of a low reading profile, or the extent of cultural literacy. On the other hand, if the child has already been labeled as having a learning disability in oral expression, listening comprehension, written expression, basic reading skills, reading comprehension, mathematical calculation, or mathematical reasoning, set up a language sample that will add to your knowledge of how the language problem specifically affects performance in each area.

You must also become aware of the changing demands and alterations in basic teaching methods that take place in the curriculum across the years, often an area of weakness for the inexperienced speech–language pathologist. Even if there is growth in a student's language skills, it frequently does not keep pace with the new skills needed to learn curricular material. Bashir (1989) stated that as the nature of a language disorder changes, it can ultimately affect a young child's academic, social, and vocational growth. As professionals in the field of speech and language, we must be able to adapt the student's goals to reflect the demands of a changing school environment, particularly as they apply to developing literacy.

Chapter 7 details the ways in which students' language skills relate to their learning how to read and write. In this section, we suggest how a language sample can provide valuable information about language deficits that are limiting literacy and educational growth. First, we must recognize how teacher expectations of students' basic language competence (oral, written, receptive, and expressive) change from early elementary grades through high school. Bashir (1989), Bashir and Scavuzzo (1992), Nippold (1998), and Westby (1999), among others, indicate that in the early grades, students are expected to understand and follow directions, and use their oral skills to generate early narratives, speak in small groups, tell themselves what to do (self-regulation), and establish and maintain social status. Reading skills in these grades require them to learn the relationship between phonology and decoding. As students progress to the middle elementary grades, their oral language skills reflect an increase in sentence length, complexity, and low-frequency syntactic structures. During these years, reading makes a shift from simple decoding to understanding content with all that this implies: gradual growth in receptive vocabulary; a shift from literal and factual understanding to making inferences; understanding idioms, sarcasm, and ambiguity; drawing conclusions and appreciating and using the organizational structure of written material (e.g., titles, appendices, subheadings). As implied earlier, students are expected to combine cognitive ability—for example, problem-solving skills—with language prowess. Orally, they are expected to apply information derived from reading to classroom discussions, dialogues, and conversation. Their academic writing becomes increasingly marked by literate language.

In the upper elementary and middle school grades, in addition to continued growth in the areas noted above, students are expected to become much more adept at adapting to the different language styles of instructional language that are present in lectures; to adjust to the vastly expanded language demands of multiplying subject areas (e.g., different kinds of science); and to read the technical material contained in their courses independently. Often the syntax found in their textbooks is far more complex than that used during conversation. Expressively, students share responsibility for acquiring information through dialogue with peers and teachers, as well as creating different types of products: summaries, research papers, and poetry, for example. Socially, language is used to maintain social bonds. Executive function demands increase as students organize their work, including their developing effective study and note-taking skills.

At the high school level, oral and written language begins to approach the adult level: Sentence length and complexity increase, particularly in written work. Persuasive and argumentative skills are used in the classroom, and knowledge of subtle stress changes and morphophonological rules allow increasing communicative sophistication both receptively and expressively.

Choosing the Area of the Limited Sample. Keep in mind the reason for this digression into the work of language researchers: You are deciding where and under what conditions to elicit a language sample. The work of language researchers suggests the role of the curriculum in your choice—that is, the language skills required to succeed academically. However, there is another way to select the means and area of your language sample: areas of weakness. A brief review of the "symptoms" of school problems and their relation to basic causes can also be helpful in deciding what area of language to target in language sampling and other testing. Globally, "the single most significant deterrent to educational growth remains the inability to use oral and written language, to speak and to read" (Stark & Wallach, 1980, p. 6). Within that inability lie the classic divisions you have learned by heart: phonology, morphology and syntax, semantics (including discourse), and pragmatics. Nelson (1989) added that a student's processing capabilities (receptive skills) should include metalinguistic skills—that is, the ability to analyze, discuss, and manipulate language. As a school speech–language professional, however, do not forget that the reason for addressing underlying language weaknesses is to enable the student to improve performance within the educational environment. You must also consider the relationship among and within the language areas. It is possible for a child to use a syntactically complex construction (embedded clauses) at the same time he exhibits very limited use of morphemes or basic verb construction, as in "I don't know he be on yet" for "I don't know if he has been on yet" (Wood, 1982, p. 14). Although the information in Appendix 3.F is hardly exhaustive, it represents a compilation of typical problems experienced by children with language-based learning problems. Incidentally, it would be rare for a student to display all the behaviors under any single heading.

Eliciting the Sample. Now to elicitation. Between preschool and high school come all the other grades, each with its own set of language expectations. Prior to student teaching, you, like many clinicians, may have had experience taking language samples from mostly preschool children. After a few times, you probably became relatively comfortable engaging in conversation while playing with a Fisher-Price Airport set. You also developed a sense of what to listen for, such as Brown's morphemes or simple syntactical structures. Facing a slouching, uncommunicative 14-year-old across the table is a distinctly different experience. Over the past decade, however, the literature has featured excellent examples of different ways to elicit samples that do relate to children in kindergarten through high school, as well as reports of the effects on obtaining a representative sample of such variables as contextual support, listener's knowledge of information, age, and mental capacity. A language sample can also serve as the basis for dynamic assessment and later mediated learning of a specific area of language. Miller, Gillam, and Pena (2001) have developed a program based on narratives that includes elicitation directions and criteria to evaluate the ability of children in this area. This information is used as a first step in understanding and choosing the supports the student will need to improve this crucial skill.

It is beyond the scope of this chapter to detail specific stories, techniques, and rationales, but the literature abounds with valuable suggestions like this treasure from Masterson and Kamhi (1991): Hold two balloons of different colors and sizes in front of the student. The larger balloon is filled with helium and the smaller with air. You hold one in each hand and then release them. The student must tell you what happened and then describe it to a classmate who was not in the room at the time. Among other results, the authors reported that more complex language occurred when the child explained what had happened to someone who was not a participant (absent referents) than when the child explained it to someone who was. The authors also gave examples of specific stories that clinicians can employ and ways that explanations can be used to elicit a good sample. Paul (2001) combines questions created by Evans and Craig to elicit a language sample from a student with learning disabilities with leading questions developed by Nelson—for example, initial question: "Are you in school? Tell me about it," followed after a few minutes of conversation by, "Did your teacher ever do anything that really bugged you?" (p. 426). If you are inexperienced in eliciting samples, be sure to consult the literature for techniques that match the age and interests of your student. The references at the end of this chapter and at the end of any article on language sampling will include some that may be exactly what you need. Note: If you have not already done so, now is the time to make the transition from seeing a journal article as something you take a test on (the student mode) to valuing it as a source of information you can use tomorrow (the professional mode).

One aspect of this complex procedure is worth noting. Practice helps enormously; trust me: The more you do it, the easier it becomes. If you have not worked around children the ages you will be working with in your student teaching, run, do not walk, to the nearest school, day care center, or Girl Scout troop and volunteer. It is not necessary to work with children who have a disability; just learning how to talk with children of different ages alone or in groups will remove some of your anxiety. Watch children's shows on television and go to G-rated movies. What cartoons or TV programs are "in"? If you are still talking about Power Rangers when first graders are crazy about Sponge Bob, you enter a conversation with two strikes against you. For older students, browse through teen or sports magazines. In case evaluation appears utterly overwhelming, remember, you do not have to do it all at once. Assessment continues to take place long after formal evaluation is over. Indeed, a competent speech–language professional continues to create hypotheses during every intervention session. This fact, incidentally, is one of the underlying assumptions of authentic assessment that is discussed later in this chapter.

Obviously, the reason you take a sample is to investigate some particular aspect of spontaneous language. But I cannot stress strongly enough that dividing language into rather arbitrary "components" for assessment purposes is potentially dangerous, whether for a language sample or otherwise. It is easy to lose sight of the effect of communicative intent, nonverbal cues, and use of scripts on overall language competence. That said, most clinicians find it helpful to provide a profile of the student's strengths and weaknesses and to include categories like "syntactic complexity," "discourse skills," and "age-inappropriate phonological processes."

Where do I stand on the issue of language samples? Although they are not routinely used in the school population except in the preschool group, and although most districts do not require them, I think that a speech–language professional, at the very least, must make notations about semantic strengths and weaknesses, presence or lack of syntactical complexity, narrative and expository discourse skills, and morphological implications of the student's spontaneous language. Problems in pragmatics should also be described. The results of a sample can be especially beneficial in helping teachers deal with specific deficits in the oral and written language of students whose first or primary means of communication is not English. Lists of structures for checking morphology and syntax are given in the sections that follow. In lieu of lists like these, you may prefer to feature "typical" utterances. In any case, samples based on oral language should also be compared with the student's written work, particularly in the upper grades. These suggestions are made with full knowledge that they do not represent the ideal or even the preferred mode. They do, however, reflect the reality of school practice, warts and all.

The kind of language interpretation that follows is not meant to be used as proof that the student should be labeled. It is more narrow. It only helps to discover the child's strengths and weaknesses as he approaches a specific verbal task required as part of his classwork. It therefore points us toward intervention that addresses any academic problems that are syntactically based. It is also quite possible that you could use a language sample primarily to investigate the child's pragmatic abilities as he interacts with peers. A month or two later, you might want to look at the child's semantics and narrative ability as he reports causes and effects while describing a third-grade science experiment. In actuality, you are continuing to assess the student long after the formal evaluation is over, creating and testing ongoing hypotheses as you work with the child.

To illustrate language sampling, I will present one way to sample a specific area. Let us assume that the student has problems using form, that is, morphology and syntax. Syntax, once a favorite topic in speech pathology, has received less emphasis in many college programs in the last decade or so. In a comment to an article by Hirschman (2000) on metalinguistic intervention for high school students, however, the editors of *Word of Mouth* (2001) added this comment, with which I heartily concur: "It is important for SLPs to understand complex sentence structure if [they] are going to teach it."

I will present an adaptation and expansion of a procedure based on Fujiki and Willbrand's (1982) suggestion that "a combination of spontaneous language sampling and sentence completion or elicited imitation" is likely to be most effective in clinical language evaluation (p. 48). You will first decide the most pertinent setting, "whether the student should be alone in the intervention room or part of a group in his class," and then arrange your chosen materials to engage the student as you take the sample (p. 48). From your sample you will note the form, content, and use your student makes of language. On the basis of that information, you can probe for elements that appear to be omitted or in error. If later you think you are still missing a key part of the puzzle, you may have to set up a means to check, preferably through a naturalistic approach.

Analyzing and Interpreting Morphological Structures in a Language Sample.
Our first task will be to review some basic morphological terms. (Although syntax and morphology analyses are usually combined, for clarity we will separate them.)

Morphology Terminology

Inflectional morpheme: Adds grammatical information to free morphemes, e.g., number, tense, possession (*goes, walked, Mama's*).

Derivational morpheme: Signals a change in part of speech (*run* [verb] + *er* = *runner* [noun]) or meaning (*tie* + *un* = *untie*, the opposite). For the older student with a language learning disability, derivational morphemes are the more difficult, but, combined with the semantic information garnered from the root of a word, they represent a means to acquire more advanced vocabulary (Templeton, 2002).

Prefix/suffix: Morphemes added at the beginning (*un-, sub-, mis-*) or end (*-ful, -ence, -ment*) of a root word. These are very difficult for the older student with LLD, who often fails to recognize independently the connection between microscope, microbiology, and microwave or fruitful, beautiful, and dreadful.

The next list contains the most common morphological and syntactical structures that are assessed in chronologically or developmentally younger students. Those marked with an asterisk are listed in Brown's 14 Morphemes

(Brown, 1973) and form the basis of morphological analysis for those in preschool or at that stage of language development. Brown's stages are frequently used as normative data, although the sample size on which they were based is extremely small.

The following refer to *verbs*:

*Copula: A linking verb that usually joins a subject to a complement, often a form of *to be*. The other copular forms are the verbs of the senses (*look, hear, taste, smell, sound*) and those like *appear, seem, become, grow, prove,* and *remain* that can be substituted in a sentence by some form of *be* and still make sense (It looks good = It *is* good; The rumor proved true = The rumor *is* true). Brown also categorized a copula on the basis of whether it could be shortened (e.g., *It's* hungry [contractible] vs. It *was* hungry [uncontractible]). This distinction is ignored in most language samples.

*Auxiliary: A helping verb used with a main verb to indicate action or tense (*is* going, has *been* running). Auxiliaries can also be characterized as contractible or uncontractible (e.g., *he's* going vs. he *was* going).

*Regular past tense: Completed action formed with the suffix *ed* (*walk* + *ed* = *walked*).

*Irregular past tense: Completed action without the suffix *ed*. Can be formed by changes in the vowel (*run/ran*), consonant (*leave/left*) or whole word (*go/went*). Students with LLD have difficulty with these, particularly the spelling rules associated with them.

*Present progressive: Continuing action formed with the suffix *ing* (*walk* + *ing*). Can be omitted in the younger child, used in place of more complex forms in the older. Students with LLD may omit the auxiliary that goes with it.

*Third-person singular: Present tense (she *eats*); action that requires *s* to be added to the third-person singular (he *walk* + *s*); often omitted in dialectical variations.

Lexical: A kind of verb that adds content or meaning to the utterance, the type you usually mean when you say that verbs show action or a state of being. The complication for students with LLD comes when they confuse the perfective auxiliary (all the forms of *have*) or the *do* auxiliary (including *does, did*) with the lexical form (I *have* six cats [lexical] vs. I *have fed* six cats [auxiliary]; I *did* the dishes [lexical] vs. I *did want* that new dress [auxiliary]). The subtle difference in meaning between "He *has* gone" and "He *had* gone" can cause problems in reading comprehension at the middle and high school levels.

Catenative: Early infinitive or modal form (*gonna, wanna, gotta, hafta*); its use persists in slang and even in formal language used by the student with LLD.

Participle: Verb form that functions as an adjective (*broken* branch, *running* shoe). Metalinguistically, this is difficult for students with LLD.

Gerund: Verb form that functions as a noun (*Swimming* is fun; *Running* can be exhausting). This form is also a metalinguistic puzzle for students with LLD.

The remaining terms deal with other parts of speech:

*Article: A noun modifier that denotes specificity. In young children it is often omitted; in older students with LLD, *an* may be omitted before a word beginning with a vowel, or *a* and *the* may be confused, that is, the student may not understand the difference between *a* book and *the* book.

*Plural: Denotes more than one. This can be omitted, particularly in certain dialects. Errors persist in the irregular forms in students with LLD (e.g., the plural *deer*). Correct spelling can also present a problem (e.g., using *cat's* instead of *cats* or *it's* for *its*).

*Possessive: Denotes ownership. Spelling confusion is common here also.

Adverb: Supplies information about time, place, manner, degree, or cause of action. The *ly* suffix is rarely used by the student with LLD.

Preposition: Connects nouns or pronouns with other parts of the sentence. The idiomatic use of these causes problems (e.g., *on time, in a hurry*).

*"In" and *"on."* Part of Brown's 14 morphemes.

Adjective: Descriptive words. The order of these may be confused by students with LLD, or they may overuse a few favorite terms.

Conjunction: A class of connectors that indicate the relationship between the joined parts of an utterance. Typical of the child with LLD is the overuse of *and,* as well as the lack of more sophisticated conjunctions, such as *although* and *however.* Comprehension of what these words "signal" in terms of lexical cohesion is also a problem in older students with LLD.

Comparatives and superlatives: A means of comparison. Irregular forms (e.g., *best*) cause problems for the child with LLD.

MLU: Mean length of utterance, used to compute the average length of the child's utterance by either the number of morphemes or the number of words divided by the total number of utterances. In the older student, the count is usually in T-units or C-units rather than morphemes. Instructions for how to calculate T-units and C-units appear later in this chapter.

Following is an illustrative language sample subjected to morphological analysis; the sample represents a younger child:

SLP	Billy
Hi, Mike, what did you do this weekend?	Billy and me goed to zoo.
What fun! Who's Billy?	Billy mine brother, mine little brother. He two.

What did you see?	We seed three lion. And two tiger. But no monkeys.
What did you do?	We climb way, way, way up.
Where?	On a ur, um, uh, hill.
Where was the hill?	In zoo.
Was something there?	Yeah, elephants up there. They feeding the baby. The baby mama mean! She runned at fence. She goed, "ROWRRRRR!"
Wow, that's exciting!	Bill and me afraid.
Do you want to go back again?	We can't.
Really?	Daddy say we can go when Grandma come.

I have entered the results of the analysis on a simple chart under these headings: mean length of utterance (MLU), morphological structures correctly used, structures omitted, and structures in error. At this point we can decide if there are other structures we need to check. Following this, we can decide if there are other structures we need to elicit, for example, the correct use of the regular past tense marker *ed*. Mike used this suffix as a substitute for the irregular past (*goed*), but did not use it when it was required to make *climbed* (*climb*).

MLU
◀▶ 76 morphemes, divided by 17 utterances = 4.47
  (age appropriate)

Morphological Structures Correctly Used in Obligatory Context
- present progressive
- *in, on*
- plural (inconsistently)
- article—*a* (inconsistently)

Structures correctly used in obligatory context include grammatical structures required in English (e.g., adding *s* to *cat* to say "a bunch of cats").

Structures Omitted
- copula
- possessive
- article—*the, a* (inconsistently)
- auxiliary—*were*
- regular past
- third person singular present tense, also called *s* verb marker

Omitting a structure, as opposed to substituting an incorrect form, is generally of greater concern because omission may indicate that the child is unaware of the structure or does not appreciate its importance.

Structures in Error
- substitution of regular for irregular past
- pronoun substitution: *mine* for *my; me* for *I*

Appendix 3.A contains a list of standardized tests that can be used in part or in their entirety if you need the standardized "numbers" for a report. Those included in the following list measure some aspect of morphology. (An asterisk marks those tests with a chart for African American English [AAE] use.) Using only a portion of a test can save time and allow you to focus only on those test items that are likely to appear as intervention goals. After assessing these limited targets, we can describe the child's strengths and weaknesses in the general area of morphology but only under the conditions and limitations that existed at the time the sample was taken. In Chapter 7, we discuss the implications of morphological limitations as they apply to the older school-age child, particularly their connection to spelling and advanced vocabulary growth. Chapter 5 will feature intervention.

In some morphological analyses, you calculate the exact percentage of times that the child used each structure. If you do not do this, at least note whether inconsistencies exist. These are often the clue to what "rule" the child is using, as, for example, the regular and irregular past tense markers in the preceding example of Mike.

Evaluation Instruments That Address Morphology
Clinical Evaluation of Language Fundamentals–4 (Semel, Wiig, & Secord, 2003), *Word Structure Subtest. Irregular and regular plurals, regular and irregular past tense, possessives, 3PS, comparatives and superlatives, auxiliaries + ing, copulas and auxiliaries, derivations of nouns and adjectives, reflexives, possessives, subjective and objective pronouns.

Bankson Language Test–2 (Bankson, 1990). Pronouns, present progressives, regular and irregular past tense, 3PS, auxiliaries, copulas.

Patterned Expressive Syntax Test with Morphophonemic Analysis–Revised (Young & Perachio, 1993). All of Brown's 14 morphemes, arranged developmentally, plus others more advanced.

**Structured Photographic Expressive Language Test–Preschool* (Dawson et al., 2004).

**Structured Photographic Expressive Language Test–3* (Dawson & Stout, 2003). Auxiliaries, copulas, plurals, present progressives, regular and irregular past tense, third-person singular.

Clinical Evaluation of Language Fundamentals–Preschool–2nd edition (Wiig, Secord, & Semel, 2004). Plurals, possessives, 3PS, regular and irregular past tense, present progressives, copulas, auxiliaries, pronouns.

Test of Language Development III–Primary (Newcomer & Hammill, 1997b), Grammatic Completion Subtest. Possessives, 3PS, regular and irregular past tense, plurals, present progressives, comparatives and superlatives.

Preschool Language Scale–4 (Zimmerman, Steiner, & Pond, 2002). Regular and irregular plurals, possessives, *in, on,* regular and irregular past tense, present progressives, auxiliaries, copulas.

Test for Examining Expressive Morphology (Shipley, Stone, & Sue, 1983). Uses cloze; present progressives, regular and irregular past tense, plurals, 3PS. Age ranges given for each structure.

Test for Auditory Comprehension of Language–3 (Carrow-Woolfolk, 1999b). Subtest 2 addresses receptive morphology. Can be used beyond age range for criterion testing.

After you complete an initial analysis, attempt to elicit all omitted or substituted structures using portions of the tests listed here or your own informal elicitation techniques.

Illustration: Sampling for Syntactic Analysis

Our next step is to perform the same type of analysis, but featuring syntax rather than morphology. In a real sample, these two linguistic areas are usually combined; they are separated here only for teaching purposes. Again, it will first be helpful to review some syntactic terms.

Sentence Types. There are four basic types of sentences:

Simple: Contains a single independent clause (My cat Zach is black).

Compound: Contains two independent clauses joined by certain words called *coordinating conjunctions*—for example, *and, but, or* (Zach is black, but his mother was a Siamese).

Complex: Contains one independent clause and a minimum of one dependent clause joined by a *subordinating conjunction*—for example, *because, until, if* (My cat won a ribbon because he was affectionate with the judge). Nippold (1998) also characterizes as complex sentence types those featuring an independent clause plus an infinitive (We wanted *to see* all the exotic breeds at the cat show) and those containing an independent clause and a gerund (Going to a cat show makes for a long day) or a participle (*Purring,* Zach snuggled into the judge's neck).

Compound–complex: Contains a minimum of two independent clauses plus at least one dependent clause (Zack didn't win Best in Show, but he won Best in my Heart because he is such a smooch).

Nippold (1998) indicates that understanding the meaning of the various types of conjunctions differentiating these sentence types is "important to the development of literacy and … [we] should pay attention to children's understanding of these words" (p. 164).

Parts of Sentences

THE NOUN PHRASE. Most SLPs include five components in the noun phrase. All but the noun itself (sometimes called the *head*) are optional. In the utterance, "Daddy come!" *Daddy* is a noun phrase. These components appear in a predetermined order:

◀▶ **initiator + determiner + adjectival + noun + post modifier**

The first three components come before (in front of) the noun, but they all modify the noun:

> *Initiator:* A special class of qualifier that can precede a determiner (*only, just, almost, nearly …*).
>
> *Determiner:* Denotes specificity; can be a quantifier (*both, some, any*), an article, a possessive pronoun (*our, my*), a demonstrative pronoun (*this, those*), or a number.
>
> *Adjective of any type:* A noun marked for possession (*Mommy's*), an ordinal number (*first, third*), a noun used as an adjective (*truck* stop, *turkey* farm).

Next comes the noun itself (e.g., *students*). After the noun comes the post noun modifier, which can include the following:

> Prepositional phrase (*in the snow, up a tree*)
> Relative clause (*that I used to know, that Mom always gave me*)
> Adverb (*here, there*)
> Appositive (Judy, *our leader*)

A noun phrase may be as simple as a single word, or as complicated as "half that scrumptious, calorie-laden chocolate cream pie they served me" or "only his incredible fire-engine-red convertible in the driveway." Noun phrases become more elaborate as a child's syntax becomes more sophisticated. All the elements listed above can occur in a child by Brown's Stage V (Brown, 1973).

THE VERB PHRASE. Like a noun phrase, a verb phrase can be composed of a single word; *go* in "Daddy go" is a verb phrase. Like a noun phrase, the verb phrase also has a head; in "Daddy go" the verb "go" is the head; the head can also be called the *main verb.* It is important to note that the copula, if one exists in a sentence, serves as the head, that is, the main verb. Optional categories that can be added to the main verb are a modal auxiliary, perfective auxiliary,

auxiliary (*be* form), negative, passive, and post verb modifier. Therefore, any of the following can come in front of the main verb:

Modal: A kind of auxiliary verb that expresses an attitude or intention (*can, may, will, shall, should, would, could, might, must*). Not understanding subtle differences in meaning between modals can reduce comprehension of both oral and written material (e.g., I *will* ski vs. I *can* ski).

Perfective: The forms of *have* verbs that denote action that has been or will be completed by a certain time (*have gone*).

"Be" auxiliary: Includes singular and plural present and past tense forms (*am, is, are, was, were, be, been*). Children with language weaknesses often omit auxiliaries ("he *is* going" becomes "he *going*"). It is also difficult for many students to differentiate between the copula and the auxiliary *be* forms: "She *is* (copula) a student" vs. "She *is* (auxiliary) going to school." SLPs must be accurate in their designation because auxiliary use is typical of later developing forms.

Negative: Not or its contracted form, *n't*. The negative comes between the modal and perfective forms (*could not have gone*).

Passive: In its simplest explanation, the passive represents a two-step process: First, it is marked by *been* or *being* (he has *been*); second, it is marked by an addition to the head, usually *ed* or *en* ("he has *been eaten* by cannibals," "he is *being nibbled* to death by ducks"). The passive is difficult for students with a language weakness to comprehend, because it changes the typical active order of subject–verb–direct object, in which the subject is the active agent (e.g., The car hit the dog) and makes the subject the object of the verb (e.g., The dog was hit by the car).

After the verb comes the post verb modifier, which can include

- prepositional phrases (e.g., *in the bucket*)
- noun phrases (e.g., *a new coat*)
- adverbial phrases (e.g., *too late, far away*)

So, a verb phrase can be as simple as the word *go* or as complicated as "might have been studying in the bedroom all night" or "would not have been eaten by the children."

NEGATIVES. Negation can include any form of negation (e.g., *no, don't, not*). It does not appear in a set sequence like noun and verb phrases. If a sentence contains auxiliaries of any type, the negative comes after the first element in a verb phrase (he is *not* happy; the cat should *not* have been let loose). When there is no auxiliary, that rule does not work (I type *not*), and we have to add a form of the auxiliary *do* in front of the main verb (I *don't* type; I *do not* type). Dialectical variations are common (e.g., *ain't* and double negative: I *don't* want *no* more cake).

QUESTION FORMS. There are three forms of questions: *yes/no* (Y/N), *WH* (what, who, when, where, why, how), and *tag* (a question added to the end of a declarative sentence, intended to seek agreement rather than information). The order of acquisition of question forms, based on Brown's stages, with examples of each is as follows:

Stage I: Intonation only (*Go? Mama?*); WH form as a single word question (*what?*).

Stage II: Y/N with intonation but no auxiliary verb (*Doggie nice? Mama go?*); use of *why* and *where*.

Stage III: Y/N with auxiliary and inversion (*Is Doggie nice?*); WH with no inversion of auxiliary (*Where she is going?*).

Stage IV: WH with inversion of auxiliary (*Where is she going?*); inversion of subject and either the main or auxiliary verb in positive questions only; use of *when, how,* and *why* completely correct.

Stage V: Inversion of subject or auxiliary with negative questions, also (*Can't I go? Isn't she going?*); use of tag questions (*She's going, isn't she?*); use of obligatory *do* in questions (*Do you want to go?*). Students with LLD often confuse the order of questions much beyond the ages expected.

CONJUNCTIONS. As stated previously, conjunctions are enormously important because they are required in more advanced clause structures. Consequently, their correct use indicates a student's ability to express a complex thought. Interpreting the precise meaning that specific conjunctions impart to the clauses they connect can be a factor in comprehending the typically longer and more complex structures found in textbooks and document-based questions. Ways to help students understand different types of conjunctions will be discussed in Chapter 7.

CLAUSES. Each clause must contain both a subject and a verb, except for infinitive, gerund, and participle types, as noted previously. There are a number of different types, and several can be combined within a single sentence.

Simple: Contains only a subject and a verb (e.g., "She's going").

Simple with compound subject ("*The girl and boy* are going), *verb* ("She *ran but fell*"), or *object* ("She likes *burritos or tacos*"). The subject, verb, or object contains two or more words, joined by *and, but,* or *or.*

Compound clause: Contains two clauses, each with a subject and a verb, joined by *and, but,* or *or.*
"The girl is running, and the boy is hopping."
"The man laughed, but the boys frowned."
"She is laughing, or she is crying."

Object clause: Uses verbs like *hope, know, think, feel, hate, like, remember;* answers the question "what?"; also called *propositional complement.*
"She knew *that they did it.*"
"I hope *that you are ready to go.*"
"I like *how you did that.*"
"I think [*that*] *I want this one.*" (*that* can be present or absent)

Relative clause, right embedded: Clause modifies a noun that appears at the end of the first clause.

"The boy hit the door *that had been left open.*"

"I want the puppy *that we saw last night.*"

Relative clause, center embedded: "Interrupts" the main clause; modifies a noun.

"The puppy *that you wanted* was sold."

"The girl *who has long red fingernails* won't wash any dishes."

Embedded question: Contains WH words but *not* in a sentence that asks a question; also called *WH clause.*

"I like *how you did that.*"

"She told him *why she wanted to go.*"

"I hope you know *when your homework is due.*"

{Complex}/[compound]: Contains both a compound and a complex clause

{She went shopping, and then she took in the movie} [that was playing at the mall].

{They ran, but they missed the bus} [that had already left].

{I know [that you wanted a scholar], but I hate school.}

Multiple clauses of other types:

"I think I know what you mean." Embedded question within object clause.

"Since I went to college, I have watched little television except when the Olympics are on." Adverbial clause, main clause (independent), embedded question.

Subordinate (dependent) clause: Can include

relative clauses

object clauses

Infinitive clauses: Generally does not include the early infinitive forms (contentatives) such as *gonna, wanna,* and *gotta.* In early stages the subject is the same as the main sentence and is often deleted ("I want to go" means "I want me to go"; *me* is deleted). Later stages feature embedded clauses that have a different subject from the main clause ("I want it to go chug" in which *it,* not *I,* will go chug).

Adverbial clauses: Dependent clauses that contain a subject and a verb that explains when, where, why, or how ("after he comes back," "where he told me to," "because I am over 21," "as if he were feeling sad").

Adverbial constructs: Linguistic devices that indicate cohesion between sentences or paragraphs; their use is an example of a student's intersentential growth. Understanding the relationship they mark is necessary to comprehend both oral and written material at the upper levels. Examples include *meanwhile, nevertheless, subsequently, thus.*

This list represents only the bare bones of information you can use to describe syntactical form. For older students and for written examples, you will need more sophisticated information—for example, Nippold's chapter on syntax (1998). Understanding and expanding different syntactic divisions is necessary to communicate the increasingly complex thoughts required in the curriculum of the upper grade levels. Remember, you are a speech–language professional, and operating without a solid metalinguistic foundation is like sailing across the ocean without charts or a GPS. On very old maps, unexplored oceans were marked, "There be dragons." Our particular dragon is labeled "misdiagnosis," and it is a frightening prospect indeed.

As a school speech–language pathologist, you will probably find it most helpful to note a student's skill at both the intrasentential and intersentential levels. Intrasentential growth occurs within the sentence; intersentential refers to changes in how sentences are joined. The latter is a more important consideration for upper middle school and high school students, particularly in written assignments. All students, however, regardless of grade level, must comprehend the meaning of intersentential terms in order to understand literate academic language.

You can document a student's intrasentential growth by checking five general areas: (a) the elaboration of noun phrases, (b) the elaboration of verb phrases, (c) the use of negatives, (d) correct use of Y/N and WH question forms, and (e) increased complexity as determined by conjunctions. For younger children, or those delayed to that level, all language development texts contain the developmental order of each of these areas through Brown's Stage V++. For students in the upper grades, calculate T-units (terminable units) and C-units (communication units), described later in this section.

Developing a representative list of standardized instruments for syntax, similar to that shown earlier in this chapter for morphology, is a valuable exercise. Instruments can be used whole or in part to gain more information about error structures identified in the sample.

Now, looking at the sample below, identify those syntactic structures that are omitted, contain errors, or do not appear (are not obligatory) in the context of the sample.

Head Start Teacher	**Client**
Hi, Luis, what did you do over the weekend?	Saturday I walk to store to get some pants that aren't dumb.
What do you mean?	My Aunt Angela give me pants on my birthday, but they are ugly.
Ugly?	Yeah.
	With stripes.
	And they is more ugly than ur, uh, warts.
	Nobody like them.
Did you find some you like?	Yeah, jeans. (Points to ones he has on) See?
(Looks at them) They *are* nice. Did you look at anything else?	Yeah, at boots.

Did you get some?

We couldn't.
My mama say that they are
too much money, so we go
home.

I'm sorry; maybe next time.

Where you shop?

I like catalogs. I was shopping just
before you came in to see me.

How you are shopping in them?

I look at pictures to find something
I like, and then I look at how much
it costs. (Points to page) Here, you
look. Do you like this shirt?

No. I no like that one. My sister
maybe would like it.

(Teacher starts to turn page)

No turn yet. (Luis points to
another shirt) My sister like big
shirts. Bought some with her
own money. (Indicates a blue
one) This is the shirt of my
sister.

Below is the analysis and interpretation of the sample.

◆▶ MLU by morphemes = 5.35 (age appropriate)

Present in Sample: Noun Phrase Elaboration
- a few adjectives
- increasing length of noun phrase
- object clauses
- post noun modifiers
- relative clauses

Verb Forms Used in Obligatory Context
- present progressive
- copula (but error in number)
- modal (*would*)
- uncontractible auxiliary (*are*)
- relative clauses

Verb Forms in Error
- irregular past
- regular past
- third-person singular verb marker

Negative Forms Used in Obligatory Context
- *no* and *no* plus verb
- *aren't, couldn't, nobody*

Negative Forms in Error
- *no* substituted for *don't*

Question Forms Used
- Intonation for Y/N
- *where, how*

Question Forms in Error
- no inversion of subject and auxiliary verb
- no inversion for WH questions
- no obligatory *do* in questions

Conjunctions Used
- *and*
- *but, so* joining clauses

Other Errors
- possessive, articles
- omission of pronouns

An interesting aspect of this sample is that Luis's use of English may be influenced by his Hispanic background and his first language, Spanish. In the background information, it was revealed that his mother does not speak English. Consequently, you will want to make a differential diagnosis between morphemes and grammatical structures that may reflect Spanish language influence versus those that may indicate a language problem. After you have elicited these structures, check the results against a standard list of morphological–syntactic differences common to Hispanic speakers. These include but are not limited to lack of a possessive marker ("the shirt of my brother" vs. "my brother's shirt"), substitution of the regular past *ed* ending for the irregular form, omission of the third-person singular, lack of the obligatory *do,* and omission of articles. You can find charts that show dialectical differences common in speakers who are of an Asian, Black English, or Hispanic background in Lund and Duchan (1993), Owens (1995), Shipley and McAfee (1998), and Roseberry-McKibbin (1995), among others.

An increase in the complexity and length of both spoken and written language (linked to semantic meaning) is the hallmark of a competent language user in the schools. Often a deficit in this area is not obvious because students may not make noticeable errors during conversational speech. If their spoken language generally is simpler in structure, uses fewer abstractions, is less organized and less elaborate than that of their peers, however, it may provide "an insufficient base both for the understanding of literate language and for age-appropriate writing skills" (Paul, 1995, p. 410). Leaving semantics, discourse, and pragmatics aside for the moment, let us consider syntax. Once a student is beyond Brown's Stage V, you must develop new means to describe the length and complexity of her sentences. Based on the work of Loban (1976), Scott

(1988), Scott and Stokes (1995), Nippold (1998), and Paul (1981, 1995), I suggest the following steps:

- calculate MLU in words (not morphemes) using T-units or C-units of both spoken and written samples;
- divide the T-units or C-units into complex, coordinating, and simple segments;
- using those segments, calculate the subordination index;
- divide clauses into early or late types;
- calculate the number of disruptions;
- determine whether the results indicate general age-appropriate development; and
- compare oral and written language complexity and length.

Because Paul indicates that "using MLU per T-unit rather than per sentence will provide a more valid assessment of utterance length" (2001, p. 514), the first step will be to divide the sample into T-units. In brief, a T-unit is one main clause with all the subordinate (dependent) clauses and nonclausal phrases attached to or embedded in it. All coordinated clauses (those connected by *and, but, or*) are separated into T-units, unless they contain a coreferential subject deletion in the second clause. For example, compare these two ways of constructing an utterance: "He runs, and he drops it" (two T-units) vs. "He runs and drops it" (one T-unit because the second *he,* the subject of *drops,* has been deleted). Breaking down an utterance into T-units helps avoid overestimating the length of an utterance separated primarily by "and … and … and …." The *subordination index,* a measure of syntactic complexity, is the average number of dependent and main clauses per T-unit, usually ranging from 1 to 4.

In analyzing the oral narrative below, we will divide it into T-units, identify how many clauses are contained in each T-unit, count the number of words (not morphemes) within each T-unit, and calculate the subordination index. I am including a few rules for counting words employed by Loban (1976). Loban notes that although other researchers may have slightly different rules, your results will not be affected if you have an adequate sample. The rules follow:

- Count as one word *maybe, okay, ain't.*
- Count words according to their adult equivalent; for example, count as two words:
  usta (used to),
  John Smith
  kinda (kind of)
  hafta (have to)
  gonna (going to)
  wanna (want to)
  musta (must have)
  other common contractions: *don't, can't, won't*
- Count as four words: *dunno* (I do not know)

And here is the oral narrative to analyze:

Today we're gonna go to Disney Land and my mom and dad are gonna go too and my cousin George is gonna come later after his dad gets off work but he's a real pain and he always wants his own way and he has to go to the bathroom all the time and one time we were at the movies and it was the best part and my mom made me take him to the men's room and boy was I mad because when we got back the movie was all over except for the mushy stuff.

The numbers of clauses and words, respectively, appear within parentheses:

T-1   Today we're gonna go to Disney Land (1, 9)
T-2   and my mom and dad are gonna go too (1, 10)
T-3   and my cousin George is gonna come later after his dad gets off work (2, 15)
T-4   but he's a real pain (1, 6)
T-5   and he always wants his own way (1, 7)
T-6   and he has to go to the bathroom all the time (1, 11)
T-7   and one time we were at the movies (1, 8)
T-8   and it was the best part (1, 6)
T-9   and my mom made me take him to the men's room (1, 11)
T-10 and, boy, was I mad, because when we got back, the movie was all over except for the mushy stuff (3, 20)

Sum of T-units: 10
Sum of words: 94
Sum of clauses: 13
Average length of T-units in words (94/10) = 9.4
Subordination index (sum of the clauses divided by the number of T-units, 13/10) = 1.3

Owens uses C-units as well as T-units to describe length and complexity, and they can be particularly helpful in evaluating the younger elementary child (Owens, 1995). C-units are similar to T-units, but they include incomplete (partial) sentences in answer to questions and aphorisms. Using the preceding example, you can count each of the 10 T-units as a C-unit also. If more utterances that count as C-units are added to the sample, you can see the difference:

CLINICIAN:	How old is George, Larry?
LARRY:	Eight. (0 T-units, 1 C-unit)
CLINICIAN:	What movie did you go to see?
LARRY:	It had Bruce Willis, but I don't remember the name. (2 T-units, 2 C-units)
CLINICIAN:	How was it?
LARRY:	Totally, completely awesome, man! (0 T-units, 1 C-unit)

Both T- and C-units become longer as verb and noun phrase elaboration take place (e.g., "run" vs. "would have been running like mad" or "cat" vs. "the short-haired gray cat with the folded-down ears and stumpy tail").

The next step is to analyze the complexity of the T-units themselves by separating simple utterances from those that are complex or coordinated. Paul divides complexity into early and late types. The early ones (MLU 3.0–4.0) include simple infinitive clauses with the same subject (*He wants to go*), object clauses (prepositional complements), embedded questions without infinitives (WH clauses), simple conjoinings, multiple embeddings, and embedded plus conjoined sentences. Later occurring types (MLU 4.0–5.0) include infinitive clauses with different subjects (*He wants me to go*), relative clauses, gerunds, embedded questions with infinitives (*He knows where to go*), and unmarked infinitives (*to* is deleted: *Look at him go*).

Because space limitations in this chapter prohibit a detailed discussion of disruptions, such as false starts and excessive revisions, I refer you to the original reference for calculating disruptions, "A Procedure for Classifying Disruptions in Spontaneous Language Samples," by Dollaghan and Campbell (1992). This would be well worth your time to investigate if your student appears to have word-finding problems or just "gets tangled up" when he or she speaks. As a general rule of thumb, the authors report that in a 100-word sample, the number of pauses and mazes, or other interruptions, produced by a typical student was 5.9 with a standard deviation of 1.8. They suggest that the possibility of word-finding deficits be investigated if a student's sample exceeds 7 or 8 disruptions.

Intersentential growth can be documented in written work or in a language sample by noting the use of adverbial constructs and lexical cohesion—for example, a student's use of synonyms. It is crucial that students understand the meaning of the different constructs they encounter in their textbooks and other materials.

After your calculations, how can you tell if your student is exhibiting adequate length or complexity for his age or grade? Although researchers have published data on T-units, C-units, and the subordination index, often their methodology, number of subjects, and definition of basic terminology differed enough to make comparisons and compilation into charts difficult. One researcher, for example, divided T-unit data into narrative, or expository, categories. Table 3.1, therefore, should be viewed as representing only a general developmental progression, not as a source of specific numerical values (Loban, 1976; Owens, 1995; Paul, 1995; Scott, 1988; Scott & Stokes, 1995).

Not included in Table 3.1 are the results of investigations by Crowhurst and Piche in 1979 and Crowhurst in 1980. In both studies, the researchers concluded that the number of T-units in a written persuasive essay were larger than T-units for a written narrative. As I stated at the beginning of this chapter, I think lists often can be more helpful than detailed reports of research. Therefore, I will close this section with some general guidelines to help you assess, understand, and describe the effects of increasing length and complexity in oral and written language.

Table 3.1 T-Units, C-Units, and Subordination Index by Grade

Grade	Length of T-Units in Words		Length of C-Units in Words		Subordination Index	
	Spoken	Written	Spoken	Written	Spoken	Written
3–4	7.6–9.0	5.2–8.6	—	—	1.2–1.3	1.0–1.3
5–6	8.1–9.6	7.3–9.0	9.8	9.0	1.3–1.4	1.2–1.4
7–8	9.7–10.7	8.9–10.4	—	—	1.3–1.4	1.3–1.5
9–10	10.7–10.9	10.1–11.8	10.9	10.1	1.3–1.5	1.4–1.5
11–12	11.1–11.7	10.7–14.4	11.7	13.3	1.5–1.6	1.5–1.7

Scott (1988) showed that MLU per T-unit increases slowly throughout the school years. Loban's research indicates that important differences exist between oral and written length. In the sixth and seventh grades, the oral T-units are longer than those in the student's written samples; in the eighth and ninth grades, they are about equal; but by the tenth through twelfth grades, T-units of written work are longer than oral ones (Loban, 1976). In sum then, if this gradual change is not taking place, during intervention you may need to work on expanding complex forms.

By the time a typically developing child is age 4 or 5, 20% of her spontaneously produced sentences contain complex structures. Therefore, you can compute or estimate the percentage as a quick check of syntactic elaboration. If your student is producing complex structures, Paul points out that you have to transcribe only those portions that contain complexity of some sort, compute the approximate percentage, and classify the forms into late or early types as listed earlier. By the time students enter school, they should be using an average of six to eight different conjunctions (usually including *and, if, because, when,* and *so*) within a 15-minute sample (Paul, 1981, 1995). If these structures, which result in clauses, are not present in a spontaneous sample, try to elicit those that are absent using part of a standardized test or other elicitation procedures.

Finally, Greenhalgh and Strong (2001) emphasize the importance of indicating the presence or absence of literate language features in spoken narratives. Because their use contributes to academic success, the researchers recommend coding the following: adverbs; coordinating, subordinating, and intersentential conjunctions; elaborated noun phrases; mental and linguistic verbs (e.g., *think, know, assume*); and words denoting emotional states (e.g., *dubious, anxious*).

Pragmatics, Semantics, Discourse, Fluency, Voice, and Metalinguistics: A Note on Assessment

Because of space limitations, I cannot provide detailed procedures for assessing narrative and expository discourse, pragmatics, semantics, voice, and fluency. Excellent programs addressing discourse deficits, including both assessment and intervention of narrative and expository types, now exist (Miller, Gillam,

& Pena, 2001; Scott, 1999; Strong, 1998; Westby 1998, 1999). The written aspects of discourse, including spelling, are discussed in Chapter 7. Voice and fluency are best addressed through specific measures and techniques found in detail in texts covering those topics. Because episodes of dysfluency are often intermittent, you should always check for its presence in multiple locations and at different times. Semantics and pragmatics can be approached much as we approached the syntactic analysis we have just completed; that is, first determine the hallmarks of normal development, typical error patterns, and implications of the student's performance in the area within the classroom using Appendix 3.B, 3.C, or 3.F. If you require standard scores, there are tests available that measure many aspects of semantics—for example, figurative language and single-word vocabulary.

Because students must also develop a conscious understanding of the linguistic code, it is crucial to evaluate the whole area of metalinguistics when dealing with the school-age population. *Metalinguistics* can be defined in simplest terms as the understanding of and ability to use language to discuss and manipulate the forms of language. This includes understanding and altering phonological segments as children learn early decoding skills, and later explaining and applying the rules of spelling, subject–verb agreement, topic sentence, dependent clause construction, and so forth. Not only are these abilities essential in learning to read, but as the student reaches upper grade levels, the skills must become increasingly sophisticated. Often included under the same heading, but sometimes considered separately are the allied skills of metacognition and metapragmatics. *Metacognition* deals with students' defining how they think ("Let's see, first I have to multiply, then subtract, and then bring down the next number"); *metapragmatics* involves a conscious knowledge of the often subtle rules of social communication ("Teacher, he's pushing into line and says it's his turn when he knows it's mine!"). Teaching written expression as a developmental process can be considered an entirely metalinguistic task. Often, the most direct way to assess a student's abilities in this area is by observation or by asking the student to explain what he is doing and why. Metalinguistics is an integral part of dynamic assessment, discussed later in this chapter under "New Approaches to Assessment."

After you review screening and school records, complete your interviews and observations, and plan an effective means to sample the student's language. On the basis of those data, choose standardized measures to fill in the blanks and provide the "numbers" that may be required by your state or district. You may find that you can combine that with your analysis of syntax or phonology, but not necessarily.

CASE SELECTION: NEW APPROACHES TO ASSESSMENT

This section contains information that emphasizes ongoing assessment, although the procedures described may also be used during periodic reviews.

Given the amount of information presented so far, you may find it hard to believe that there are additional ways to approach assessment. From a student perspective, you may well be wondering if we need more. In my experience, we do, but the reason is neither simple nor straightforward. According to Westby, Stevens-Dominguez, and Oetter (1996) and Idol, Nevin, and Paolucci-Whitcomb (1996), much of the information gained through the traditional procedures outlined earlier in this chapter is quantitative and of little use in guiding intervention. Therefore, drawing on research from the psychology of learning, professionals in our field are creating new methods of assessment, in which the line between intervention and evaluation is blurred. Although I have written this section of the chapter to underscore the differences between traditional assessment approaches and "new" approaches, the separation is largely artificial, because new theories always owe something to their predecessors. In fact, I hope you will discern that many of the concepts and procedures discussed in this section are ones you have met before dressed in new clothes. After a brief history and rationale for using these new approaches, Nanette Clapper will discuss how authentic assessment works in the real world of the classroom.

Authors have created various names to describe new concepts of assessment: dynamic, interactive, observational, judgmental, ecological, portfolio, Response to Intervention (RTI), or, when applied to the school population, curriculum-based. Space does not permit a detailed description of every type, or its place in the developmental history of these approaches, but the sources cited throughout this section contain definitions, discussion, and examples of each if you need more specific information. For clarity, my descriptions will refer to them as if they were all developed to be used in the school environment; in actuality, many were not originally designed with the school-age population in mind. The feature they share, however, is a multistage, ongoing analytical procedure. In one form or another, the proponents of each type look at a student's language as it relates to the communication expectations of the classroom but do not stop at this point. They continue to identify points of match and mismatch between the ability of the student, the demands he faces, and the specific strategies that support his attempts to learn. These steps of testing, teaching, and retesting are repeated with a conscious, concerted effort to decrease dependence on the clinician's help (Nelson, 1994; Palincsar, Brown, & Campione, 1994; Schneider & Watkins, 1996; Westby et al., 1996). Obviously, two of the substantial differences from traditional assessment involve the ongoing nature of the process—that is, assessment has no real end point—and an acceptance that "the focus of assessment should shift from identifying the conditions that cause failure to identifying those that are likely to lead to academic success" (Paratore, 1995, pp. 67–68). Finally, Miller, Gillam, and Pena (2001) asserted that "dynamic assessment, unlike most other approaches, leads directly into intervention in a clear and comprehensive manner" (p. 2).

Before we delve into the historical roots of interactive assessment, let us look at why it has been so appealing for the school-based speech–language professional. First, the general concept of curriculum-based assessment has itself grown out of an increased use of the collaborative intervention model that you will find discussed in detail in Chapter 5. In simplest terms, the previous practice of removing students from the regular classroom (pull-out) was based on the assumption that professionals could "fix" the child's deficits outside class by using intervention approaches specific to the handicapping conditions. By definition, the techniques were quite different from those used to teach typical children. As a result of this appropriate therapy, proponents predicted, failure would be prevented, and students could reenter the class when they had caught up with their peers. Problem: For many students, it simply never happened.

As a result, many speech–language professionals have endeavored to provide speech–language services within the regular classroom to the greatest extent possible (push-in), using the regular curriculum as "therapy" material. Advantages and disadvantages of this intervention approach are discussed in Chapter 5. To return to our subject of assessment, however, it appears logical that if you expect a student to succeed using a specific curriculum, then the curriculum itself must be part of the evaluation process. For the student with language-based learning disabilities, "Curriculum-based language intervention … involves starting with an inventory of areas where change is needed most" (Nelson, 1994, p. 106). Nelson listed and defined the different curricula that language can affect, namely "official," "cultural," "de facto," "school culture," "hidden," and "underground." She recommended identifying "zones of significance," contextually based areas that at least two informants have selected as priorities. The following methods are all used to identify zones of significance:

- interviewing the participants (teachers, parents, the students themselves) to elicit intervention priorities;
- carefully studying artifacts (written language samples);
- observing students in the classroom to determine strengths and weaknesses as they relate to the linguistic, communicative, and cognitive demands of the curriculum; and
- closely observing students as "scaffolding" and "miscue analysis" (Goodman, 1983) take place.

As mentioned previously, "new" concepts build on those that have come before. The basic premise of reading miscue analysis, for example, states that the errors a student makes while reading aloud are not accidental; that is, the inaccuracies reflect the decoding process gone awry in a specific way. Therefore, by analyzing errors as a student reads curriculum-level material aloud, you can gain insights into areas that should be addressed during intervention. Another of the underlying assumptions of curriculum-based assessment is that scaffolding is effective.

Scaffolding can be thought of as focusing on a level of understanding just slightly more advanced than the low-achieving student is presently capable of. In a nascent model developed in 1969, Feuerstein proposed the concept of mediated learning, a means by which an experienced adult selects, focuses, and feeds back a learning experience to children, leading to the child's gradual internalization of the structure as her own. Feuerstein developed the concept of the learning potential assessment device (LPAD) to measure a low-achieving student's ability to profit from such instruction. It is, in effect, a way to "depict the modifiability of cognitive structures and the source of difficulties in learning" (Palincsar et al., 1994, p. 133). Although later researchers acknowledged their debt to Feuerstein, they were not fully satisfied with the model because it did not involve the curriculum in any meaningful way: LPAD was "divorced from the content and context of classrooms" (p. 134).

Some 35 years earlier, in 1934, Vygotsky postulated a seminal theory based on the importance of social interaction in learning. He developed the concept of a zone of proximal development (ZPD), defined as "the difference between a child's actual developmental level as determined by independent problem solving and the level of potential development as determined through problem solving under adult guidance or in collaboration with more capable peers" (Vygotsky, 1978, p. 86). Assuming this, then if we are to understand the child's present level of development, we cannot use a "static" test; we must look at those processes that are in a state of flux, of maturation. Predictably, other researchers refined the theories of Vygotsky and Feuerstein; Carlson and Weidl modified specific test procedures to include an interactive component, and Campione and Brown focused on determining how easy it was for students to learn from others and the amount of flexibility they displayed in transferring their new skills to similar situations (Palincsar et al., 1994).

Westby et al. (1996) suggested that we use ecological assessment, which considers the combined effects of physical, social, and psychological context on a student's classroom performance and therefore includes "insights, knowledge and impressions of professionals and parents who work with the children" (p. 145). Such assessment should be conducted in multiple natural, familiar settings (home, school) and should include multiple domains (e.g., speech–language, sensory, motor, cognitive, social–emotional, temperament). Because professionals representing different backgrounds have distinct insights, the overall picture that emerges will lead to an intervention plan that should address all the child's needs. Westby et al. described in detail the NEW TeamS model; although it was originally developed for preschoolers and below, she suggested that the principles would apply to an individual of any age. The goals of this program all reflect an awareness of a child's ZPD. According to Westby et al., using intervention within ZPD maximizes the development of the child's competence and confidence. Implicit in the application of this transdisciplinary approach to the school environment is the presence of language-based tasks that are directly related to the curriculum.

One of the concerns of speech–language professionals unfamiliar with curriculum-based intervention is that they will become tutors. Admittedly, with a deadline for an assignment approaching rapidly, the temptation to help one of your students get a passing grade is a real one. But a restatement of the saying "Give the man a fish, and he eats for a day; teach a man to fish and he eats for a lifetime" is clearly applicable here. The intent of these assessment–intervention procedures is in their sequence. First, we must discover what the student's abilities are at present as he struggles to complete a particular task. Then we want to determine how much and, most important, what kind of help (support, scaffold, model, strategy) the particular student needs to be able to succeed at a more advanced stage of the activity. After this step comes the one that differentiates this view of assessment from previous ones; as we guide the student, we work to discover his potential to change his approach to the task. Our assessment–intervention continues until the student can use the strategies he has learned independently in an untrained but related situation. In essence, we have taught him how to fish. If this sounds like the definition of generalization, it is, but our focus is on discovering and working within the ZPD, not in using assessment information (weaknesses) to apply a diagnostic label, compare the student's results to a norm, or determine if he qualifies for services within our area of professional expertise. As Miller, Gillam, and Pena (2001) explain, "The focus is on how modifiable [the child is] during the teaching and intervention phase ... to discover ... how he responds to and uses information ... [and] the quantity and quality of effort necessary to teach new information and to induce change" (p. 3).

Another reason speech–language professionals have become increasingly interested in trying these new assessment approaches is that the reading and writing processes are so clearly an appropriate application (see Chapter 7). Wallach and Butler (1994a) note that "learning to read and write is part of, not separate from, learning to speak and comprehend language" (p. 11). Reading can be, and has been, divided into a series of subskills, often taught in a bottom-up fashion, with children learning letter–sound correspondence and then decoding words containing different syllable types. Several grades later, the reading process, now largely applied below the level of consciousness, is used to comprehend the meaning of passages, paragraphs, and chapters. Researchers have become particularly interested in two aspects of language-based strategies: first, teaching students how to recognize the opportunity for using one or more of them; and, second, helping them discover specific ways to apply the strategies to new, different material or subjects. These strategies can include understanding how to activate prior knowledge, use text structure and schemas, and connect ideas to infer meaning. In reciprocal teaching, students and instructors take turns in discussing a shared text. A similar sequence exists for evaluating and teaching the writing process. One of the ways to evaluate and teach writing skills is through portfolio assessment, defined as "a purposeful collection of student work and records of progress and achievement assembled over time ... permit[ting] the documentation of children's performances across a range of literacy tasks, texts, and settings ... [and allowing] students to display their literacy knowledge under the real conditions of daily classroom demands" (Paratore, 1995, p. 68). This clear connection between intervention and evaluation is the differentiating characteristic and strength of dynamic assessment. In your role as a speech–language professional, you determine the student's level, teach, retest, move the level up a notch, teach, retest, and repeat the sequence over and over again.

While Response to Intervention clearly belongs in the category of dynamic assessment, what differentiates it from other approaches is its focus on prevention. RTI usually begins by providing all children with a theoretically sound instructional technique—for example, phonological awareness training. At periodic intervals, teachers or therapists identify any students who are experiencing difficulty. These children are provided with *additional* help while remaining in their original peer group. Only if they fail to progress are they singled out for special and perhaps different instruction. The intent is to provide help before a child has fallen far behind others in her class. As in any new procedure, questions about applicability have been raised—for example, in the National Research Center on Learning Disabilities (NRCLD) investigation of using RTI as a means of LD indentification (NRCLD, 2004).

Some critics have complained that these approaches rely too heavily on the skill of the clinician and the "intuitive nature" of the assessment (Palincsar et al., 1994, p. 134). Although the criticism may be justified, any approach that demands careful observation should have a place in evaluation. In the first part of this chapter, I stated repeatedly that assessment is not a one-time event, that each time you meet with a student you should gain new insights and make new hypotheses. The skill to do this will grow as you gain experience. Theoretical knowledge will gain new meaning as you apply new ideas and techniques to the assessment and intervention processes; it is one of the reasons you will never be bored.

AUTHENTIC ASSESSMENT: NANETTE CLAPPER

For years, professionals in the public schools, including speech pathologists, school psychologists, and occupational and physical therapists, as well as members of the Committee on Special Education (CSE), as it is called in New York State, have depended on a student's performance on standardized tests to determine whether that child would receive special services. Standardized tests were held in such high regard that in most cases they not only represented the means to place a student in special education, but also determined specific therapy services. In addition, the instruments were used as pretests and posttests to measure a child's growth in a particular area.

Standardized testing served to compare a particular child's performance in a particular subject area to the performance of his peers (those sharing the same age range and grade level). While the tests provided the child's ranking among his peers, they did not always present the whole story. In resource team meetings, members listened to psychologists' accounts of classroom observations and teachers' and therapists' accounts of how the student actually performed in the classroom, but the preponderance of decision making was based on the child's performance on standardized tests. Teachers, therapists, and parents often left meetings feeling frustrated when the results of the child's performance on standardized tests did not agree with the child's performance in the classroom setting.

Those working in the educational system, particularly staff involved in evaluation and instruction, have debated the value of standardized testing for years. In *The Mindful School: How To Assess Authentic Learning,* Burke (1994) includes this statement:

> Charges that standardized tests do not measure significant higher learner outcomes, do not measure growth and development, and do not accurately reflect what students can and cannot do have been made over and over again. Yet, despite the research and the critics of standardized tests, policy makers, parents, and the general public base much of their perception of the educational system on the publication of standardized test scores and the comparisons of the scores in schools, districts, and states.

The bottom line? Standardized testing for evaluation purposes has its problems, but it is the best we have. That is, until now.

Changes in how we assess a student's achievements are emerging, following an already changed set of expectations for young people entering the workplace. Although there is no argument against the requirement of teaching and learning the basic skills in "reading, writing and arithmetic," educators are recognizing not only the importance, but the necessity, of assessing both what a student has learned and how she can apply it in everyday life situations. Bond (1995) states,

> As society shifts from an industrial age, in which a person could get by with basic reading and arithmetic skills, to an information age, which requires the ability to access, interpret, analyze, and use information for making decisions, the skills and competencies needed to succeed in today's workplace are changing as well. In response to these changes, content standards—the knowledge, skills, and behaviors needed for students to achieve at high levels—are being developed at the national and state levels. In this atmosphere of reform, student assessment is the centerpiece of many educational improvement efforts. (p. 1)

Authentic assessment (also known as alternative assessment, direct assessment, and performance assessment) is an alternative, as well as a supplement, to standardized testing. It is a relatively new approach in the field of educational evaluation. Although it is still in the developmental stages, there is a general consensus as to the characteristics of authentic assessment. Sources of information are readily available online, for example, *Approaches to Authentic Assessment, What is Authentic Assessment?* and *Select or Design Assessments that Elicit Established Outcomes* (Herman, Aschbacher, & Winter, 1992). The approach requires a student to *create* a response rather than *choose* a response. Its purpose is to assess a student's performance in actual situations, in his everyday classroom setting, and to see how that child is able to communicate his knowledge, as well as apply it to real-life situations. Authentic assessment allows the "examiner" to evaluate the child's performance in tasks that hold everyday meaning for him. This approach allows the student to express his knowledge of a subject through various means, typically over a period of time, with expectations (criteria) clearly enunciated before the student begins his tasks. Many teachers and therapists use a portfolio that includes a variety of samples of the work that a student has completed over a period of time, often representing improvement (self-assessment in portfolios online). This procedure is in contrast to standardized testing, which measures a student's performance on a particular test on one particular day.

Approaches to Authentic Assessment defines *authentic assessment* as "the measurement of actual performance in a subject area" and argues that it is both valuable and appropriate:

> Authentic assessment was developed in the arts and in apprenticeship systems, where assessment has always been based on performance. It is impossible to imagine evaluating a musician's ability without hearing her sing or play an instrument, or judging a woodworker's craft without seeing the table or cabinet the student has built. It is also impossible to help a student become a better woodworker or musician unless the instructor observes the student in the process of working on something real, provides feedback, monitors the student's use of the feedback, and adjusts instruction and evaluation accordingly. Authentic assessment extends this principle of evaluating real work to all areas of the curriculum. Standardized multiple-choice tests, on the other hand, measure test-taking skills directly and everything else either indirectly or not at all.

The Mindful School cites Stefonek's compilation of the following aspects of authentic assessment (Burke, 1994):

- methods that emphasize learning and thinking, especially higher-order thinking skills such as problem-solving strategies;
- tasks that focus on students' abilities to produce a quality product or performance;
- disciplined inquiry that integrates and produces knowledge, rather than reproduces fragments of information others have discovered;
- meaningful tasks at which students should learn to excel;
- challenges that require knowledge in good use and good judgment;
- a new type of positive interaction between the assessor and the assessee;
- an examination of differences between trivial school tasks (e.g., giving definitions of biological terms) and more meaningful performance in nonschool settings (e.g., completing a field survey of wildlife); and
- involvement that demystifies tasks and standards.

How frustrating it has been for educators and clinicians to see deflated standardized scores when their observation of the student in the classroom indicated a much more positive picture. The teacher–observer bases his assessment of the student's achievements on the student's responses to classroom projects, assignments, and so forth. The following case provides an example.

When a task or goal was presented in a rubric format with expectations and criteria clearly delineated, a student we'll call Maria demonstrated her comprehension of the facts, as well as her ability to transfer the information to everyday life situations. She enthusiastically shared her science project with peers and the teacher–observer in the classroom environment, explaining the differences between gases, liquids, and solids. She used advanced descriptive attributes as well as comparative and superlative forms as she demonstrated the differences between the forms. She also employed visual aids of her own making, which charted similarities and differences between gases, liquids, and solids and included pictures she had drawn of how each form appears. She demonstrated the relevance of her project to an everyday life situation by illustrating how different forms of the same element can change our environment. She explained how, as water freezes and expands, it can break, split, or widen the container it is in (e.g., cracks in the streets that expand into holes, pipes that burst). The teacher–observer concluded that this student used curriculum vocabulary correctly and clearly demonstrated her understanding of what was taught. However, her performance on traditional vocabulary and language tests that looked only at a particular skill in isolation was poor and showed little improvement.

The authentic assessment approach is especially valuable in the field of special education. Standardized tests are particularly vulnerable to missing the mark for those children who are classified, or soon to be classified, for example, those with mental retardation or multiple handicaps. It is painful to sit at a resource team meeting and hear a clinician describe to parents who are perhaps hearing bad news for the first time, or suspected bad news confirmed, the results of their child's performance on standardized testing. Clinicians will often begin such a report by sharing the child's standardized scores, explaining how far below the norm the student is in terms of standard deviations. They go on to explain what areas were particularly challenging for the student and give examples of his errors. The clinician may end by recommending any variety of therapeutic interventions and special classroom placements. When a child's performance on standardized testing is presented alone, in the absence of a description of the child's abilities in real-life situations, the information shared with the parents often lands on deaf ears or stirs in parents an immediate defensive response. They will not validate findings regarding their child if the assessment has failed to recognize what the child can do, and how he functions in his immediate environment.

It is not easy to give bad news or to face the reality or probability that a student may be cognitively challenged. It is imperative, therefore, to assess what that student is able to do and what that child is able to do well. Authentic assessment is particularly sensitive to this need as it applies to the special education population. In *Performance-Based Learning and Assessment* (2000), a group of educators in Connecticut indicated that standardized tests asks, "Do you know it?" whereas authentic assessment asks, "How well can you use what you know?"

Let's look again at the meeting scenario noted above. The speech–language professional might begin by illustrating the different assessment approaches that were used in evaluating the student's performance. She might explain that both authentic and standardized assessments were used and briefly share with the family what they are and how each approach complements the other. Both approaches are used to glean information concerning the student's strengths and the areas that are challenging to him. The clinician might share, for example, that on standardized testing their youngster struggled trying to follow novel directions. Observing and interacting with the student in the classroom, however, revealed that he was able to follow directions presented within a context or routine or that followed a logical or anticipated sequence (e.g., "Put your books in your desk and line up at the door for gym"). Although the child did poorly reproducing or repeating unrehearsed sequences on the standardized tests, he was able to demonstrate in the classroom that he understood the morning routine (jacket in the cubby, notes on the teacher's desk, personal supply box on the desk top, quiet reading at his desk, etc.); the sequence of seating (Bobby's chair is first in the row, Teresa's is second, etc.); and "helper" routines (bring the attendance to the main office and the notes to the nurse's office).

There are several benefits to sharing the results of your authentic assessment. When you present the findings of the "How well can you use what you know" approach (authentic assessment), you validate for parents that you recognize and value what their child has to offer despite his cognitive challenges. Most important, however, authentic assessment findings serve to offer those working directly with the student a baseline or foundation for developing future skills. Observing the child as you work with him offers information on what modalities stimulate his understanding and what modalities he prefers to use to express himself. The format for an authentic assessment allows the examiner to intervene, making task and modality modifications as necessary, to see if different approaches enhance the student's understanding.

The atmosphere in which a student's achievements are assessed can also affect how a child performs. Teachers and clinicians who have had children with auditory processing difficulties have struggled with the results of standardized tests for years. In the classroom these students may display the multiple characteristics of auditory processing deficits, but they frequently perform within the average range on standardized tests. In the quiet evaluation room, the tests are presented one on one, face to face with the person presenting the auditory information. There is no competition from background noise, the chatter of other students, or the rustling of papers. In short, the testing atmosphere is a sterile, unrealistic environment. Consequently, many of these students perform better on the tests than on similar tasks in the classroom or home environment. This becomes an issue when needed suggestions, recommendations, and services are not provided to help the student because his weaknesses were not evident in the environment in which the standardized testing was completed.

Conversely, the environment in which standardized tests are given can negatively affect a student's confidence and performance. Some students demonstrate physical changes as they become anxious about the testing situation. Despite the calming reassurance of the examiner, some students share how nervous they are; others rock in their chairs or develop a nervous cough, laugh, or frequently need to use the bathroom. When out of the natural environment of their classroom, students, particularly older ones, are keenly aware of the testing process and the importance of doing well on the instruments in question. The anxiety of many students intensifies as they reach areas in the tests that are particularly challenging for them (ceiling levels). Most standardized tests do not permit extraneous comments, changes in the way the examiner presents material, or alternate responses. In contrast to that traditional approach, authentic assessment encourages the examiner to present the goal to the student up-front. The student is given the target task, full information about the areas that will be assessed, and the criteria necessary for her to achieve a specific standard of excellence. She is told from the onset that if she begins to struggle, different strategies will be offered to make the material easier for her to understand. Starting off with this reassurance can have a calming effect on the student and ultimately may facilitate her best performance.

Authentic assessment, now in its developmental stages, offers a new approach to evaluate a student's performance. As with anything new, it is subject to trial and error and inevitable but necessary "growing pains." There are still hurdles we must jump to develop this approach as a viable and reliable means of assessment. Authentic assessment offers a description of how a single student's performance compares to the performance of her peers in the same class, grade, and even school district, but it is more difficult to use this approach at state and national levels. Fuchs (1995) sums up another concern expressed by those already experimenting with this approach on a daily basis:

> Performance assessment can require large amounts of teacher time to design and administer assessments and to scrutinize student performances. It is easy to see how this type of assessment could generate so many different plans for intervention strategies for different students that teachers in a classroom situation with 20 to 30 students would be unable to manage. Performance assessment developers need to solve the problem of how to implement plans based on performance assessments within the constraints of classroom life.

In sum, authentic assessment should be considered not as a replacement for standardized testing but rather as a complement or addition to it. Both approaches offer valuable information about a student's performance.

CASE STUDIES

By necessity, much of the information covered so far in this chapter has been contained in general statements; it has been my experience, however, that students absorb information better if they can apply general information to a specific case. Therefore Eileen Gravani, the coeditor of this book and the author of Chapters 1 and 4, and I have developed four profiles to illustrate steps to follow as you (a) plan and implement assessment procedures, (b) develop IEP goals, and (c) suggest how to address them in intervention. The students you are introduced to in this chapter will appear again in Chapters 4 and 5. The cases described here were chosen to represent common patterns of deficits. I am sure you realize, however, that in the real world every student and case is unique. Therefore, approach the four cases as illustrative models only; they should not be taken as a checklist to use for every similar student. As new instruments become available and as new research provides insights and methods to improve the quality of assessment, adopt them.

For each case, we have used the first person and described the student as if a school-based SLP were relaying the information verbally. Using what you have learned in this chapter, your job is to take a few minutes to think about what you would do to assess this student. Try to cover all the bases: Think how the apparent problems could affect classroom performance, and decide what information you need and could get from records, interviews, observation, and less formal means. Although I will give you one set of possible outcomes of the assessment process, be aware that there are probably dozens of other solutions that could address the issues just as effectively. Most texts warn you not to use a "cookbook" approach when you plan an evaluation, and I agree. As someone who has cooked, literally as well as figuratively, for a long time, a cookbook is not a bad analogy. If you want to bake a cake, there are whole books full of good recipes to consult, but it remains up to you to consider your budget, what the occasion is, how much time you have, what is in the cupboard, who is allergic to nuts, whether the cake is a good "keeper," who is on a diet, or even if a pie would be a better choice. Therefore, as you read my solution for each of the first three cases, keep in mind that you may well come up with a better recipe.

Case One: Zachary

Zachary, called "Mr. Smiles" by his kindergarten teacher, Ms. Warren, was referred to you in late February by Ms. Cato, his first-grade teacher, because he has been struggling academically all year, particularly in reading and spelling. Ms. Cato describes him as a delightful, hard-working, popular child who appears somewhat younger than his age because of his slight build. Ms. Cato is an experienced teacher with a master's degree in reading. She regularly takes courses and attends workshops on the needs of the underachieving child because she enjoys the challenge of working with students in her lowest reading group, which this year includes Zachary. Even compared with those classmates, he is making limited progress. In her written referral for a possible evaluation, she states that she is undecided as to whether she should recommend that Zachary be retained in first grade. It has been my experience that January and February are very heavy months for referrals. With the excitement of the holidays over, teachers begin to think about possible retentions. We will assume that no full-scale meeting of an evaluation (or preevaluation) team was deemed necessary until I had done some initial investigation. My first task as a speech–language pathologist (and yours) is to figure out what I know and what I need to find out.

Without letting your eyes cruise down the page, think: What questions would you ask Zachary's teacher? His parents? Zachary himself? What other sources of information could you tap? Is there anything specific you might look for during your classroom observation? On the basis of these accumulated data, what procedures or instruments would you then plan to test his language?

Here are my answers: Although I had planned to begin by conferring with Ms. Cato, she was not available, so I checked Zachary's records, instead. According to his kindergarten screening results, his vision, hearing, and gross motor skills were within normal limits, but he had been placed on a "watch" list because of borderline scores on the articulation and sentence-repetition tasks of the language section of the screening. It is frequently instructive to check individual items that were in error, but only the scores of the speech–language screening had been retained; the actual protocol (test sheet) for this part of the screening had been discarded. The SLP who administered the screening had resigned midyear and moved to another state, so no details were available. The "school readiness" portion of the screening administered by the kindergarten teachers was intact, however, and indicated that Zachary counted to 20, knew eight colors, and recounted personal information (name, age, etc.) but could not identify any upper- or lower-case letters.

A routine hearing screening of everyone in Zachary's first-grade class 2 months before Ms. Cato's referral indicated that Zachary's results were, as before, unremarkable. His attendance in both grades had been excellent. In this particular school district, end-of-the-year tests are not used in kindergarten, and those administered to first graders are not scheduled until June, some 4 months in the future.

My interview with Ms. Cato began with a discussion of those borderline kindergarten screening scores. Zachary's kindergarten teacher had told her that even with lots of practice, Zachary didn't seem to "get" sound–symbol relationships. Note this exchange because, in schools, much information is shared informally. It is very common for one teacher to check for insights into a student's problems with a colleague from the preceding year. Often, this information does not appear in written form, so you have to ask.

Discussing current problems, Ms. Cato commented that while most first graders use at least two related sounds (phones) as they attempt to spell an unfamiliar word, Zachary used only one, always in the initial position. The other letters he printed bore little relation to the sounds in the word (e.g., "dabat" for "dinosaur"). Actually printing letters did not appear to be difficult for him. Although he always paid attention, from September to December he often copied his friend's work in language arts as if he were not sure what to do. When Ms. Cato moved his seat away from his friend after Christmas vacation, Zachary seemed lost, and his performance worsened. His spelling tests earned low-average marks. Ms. Cato remarked that the grades represented Zachary's hard work memorizing the simple words at home; 3 weeks later, he could not pass the identical test. During this period, she recommended that Zachary be considered for Title I reading assistance. He was placed in a small class with the Title I teacher, Ms. Ruiz, who reports that she is continuing to evaluate his skills. The class that includes him is currently working on sound–letter correspondence. So far Zachary has shown limited progress, particularly in his ability to "hear" sounds in words.

Because the borderline scores occurred in articulation and receptive language, I asked specifically about Zachary's ability to pronounce sounds in words during spontaneous conversation. Ms. Cato responded that some sounds, mostly *r*'s, were "a little funny," and that Zachary "gets his tongue tangled up when he tries to pronounce a long word with lots of syllables." Occasionally, she could not understand him. Because I wondered about the reason for Zachary's poor performance on the sentence-repetition task, I asked Ms. Cato if she had noticed any memory problems. She reported she wasn't sure; he seemed to follow directions for art projects and science experiments fairly well, but at other times he appeared very confused. Ms. Cato added that he remembered classroom rules and followed them better than many of his classmates.

Before making an appointment to observe Zachary, I determined the subjects in which and times during the day when his deficits were most likely to be evident. Later that week, I observed him first during his reading instruction and then as he took part in a language arts writing activity. He attended well during the reading lesson. He experienced real difficulty, however, in sounding out words, even though Ms. Cato reviewed most of the sounds before each child read a short passage aloud. There appeared to be no pattern to his errors when he guessed a word. I noted that he looked very carefully at the pictures on the page and also listened intently to the questions Ms. Cato asked that gave clues about what was coming next.

The language arts lesson featured pictures representing the main points of the story the class had just finished. The pictures had been cut apart, and the children were told to put them into the correct sequence. After this had been accomplished, Ms. Cato called on Zachary to retell the story from the pictures. His rendition demonstrated correct sequencing and appropriate vocabulary but contained some errors in morphology; overall the retelling was adequate, if brief. Although his attempts at clarifying questions were not always successful, his pragmatics were appropriate. He had far less difficulty with this activity than the previous one, and his obvious fatigue at the end of the reading lesson disappeared.

Before the observation, I had interviewed Zachary's kindergarten teacher, Ms. Warren, who agreed that Zachary was a child who tried hard every minute. She reiterated that he just didn't seem to grasp the sound–symbol connection and added that his parents were concerned. At their request, another hearing test had been completed. Ms. Warren said that Zachary really liked finger plays but didn't remember the words, although he knew all the actions. The "watch" status had not been pursued because of the SLP's departure in January. I interviewed Zachary's art and physical education teachers briefly, also; both felt that his memory was fine and described him as a charming, popular child.

Zachary's parents appeared tense during their interview, alternating between expressing fear that something was wrong with their son and commenting that they were sure he would catch up soon because he tried so hard, particularly since he was getting extra help in the Title I class. They confirmed that all of Zachary's developmental milestones had been met at typical times, except speech, which was "a little slow in coming." There was no family history of language problems. Mom volunteered that although Zachary would "sit for hours" playing Legos, he was easily frustrated when they tried to teach him a few letters. He loved looking at books by Dr. Seuss but didn't seem to understand the concept of rhyme. Both his behavior and his health were good, but he was usually exhausted when he came home from school. At the close of the meeting, the parents asked that Zachary be tested. After appropriate meetings and procedures outlined earlier, I audiotaped a brief language sample during recess. An informal analysis revealed somewhat restricted vocabulary, some articulation errors, a few morphological omissions in longer sentences, and not many examples of syntactic complexity.

When I talked with Zachary, he reported that although he liked school, "reading is really, really hard." He stated that he tries to sound out words, but when he attempts to put sounds together to make a word, he just can't figure out how they go. He added that sometimes he forgets what sounds go with what letters.

Now, what standardized evaluation instruments do you recommend for this case? Make a list before reading on.

On the basis of information gained through observations, interviews, and screenings, the Committee on Special Education recommended that a core evaluation take place. I administered the following standardized tests—except for the PPVT–3, which was administered by the school psychologist—for the reasons noted:

Instrument	Taps Information Concerning
Clinical Evaluation of Language Fundamentals–Preschool–2nd Edition (CELF–Preschool–2; Wiig, Secord, & Semel, 2004)	Word structure and receptive morphology and syntax (to determine whether he can understand complex forms)
Expressive One-Word Picture Vocabulary Test–Revised (EOWPVT–2000; Gardner, 2000)	Single-word expressive vocabulary

Structured Photographic Expressive Language Test–3 (SPELT–3; Dawson & Stout, 2003)	Morphology/syntax-based omissions/errors in language sample, and confirmation of errors in the CELF–Preschool
Goldman–Fristoe Test of Articulation–2 (GFTA–2; Goldman & Fristoe, 2000)	Articulation errors
Peabody Picture Vocabulary Test–3 (PPVT–3; Dunn & Dunn, 1997)	Single-word receptive vocabulary
Phonological Awareness Test (Robertson & Salter, 1997) and *Comprehensive Test of Phonological Processing* (CTOPP; Wagner, Torgesen, & Rashotte, 1999)	Deficits in early decoding skills and phonological memory

No fluency, voice, or formal pragmatics assessment appeared necessary. The *Weschler Intelligence Scale for Children–Third Edition* (WISC–III; Wechsler, 1997) revealed overall intelligence within normal limits, with performance subtests significantly better than verbal ones. You will find a complete psychological report concerning Zachary in Chapter 12, written by a school psychologist; be sure to read it, as it gives another professional's view of the student, as well as the psychologist's description of the PPVT–3.

In addition to the standardized tests, I transcribed two brief language samples: The first was Zachary's retelling of a story featuring rhyme that his teacher had read aloud to the class that morning. In the second, he described a science experiment that had taken place the day before.

A speech–language diagnostic report can take various forms, depending on your school district's requirements, whether it is an initial report, and to whom the report is addressed. We have included examples of two different types of reports in this chapter. The first one, based on Zachary's case, appears as Appendix 3.G. Compared with university or hospital clinic evaluation reports, it may appear abbreviated. When I was first employed in the schools, my reports were detailed, comprehensive, and lengthy—very lengthy. One day during a meeting of our Committee on Special Education, the chair asked me a question, the answer to which had been covered in my report. When I referred to that fact, the chair responded, "I don't have the time to read your reports; I only read your recommendations." Although my initial reaction was annoyance, I came to realize that if my report was so long that nobody (teachers, administrators, other specialists) was reading it, then I was defeating my own purpose. Teachers wanted to know what I had discovered; it was my job to make my explanation as brief as the case would allow. After that, only if another SLP needed exhaustive detail did I provide it. You will see that the report in Appendix 3.G includes some of the information you have just read. Other details, however, have been omitted or condensed. The second report, Appendix 3.H, concerns a high school student and is much more thorough. It can be used as a guide if your district requires more detail. As you work through the succeeding cases, write a report for each of them, using your district's guidelines if possible, or discuss with another student what should be included.

 ## Case Two: James

James is a youngster in third grade, the child of an African American military family who just moved into the district from another state. Because he is a transfer student, I administered the *CELF–3 Screening Test* (Semel, Wiig, & Secord, 1996); his score fell below the cutoff score established by the district. As a quick check of articulation, I asked him to count to 20 and recite the days of the week and the months of the year. He started the recitation of the days of the week with Wednesday, named the months of the year in random order, omitting October and February entirely, and employed some articulation characteristics of African American English (AAE) dialect. In spontaneous conversation, he was shy and hesitant, frequently used interjections (*err, ah, um*), and appeared to apply some morphological and syntactic rules of AAE, such as eliminating the plural marker if a number was given ("two shoe") and eliminating the third-person-singular present-tense verb ending ("he walk"). Second-grade records from his previous school revealed that he was a slightly below-average student; older files were not available because they had been lost during transfers between earlier schools. His older brother Douglas's screening results were unremarkable, although I noted he also used some AAE forms; Douglas is in fourth grade.

In this quite different case, what questions would you ask James's teacher, Ms. Dwyer? His parents? James himself? What other sources of information could you tap? Is there anything specific you might look for during your classroom observation? In James's case, Ms. Dwyer will have limited information, but she (or the reading specialist) will have reviewed what past records are available and completed enough testing to place him in an appropriate reading group. In our conference, she noted that his oral reading skills seemed "about average"; she also related this additional information based on his "permanent record": Standardized tests given at the end of second grade resulted in scores 1 standard deviation below the mean in reading comprehension. Because this score falls within normal range, albeit low average, James would not qualify for special reading services. Mathematical computation, spelling, and basic decoding skills in reading were all also within normal limits. Note that you can often save yourself time by checking with the classroom teacher concerning previous years' accomplishments, particularly if you do not understand what the scores or subtests of these educational instruments imply (i.e., what they measure).

Ms. Dwyer reported that "so far" James appears to be a quiet, almost shy child who rarely asks for help, even though he seems to have problems following directions some of the time. Her class is divided into heterogeneous groups, and although he hasn't made any close friends yet, he gets along well with the other children, and his "different way of talking" doesn't seem to matter. Right now you should be asking yourself what she meant by that statement; it is typical of information that sometimes just materializes during an interview. In clarifying the comment, Ms. Dwyer appeared to be referring to elements of AAE in both articulation and language. She added, however, that James often seems to have a hard time finding the word he wants and almost acts as if he were stuttering.

I observed James during a science lesson and later as part of a small group working on map skills (social studies). He was attentive during the lesson but did not volunteer any answers. He experienced difficulty with a worksheet of definitions based on the science lesson but did not seek help. During the other small-group activity, the students were required to follow directions and find a "hidden treasure" on a map of the United States. James consistently struggled with left–right concepts and compass directions. He spoke little and did not ask clarifying questions; there were few hesitations or interjections. The school nurse's records indicate that he passed the hearing screening; he has never appeared at her office because of illness.

Neither parent was available during the day for a meeting (a not uncommon occurrence), but a telephone conference with James's mother revealed that she was concerned about his past educational progress, particularly because Douglas had never had any problems in the same school. She said that James had always been a healthy child, had met all developmental milestones at age-appropriate levels, but often looked to his brother for help with his homework or to interpret events in general. When asked about possible stuttering behavior, she said that it seemed to her that James had trouble figuring out what word he *wanted*, not in trying to "get a word out." She described her son as a likable child who rarely got into trouble. Now, based on the above, what procedures or instruments would you choose to evaluate his speech and language?

During an interview, James said that "school was okay" and that his favorite subjects were math and "sometimes science"; reading was "okay," if he liked the story. His conversation again included multiple instances of sentence revisions, hesitations, fillers, and circumlocution.

One of the key issues here is James's apparent use of African American English (AAE). All standardized instruments must be carefully checked to be sure they were normed on a substantial number of male African American students his age. The possibility of stuttering will require multiple observations and samples, because dysfluency can occur intermittently. A language sample taken early in the assessment process should give a general idea of what areas of language to test formally.

One language sample was recorded during a planning session for a school party; James and two other students had to think of several ideas for a theme and a list of items to be purchased. I elicited a second sample on a Friday afternoon when I played a game with James and three other boys, one of whom was on my caseload. James's use of interjections, circumlocutions, hesitations, and proforms (nonspecific words like *whatzit, thing, whatchamacallit*) was particularly noticeable during the planning session as he attempted to name items like party favors, cupcakes, and Hi-C. To the nonprofessional, some of these behaviors could indeed be mistaken for stuttering, but no hallmarks of that disorder—such as repetition of sounds, syllables or phrases; long hesitations; or "blocking"—were present. Occasionally, he seemed confused with the planning time line—for example, not understanding when "a week from Friday" was.

His use of some AAE morphological, syntactical, and phonological forms was consistent but not pervasive; that is, he did not use many dialectical forms, but the ones present were used in all applicable cases. His vocabulary appeared limited and his syntax somewhat simplified; his MLU by words appeared inflated by circumlocutions. Both Ms. Dwyer and his mother confirmed that these samples "sounded like the way James talked," a useful quick check for the validity of a specific language sample. Given this additional information, I ask again, what procedures or instruments would you choose to test James's speech and language?

On the basis of the information gained through observations, interviews, and screenings, I administered the following standardized tests for the reasons noted:

Test	Taps Information Concerning
Test of Language Development– Primary–Third Edition (TOLD– P–3; Newcomer & Hammill, 1997)	Overall receptive and expressive language; syntax and sentence repetition for morphology errors (AAE?)
Comprehensive Receptive and Expressive Vocabulary Test–2 (CREVT–2; Wallace & Hammill, 2002)	Additional single-word receptive and expressive vocabulary to confirm TOLD–P–3; ability to define single words: word-finding problems? Test has AAE norms.
Test of Word Finding–Second Edition (TWF–2; German, 2000)	Word-finding plus problems, general
Clinical Evaluation of Language Fundamentals–4 (CELF–4; Semel et al., 2003), Rapid Automatic Naming (RAN) subtest	Word-finding problems, familiar subjects

Clinical Evaluation of Language Fundamentals–Fourth Edition (CELF–4; Semel, Wiig, & Secord, 2003), Familiar Sequences subtest	Word-finding problems, automaticity
Clinical Evaluation of Language Fundamentals–Fourth Edition (CELF–4; Semel, Wiig, & Secord, 2003), Word Structure subtest	AAE influence on morphology using Word Structure subtest
Goldman–Fristoe Test of Articulation–2 (GFTA–2; Goldman & Fristoe, 2000)	Articulation errors; check against AAE dialectical forms
Comprehensive Assessment of Spoken Language, Carrow-Woolfolk, 1999a), Basic Concepts subtest. *Clinical Evaluation of Language Fundamentals Preschool–Second Edition* (CELF-Preschool 2, Wiig, Secord and Semel, 2004), Linguistic Concepts subtest	Spatial, temporal, and other common school concepts

No voice or formal pragmatics assessment appeared necessary. A *Weschler Intelligence Scale for Children–Third Edition* revealed overall intelligence within normal limits, with performance subtests superior to verbal ones. James's scores and their interpretation are reported below. Average standard scores based on 10 fall between 7 and 10; a moderately low score falls between 7 to 4; and an extremely low score is below 4. Average standard scores based on 100 fall between 85 and 115; a moderately low score falls between 70 to 85; and an extremely low score is below 70.

Test	Subtest	Standard/ Scaled Score
TOLD–P–3	Picture Vocabulary	10
	Relational Vocabulary	8
	Oral Vocabulary	6
	Grammatic Understanding	9
	Sentence Imitation	7
	Grammatic Completion	7
	Word Discrimination	12
	Word Articulation	7
	Listening (Composite Score)	97
	Spoken Language (Composite Score)	85
	Speaking (Composite Score: Oral Vocabulary plus Grammatic Completion)	45

CREVT–2	Receptive	92
	Expressive	75
	General	80
TWF–2	Total Score	76
	Word Finding Profile	Slow and inaccurate namer
CELF–4	Word Structure	4(9)*
	Familiar Sequences	5
	Rapid Automatic Naming	Non-normal score**
GFTA–2		All errors attributable to AAE dialect
CASL, Basic Concepts subtest. CELF-Preschool–2, Linguistic Concepts subtest		Some spatial and temporal concepts in error; can affect sequencing accuracy

---

* First score represents standard American English; score in parentheses allows credit for AAE differences (Semel et al., 2003, pp. 312–313).
** Reflects performance that "suggests a need for follow-up assessment … includ[ing] testing for word finding problems" (Semel et al., 2003, p. 139).

I should explain that some of the instruments were not chosen before testing began. The first tests to be administered were the CREVT–2 and the TOLD–P–3. James's performance on the receptive portion of the CREVT–2 was within normal limits. However, during the expressive subtest of that instrument, it was obvious that he struggled to find words to define items he clearly knew. With the exception of the Oral Vocabulary and Relational Vocabulary subtests, the TOLD–P–3 results appeared to indicate that his overall language skills were roughly within normal limits, providing his use of AAE morphological, phonological, and syntactic substitutions was taken into consideration. His performance on the Oral Vocabulary and Relational Vocabulary subtests indicated the same behaviors as on the CREVT–2; on the Oral Vocabulary subtest in particular he lost credit because he gave up before he could find the words to describe a required second characteristic. I administered the Rapid Naming Subtest of the CELF–4 to determine if word familiarity would improve his performance; it did not. Therefore, combined with other reported indications of probable anomia, the *Test of Word Finding–2* was administered. Its results confirmed word-finding deficits. This test, however, does not address automatic recall of common sequences like the days of the week, a problem during initial screening. Therefore, I administered the Familiar Sequences subtest of the CELF–4; the results clearly identified automaticity as weak, also.

Addressing factors that could affect James's ability to comprehend directions, the Linguistic Concepts subtest of the *Clinical Evaluation of Language Fundamentals–Preschool, Second Edition* and the Basic Concepts subtest of the *Comprehensive Assessment of Spoken Language* were administered informally. Standard scores could not be reported because James had surpassed the upper age limit of both tests. His errors appeared only in spatial and temporal concepts, specifically left–right, ordinal numbers, and before–after. Finally, to confirm that AAE usage did account for the marginal scores in articulation, I administered the *Goldman–Fristoe Test of Articulation–2*; as suspected, all articulation errors were so identified. I also checked James's spelling capabilities and found that they were entirely grade appropriate; that is, his articulation difference did not appear to affect a related classroom subject. Note that the results of one test lead to using another; if you have a battery of tests you "always" administer, you can miss important information. Playing chess is a good analogy for the diagnostic process: At the beginning of the game, you may have a general plan of attack, but your specific moves depend on what happens at each stage of the game. Therefore, learn to ask yourself at every stage of the evaluation process, Where do I go next? Now, using the information above, write a summary statement: How would you characterize James's use of language in the classroom?

I classified James's errors in morphology, syntax, and articulation as a language *difference* not a language deficit. Equally on the basis of the scores of the standardized instruments and the interpretation of nonstandardized procedures, I concluded that his most serious deficit appeared to stem from word-finding problems, which directly affected his scores in expressive tasks. Semantically, he demonstrated receptive weaknesses with some age-inappropriate temporal and spatial concepts. This case is an example of one in which some errors can be explained by dialect, and others represent real deficits. Therefore, see this case as a cautionary tale: Just because you recognize the use of dialect, do not jump to the conclusion that it represents the sole explanation for every deficit you identify.

Case Three: Christine

Christine is 15 and is in the second semester of her sophomore year in high school. In late March, she was referred because of declining grades in several subjects since September. She has been a student in the same district since kindergarten, so her records are complete. In grade school (K–5), she received mostly C's and low B's. She was in the lowest reading group in first grade; as a result of her slow progress, she received Title I reading assistance during second grade. In middle school (Grades 6–8), her average was C to C–. During the fall semester of her freshman year, her average slipped to C– to D+. She had been placed on the watch list by her 9th-grade team when she passed, barely, into 10th grade. The team did not recommend retention, because it is not uncommon for students to experience problems during the transition from middle school to high school, with its seven academically challenging classes and seven different teachers each day. By March of the spring semester of the 10th grade, however, she was clearly failing several courses. Her team members report that she works hard, often completing extra-credit assignments, but experiences difficulty understanding complex material from either lectures or textbooks. Her outlining skills are poor; she does not analyze or synthesize curriculum material adequately, even compared with those classmates who exhibit generally low-average ability. What would you ask these teachers? Her parents?

Entering a high school as a speech–language pathologist means going into an entirely new world. Ehren (2002) identifies instructional demands related to

> a student's ability to acquire, manipulate, store, and use large amounts of information from sources that often do not consider the learning inefficiencies demonstrated by students with disabilities.... [Classes] require students to gain information from textbooks that are often both poorly organized and written, on the average, at the 11th grade level.... [plus] students are required to gain large amounts of information from classroom lectures that often lack explicit organization, appropriate instruction on prerequisite vocabulary and sufficient repetition of key information. (p. 64)

Teachers usually consider themselves specialists within their area (e.g., math, English, biology), and many find it difficult to adapt curriculum material to meet the needs of students with language-based learning problems. In this era of "standards," teachers are frequently sensitive to possible criticism that they passed a student who clearly did not have a grasp of the material. In extreme cases, they can be blunt: "Look, I teach ____; if students can't do the work, they don't belong in my class." The focus for the SLP shifts to student survival—and keeping the youngster from dropping out. To compound matters, for every student you serve, you must also interact with five to seven instructors. Because scheduling can be daunting, it is extremely helpful if teachers meet in teams. Typically, they meet early in the morning, and your time for questions will be brief.

In this atmosphere, I learned that her teachers considered Christine "a really nice girl" who is interested in the content of her science and social studies courses, works hard, and wants to do better than she does. She appears to get along fine with classmates, but since she is quiet, it is hard to tell. Her parents had met with the team three times and, although willing to help, said that Chris had already dropped all extracurricular activities and the babysitting she enjoyed, spent

3 to 4 hours a night on homework, and was getting very discouraged. She consistently received after-school help from a number of her teachers and had also worked with a peer tutor. That assistance was discontinued when the other student reported that Christine's notes from class were so disorganized, it took most of their assigned time just trying to make heads or tails of what she had managed to get down on paper. When none of the typical remedies seemed to help, Christine was referred for possible evaluation.

School records indicated a steady downhill slide in grades and an increase in teachers' comments that Christine was struggling to understand cognitively difficult or "dense" material, even though her guidance counselor had switched her from a precollege program to one in general education to lessen classwork complexity. End-of-year test results in reading comprehension were in the very-low-normal range, and her comprehension of 10th-grade texts and lectures appeared limited, particularly if she felt rushed. When I observed her in class, she rarely volunteered to speak. When she was forced to respond to a direct question, her answers were disorganized, marked by irrelevant remarks and a failure to integrate information into a cohesive whole. Her performance improved, however, when she was part of a small discussion group or when the assignment reflected a series of steps to follow. I reviewed a number of written assignments, and although her spelling and grammar were correct, her writing usually featured simple vocabulary and structure, mostly declarative subject–verb sentences with few dependent clauses and a complete lack of intersentential connectives. Because written assignments took her so long to complete, several of her teachers had allowed her to make oral reports, instead. They, too, were substandard. Both expository and narrative oral discourse were marked by the same features that characterized her answers to teachers' questions: disorganization, limited support for opinion, lack of intersentential connectives, meager descriptive detail, and absence of a clear main idea. She earned passing grades in math but could not explain the process she used to get a correct answer. During middle school, her seventh-grade English teacher suggested that she be tested for a learning disability, but there was no indication that any testing had been undertaken.

A parent conference indicated that although Christine's development was average and she has had no medical problems, she was a "late talker." She attended a university clinic for language when she was 3 and 4 years old. She received Title I reading help from the second through fifth grade, and then again in seventh grade, when it focused on reading comprehension. Her mother said that "it broke her heart" to see that no matter how hard Christine worked, she is still failing. A popular babysitter in their neighborhood, Chris has limited the hours she spends taking care of children in order to complete her homework and study for tests. Because she has also dropped all but one of her extracurricular activities (the Food Club), her social life has changed, and she is now alone much of the time and often "depressed." She spends an average of 4 hours each night on homework assignments. Chris's mother is a high school graduate, but her dad left school at the end of 10th grade because it "got too hard." He was concerned that his daughter would end up the same way and would not be able to get a good job. When I asked about the recommendation for testing, the parents said that Chris had objected, so she went to summer school instead and passed seventh-grade English that way. They expressed a desire to work on classwork with her and to continue with tutoring if that seemed advisable.

I observed Chris in her social studies class while I was working with another student on a project. She was attentive but frequently checked with her neighbor during the short lecture; twice I heard her ask, "What did he say?" Her difficult-to-read notes filled the page, margin to margin. There was no sign of "chunking" of information, such as headings or outline configuration. A free study period followed the lecture, and Chris was clearly having a problem finding the answers to chapter review questions in her book. Mr. Baker, the social studies teacher, showed me an essay question from her last test. It was short, and internal paragraph development was inadequate, with no transitions between paragraphs. Overall, her answer did not support any discernible argument. Mr. Baker commented that this example was actually a little better than most of her work. He confirmed that Chris was a hard worker but just did not seem to "be with the program."

Later, in my room, when I asked about her problems in school, Christine said that she had to read assignments "over and over" before she could figure out what they meant. She added that "long sentences that start and stop" bothered her the most. She used to like to write, but in high school they wanted "pages and pages and pages," and she did not know what to say or how to "put stuff together." When she borrowed a friend's notes from class, it helped her to study; using her own did not help at all. When I asked about strategies such as semantic maps, she responded that no one had ever mentioned them. She volunteered that even though science was hard, she enjoyed the experiments, partly because the teacher provided a list of steps to follow. She commented that it was also easier to answer questions on science tests based on the experiments, because she could think back on what she did, and that helped her to remember.

Outside school, Christine said that she loved to babysit when she could find the time, and she also liked to cook, especially baking. She reported sadly that she didn't have much time for either because of all the time she had to spend on homework after school and weekends.

The school psychologist determined that Christine's overall IQ was 91, with a 12-point discrepancy between her verbal score (84) and her performance score (96); the psychologist suggested that language testing be completed before any decisions were made about a possible label.

So, now it is up to you. How will you evaluate Christine? I hope you feel a sense of urgency about this third case; when a student is 15, depression about school can have serious repercussions.

Tests	Taps Information Concerning
CELF–4	Overall receptive and expressive language (four subtests of Core Language Battery will be given first; based on that score and other information, more subtests may be administered)
PPVT–3	Receptive vocabulary
Evaluating Communicative Competence–Revised, (ECC–R; Simon, 1994)	"School" language skills

No voice, formal pragmatics, fluency, or articulation assessment appeared necessary. Christine's scores and their interpretation are reported in the diagnostic report that represents the longer form in Appendix 3.H.

You will meet Zachary, James, and Christine again in Chapter 4, when we develop an IEP for each of them, and finally in Chapter 5, when we discuss intervention plans.

Case Four: Megan

For this case, you are on your own. I will describe Megan, but you will develop assessment procedures, choose evaluation instruments, and fabricate probable test results. On the basis of these, you will write an IEP and describe some appropriate intervention goals. At each stage, you may want to check with classmates in a cooperative learning group and discuss your results, conclusions, and plans with your instructor.

Megan, a redhead with big brown eyes, is 13 and in the sixth grade. She was labeled as mentally retarded when she entered school, based initially on *Wechsler Preschool and Primary Scale of Intelligence* (WPPSI; Wechsler, 2002) results and confirmed later by *Wechsler Intelligence Scale for Children–Third Edition* (WISC–III; Wechsler, 1991). Her parents, aware of her mental status since birth, were actively involved in all aspects of an early intervention program. Megan was a student in a typical preschool for 3 years, with speech–language services integrated into her daily routine. She has been mainstreamed since first grade. Considering her combined IQ of 70, with verbal–performance scores of 70 and 71, respectively, she has held her own very well. Her most recent report card (modified program) features grades mostly in the B range in science, social studies, language arts, and math. Achievement scores in those subjects place her at the early fourth-grade level. She is pragmatically appropriate in social situations, although in recent years she has interacted more successfully with adults than with her peers. Her mouth breathing and sometimes careless hygiene may be part of the reason that sixth-grade students do not seek her out. In addition, her classmates' behavior reflects the language and interests of early adolescence, and Meg is still very much a child. She often seeks out younger students to talk with during lunch and recess.

Her teacher, Mr. Walters, reports that Megan appears to enjoy school and works hard. As noted above, most of her subject areas reflect at least a 2-year lag, but he comments that there are a number of other students whose skills place them in "the low group," too. All "solid" subjects are taught in the classroom by Mr. Walters; with the rest of the class, Megan leaves the room for art, music, and physical education. She is an average student in music and does fairly well in art if the lesson deals with crafts but struggles if the activity features something like perspective. She is having increasing difficulty in gym class as her classmates develop more skill, but her teacher at this time does not recommend adaptive P.E. Megan has a very difficult time taking notes and relies on teacher-designed study questions to prepare for examinations. Her parents report that they spend an hour or two every night helping her with her homework or studying for tests.

Math was Megan's favorite subject until fifth grade. Her good rote memory made simple addition, subtraction, and multiplication tasks easy for her. Long division and double-digit multiplication, however, present difficulty, exacerbated by Megan's failure to keep columns of figures straight on her paper. Word problems have always been hard and are getting harder. Following directions has become more difficult, too. If they are single-step, logical, and clearly laid out, she can cope, but when they are long or contain words like "if" and "except," she flounders. Semantically, she exhibits problems comprehending figurative language, multiple-meaning words, comparisons, and inference in written material; understanding oral language containing those same elements appears easier. Her basic decoding and spelling skills are adequate, representing third- to fourth-grade skills. Automatic series, such as days of the week and months of the year, are fine. Her spontaneous writing consists of simple one-clause declarative sentences containing few complexities and using straightforward sequence as the only form. In her narratives, mostly stories about her family, there is little sense of motivation, detail, concept of a plot, or use of intraparagraph connectors. Her speech is intelligible, but a persistent gliding of liquids, now more of a distortion, as well as problems with multisyllabic words, sometimes makes her hard to understand, particularly to someone who does not know her.

Megan's organization skills leave much to be desired; her desk is a disaster, with papers stuffed everywhere. Her glasses, which she needs to read, are often "lost." Mr. Walters is not sure if she really does forget where she has taken them off or just does not like to wear them because they constantly slide down her nose. Students around her have learned to keep extra pencils and paper handy because Megan can never find hers.

Megan is due for a triennial evaluation in a month or so. Her parents and Mr. Walters are worried about her ability to function in the seventh grade. They are particularly concerned about her changing classes each period, the increased amount and complexity of the material in upper middle school, and her ability to switch from one teaching style to another, particularly when the teachers at that level see themselves as being responsible for covering a specific amount of material in their subject area. Mr. Walters and Megan's parents have also expressed concern about the availability of assistance for Megan, as well as a possible lack of coordination among her teachers.

The following is an excerpt from Megan's oral language sample:

My family is going camping. It is fun! We will drive to Pennsylvania and then go the campground. First we will unload the car and set up our tent. Then we can go for a hike. We will probably go to the big pond. I like to go there because I catch salamanders and see some little fish. The baby salamanders are small and very fast. They're orange. At dinnertime, we cook hamburgers and hot dogs. We also cook potatoes and corn. Later we sing around the campfire and eat s'mores. We stay at the campfire until it's time for bed. Camping is a lot of fun. I like it.

The following is an excerpt from Megan's spontaneous written sample:

My sister Jess has a dog. His name is Sam. Sam is a little black puppy. One day he made a hole under the fens. He squesed through. He ran down the street. He fell into a hole. The hole was very deep. He tried to get out but he couldn't. Jess came out to get him. My mom and Jess looked for him. Jess herd barkking and she falloed the sound. She saw Sam. They reskued him. We were happy. The end.

On the basis of an analysis of the two samples and the information contained in the case history, what are your standardized testing recommendations for Megan? Remember, with a student who is mentally retarded, the published age range on instruments should match her approximate mental age (MA), not necessarily her chronological age (CA). Appendix 3.A lists instruments commonly available in most schools. Typically, the total time you have available for administering standardized measures in the schools is about 2 hours. Therefore, choose instruments that meet your purposes but whose administration time fits into that time frame. Be prepared to provide well-thought-out, specific reasons for your choices. Check with your instructor before proceeding to the next step. After choosing the instruments, project probable scores. At the close of Chapter 4, you will be asked to develop an IEP for Megan.

CONCLUSION

Before leaving this chapter, we have final words of both caution and consolation. First the consolations: Regardless of whether the assessment model you adopt falls into the traditional or new category, assessment and evaluation are an ongoing process; each time you work with a student, you will discover something about what she knows or how she learns that will affect your future plans. Therefore, if you have missed something in the initial assessment, you will have ample opportunity to evaluate new information and state a new hypothesis. In addition, as you gain experience, you will begin to see patterns and gain insights that will assist you in reaching conclusions more quickly and surely. Now the caution. Be aware that each time you interact with a student, whether you are formally evaluating him or providing therapy, a yellow light should always be blinking in your head: Attention, attention, important new evaluation information lies ahead.

STUDY QUESTIONS

1. What does standardized testing include? What are the advantages and disadvantages of standardized testing?
2. Describe the differences between case finding and case selection.
3. What factors are important in choosing an appropriate standardized instrument for a particular student? In purchasing a particular test for your district?
4. What is the role of the interview in the public school setting? What different kinds of interviews are you likely to complete?
5. Your principal has put you in charge of the speech and language testing for kindergarten screenings to be held in May. What factors will you consider in your plans?
6. What is the role of school records of various types in assessment and evaluation?
7. Make a case for language sampling in the schools. What would a language sample tell you about a child's communication ability?
8. Compare and contrast "traditional" approaches to assessment using the procedures that are part of the "new" types—for example, dynamic, curriculum-based.
9. Describe the factors you would consider before recommending that a child receive a label of speech (or language) impaired.

10. Why is observing a student in the classroom setting an important part of an evaluation?
11. Explain why a knowledge of syntax has acquired new prominence in school-based practice. What is the connection between syntax and literacy (reading and writing)?

REFERENCES

Adler, S. (1991). Assessment of language proficiency of limited English proficient speakers. *Language, Speech and Hearing Services in the Schools, 22,* 12–18.

American Speech-Language-Hearing Association, Committee on Language Disorders. (1989). Issues in determining eligibility for language intervention. *Asha, 31,* 113–118.

American Speech-Language-Hearing Association. (1997). *Directory of speech–language pathology assessment instruments.* Rockville, MD: Author.

American Speech-Language-Hearing Association. (1999a). *Guidelines for the roles and responsibilities of the school-based speech–language pathologist.* Rockville, MD: Author.

American Speech-Language-Hearing Association. (1999b). *IDEA and your caseload: A template for eligibility and dismissal criteria for students ages 3 to 21.* Rockville, MD. Author.

American Speech-Language-Hearing Association. (2003). Catalog. Rockville, MD. Author.

Approaches to authentic assessment. (n.d). Retrieved September 3, 2005, from the North Central Regional Educational Laboratory Web site: http://www.ncrel.org/sdrs/areas/issues/envrmnt/stw/sw1lk8.htm

Bader, L. (2005). *Bader reading and language inventory* (5th ed.). Englewood Cliffs, NJ: Prentice Hall.

Bankson, N. (1990). *Bankson language test* (2nd ed.). Austin, TX: PRO-ED.

Bankson, N., & Bernthal, J. (1990). *Bankson–Bernthal test of phonology.* Austin, TX: PRO-ED.

Barrett, M., Huisingh, R., Zachman, L., LoGiudice, C., & Orman, J. (1992). *The listening test.* East Moline, IL: LinguiSystems.

Bashir, A. (1989). Language intervention and the curriculum. *Seminars in Speech and Language, 10,* 181–191.

Bashir, A. S., & Scavuzzo, A. (1992). Children with language disorders: Natural history and academic success. *Journal of Learning Disabilities, 25,* 53–65.

Battle, D. E. (1998). *Communication disorders in multicultural populations* (2nd ed.). Newton, MA: Butterworth-Heinemann.

Blank, M., Rose, S., & Berlin, L. (2003). *Preschool language assessment instrument* (2nd ed.). Austin, TX: PRO-ED.

Blau, A., Lahey, M., & Oleksiuk-Velez, A. (1984). Planning goals for intervention: Language testing or language sampling? *Exceptional Children, 51,* 78–79.

Boehm, A. (2000). *Boehm test of basic concepts* (3rd ed.). San Antonio, TX: Psychological Corp.

Boehm, A. (2001). *Boehm test of basic concepts–PreK* (3rd ed.). San Antonio, TX: Psychological Corp.

Bond, L. (1995). *Critical issues: Rethinking assessment and its role in supporting educational reform.* Retrieved September 1, 2005, from the North Central Regional Educational Laboratory (NCREL) Web site: http://www.ncrel.org/sdrs/areas/issues/methods/assessment/as700.htm

Bowers, L., Barrett, M., Huisingh, R., Orman, J., & LoGiudice, C. (1991). *Test of problem solving–adolescent.* East Moline, IL: LinguiSystems.

Bowers, L., Huisingh, R., LoGiudice, C., & Orman, J. (2002). *Test of semantic skills–primary.* East Moline, IL: LinguiSystems.

Bowers, L., Huisingh, R., LoGiudice, C., & Orman, J. (2004). *The word test 2: Elementary*. East Moline, IL: LinguiSystems.

Bowers, L., Huisingh, R., LoGiudice, C., & Orman, J. (2005). *The word test 2: Adolescent*. East Moline, IL: LinguiSystems.

Bracken, B. (1998). *Bracken basic concept scale–revised*. San Antonio, TX: Psychological Corp.

Bracken, B. (2002). *Bracken School Readiness Assessment*. San Antonio, TX: Psychological Corp.

Brinton, B., & Fujiki, M. (1992). Setting the context for conversational speech sampling. *Best Practices in School Speech–Language Pathology, 2,* 9–19.

Brown, R. (1973). *A first language: The early stages*. Cambridge, MA: Harvard University Press.

Brown, V. L., Hammill, D. D., & Wiederholt, J. L. (1995). *Test of reading comprehension* (3rd ed.). Austin, TX: PRO-ED.

Bryant, B. R., Wiedenholt, J. L., & Bryant, D. P. (2004). *Gray diagnostic reading tests–Second edition*. Austin, TX: PRO-ED.

Burke, K. (1994). *The mindful school: How to assess authentic learning*. Palatine, NY: IRI/Skylight. Retrieved November 1, 2004, from http://www.businessl.com/IRI_sky/Assess/htaali.htm

Butler, K. G. (1999). From oracy to literacy: Changing clinical perceptions. *Topics in Language Disorders, 20,* 14–32.

Carrow-Woolfolk, E. (1996). *Oral and written language scales*. Circle Pines, MN: American Guidance Service.

Carrow-Woolfolk, E. (1999a). *Comprehensive assessment of spoken language*. Circle Pines, MN: American Guidance Service.

Carrow-Woolfolk, E. (1999b). *Test for auditory comprehension of language* (3rd ed.). Austin, TX: PRO-ED.

Congress Reauthorizes IDEA. (2004). *ASHA Leader* 9(22), 27.

Creaghead, N., & Tattershall, S. (1985). Observation and assessment of classroom pragmatic skills. In C. S. Simon (Ed.), *Communication skills and classroom success: Assessment of language-learning disabled students* (pp. 105–134). San Diego, CA: College Hill.

Critical Issue: Rethinking assessment and its role in supporting educational reform. Retrieved July 18, 2005, from the North Central Regional Educational Laboratory Web site: http://www.ncrel.org/ncrel/sdrs/areas/issues/methods/assment/as700.htm

Crowhurst, M. (1980). Syntactic complexity in narration and argument at three grade levels. *Canadian Journal of Education, 5,* 6–13.

Crowhurst, M., & Piche, G. L. (1979). Audience and mode of discourse effects on syntactic complexity in writing at two grade levels. *Research in the Teaching of English, 13,* 101–109.

Crumrine, L., & Lonegan, H. (2000). *Phonemic awareness skills screening*. Austin, TX: PRO-ED.

Damico, J. (1985). Clinical discourse analysis: A functional language assessment technique. In C. S. Simon (Ed.), *Communication skills and classroom success: Assessment of language-learning disabled students* (pp. 165–206). San Diego, CA: College Hill.

Damico, J., & Hamayan, E. (1992). *Multicultural language intervention: Addressing cultural and linguistic diversity*. Buffalo, NY: EDUCOM Associates.

Dawson, J., & Stout, C. (2003). *Structured photographic expressive language test* (3rd ed.). San Antonio, TX: Psychological Corp.

Dawson, J., Stout, C., Eyer, J., Tattersall, P., Fonkalsrud, J., & Crowley, K. (2004). *Structured photographic expressive language test–Preschool 2*. San Antonio, TX: Harcourt Assessments.

DiSimoni, F. (1978). *Token test for children*. Chicago: Riverside.

Dollaghan, C. A., & Campbell, T. F. (1992). A procedure for classifying disruptions in spontaneous language samples. *Topics in Language Disorders, 12,* 53–68.

Duchan, J. F. (1982). The elephant is soft and mushy: Problems in assessing children's language. In N. Lass, L. McReynolds, J. Northern, & D. Yoder (Eds.), *Speech, language and hearing.* Philadelphia: W.B. Saunders.

Duncan, S., & DeAvila, E. (1994). *Language assessment scales–reading and writing.* Monterey, CA: CET-McGraw-Hill.

Dunn, L., & Dunn, L. M. (1981). *Peabody picture vocabulary test–revised.* Circle Pines, MN: American Guidance Service.

Dunn, L., & Dunn, L. M. (1997). *Peabody picture vocabulary test* (3rd ed.). Circle Pines, MN: American Guidance Service.

Edmonston, N., & Thane, N. (1993). *Test of relational concepts–revised.* Tucson, AZ: Communication Skill Builders.

Ehren, B. J. (2002). Speech–language pathologists contributing significantly to the adademic success of high school students: A vision for professional growth. *Topics in Language Disorders, 22*(2), 60–80.

Feuerstein, R. (1969). *The instrumental enrichment method: An outline of theory and technique.* Jerusalem, Israel: Hadassah-W120-Canada Research Institute.

Fisher, H., & Logemann, J. (1971). *Fisher–Logemann test of articulation competence.* Boston: Houghton Mifflin.

Fluharty, N. (2000). *Fluharty preschool speech and language screening test* (2nd ed.). San Antonio, TX: Psychological Corp.

Francis, D., Fletcher, J., Shaywitz, B., Shaywitz, S., Rourke, B., & Sabers, D. (1996). Defining learning and language disabilities: Conceptual and psychometric issues with the use of IQ tests. *Language, Speech, & Hearing Services in Schools, 27,* 132–143.

Fressola, D., & Hoerchler, S. (1989). *Speech and language evaluation scale.* Columbia, MO: Hawthorne Educational Services.

Fuchs, L. (1995). Connecting performance assessment to instruction: A comparison of behavioral assessment, mastery learning, curriculum-based measurement, and performance assessment. *ERIC clearinghouse on disabilities and gifted children, ERIC Digest E 530.* (online) Retrieved September, 1, 2005 from http://www.ed.gov/databases/ERIC_Digests/ed381984.html

Fudala, J. (2000). *Arizona articulation proficiency scale* (3rd ed.). Los Angeles: Western Psychological Services.

Fujiki, M., & Willbrand, M. (1982). A comparison of four informal methods of language evaluation. *Language, Speech, & Hearing Services in Schools, 13,* 42–52.

Garcia, G. (1992). Ethnography and classroom communication: Taking an "emic" perspective. *Topics in Language Disorders, 12,* 54–66.

Gardner, M. (1994). *Test of auditory perceptual skills: Upper level.* Austin, TX: PRO-ED.

Gardner, M. (2000). *Expressive one-word picture vocabulary test–revised.* San Antonio, TX: Psychological Corp.

Gardner, M., & Brownell, B. (2000). *Receptive one-word picture vocabulary test–2000.* San Antonio, TX: Psychological Corp.

Gauthier, S., & Madison, C. (1998). *Kindergarten language screening test* (2nd ed.). Austin, TX: PRO-ED.

German, D. (1990). *Test of adolescent/adult word finding.* Austin, TX: PRO-ED.

German, D. (1991). *Test of word finding in discourse.* Austin, TX: PRO-ED.

German, D. (2000). *Test of word finding* (2nd ed). Austin, TX: PRO-ED.

Goldman, R., & Fristoe, M. (1986). *Goldman–Fristoe test of articulation.* Circle Pines, MN: American Guidance Service.

Goldman, R., & Fristoe, M. (2000). *Goldman–Fristoe test of articulation* (2nd ed.). Circle Pines, MN: American Guidance Service.

Goodman, K. S. (1983). Analysis of oral reading miscues: Applied psycholinguistics. In F. Smith (Ed.), *Psycholinguistics and reading* (pp. 158–176). New York: Holt, Rinehart & Winston.

Greenhalgh, K., & Strong, C. (2001). Literate language features in spoken narratives of children with typical language and children with language impairments. *Language, Speech, and Hearing Services in Schools, 32,* 114–125.

Gummersall, D. M., & Strong, C. J. (1999). Assessment of complex sentence production in a narrative context. *Language, Speech, and Hearing Services in Schools, 30,* 152–164.

Hammill, D., Brown, V., Larsen, S., & Wiederholt, J. (1994). *Test of adolescent and adult language* (3rd ed.). Austin, TX: PRO-ED.

Hammill, D., Larsen, S., & Wiederholt, J. (1996). *Test of written language* (3rd ed.). Austin, TX: PRO-ED.

Hammill, D., Mather, N., & Robert, R. (2001). *Illinois test of psycholinguistic abilities.* Austin, TX: PRO-ED.

Hammill, D., & Newcomer, P. (1997). *Test of language development–Intermediate* (3rd ed.). Austin, TX: PRO-ED.

Herman, J., Aschbacher, P., & Winters, L. (1992). *Select or design assessments that elicit established outcomes.* Retrieved September 4, 2005 from the North Central Regional Education Laboratory Web site: http://www.ncrel.org/ncrel/sdrs/areas/issues/methods/assment/as7sele2.htm

Hill, S., & Haynes, W. (1992). Language performance in low-achieving elementary school students. *Language, Speech, and Hearing Services in Schools, 23,* 169–175.

Hirschman, M. (2000). Language repair via metalinguistic means. *International Journal of Language & Communication Disorders, 35*(2), 251–268.

Hodson, B. (1986). *Assessment of phonological processes–revised.* Austin, TX: PRO-ED.

Hodson, B., & Paden, E. (1991). *Targeting intelligible speech: A phonological approach to remediation* (2nd ed.). Austin, TX: PRO-ED.

Hresko, W., Reid, D. K., & Hammill, D. D. (1999). *Test of early language development* (3rd ed.). Austin, TX: PRO-ED.

Hresko, W., Herron, S. R., & Peak, P. K. (1996). *Test of early written language* (2nd ed.). Austin, TX: PRO-ED.

Huisingh, R., Bowers, L., & LoGiudice, C. (2005). *Test of problem solving: Elementary* (3rd ed.). Austin, TX: PRO-ED.

Huisingh, R., Bowers, L., LoGiudice, C., & Orman, J. (2004). *Test of semantic skills–intermediate.* East Moline, IL: LinguiSystems.

Hutchinson, T. (1996). What to look for in the technical manual: Twenty questions for users. *Language, Speech, & Hearing Services in Schools, 27,* 109–121.

Hux, K., Morris-Friehe, M., & Sanger, D. (1993). Language sampling practices: A survey of nine states. *Language, Speech, & Hearing Services in Schools, 24,* 84–91.

Idol, L., Nevin, A., & Paolucci-Whitcomb, P. (1996). *Models of curriculum-based assessment* (2nd ed.). Austin, TX: PRO-ED.

Individuals with Disabilities Act of 1997. (1997). Public Law 101-336.

Individuals with Disabilities Improvement Act. (2004). Public Law 108-446.

Johnston, E., & Johnston, A. (1990). *Communication abilities diagnostic test.* Chicago: Riverside.

Kamhi, A. (1993). Assessing complex behaviors: Problems with reification, quantification, and ranking. *Language, Speech, & Hearing Services in Schools, 24,* 110–113.

Kaufman, N. (1992). *Kaufman speech praxis test for children.* Austin, TX: PRO-ED.

Kelly, D., & Rice, M. (1986). A strategy for language assessment of young children: A combination of two approaches. *Language, Speech, & Hearing Services in Schools, 17,* 83–94.

Khan, L., & Lewis, N. (2002). *Khan–Lewis phonological analysis* (2nd ed.). Circle Pines, MN: American Guidance Service.

Kinzler, M., & Cowing Johnson, C. (1993). *Joliet 3-minute speech and language screen.* San Antonio, TX: Harcourt Brace Educational Measurements.

Larsen, S., Hammill, D., & Moats, L. (1999). *Test of written spelling* (4th ed.). Austin, TX: PRO-ED.

Larson, V., & McKinley, N. (1995). *Language disorders in older students.* Eau Claire, WI: Thinking Publications.

Lee, L. (1971). *Northwest syntax screening test.* Evanston, IL: Northwestern University Press.

Lindamood, C., & Lindamood, P. (2004). *Lindamood auditory conceptualization test* (3rd ed.) Austin, TX: PRO-ED.

Lippke, S., Dickey, S., Selmar, J., & Soder, A. (1997). *Photo articulation test* (3rd ed.). Danville, IL: Interstate.

Loban, W. (1976). *Language development: Kindergarten through grade twelve.* Urbana, IL: National Council of Teachers of English.

Lombardino, L., Lieberman, J., & Brown, J. (2005). *Assessment of literacy and language.* San Antonio, TX: Harcourt Assessments.

Lund, N., & Duchan, J. (1993). *Assessing children's language in naturalistic contexts* (3rd ed.). Englewood Cliffs, NJ: Prentice Hall.

Martin, M., & Brownell, R. (2005). *Test of auditory processing skills* (3rd ed.). Austin, TX: PRO-ED.

Masterson, J., Apel, K., & Wasowicz, J. (2002). *Spelling performance evaluation for language and literacy.* San Antonio, TX: Psychological Corp.

Masterson, J., & Kamhi, A. (1991). The effects of sampling conditions on sentence production in normal, reading-disabled, and language-learning-disabled children. *Journal of Speech and Hearing Research, 34,* 549–558.

McCauley, R. (1996). Familiar strangers: Criterion-referenced measures in communication disorders. *Language, Speech, & Hearing Services in Schools, 27,* 122–131.

McCormick, L., & Schiefelbusch, R. (1984). *Early language intervention: An introduction.* Columbus, OH: Merrill.

McDonald, E. (1968). *Deep test of articulation.* Pittsburgh, PA: Stanwix House.

McFadden, T. (1996). Creating language impairments in typically achieving children: The pitfalls of "normal" normative sampling. *Language, Speech, and Hearing Services in Schools, 27,* 3–9.

McGhee, R., Bryant, B., Larsen, S., & Rivera, D. (1995). *Test of written expression.* Austin, TX: PRO-ED.

Miller, L., Gillam, R. B., & Pena, E. D. (2001). *Dynamic assessment and intervention: Improving children's narrative abilities.* Austin, TX: PRO-ED.

Morgan, D., & Guilford, A. (1984). *Adolescent language screening test.* Austin, TX: PRO-ED.

Muma, J. (1978). *The language handbook: Concepts, assessment, intervention.* Englewood Cliffs, NJ: Prentice Hall.

Muma, J., Lubinski, R., & Pierce, S. (1982). A new era in language assessment: Data or evidence. In N. Lass (Ed.), *Speech and language: Advances in basic research and practice* (vol. 7, pp. 135–147). New York: Academic Press.

Naremore, R., Densmore, A., & Harman, D. (2001). *Assessment and treatment: Manual of school-age language disorders: A resource manual.* San Diego, CA: Singular.

National Research Center on Learning Disabilities. (2004). *Executive summary of the NRCLD symposium on responsiveness to invervention* (Brochure). Lawrence, KS: Author.

Nelson, K. (1985). *Making sense: The acquisition of shared meaning.* New York: Academic Press.

Nelson, N. (1989). Curriculum-based language assessment and intervention. *Language, Speech, and Hearing Services in Schools, 20,* 170–184.

Nelson, N. (1990). Only relevant practices can be best. *Best Practices in School Speech–Language Pathology, 1,* 15–27.

Nelson, N. (1994). Curriculum-based language assessment and intervention across the grades. In G. Wallach & K. Butler (Eds.), *Language learning disabilities in school-age children and adolescents* (pp. 104–131). New York: Macmillan.

Newcomer, P., & Barenbaum, E. (2003). *Test of phonological awareness skills.* Austin, TX: PRO-ED.

Newcomer, P., & Hammill, D. (1997). *Test of language development–primary* (3rd ed.). Austin, TX: PRO-ED.

Nippold, M. (1998). *Later language development: The school-age and adolescent years* (2nd ed.). Austin, TX: PRO-ED.

Owens, R. (1995). *Language disorders: A functional approach to assessment and intervention* (2nd ed.). Needham Heights, MA: Allyn & Bacon.

Palincsar, A., Brown, A., & Campione, J. (1994). Models and practices of dynamic assessment. In G. Wallach & K. Butler (Eds.), *Language learning disabilities in school-age children and adolescents* (pp. 132–144). New York: Macmillan.

Paratore, J. R. (1995). Assessing literacy: Establishing common standards in portfolio assessment. *Topics in Language Disorders, 16,* 67–82.

Paul, R. (1981). Analyzing complex sentence development. In J. F. Miller (Ed.), *Assessing language production in children: Experimental procedures* (pp. 33–40). Needham Heights, MA: Allyn & Bacon.

Paul, R. (1995). *Language disorders from infancy through adolescence: Assessment and intervention.* St. Louis, MO: C.V. Mosby.

Paul, R. (2001). *Language disorders from infancy through adolescence: Assessment and intervention* (2nd ed.). St. Louis, MO: C.V. Mosby.

Performance based learning and assessment. (2000). Alexandria, VA: Association for Supervision and Curriculum Development.

Peterson, H., & Marquardt, T. (1990). *Appraisal and diagnosis of speech and language disorders* (2nd ed.). Englewood Cliffs, NJ: Prentice Hall.

Phelps-Terasaki, D., & Phelps-Gunn, T. (1992). *Test of pragmatic language.* Austin, TX: PRO-ED.

Phonological awareness literacy screening. (2004). Curry School of Education, University of Virginia, Charlottesville, VA. Retrieved September 1, 2005 from http://pals.virginia.edu/PALS-Instruments/PALS-K.asp

Plante, E., & Vance, R. (1994). Selection of preschool language tests: A data-based approach. *Language, Speech, and Hearing Services in Schools, 25,* 15–24.

Reid, D., Hresko, W., & Hammill, D. (2001). *Test of early reading ability* (3rd ed.). Austin, TX: PRO-ED.

Rhyner, P., Kelly, D., Brantley, A., & Drueger, D. (1999). Screening low-income African American children using BLT–2S and SPELT–P. *American Journal of Speech–Language Pathology, 8,* 44–52.

Richard, G., & Hanner, M. (2005). *Language processing test–Elementary* (3rd ed.). East Moline, IL: LinguiSystems.

Richard, G. J., & Hoge, D. R. (1999). *The source for syndromes.* East Moline, IL: LinguiSystems.

Richard, G. J., & Hoge, D. R. (2000). *The source for syndromes* (2nd ed.). East Moline, IL: LinguiSystems.

Riley, A. M. (1984). *Evaluating acquired skills in communication–revised.* Austin, TX: PRO-ED.

Robertson, C., & Salter, W. (1997). *Phonological awareness test.* East Moline, IL: LinguiSystems.

Roseberry-McKibbin, C. (1995). *Multicultural students with special language needs: Practical strategies for assessment and intervention.* Oceanside, CA: Academic Communication Associates.

Sabers, D. (1996). By their tests we will know them. *Language, Speech, and Hearing Services in Schools, 27,* 102–108.

Schneider, P., & Watkins, R. (1996). Applying Vygotskian developmental theory to language intervention. *Language, Speech, and Hearing Services in Schools, 27,* 157–170.

Scott, C. (1988). Spoken and written syntax. In M. Nippold (Ed.), *Later language development* (pp. 49–96). Boston: College-Hill Press.

Scott, C. (1999). Learning to write. In H. Catts and A. Kamhi (Eds.), *Later language development* (pp. 224–258). Boston: College-Hill Press.

Scott, C., & Stokes, S. (1995). Measures of syntax in school-age children and adolescents, *Language, Speech, and Hearing Services in Schools, 26,* 309–317.

Secord, W. (1981). *Test of minimal articulation competence.* San Antonio, TX: Psychological Corp.

Self-assessment in portfolios. Retrieved July 18, 2005, from the North Central Regional Educational Laboratory Web site: http://www.ncrel.org/sdrs/areas/issues/students/learning/lr-2port.htm

Semel, E., & Wiig, E. (1980). *Clinical evaluation of language fundamentals.* San Antonio, TX: Psychological Corp.

Semel, E., Wiig, E., & Secord, W. (1987). *Clinical evaluation of language fundamentals–Revised.* San Antonio, TX: Psychological Corp.

Semel, E., Wiig, E., & Secord, W. (1995). *Clinical evaluation of language fundamentals* (3rd ed.). San Antonio, TX: Psychological Corp.

Semel, E., Wiig, E., & Secord, W. (1996). *Clinical evaluation of language fundamentals–3 screening test.* San Antonio, TX: Psychological Corp.

Semel, E., Wiig, E., & Secord, W. (2003). *Clinical evaluation of language fundamentals* (4th ed.). San Antonio, TX: Psychological Corp.

Seymour, H., Roeper, T., & deVilliers, J. (2003). *Diagnostic evaluation of language variation–criterion referenced.* San Antonio, TX: Psychological Corp.

Seymour, H., Roeper, T., & deVilliers, J. (2003). *Diagnostic evaluation of language variation–Screening test.* San Antonio, TX: Harcourt Assessments.

Seymour, H., Roeper, T., & deVilliers, J. (2005). *Diagnostic evaluation of language variation–Norm referenced.* San Antonio, TX: Harcourt Assessments.

Shipley, K., & McAfee, J. (1998). *Assessment in speech language pathology: A resource manual* (2nd ed.). San Diego, CA: Singular.

Shipley, K., Stone, T., & Sue, M. (1983). *Test for examining expressive morphology.* Austin, TX: PRO-ED.

Shprintzen, R. J. (2000). *Syndrome identification for speech–language pathology: An illustrated pocket guide.* San Diego, CA: Singular.

Siegel, G., & Broen, P. (1976). Language assessment. In L. Lloyd (Ed.), *Communication assessment and intervention strategies* (pp. 73–122). Baltimore: University Park Press.

Simon, C. (Ed.). (1985). *Communication skills and classroom success: Assessment of language-learning disabled students.* San Diego, CA: College Hill.

Simon, C. (1987). *Classroom communication screening procedures for early adolescents: A handbook for assessment and intervention.* Tempe, AZ: Communi-Cog.

Simon, C. (1994). *Evaluating communicative competence–Revised* (2nd ed.). Tempe, AZ: Communi-Cog.

Simon, C. (1998). *Assessment of classroom communication and study skills.* Tempe, AZ: Communi-Cog.

Snyder, N. (2004). Congress reauthorizes IDEA. *Asha Leader, 9*(22), 26–27.

Sommers, R. (1987). *STIM-CON: Prognostic inventory for misarticulating kindergarten and first grade children.* Washington, DC: United Educational Services.

Speech-Ease screening inventory (K–1). (1985). Austin, TX: PRO-ED.

Stark, J., & Wallach, G. (1980). The path to a concept of language-learning disabilities. *Topics in Language Disorders, 1,* 1–14.

Strong, C. J. (1998). *The Strong narrative assessment procedure.* Eau Claire, WI: Thinking Publications.

Swank, L. (1994). Phonological coding abilities: Identification of impairments related to phonologically based reading problems. *Topics in Language Disorders, 14*(2), 56–71.

Tallal, P., Ross, R., & Curtiss, S. (1989). Familial aggregation in specific language impairment. *Journal of Speech and Hearing Disorders, 54,* 167–173.

Temple, C., & Gillet, J. (1984). *Language arts learning process and teaching practices.* Boston: Little, Brown.

Templeton, S. (2002). Spelling: Logical, learnable and critical. *ASHA Leader, 7*(3), 4–5, 12.

Templin, M., & Darley, F. (1969). *Templin–Darley tests of articulation.* Iowa City: University of Iowa, Bureau of Educational Research and Service.

Thorum, A. (1986). *Fullerton language test for adolescents* (2nd ed.). Austin, TX: PRO-ED.

Tomblin, B. (1991). Familial concentration of developmental language impairment. *Journal of Speech and Hearing Disorders, 54,* 587–595.

Torgesen, J., & Bryant, B. (2004). *Test of phonological awareness.* (2nd ed.: PLUS) Austin, TX: PRO-ED.

Torgesen, J., Wagner, R., & Rashotte, C. (1999). *Test of word reading efficiency.* Austin, TX: PRO-ED.

Trivette, C., Dunst, C., Deal, A., Hamer, A., & Propst, S. (1990). Assessing family strengths and family functioning style. *Topics in Early Childhood* (special ed.), *10,* 13–35.

van Kleeck, A. (1994). Metalinguistic development. In G. Wallach, & K. Butler (Eds.), *Language learning disabilities in school-age children and adolescents: Some principles and applications* (pp. 53–98). New York: Macmillan.

Vygotsky, L. S. (1978). *Mind in society: The development of higher psychological processes.* Cambridge, MA: Harvard University Press.

Wagner, R., Torgesen, K., & Rashotte, C. (1999). *Comprehensive test of phonological processing.* Austin, TX: PRO-ED.

Wallace, G., & Hammill, D. (2002). *Comprehensive receptive and expressive vocabulary test* (2nd ed.). Austin, TX: PRO-ED.

Wallach, G., & Butler, K. G. (1994a). Creating communication, literary, and academic success. In G. P. Wallach & K. G. Butler (Eds.), *Language learning disabilities in school-age children and adolescents: Some principles and applications* (pp. 2–26). New York: Macmillan.

Wallach, G., & Butler, K. (Eds.). (1994b). *Language learning disabilities in school-age children and adolescents: Some principles and applications.* New York: Macmillan.

Warden, M., & Hutchinson, T. (1992). *The writing process test.* Austin, TX: PRO-ED.

Washington, J., & Craig, H. (1992). Performances of low-income, African-American preschool and kindergarten children on the Peabody Picture Vocabulary Test–Revised. *Language, Speech, and Hearing Services in Schools, 23,* 329–333.

Wechsler, D. (1991). *Wechsler intelligence scale for children* (3rd ed.). San Antonio, TX: Psychological Corp.

Wechsler, D. (2002). *Wechsler preschool and primary scale of intelligence* (3rd ed.). San Antonio, TX: Psychological Corp.

Wechsler, D. (2004). *Wechsler intelligence scale for children–Integrated* (4th ed.). San Antonio, TX: Harcourt Assessments.

Weiss, C. (1980). *Weiss comprehensive articulation test.* Austin, TX: PRO-ED.

Westby, C. (1994). Multicultural issues. In J. Tomblin, H. Morris, & D. Spriestersbach (Eds.), *Diagnosis in speech–language pathology.* San Diego, CA: Singular.

Westby, C. (1998). Communicative refinement in school age and adolescence. In W. Hayes & B. Shulman (Eds.), *Communication development: Foundations, processes, and clinical applications* (pp. 311–360). Baltimore: Williams & Wilkins.

Westby, C. (1999). The right stuff for writing: Assessing and facilitating written language. In H. Catts and A. Kahmi (Eds.), *Language and reading disabilities* (pp. 259–324). Boston: Allyn & Bacon.

Westby, C., Stevens-Dominguez, M., & Oetter, P. (1996). A performance/competence model of observational assessment. *Language, Speech, and Hearing Services in Schools, 27,* 144–156.

Wiederholt, J., & Blalock, G. (2000). *Gray silent reading tests.* Austin, TX: PRO-ED.

Wiederholt, J., & Bryant, B. (2001). *Gray oral reading tests* (4th ed.). Austin, TX: PRO-ED.

Wiig, E., & Secord, W. (1989). *Test of language competence* (expanded ed.). San Antonio, TX: Psychological Corp.

Wiig, E., Secord, W., & Semel, E. (2004). *Clinical evaluation of language fundamentals–preschool* (2nd ed.). San Antonio, TX: Psychological Corp.

Wiig, E., & Semel, E. (1992). *Test of word knowledge.* San Antonio, TX: Psychological Corp.

Willabrand, M., & Iwata-Reuyl, G. (1994). Gender bias in language testing. *Asha, 36,* 50–52.

Williams, K. (1997). *Expressive vocabulary test.* Circle Pines, MN: American Guidance Service.

Wood, M. L. (1982). *Language disorders in school-age children.* Englewood, NJ: Prentice Hall.

Word of Mouth. (2001). *Reviews and comments, 12*(5), 4.

Word of Mouth: A newsletter dedicated to speech & language in school-age children. Austin, TX: PRO-ED Journals.

Young, E., & Perachio, J. (1993). *Patterned elicitation of syntax test–revised with morphophonemic analysis.* San Antonio, TX: Psychological Corp.

Zimmerman, I., Steiner, V., & Pond, R. (2002). *Preschool language scale* (4th ed.). San Antonio, TX: Psychological Corp.

Appendix 3.A

◆ ◆

Sampling of Evaluation Instruments for the School-Aged Child Pre-K–Grade 12

A/G = age/grade; R = receptive measure; E = expressive measure; Ph = phonology; M = morphology; Sx = syntax; Sm = semantics; Pr = pragmatics; L = literacy, e.g., phonological awareness, writing, reading, spelling; * = primarily a screening instrument

Instrument	Comments	A/G	R	E	Ph	M	Sx	Sm	Pr	L	Date
*Adolescent Language Screening Test (ALST): Morgan & Guilford	7 subtests; less than 15 minutes to administer	11–17	X	X	X	X	X	X	X	—	1984
Arizona Articulation Proficiency Scale (3rd ed.; AAPS–3): Fudala	Contains quick screening; black and white pictures; each phoneme listed by age; gender-specific norms to age 6	3–7	—	X	X	—	—	—	—	—	2000
Assessment of Literacy and Language (ALL): Lombardino, Lieberman, & Brown	Language disorders related to reading problems; 6 areas: print concepts, phonological awareness, alphabetic principles, reading fluency, language, and comprehension	pre K–1	X	X	X	—	X	X	—	X	2005
Assessment of Phonological Processes–Revised (APP–R): Hodson	For severe disorders; uses objects to assess phonological processes directly	Early elem	—	X	X	—	—	—	—	—	1986
*Assessment of Classroom Communication and Study Skills (ACCSS): Simon	Metalinguistics, oral directions, comprehension, analysis of text	10–18	X	X	—	X	X	X	X	—	1998
Bader Reading and Language Inventory (5th ed.): Bader	Assesses semantics, phonology, and syntax skills as they relate to reading	7–adult	X	X	—	X	X	X	—	X	2005
Bankson–Bernthal Test of Phonology (BBTOP): Bankson & Bernthal	Tests directly for 10 phonological processes; 80 plates; initial and final consonant inventory	3–9	—	X	X	—	—	—	—	—	1990

Test	Description	Age range								Year
Bankson Language Test (2nd ed.; BLT–2): Bankson	Assesses 3 language categories; cortical for intervention; individually administered; standard scores	3–7	X	X	—	X	X	X	X	1990
Boehm Test of Basic Concepts (3rd ed.): Boehm	25 concepts; administer to group or individually	K–2	X	—	—	X	—	X	—	2000
Boehm Test of Basic Concepts–Preschool (3rd ed.): Boehm	Can be used with younger children; separate norms for Spanish speakers	3–6	X	—	—	X	—	X	—	2001
Bracken Basic Concept Scale (Revised; BBCS–R): Bracken	11 school concepts including letters, shapes, and self/social awareness; administer to small group or individual in 30 minutes	2:6–8	X	—	—	X	X	X	X	1998
Bracken School Readiness Assessment: Bracken	First 6 subtests of the BBCS–R comprise readiness composite for screening	2:6–8	X	X	X	X	—	X	—	2002
Classroom Communication Screening Procedures for Early Adolescents: Simon	Follow oral and written directions; definitions, metalinguistics, synonyms, classroom focus	9–14	X	X	—	X	X	X	—	1987
Clinical Evaluation of Language Fundamentals–Preschool, (2nd ed.; CELF Pre–2): Wiig, Secord, & Semel	9 subtests, including phonological awareness and preliteracy scale; composite scores; colorful pictures	3–7	X	X	—	X	X	X	X	2004

(continues)

A/G = age/grade; R = receptive measure; E = expressive measure; Ph = phonology; M = morphology; Sx = syntax; Sm = semantics; Pr = pragmatics; L = literacy, e.g., phonological awareness, writing, reading, spelling; * = primarily a screening instrument *Continued.*

Instrument	Comments	A/G	R	E	Ph	M	Sx	Sm	Pr	L	Date
Clinical Evaluation of Language Fundamentals (4th ed.; CELF–4): Semel, Wiig, & Secord	Standard scores on each of 11 subtests plus receptive, expressive, total language and 5 other composite scores; phonological awareness subtest; scoring software available	5–21	X	X	—	X	X	X	X	X	2003
Clinical Evaluation of Language Fundamentals Screening Test (3rd ed.; CELF–3 Screening): Semel, Wiig, & Secord	Criterion scores on 4 or 6 subtests; includes storytelling and written skills	5–21	X	X	—	X	X	X	—	—	1996
Comprehensive Assessment of Spoken Language (CASL): Carrow-Woolfolk	21 subtests including inference, ambiguity, idioms; 2 age forms; composite scores	3–21	X	X	—	X	X	X	X	—	1999
Comprehensive Receptive and Expressive Vocabulary Test (2nd ed.; CREVT–2): Wallace & Hammill	10 color photos; series of increasingly difficult words (receptive); definitions (expressive); 2 forms	4–17	X	X	—	—	—	X	—	—	2002
Comprehensive Test of Phonological Processing (CTOPP): Wagner, Torgesen, & Rashotte (5–6 years)	7 core plus 1 supplemental subtests, for ages 5–6; measures many aspects of skills related to reading	5–6	X	X	X	—	—	—	—	X	1999
Comprehensive Test of Phonological Processing (CTOPP): Wagner, Torgesen, & Rashotte (7–24 years)	6 core plus 6 supplemental subtests, for ages 7–24; measures many aspects of skills related to reading	7–24	X	X	X	—	—	—	—	X	1999
Deep Test of Articulation: McDonald	To determine facilitation contexts; not for initial diagnosis; pictures or sentences	3–12	—	X	X	—	—	—	—	—	1968

Test / Author	Description	Age Range								Year
Diagnostic Evaluation of Language Variation–Criterion Referenced (DELV–Criterion Referenced): Seymour, Roeper, & deVilliers	Neutralizes effect of variations on mainstream American English to make accurate diagnosis of language deficits	4–9	X	X	X	X	X	X	—	2003
Diagnostic Evaluation of Language Variation–Norm-Referenced (DELV–Norm-Referenced): Seymour, Roeper, & deVilliers	Similar to criterion-referenced version, but provides scaled scores in syntax, pragmatics, semantics, and phonology	4–12	—	—	X	X	X	X	—	2005
Diagnostic Evaluation of Language Variation–Screening Test (DELV–Screening): Seymour, Roeper, & deVilliers	Criterion referenced; degree of language variation; degree of risk for language disorder	4–12	X	X	X	X	X	X	—	2003
Dynamic Assessment and Intervention: Miller, Gillam, & Pena	Features narrative dynamic assessment and mediated learning techniques	K–8	X	—	—	—	X	X	X	2001
Evaluating Acquired Skills in Communication–Revised (EASIC–R): Riley	Verbal, sign, and alternative and augmentative communication for severely impaired students	3 mo–8 yrs	X	X	X	X	X	X	—	1984
Evaluating Communicative Competence (Revised; ECC–R): Simon	Metalinguistic skills, functional use of receptive and expressive school language skills; criterion referenced; 21 areas	9–17	X	—	X	X	X	X	X	1994
Expressive One-Word Picture Vocabulary Test–2000 (EOWPVT–2000): Gardner	Measures single-word vocabulary; 100 items; includes category words	2–19	X	—	—	—	X	—	—	2000
Expressive Vocabulary Test (EVT): Williams	Measures single-word vocabulary; can be used with PPVT–3 to compare receptive and expressive vocabulary; requires synonyms	2:6–adult	X	—	—	X	X	—	—	1997
Fisher–Logemann Test of Articulation Competence: Fisher & Logemann	Word and sentence forms; dialect table; includes screening form; 35 plates	3–adult	X	X	—	—	—	—	—	1971

(continues)

A/G = age/grade; R = receptive measure; E = expressive measure; Ph = phonology; M = morphology; Sx = syntax; Sm = semantics; Pr = pragmatics; L = literacy, e.g., phonological awareness, writing, reading, spelling; * = primarily a screening instrument *Continued.*

Instrument	Comments	A/G	R	E	Ph	M	Sx	Sm	Pr	L	Date
*Fluharty Preschool Speech and Language Screening Test (2nd ed.): Fluharty	5 subtests; describes actions, sequences events	3–7	X	X	X	X	X	X	—	—	2000
Fullerton Language Test for Adolescents (2nd ed.; FLTA–2): Thorum	8 subtests including idioms, syllabification, auditory synthesis; discriminates between achieving and nonachieving students; remediation suggestions	11–adult	X	X	X	X	X	X	—	X	1986
Goldman–Fristoe Test of Articulation (2nd ed.; GFTA–2): Goldman & Fristoe	Uses single words, words in sentences; 35 color plates; stimulability subtest	2–16	—	X	X	—	—	—	—	—	2000
Gray Diagnostic Reading Tests (2nd ed.; GDRT–2): Bryant, Wiederholt, & Bryant	4 core subtests: letter/word identification, phonetic analysis, reading vocabulary, meaningful reading; 3 supplemental tests: listening, rapid naming, and phonological awareness	6–14	X	X	—	—	—	X	—	X	2004
Gray Oral Reading Tests (4th ed.; GORT–4): Wiederholt & Bryant	Provides fluency and comprehension scores: 14 developmentally sequenced passages	6–19	X	X	—	—	—	—	—	X	2001
Gray Silent Reading Test (GSRT): Wiederholt & Blalock	13 developmentally sequenced passages assess reading ability	7–25	X	X	—	—	—	—	—	X	2000
Illinois Test of Psycholinguistic Abilities (3rd ed.; ITPA–3): Hammill, Mather, & Roberts	An updated version of an original language diagnostic test battery; 12 subtests for oral and written language	5–13	X	X	X	X	X	X	—	X	2001

Test	Grade/Age								Year
*Joliet 3-Minute Speech and Language Screen–Revised: Kinzler & Cowing Johnson	Grades K, 2, 5	X	X	X	X	X	X	—	1992
Kahn–Lewis Phonological Analysis (2nd ed.; KLPA–2): Khan & Lewis	2:5–11	—	X	—	—	—	—	—	2002
Kaufman Speech Praxis Test for Children: Kaufman	2–6	X	X	—	X	X	—	—	1992
*Kindergarten Language Screening Test (2nd ed.; KLST–2): Gauthier & Madison	3:6–7	X	—	X	X	X	X	—	1998
Language Assessment Scales–Reading and Writing (LASR/W): Duncan & DeAvila	Grades 4–6 7–9	X	—	X	X	X	X	X	1994
Language Processing Test–Elementary (3rd ed.; LPT–3): Richard & Hanner	5–12	X	X	—	—	X	—	X	2005
Lindamood Auditory Conceptualization Test (3rd ed.; LAC–3): Lindamood & Lindamood	Pre-K to adult	X	X	X	—	—	—	X	2004
The Listening Test: Barrett, Huisingh, Zachman, LoGiudice, & Orman	6–12	X	X	—	—	X	X	—	1992
*Northwest Syntax Screening Test (NSST): Lee	3–8	X	—	X	X	X	X	—	1971

Comments:
- Joliet 3-Minute Speech and Language Screen–Revised: Used for kindergarten, 2nd, and 5th grades
- Kahn–Lewis Phonological Analysis: Use after completing GFTA–2 to identify 15 phonological processes
- Kaufman Speech Praxis Test for Children: Assesses developmental apraxia
- Kindergarten Language Screening Test: 5-minute test; typical school language tasks
- Language Assessment Scales–Reading and Writing: Measures reading and writing of students whose first language is not English; 2 forms for different grade levels
- Language Processing Test–Elementary: 6 subtests, all school related including similarities/differences, multiple meanings, categorization, attributes
- Lindamood Auditory Conceptualization Test: Measures ability to segment words into phonemic units by manipulating discs; requires practice to administer
- The Listening Test: 5 subtests related to school functions: main idea, details, reasoning, story comprehension
- Northwest Syntax Screening Test: Uses picture pointing and sentence repetition; can differentiate between receptive and expressive knowledge of structures

(continues)

A/G = age/grade; R = receptive measure; E = expressive measure; Ph = phonology; M = morphology; Sx = syntax; Sm = semantics; Pr = pragmatics; L = literacy, e.g., phonological awareness, writing, reading, spelling; * = primarily a screening instrument *Continued.*

Instrument	Comments	A/G	R	E	Ph	M	Sx	Sm	Pr	L	Date
Oral and Written Language Scales (OWLS): Carrow-Woolfolk	Measures student's ability to communicate orally and in writing	5–21	—	X	—	—	X	X	—	X	1996
Patterned Elicitation of Syntax Test–Revised with Morphophonemic Analysis (PEST–R): Young & Perachio	Delayed-imitation format used to identify structures listed in developmental order	3–7:6	—	X	—	X	X	—	—	—	1993
Peabody Picture Vocabulary Test– (3rd ed.; PPVT–III): Dunn & Dunn	Monotone pictures; 2 forms used to identify single-word vocabulary only	2:6–	X	—	—	—	—	X	—	—	1997
**Phonemic-Awareness Skills Screening* (PASS): Crumrine & Lonegan	15-minute test identifies weaknesses in 8 areas of phonological awareness	Grades 1 & 2	X	X	X	—	—	—	—	X	2000
Phonological Awareness Test: Robertson & Salter	Measures discrimination and identification of graphemes, decoding, segmentation, deletion, substitution, blending	5–9	X	X	X	—	—	—	—	X	1997
**Phonological Awareness Literacy Screening* (PALS) http://www.pals.virginia/edu/PALS-InstrumentalPALS-k.asp	Subtests measure phonological awareness, alphabet & sound recognition, concept of words, knowledge of letter sounds and spelling	Grade K	X	X	X	—	—	—	—	X	2004
Photo Articulation Test (3rd ed.; PAT–3): Lippke, Dickey, Selmar, & Soder	Uses color photographs	3–12	—	X	X	—	—	X	—	—	1997
Preschool Language Assessment Instrument (2nd ed.; PLAI–2): Blank, Rose, & Berlin	Based on discourse model; designed for school language demands; 60 questions	3–6	—	X	X	—	—	X	—	—	2003

Test	Description	Age									Year
Preschool Language Scale (4th ed.; PLS–4): Zimmerman, Steiner, & Pond	Concepts, cloze, sentence repetition; includes articulation screen, language sample checklist, phonological awareness, family interview; provides receptive, expressive, and total language scores	Birth–7	X	X	X	X	X	X	X	X	2002
Receptive One-Word Picture Vocabulary Test–2000 (ROWPVT–2000): Gardner & Brownell	Single-word vocabulary; color plates; use with EOWPVT–2000 for comparison of single-word receptive and expressive vocabulary	2–19	X	—	—	—	X	—	—	—	2000
Speech and Language Evaluation Scale: Fressola & Hoerchler	Uses teacher rating scales; includes fluency and voice	Adoles. 4.5–18	X	X	X	—	—	—	X	X	1989
Speech-Ease Screening Inventory	Covers most linguistic areas plus articulation and auditory recall	K–1	X	X	X	X	X	X	—	—	1985
Spelling Performance Evaluation for Language and Literacy (SPELL): Masterson, Apel, & Wasowicz	Software; analysis of spelling	3–6	—	X	—	—	—	—	—	X	2002
STIM-CON: Prognostic Inventory for Misarticulating Kindergarten and First Grade Children: Sommers	Identifies students whose articulation is not likely to improve without intervention	K–1	—	X	—	—	—	—	—	—	1987
Structured Photographic Expressive Language Test–Preschool (2nd ed.; SPELT–P2): Dawson, Stout, Eyer, Tattersall, Fonkalsrud, & Crowley	Earlier developing morphemes and syntax; color photos; cloze procedure; use for eliciting forms	3–6	—	X	—	—	—	—	—	X	1983
Structured Photographic Expressive Language Test (3rd ed.; SPELT–3): Dawson & Stout	Analyzes specific morphemes and syntactic structures; color photos; cloze procedure; has AAE scoring guide	4–10	—	X	—	—	—	—	—	X	2003

(continues)

A/G = age/grade; R = receptive measure; E = expressive measure; Ph = phonology; M = morphology; Sx = syntax; Sm = semantics; Pr = pragmatics; L = literacy, e.g., phonological awareness, writing, reading, spelling; * = primarily a screening instrument *Continued.*

Instrument	Comments	A/G	R	E	Ph	M	Sx	Sm	Pr	L	Date
Templin–Darley Tests of Articulation: Templin & Darley	Contains Iowa Pressure Articulation Test, which assesses velopharyngeal closure	3–8	—	X	X	—	—	—	—	—	1969
Test for Auditory Comprehension of Language (3rd ed.; TACL–3): Carrow-Woolfolk	3 subtests: semantics, syntax, and morphology; can be used with older students to identify lack of comprehension of embedded structures	3–11	—	X	—	X	X	—	—	—	1999
Test for Examining Expressive Morphology (TEEM): Shipley, Stone, & Sue	Cloze format; score sheet separates irregular forms	3–8	—	X	—	X	X	X	—	—	1983
Test of Adolescent and Adult Language (3rd ed.; TOAL–3): Hammill, Brown, Larsen, & Wiederholt	Includes 10 areas including reading, writing, and oral language; scoring software available	12–25	X	X	—	X	X	X	—	X	1994
Test of Auditory Processing Skills (3rd ed.; TAPS–3): Martin & Brownell	6 subtests of auditory memory: auditory discrimination, reasoning	4–19	X	X	—	—	X	X	—	X	2005
Test of Auditory Perceptual Skills– Upper Level (TAPS–UL): Gardner	Short test for older students	12–18	X	X	—	—	X	X	—	X	1994
Test of Early Language Development (3rd ed.; TELD–3): Hresko, Reid, & Hammill	2 subtests (receptive and expressive language); measures syntax and semantics	2–8	X	X	—	X	X	X	—	—	1999
Test of Early Reading Ability (3rd ed.; TERA–3): Reid, Hresko, & Hammill	Measures mastery of reading skills; alphabet; conventions of print; meaning	3:6–8:6	X	X	—	—	—	—	—	X	2001

Test	Description	Ages							Date
Test of Early Written Language (2nd ed.; TEWL–2): Hresko, Herron, & Peak	Extends TOWL–3 downward; story in the writing area: students construct using picture prompts; 2 forms	3–11	X	X	X	—	X	X	1996
Test of Language Competence–Expanded Edition (TLC–Expanded): Wiig & Secord	Addresses higher-level language and metalinguistic functions; includes ambiguity, memory; figurative language; making inferences; 2 age-level test batteries; screening composite	5–9 & 10–18	X	X	X	X	X	X	1989
Test of Language Development–Intermediate (3rd ed.; TOLD–I:3): Hammill & Newcomer	6 subtests plus composite scores; includes malapropisms and abstract relationships	8:6–11:6	—	X	X	—	X	X	1997a
Test of Language Development–Primary (3rd ed.; TOLD–P:3): Newcomer & Hammill	9 subtests plus composite scores; includes word discrimination and phonemic analysis	4–9	X	X	X	—	X	X	1997b
Test of Minimal Articulation Competence (TMAC): Secord	Gives developmental articulation index; includes quick screening	3–adult	—	—	—	—	X	X	1981
Test of Phonological Awareness (2nd ed.: PLUS; TOPA–2+): Torgesen & Bryant	Norm referenced; identifies students at risk for phonologically based reading problems; can be administered individually or in groups; 2 versions: kindergarten and early elementary	5–8	X	—	—	—	X	X	2004
Test of Phonological Awareness Skills (TOPAS): Newcomer & Barenbaum	Segmentation, blending, sound comparisons	5–10	—	—	—	—	X	X	2003
Test of Pragmatic Language (TOPL): Phelps-Terasaki & Phelps-Gunn	6 subtests including setting and topic maintenance	5–14	X	X	X	—	X	X	1992

(continues)

A/G = age/grade; R = receptive measure; E = expressive measure; Ph = phonology; M = morphology; Sx = syntax; Sm = semantics; Pr = pragmatics; L = literacy, e.g., phonological awareness, writing, reading, spelling; * = primarily a screening instrument *Continued.*

Instrument	Comments	A/G	R	E	Ph	M	Sx	Sm	Pr	L	Date
Test of Problem Solving–Adolescent (TOPS–Adolescent): Bowers, Barrett, Huisingh, Orman, & LoGiudice	6 areas of aspects of critical thinking present in verbal and written forms; can also be used to assess pragmatics informally (fair mindedness, affect, clarifying)	12–17	—	X	—	—	—	—	X	—	1991
Test of Problem Solving Elementary (3rd ed.; TOPS–3: Elementary): Huisingh, Bowers, & LoGiudice	6 subtests of aspects of critical thinking; can be used to assess pragmatics informally (empathizing, drawing inferences, using context)	6–12	—	X	—	—	—	—	X	—	2005
Test of Reading Comprehension (3rd ed.; TORC–3): Brown, Hammill, & Wiederholt	Holistic; cognitive and linguistic aspects of reading; 8 subtests include syntactic, semantic, and sequencing; measures math, social studies, and science vocabulary and reading directions	5–10	X	X	—	X	X	X	—	X	1995
Test of Semantic Skills–Primary (TOSS–P): Bowers, Huisingh, LoGiudice, & Orman	Identify and name items in a pictured scene; vocabulary centered on themes and includes categories, attributes, labels, functions, and definitions	4–8	X	X	—	—	—	X	—	—	2002
Test of Semantic Skills–Intermediate (TOSS–I): Huisingh, Bowers, LoGiudice, & Orman	Upper-level extension of the TOSS–P	9–13	X	X	—	—	—	X	—	—	2004
Test of Word Finding (2nd ed.; TWF–2): German	Diagnoses word-finding deficits using 4 naming sections; use with LD and TBI; difficult to administer without practice	4–13	—	X	—	—	—	X	—	—	2000

Test	Description	Age/Grade Range									Year
Test of Adolescent/Adult Word Finding (TAWF): German	5 naming sections; administer individually	12–80	—	X	—	—	—	X	—	—	1990
Test of Word Finding in Discourse (TWFD): German	Extends naming to longer passages	6:6–13	—	X	—	—	—	X	—	—	1991
Test of Word Knowledge: Wiig & Semel	2 age levels, each with core battery; definitions, synonyms, multiple meanings, conjunctions, figurative language, transition words	5–18	—	X	—	—	—	X	—	—	1992
Test of Word Reading Efficiency (TOWRE): Torgesen, Wagner, & Rashotte	Measures sight word efficiency and phonetic decoding efficiency; provides normative data	6–25	X	X	—	—	—	X	—	X	1999
Test of Written Expression (TOWE): McGhee, Bryant, Larsen, & Rivera	Assesses writing achievement	6:6–15	—	X	—	X	X	X	—	X	1995
Test of Written Language (3rd ed.; TOWL–3): Hammill, Larsen, & Wiederholt	Administer in small group or individually; essay and multiple-answer formats; 2 forms	Grades 2–12	—	X	—	X	X	X	—	X	1996
Test of Written Spelling (4th ed.; TWS–4): Larsen, Hammill, & Moats	Uses dictated word format; identifies students below grade level and demonstrates progress; 2 forms	Grades 1–12	—	X	—	—	—	—	—	X	1999
Token Test for Children (TTFC): DiSimoni	Measures auditory comprehension of spatial and temporal concepts; student manipulates colored circles and squares; takes practice to administer	3–12	X	—	—	—	—	X	—	X	1978
Weiss Comprehensive Articulation Test (WCAT): Weiss	82 pictures; stimuability test; speech sample elicitation pictures; blends; phonemes listed by frequency of occurrence	3–7	X	X	—	—	—	—	—	—	1980

(continues)

A/G = age/grade; R = receptive measure; E = expressive measure; Ph = phonology; M = morphology; Sx = syntax; Sm = semantics; Pr = pragmatics; L = literacy, e.g., phonological awareness, writing, reading, spelling; * = primarily a screening instrument *Continued.*

Instrument	Comments	A/G	R	E	Ph	M	Sx	Sm	Pr	L	Date
The Word Test–Adolescent (2nd ed.): Bowers, Huisingh, LoGiudice, & Orman	Definitions; synonyms; antonyms; associations; absurdities; multiple-meaning words	12–18	X	X	—	—	—	X	—	—	2005
The Word Test–Elementary (2nd ed.): Bowers, Huisingh, LoGiudice, & Orman	Critical semantic features: associations; synonyms; antonyms, absurdities, multiple-meaning words, definitions	6–12	X	X	—	—	—	X	—	—	2004
The Writing Process Test (WPT): Warden & Hutchinson	Evaluates writing and critical thinking; provides normative data	8–19	X	X	—	—	—	X	—	X	1992

Appendix 3.B

◆ ◆

Referral Form for Elementary Through Middle School Students

Name of student: _____

Name of person referring: _____

Course/grade: _____ Date: _____

How long have you had a concern? _____

Please mark any item below if it is of concern (+) or serious concern (++).

Articulation

- ☐ overall pronunciation hard to understand
- ☐ some sounds missing or in errror
- ☐ confuses sounds when sounding out words
- ☐ confuses sounds when spelling

Meaning of words, sentences, and longer segments

- ☐ has difficulty learning new vocabulary in curriculum
- ☐ has restricted "everyday" vocabulary
- ☐ sometimes seems to "search" for words when talking
- ☐ sometimes uses a "sound alike" or related word instead of one he/she wants
- ☐ overuses particular words, e.g., *thing, gross*
- ☐ has problems understanding more than one meaning of a multiple-meaning word
- ☐ can't identify the topic sentence in a paragraph
- ☐ can't identify the organization of a chapter, e.g., cause/effect, sequenced
- ☐ has problems with referents, e.g., pronouns
- ☐ appears confused by temporal or spatial words
- ☐ often just doesn't seem to make sense when speaking or writing
- ☐ often requires many repetitions of directions
- ☐ has more difficulty when the material is lengthy or in a different form

Grammatical form

- ☐ leaves off endings of words (walk*ed*) or entire words (he _____ walking)
- ☐ uses mostly short, simple sentences in speech or written work
- ☐ uses very simple noun and verb phrases
- ☐ appears confused by sentences containing one or more dependent clauses, e.g., "You may use the computer if you have finished your math, your lab report has been handed in, and you have returned your books to the library."
- ☐ sometimes confuses word order when asking questions or making statements
- ☐ has problems with irregular forms, e.g., *swam, mice, has*
- ☐ uses incorrect verb tenses in speaking or writing

- [ ] doesn't appear to understand meaning of tense differences such as passive or using multiple auxiliaries, e.g., *would have been* gone
- [ ] doesn't recognize grammatical errors even when pointed out
- [ ] overall, sentences sound like a younger child's

Social uses of language

- [ ] is often confused about the routines of the classroom
- [ ] doesn't properly initiate or end conversation with peers
- [ ] doesn't maintain the topic of conversation
- [ ] makes comments that are not organized; connection is difficult to understand
- [ ] stories/explanations often have no point or are disorganized
- [ ] persists in one topic of conversation when others want a change
- [ ] doesn't understand implied meaning
- [ ] frequently seems lost during conversation with peers or adults
- [ ] is socially inappropriate
- [ ] appears younger than he/she is
- [ ] doesn't play by the rules

Voice

- [ ] voice often sounds hoarse or rough
- [ ] often speaks too loudly
- [ ] often speaks too softly

Fluency

- [ ] often repeats sounds, syllables, or words when speaking
- [ ] hesitates before beginning to talk, sometimes looking distressed
- [ ] blinks, jerks shoulders, moves head before beginning to talk
- [ ] avoids circumstances in which he/she is expected to speak

Organization

- [ ] experiences problems planning a sequence of activities required to complete a task
- [ ] desk, cubby, backpack possessions are frequently missing or mislaid
- [ ] does not recognize organizational patterns of oral or written material
- [ ] does not self-monitor

General Comments: Briefly note in what areas of curriculum or instruction your concern is greatest. If you have used any modifications or other remediation with the student, note them and indicate if they seemed to help or not. Any information you can provide will be of help.

Appendix 3.C

Referral Form for Middle School Through High School Students

Name of student: _____

Name of person referring: _____

Course/grade: _____ Date: _____

How long have you had a concern? _____

Please mark any item below if deficits in the area are of concern (+) or serious concern (++).

Reading

The student usually:

☐ gains information from independent reading assignments.

☐ studies for examinations effectively.

☐ picks out the main idea in paragraphs, chapters, etc.

☐ follows written directions without asking for clarification.

☐ independently accesses information from Web sites, dictionaries, encyclopedias, and other reference material.

☐ follows the sequence inherent in written material without difficulty.

Writing

In written work, the student usually:

☐ does not ramble.

☐ is unambiguous.

☐ displays appropriate tone.

☐ displays adequate handwriting skills.

☐ displays adequate spelling skills.

☐ uses correct punctuation and capitalization.

☐ takes adequate notes.

☐ completes take-home assignments that:

  ☐ contain descriptions of acceptable quality.

  ☐ contain explanations of acceptable quality.

  ☐ contain essay questions of acceptable quality.

☐ completes a protracted assignment, e.g., a term paper, acceptably.

☐ uses correct sequencing or other patterns.

☐ applies adequate editing skills.

In a test situation, the student:

☐ produces short-answer questions with adequate written support.

☐ writes essay questions in an acceptable manner.

☐ displays skills in logic (argumentation).

☐ uses age- and grade-appropriate grammatic complexity.

Speaking

The student usually:

- ☐ speaks with no articulation errors.
- ☐ speaks fluently.
- ☐ uses correct grammar.
- ☐ uses age- and grade-appropriate complexity.
- ☐ discusses everyday topics with adequate skill.
- ☐ discusses abstract "school" topics with adequate skill.
- ☐ organizes thoughts adequately when speaking.
- ☐ displays adequate vocabulary, including homonyms and multiple-meaning words.
- ☐ makes sense.
- ☐ uses slang appropriately, does not use dated or overused expressions.
- ☐ keeps to the point, doesn't ramble.
- ☐ does not "search" for words.
- ☐ is not redundant.
- ☐ uses specific vocabulary (doesn't overuse words like *thing, whatchamacallit, you know*).

Pragmatics

The student usually:

- ☐ asks clarifying questions.
- ☐ uses humor appropriately (gets jokes, tells jokes appropriately, can use sarcasm, can kid).
- ☐ understands and uses classroom routines.
- ☐ understands implied meaning.
- ☐ uses these conversational skills appropriately:
  - ☐ initiates.
  - ☐ maintains topic.
  - ☐ does not interrupt.
  - ☐ within cultural guidelines, maintains appropriate eye contact.
  - ☐ answers questions.
  - ☐ appears to follow conversation among members of a group of four or five people.
  - ☐ can switch code between peers and adults in authority.
  - ☐ does not perseverate on a topic when conversational partner wishes to move on.
  - ☐ ends conversation appropriately.
  - ☐ uses polite forms.

☐ is tactful.

☐ reads nonverbal language accurately.

☐ can express opinions clearly.

☐ can accept another's opinion without anger.

☐ can work as part of a small group.

☐ can role-play.

☐ can play a game appropriately, following the rules of play.

Organization

The student usually:

☐ works independently in the classroom.

☐ completes homework.

☐ completes in-class assignments.

☐ takes notes that are sequenced correctly.

☐ takes notes that reflect the organizational pattern of lecture or written material.

☐ plans ahead for material or information needed to complete tasks.

☐ organizes materials in desk, locker, notebooks, and carrier (backpack).

☐ self-monitors task focus and use of appropriate strategies during extended tasks.

Listening

The student usually:

☐ follows simple oral directions the first time.

☐ follows complex oral directions the first time.

☐ follows the organizational pattern of a lecture.

☐ understands idioms, proverbs, and analogies when presented in context.

☐ gives some indication that he/she has followed part of the presentation when asking questions.

☐ can follow orally presented information contained in:

☐ films, videotape, and CD-ROM.

☐ lectures without visual material.

☐ in-class reports by peers.

☐ answers questions based on just-presented information.

☐ distinguishes between inflectional differences that alter meaning.

☐ recalls and repeats events of an orally presented story accurately.

Metalinguistics

The student usually:

☐ applies rules of pronunciation to unknown words.

☐ understands and applies prefixes and suffixes to root words.

☐ recognizes and defines parts of speech at a grade-appropriate level.

☐ understands and applies editing rules.

General comments: Briefly note in what areas of your curriculum or instruction your concern is greatest. If you have used any modifications or other remediation with the student, note them and indicate if they seemed to help or not. Any information you can provide will be of help.

Appendix 3.D

Student Observation

Student: _____ Teacher: _____

Grade/subject: _____

Date of observation: _____ Time: From _____ to _____

Number of students in class: _____

If any of the areas below are not applicable, mark a slash through the number.

1. *Position* of student in classroom:

   front ☐ back ☐ middle ☐ side ☐ circle ☐

2. Type of *activity*:

   whole-class lecture ☐ small-group lecture ☐ cooperative learning ☐

   conversational ☐ narrative ☐ students working independently ☐

   Other: _____

3. *Material read* by student:

   none ☐ text ☐ worksheet ☐ study sheet ☐ test ☐ on chalk board ☐

   Other: _____

   Student read: aloud ☐ silently ☐

4. Student followed written *directions*:

   yes ☐ no ☐ some ☐

   Comments: _____

   _____

   _____

   _____

5. *Material written* by student:

   short-answer ☐ essay ☐ copying ☐ note taking ☐

   Result was: acceptable ☐ not acceptable ☐

   Comments: _____

   _____

   _____

   _____

6. Student *attended* (listened):

   most of time ☐ part of time ☐ rarely ☐ couldn't tell ☐

7. Student followed orally presented *directions*:

   yes ☐ no ☐ some ☐

   Comments: _____

   _____

   _____

8. Student was *on task* (completed requirements, persistent):

   most of time ☐ part of time ☐ rarely ☐

   Comments: _____

   _____

   _____

9. Student *distracted other classmates:* yes ☐ no ☐

10. Student *asked questions:*

    yes ☐: clarifying ☐ asked for new information ☐

    few ☐ none ☐

11. Student *responded* appropriately to teacher *questions on material*:

    yes ☐ no ☐ part of time ☐

    Result: short sentences ☐ complex sentences ☐

    sequenced correctly: yes ☐ no ☐

    vocabulary: poor ☐ rich ☐ marginal ☐

    pragmatics acceptable: yes ☐ no ☐

    reasoning ability appeared acceptable: yes ☐ no ☐

12. Number of times student was *called on* _____ *volunteered* answer or info: _____

13. In *conversation,* student:

    initiated ☐ took turns ☐ was polite ☐ completed (did not end abruptly) ☐

    maintained topic ☐ perseverated on topic ☐

    appeared confused ☐ was confrontational or antagonistic ☐

14. Student *appeared aware of classroom routine*:

    yes ☐ no ☐ part of time ☐

    Comments: _____

    _____

    _____

15. Student's *reaction to transitions* was:

    confused ☐   smooth ☐   disorganized ☐

    Student looked to other students for help ☐

    Comments: _____

    _____

    _____

16. *Modifications present* included:

    list on board or at desk ☐   restated information ☐

    simplified syntax ☐   vocabulary or concepts retaught ☐

    modified worksheet or test ☐   restatements ☐   peer help ☐

    Distractions were reduced: visual ☐   auditory ☐

    Directions were simplified ☐

    Teacher: moved around classroom ☐

    expanded wait time ☐   gave verbal prompts ☐   modeled ☐

    gave visual prompts ☐   used mnemonic devices ☐   gave feedback ☐

17. Comments, questions, hypotheses, suggestions for follow-up:

    _____

    _____

    _____

    _____

Appendix 3.E

◆ ◆

Quick Oral Peripheral Examination

Name: _____ Date of birth: _____

Age: _____ Grade: _____ Date: _____

Examiner: _____ Reason for exam: _____

I. *Oral Cavity and Dental Structures*

    A. Occlusion of anterior teeth

        Normal ☐   Overbite ☐   Underbite ☐   Open bite ☐

    B. Alignment with dental arch

        Normal ☐   Misaligned ☐   Jumbled ☐   Spacing abnormal ☐

    C. Height and confirmation of hard palate

        Normal ☐   Unusually narrow ☐   Unusually high ☐   Flat ☐

        Palatal vault ☐

        Other _____

    D. Soft palate

        Normal ☐   Large & bulged ☐

        Other _____

        Abnormal tonsils ☐   Narrow faucial isthmus ☐

    E. Tongue

        Normal ☐   Abnormally large ☐   Short ☐

        Other _____

II. *Function of Oral Structures*

	Easy	Hard	Can't Do
A. Touch hard palate with tongue tip	☐	☐	☐
B. Bulge back of tongue to touch soft palate	☐	☐	☐
C. Thrust tongue	☐	☐	☐
D. Point tongue	☐	☐	☐
E. Groove tongue	☐	☐	☐
F. Control tongue generally	☐	☐	☐
G. Smack lips together	☐	☐	☐
H. Pucker lips	☐	☐	☐

I. Lick lips in continuous circle ☐ ☐ ☐

J. Pucker and smile alternately ☐ ☐ ☐

K. Clear throat ☐ ☐ ☐

L. Push cheek out with tongue: left & right sides ☐ ☐ ☐

M. Smile ☐ ☐ ☐

N. Tongue pulls to one side when speaking? Yes ☐ No ☐

O. Drooling? Yes ☐ No ☐

P. Open mouth posture at rest? Yes ☐ No ☐

III. *Frenum*

	Easy	Hard	Can't Do
Touch alveolar ridge with tongue tip	☐	☐	☐

IV. *Uvula*

Normal ☐ Bifid ☐

V. *Velopharyngeal Closure*

A. Prolong vowel (ah): Normal ☐ Abnormal ☐

B. Short repeated (ah): Normal ☐ Abnormal ☐

C. Gag reflex: Normal ☐ Hypersensitive ☐ Hyposensitive ☐

D. Nasality: Normal ☐ Hypernasal ☐ Hyponasal ☐

VI. *Diadochokinetic Rate:*

Normal ☐ Abnormal ☐

Comments: _____

Appendix 3.F

◆ ◆ ◆ ◆ ◆ ◆ ◆ ◆ ◆ ◆ ◆ ◆ ◆ ◆ ◆ ◆ ◆ ◆ ◆ ◆

Some Common Classroom Behaviors Resulting From Possible Language Deficits

PHONOLOGY

Student may:

- take longer than "typical" classmates to recognize that language is a code, that the code is print, and that individual sounds correspond to the smallest segments.
- have poor spelling skills, even of phonetically regular spelling words.
- confuse vowel sounds, particularly short vowels, e.g., *tin* vs. *ten*.
- have weak decoding skills in reading.
- have difficulty creating or hearing rhyme.
- not be able to identify how many syllables are in a word (clap three times for butterfly, twice for butter).
- have poor skills in sound manipulation (metaphonology), e.g., sound blending or phoneme segmentation (e.g., *t* + *ap* = *tap*; *sink* − *s* = *ink*).
- have difficulty organizing, storing, and retrieving words from memory on the basis of their phonological properties.
- have a history of a phonological disorder as a preschooler.
- in connected speech, may omit sounds or syllables in words, substitute one sound for another, or insert an extra sound.
- have difficulty imitating speech sounds, particularly in multisyllabic words or difficult phrases, e.g., "Fly free in the Air Force."

MORPHOLOGY

Student may:

- experience difficulties with irregular verb forms, e.g., *swung*.
- use incorrect verb tenses in speaking and writing.
- leave out words, e.g., "He going."
- use plurality incorrectly, particularly irregular forms.
- have problems perceiving and discriminating among various pronunciations of the plural morpheme, e.g., *cats, dogs, glasses.*
- make errors in article use.
- have difficulty with changes in spelling of irregular forms that persists into adulthood.
- have difficulty understanding and using affixes.
- have persistent problems with comparative and superlative forms.
- have persistent difficulty in spelling and pronunciation changes dictated by derivational affixes, e.g., *medicine, medical, medicinal.*

SYNTAX

Student may:

- have receptive or expressive syntactic deficits.
- use few sentence complexities (clauses or multiple verbs), instead using short, syntactically simple sentences, usually subject–verb–object.
- not elaborate noun or verb phrases beyond a simple level.
- have particular difficulty interpreting relative and adverbial clauses, e.g., those containing *if, before,* etc., after age 7 or 8.
- not use correct subject–verb agreement, e.g., "They is going."
- use incorrect pronoun forms, e.g., substituting an object pronoun for a subject pronoun, e.g., "Him and me are friends."
- confuse word order, particularly in questions.
- habitually use incomplete sentences when writing.
- have problems in perceiving, acquiring, and recalling the rules for modals and auxiliaries (e.g., *must, will, should, could, have, had,* etc.)
- confuse WH words.
- have persistent problems understanding and using the passive.
- sequence adjective strings incorrectly, e.g., "a green, big ball."
- have problems using negatives correctly.
- have difficulty understanding the relationship between direct and indirect objects.
- not understand subtle differences in tense meaning, e.g., the difference between "I study all the time," "I studied all the time," and "I will study all the time."
- repeat a grammatically correct sentence incorrectly.
- not identify as incorrect an utterance with a syntactic error.
- use poorer grammar in writing than in speaking.

Metalinguistic skills are particularly weak in this area of language, even if the student's spontaneous production appears the same as normally achieving children, e.g., student may:

- have difficulty in structured tasks requiring syntactic manipulation, such as changing a statement to a question, using a given word in a sentence, completing a sentence like, "I will go tomorrow because…"
- experience difficulty with syntactic compression, e.g., putting two statements together, such as taking "The baby fell" and "The baby cried" and combining them to make "The baby that fell cried."
- rarely use low-frequency syntactic structures such as appositives (e.g., "the woman, *a teacher at our middle school,* won a prize"), elaborated subjects, postmodification using prepositional phrases, nonfinite verbs, the perfect, and the passive (see examples in Table 3.1).

- rarely if ever use *clefting*—that is, focusing attention on a particular element of a sentence for emphasis, e.g., "Before the lecture was half over, she was bored to death" vs. the more direct "She was bored to death before the lecture was half over."

SEMANTICS

Deficits occur receptively or expressively or both. Students may:

- have a limited vocabulary.
- overuse certain words, e.g., *cool, dumb, stuff, thing.*
- have difficulty understanding and using synonyms, antonyms, and homonyms—for example, will give a word that has a similar meaning when asked for an opposite.
- not use context to differentiate meaning, e.g., *die* or *dye.*
- overuse one meaning of multiple-meaning words.
- not understand analogies.
- have problems interpreting figurative language, including common idiomatic expressions, proverbs, slang, metaphors, and similes.
- confuse WH words (e.g., when asked when he/she eats lunch may respond, "In the lunch room").
- experience difficulty understanding complex sentences, because he/she does not understand the meaning of clausal connectors, e.g., *since, nor, if.*
- have problems with reference, particularly pronouns.
- experience difficulty with abstractions, e.g., words like *democracy,* and struggle with time relationships, particularly those with shifting references, e.g., the day before yesterday, a week from Friday.
- have difficulty with spatial and temporal concepts, e.g., *on* vs. *in* (younger students) or *in time* vs. *on time* (older students).
- substitute inaccurate words, e.g., *lemon* for *orange.*
- offer limited information in verbal reports.
- exhibit symptoms of word finding problems: may ramble.
- use inexact, ambiguous, and nonspecific words; appear disorganized and hesitant; use repetitions, disjointed phrases, circumlocutions, and fillers, which may be rooted in a faulty semantic reference system.
- have inadequate understanding of relational meanings beyond single word signification, e.g., understanding either intrasentential or intersentential connectives.
- use narratives that lack a clear sequence, sufficient detail, or internal cohesion.
- experience problems with expository discourse: explanations lack clarity, uses an inappropriate form to explain concepts (semantic maps).

PRAGMATICS

Student may:

- have difficulty understanding implied messages, e.g., doesn't recognize what the teacher wants when he/she says, "This room is noisy."
- not get jokes.
- have problems understanding the need for or asking for assistance or clarification.
- have difficulty with ritualistic greetings and farewells, e.g., starts a conversation without saying hello, walks away without closing conversation.
- have problems with topic initiation and maintenance, often changing the subject or perseverating on a topic the listener wishes terminated.
- have difficulty concentrating on conversations among peers and adults.
- not alter presentation according to his/her knowledge of and relationship to listeners, e.g., their age, familiarity, social status, or sex.
- display disorganized content within or among utterances.
- express socially inappropriate emotional reactions.
- have limited interpersonal relationships.
- be inappropriately loud or passive in classroom situations.
- maintain poor eye contact that is not culturally based.
- have difficulty with implied cause-and-effect relationships.
- appear immature or silly.
- have difficulty adhering to classroom etiquette, e.g., interrupting another student to answer, shouting out an answer, answering in a disrespectful manner to teachers and administrators without any awareness.
- cheat or lie to cover up incomplete or undone class work.
- misread a speaker's signals, verbal or nonverbal, that are part of the message.
- use conflicting verbal and nonverbal messages.
- not repair communicative breakdowns.
- not honor correct turn-taking behavior either conversationally or otherwise.
- not provide the listener with necessary information.

EXECUTIVE FUNCTION

Student may:

- have difficulty working independently in the classroom.
- fail to complete homework on a regular basis.
- often leave in-class assignments incomplete.
- create notes that are sequenced incorrectly.

- take notes that do not reflect the organizational pattern of a lecture or written material.
- appear to rarely plan ahead for material or information needed to complete tasks.
- fail to organize materials in desk, locker, notebooks, and carrier (backpack).
- rarely self-monitor task focus or use appropriate strategies during extended tasks.

Appendix 3.G

Report of Speech–Language Evaluation: Short Form

Identifying Information:

Name:	Zachary Johnson	**Date of birth:**	8/28/97
Age:	6-6	**School:**	Smallville Elementary School
Address:	24 Winget Road Anywhere, Illinois	**Grade/teacher:**	First, Ms. Cato
Parents:	Susan & Samuel Johnson	**Date of speech– language evaluation:**	3/28/04–4/2/04

Background Information:

Zachary, age 6-6, was referred for a core evaluation on February 1, 2004, on the basis of academic problems reported by Ms. Cato involving the language arts curriculum, particularly reading and spelling. Both she and Ms. Warren, his kindergarten teacher, cite deficits in articulation, formation of some grammatical endings, and the lack of age- and grade-appropriate sound–symbol relationships, which are negatively affecting his learning to read and spell. Ms. Ruiz, the school's Title I teacher, notes weaknesses in Zachary's decoding skills. No prior speech–language evaluations took place before the one completed on February 25, 2004.

Zachary's developmental and medical history are unremarkable except for recurring otitis media until 2½ and surgical removal of his adenoids; he has passed two recent hearing screenings. His mother reports that he attends for long periods when building with Legos but becomes "antsy" and frustrated when she attempts reading activities with him. She states that she is concerned because there is a history of reading problems on her husband's side of the family. This examiner's observation of Zachary during reading instruction and a language arts activity confirmed Ms. Cato's description. Zachary attended well but could not sound out words that had just been taught. His story sequencing ability (narrative discourse) was adequate, featuring acceptable sequencing and good vocabulary, but his morphology and syntax during the story retelling contained age-inappropriate errors. He used picture cues and teacher "hints" effectively. He stated in a conversation that he likes school but is worried "because he can't read as well as the other kids." On the basis of these observations and the reading specialist, Ms. Ruiz's report noting sound–symbol deficiencies, the following standardized and nonstandardized procedures were chosen to assess possible deficits in word structure, articulation, and phonological awareness and memory to determine the presence or absence of a disorder. Results are listed below.

Interpretation of Standardized Measures:
- Average standard scores (based on 10) fall between 7 and 10; a moderately low score falls between 4 and 7, and an extremely low score is below 4.

- Average percentile ranks are between 16 and 84; a moderately low score falls between 5 and 15, and an extremely low score is below 5.

Instrument	Subtest	Standard Score
CELF Preschool–2	Concepts & Following Directions	9
	Basic Concepts	12
	Sentence Structure	8
	Recalling Sentences	4
	Expressive Vocabulary	9
	Word Structure	7
	Word Classes–Receptive	10
	Total	9
	Core Language Score	88
	Receptive Language Index	93
	Expressive Language Index	81
	Language Content Index	93
	Language Structure Index	79
PPVT–3*		111
		Age equivalent: 6-0
		Stanine: 4*
		*(Administered by E. Grimly, School Psychologist)
EOWPVT–R		92
		Age equivalent: 5-9
		Stanine: 4
SPELT–II		% correct: 76 —
Goldman–Fristoe–2		11th percentile
		17 errors
	Stimuability	35th percentile
Phonological Awareness Test		scores based on a mean of 100 numbers refer to standard

Note: Total subtest scores are not reported when any subtest score was zero.

	Rhyme	Total score 61
		Discrimination 65
		Production 66
	Segmentation	Total score could not be calculated
		Sentences 105
		Syllables 107
		Phonemes 0
	Isolation	Total score could not be calculated
		Initial 94
		Final 69
		Medial (zero score)
	Deletion	Total score 75
		Compounds/syllables 78
		Phonemes 77
	Substitution	Total score could not be calculated
		With manipulatives 0
		Without manipulatives 0
	Blending	Total score 71
		Syllables 78
		Phonemes 74

Graphemes	Total score could not be calculated
	Consonants 84
	Long/short vowels, consonant blends and digraphs, R-controlled vowels, vowel digraphs, diphthongs: all 0 scores
Decoding	Total score could not be calculated
	VC words 101
	CVC words 87
	Consonant digraphs, consonant blends, vowel digraphs, R-controlled vowels, CVC words, diphthongs: all 0 scores

Comprehensive Test of Phonological Processing (CTOPP) (ages 5 & 6)

Note: Only subtests evaluating phonological memory were administered.

Memory for digits	Standard score of 7 (mean of 10)
Nonword repetition	Standard score of 6 (mean of 10)
	Phonological memory composite score 79 (mean of 100)

Interpretation of Results

Articulation: Errors of individual phonemes were confined to gliding, distortion, and vocalization of /r/ and /l/, with fewer errors in single words than in words in sentences. The misarticulations in the GFTA–2 were also confirmed in Zachary's connected speech; as a time-saving measure, the language sample also served as a speech sample. Because the quality of /l/ production was somewhat superior to that of /r/, deficits in single words may represent a developmental lag in liquids.

Informal measures included Zachary's retelling a story read aloud in class and explaining a science experiment that contained some newly learned terminology (*cotyledon, capillaries, respiration,* etc.). As his teacher had noted, Zachary struggled with pronouncing most of the multisyllabic words. This may indicate a difficulty in sequencing speech sounds during processing (receptive phonology) or problems producing a complex series of phonemes (Swank, 1994). According to Hodson and Paden (1991), 6-year-olds should be significantly more successful in producing common multisyllabic words than 5-year-olds. Zachary was not able to identify many rhyming words in the story and could not produce an additional rhyming word, e.g., one that rhymes with *root*.

Based on the results of the *Test of Phonological Awareness* (Robertson & Salter, 1997), portions of the *Comprehensive Test of Phonological Processing* (CTOPP; Wagner, Torgesen, & Rashotte, 1999), and other classroom observations, Zachary's phonological awareness abilities and phonological memory are of concern. Although he identified rhyme approximately 50% of the time, successfully segmented sentences into words and two- to three-syllable words into component parts by clapping, recognized the initial sound in a word, identified printed consonants, and decoded VC and CVC words at approximately age-appropriate levels, he was unable to complete the following tasks in the manner expected of a student in the second half of first grade: produce rhyme, segment either four-syllable or longer words into syllables or words into phonemes, identify final and medial sounds, delete syllables, or delete or substitute individual phonemes within a word or blend phonemes to make a word. An underlying factor may be a weakness in phonological memory, defined by the authors of the CTOPP as the ability to code information phonologically for temporary storage in working (or short-term) memory (Wagner, Torgesen, & Rashotte, 1999, pp. 4–5). The Nonword Repetition subtest confirmed that Zachary has difficulty repeating multisyllabic words. For details, see the reported scores above. Zachary appeared anxious during these tasks.

As intervention progresses, we will want to check for any increase in Zachary's ability to segment longer words into syllables or blend segments into words. This is especially important because he must be able to store phonological representations long enough for the meaning of the word to be recognized. Limitations can impede comprehension (and consequent production) of complex morphological and syntactic forms as he grows older. Spelling concerns should be addressed partly by determining what phonological skills he is bringing to the task, that is, what stage of spelling he is in (probably early phonemic), and then moving him into the next stage, even though it may not be grade appropriate (Temple & Gillet, 1984).

Language: Zachary's narrative skills and vocabulary scores are within acceptable limits with no significant discrepancy between receptive and expressive skills. His performance on the SPELT–II indicated areas of weakness in producing both derivational and inflectional morphemes, particularly those forms that are not as salient. In a typical example, he omitted the *ed* ending from a verb when it is pronounced as "t," as in *walked;* this morpheme is harder to perceive than the regular past tense marker in *climbed* ("d") or *planted* ("ed"). In sentence repetition tasks, he left out small words, omitted endings, and reversed the order of words, again indicating that memory for sounds is weak. Being able to sequence events correctly appeared to be related to the availability of visual cues; when Zachary could observe the steps in a science experiment, see block patterns, use pictures in a book as cues or follow the movements of the art or P.E. teacher, he was much more successful than when he had to rely solely on his auditory memory.

Summary Statement: Zachary exhibits deficits in speech and language characterized by omission of word endings (morphology) and age-inappropriate skills in comprehending and remembering sounds and sound sequences, including rhyme and alliteration. He also exhibits deficits in his ability to manipulate sounds during segmentation, blending, substitution, and deletion tasks. These deficits in receptive and expressive phonology can negatively affect his learning to read (decode) and spell.

Recommendations: Zachary should be labeled as handicapped in speech and language by the appropriate district committee. (Note that this evaluation was done prior to the meeting of the labeling body; if the evaluation had been completed as a result of their deliberations, the recommendation would specify information for teachers, the kind and frequency of intervention, and whether it was to take place during individual or group sessions.)

Appendix 3.H

◆ ◆

Sample Diagnostic Report: Long Form

Southtown High School
Anytown, California
Speech–Language Evaluation Report

Name:	Christine Mason	**Grade:**	10
Date of evaluation:	March 25, 2004	**Referral source:**	TEAM
School:	Southtown HS	**Homeroom:**	18 Annex
	Anytown, CA		
Date of birth:	February 11, 1989	**C.A.:**	15-1
Type of evaluation:	Initial	**Native language:**	English
Examiner:	Jacqueline Meyer, MHS, CCC-SLP	**English proficient:**	Yes

Background Information:

Reason for referral: Christine's academic performance has been steadily declining in all subjects, with barely passing grades in several subjects.

Previous testing: Previous to this assessment, Christine has not participated in a speech–language evaluation.

Parent concerns regarding speech and language: Christine's mother reported a concern regarding her daughter's inability to keep up with the increasingly difficult demands of high school, even with "very hard work" in school and at home. Reading support through Title I services during elementary grades and again in the seventh grade proved helpful, but her mother feels that Christine's difficulty in understanding course content now includes her teachers' lectures, as well as written material.

Teacher concerns re: speech and language: Christine's teachers reported that although she works hard and completes extra-credit assignments, she has difficulty following lectures and spoken directions; her notes are disorganized and lack key information; and her written work is substandard in content, complexity, and organization. Classroom participation is limited, and when she is pressed to respond, her answers lack coherence and detail.

Student's self-evaluation re: speech and language: Christine reported that she feels her academic difficulty is due to how hard the work has become, particularly reading and writing assignments. She states that even when she reads and rereads the material, she has difficulty understanding the long sentences. She stated that she is increasingly reluctant to respond to the teacher's questions in class because her answers are rarely correct.

Medical history: Unremarkable

Current and past academic performance: Since the 1st grade, Christine's reading progress has consistently been in the below-average range (between −1 and −1.5 standard deviations below the mean, with decoding and fluency superior to reading comprehension scores). She received tutoring and Title I services during the 2nd through 5th grades. Title I services during the 7th grade emphasized reading comprehension. She was placed on the watch list by her 9th-grade team when she barely passed into 10th grade. End-of-year (9th grade) test results in reading comprehension were in the very-low-normal range. The team did not recommend retention, because it is common for students to experience problems during the transition from middle school to high school. To lessen class work complexity, Christine's guidance counselor switched her from a precollege program to one in general education at the beginning of 10th grade. She also placed her in a science class that featured increased "hands-on" assignments and had a lower teacher–class ratio. At the close of the second marking period, Christine's grades were in the D+/C− range in most courses, with the exception of a somewhat higher grade in science. Teachers' comments that Christine was struggling to understand grade-level material had increased. Grade 10 team members report that although she works hard, has taken advantage of a peer tutoring program, and often completes extra-credit assignments, she has continued to experience difficulty understanding cognitively difficult material from either lectures or textbooks. Her outlining skills are poor, and she does not analyze or synthesize curriculum material adequately, even compared with those classmates who exhibit low-average ability.

Current services and accommodations: Christine does not currently receive special education, reading, or speech–language services, although she has sought after-school help from her teachers. Peer tutoring has been discontinued.

Assessment procedures used in this evaluation: Student and teacher interviews and checklists; classroom SLP observation to assess effectiveness of speaking and listening skills; formal evaluation (see attached test descriptions and scores); informal evaluation; review of school records, report cards, and progress reports; portfolio review of writing samples.

Observations:

Pragmatics: Christine presents as a friendly but worried adolescent. She demonstrated excellent cooperation during all one-on-one sessions and appeared eager to find out "why school is so hard" for her. She initiated and maintained conversation, made appropriate eye contact, and asked a number of questions during spontaneous conversation.

Performance in class: Christine was observed within her social studies class as the teacher was giving a short lecture. She twice asked another student what the teacher had said. Her answers to the teacher's questions were inadequate. The notes that she took during this time did not demonstrate any discernible organizational format. She rarely volunteered to speak in class. When she was forced to respond to a direct question, her answers were disorganized, marked by irrelevant remarks and a failure to integrate information into a cohesive whole. Her performance improved, however, when she was part of a small discussion group and when she was following step-by-step instructions to solve a map puzzle. Because writing assignments take her so long to complete, several of her teachers had allowed her to make oral reports instead. They, too, were substandard. Both expository and narrative oral discourse were marked by the same disorganization, limited support for opinion, meager descriptive detail, and lack of a clear main idea that characterized her answers to teachers' questions.

Although her spelling and grammar were correct in her written work, her writing at both the intra- and intersentential levels usually featured simple vocabulary and structure, mostly single-clause, declarative subject–verb sentences. Christine earns passing grades in math but cannot explain the process she uses to arrive at a correct answer.

Behavioral performance during assessment: Christine presented with cooperative behavior throughout all testing sessions, although she appeared anxious. She seemed more relaxed when the examiner explained what each part of the testing would reveal about how she learned. She frequently needed verbal repetition in order to respond to the examiner's questions or requests.

Speech Evaluation: No deficiencies were observed in articulation, voice, or fluency.

Language Evaluation:

Average standard scores based on 100 fall between 85 and 115; a moderately low score falls between 70 and 85, and an extremely low score is below 70.

Average standard scores based on 10 fall between 7 and 10; a moderately low score falls between 4 and 7, and an extremely low score is below 4.

Four subtests of the CELF–4 that constituted a Core Language battery were administered first; based on that borderline score (a standard score of 85) and other factors, additional subtests were given.

Tests assessing language comprehension, reasoning, and auditory memory are listed below, including the possible impact of deficiencies on classroom performance.

Tests	**Subtest**	**Standard Score**
CELF–4	Word Classes–Receptive	8

Assesses the student's ability to perceive relationships between words by identifying two of four words that are related. Christine's ability falls in the average range. This skill is necessary to understand precise meaning, particularly within Christine's school environment, where students are expected to make connections between curriculum-based vocabulary, understanding which terms are synonyms, antonyms, or associated in some other manner.

CELF–4	Semantic Relationships	7

Assesses the ability to evaluate processing of comparative, sequential, spatial, and temporal relationships and the passive voice. Christine presents with a moderately below-average ability to understand language relationships. Therefore, she may have a limited ability to comprehend comparative, temporal, and sequential relationships. This has important implications for her classroom performance, because students are expected to understand how concepts relate in terms of similarity and differences, location, and order of occurrence. Christine may require assistance in understanding relationships as they relate to curriculum issues.

CELF–4   Understanding Spoken Paragraphs   6

Assesses the student's ability to evaluate, process, and recall content and relations in spoken paragraphs. Christine's low score and an analysis of her errors indicate that she has the ability to understand and recall the main idea of paragraph-length information but has difficulty recalling details and making inferences. This has important implications for her classroom performance, because teachers, adults, and peers generally give information verbally. Based on her performance, Christine would benefit from multiple repetitions of material and having her attention called to pertinent details.

CELF–4   Receptive Language   82

Indicates this instrument's evaluation of a student's overall ability to comprehend spoken language. Christine's score suggests that she has a below-average ability in this area, with deficits in specific areas as noted by the subtests.

Peabody Picture Vocabulary Test–3   87

Assesses understanding of vocabulary at the single-word level. Christine's understanding of single words falls in the low-average range. Therefore, she possesses a relatively solid basis for comprehending words used in the classroom, her peer group, and textbooks. However, she may require assistance in understanding complex or unfamiliar terms. A well-developed vocabulary is basic to understanding curricular content.

Evaluating Communicative Competence–Revised (Receptive Language Subtests)
Note: *ECC* is a criterion-based instrument.

Interpretation of ECC scores:
80%   good
70%   adequate
50%   marginally adequate
30%   present but inadequate
0%   not present

ECC–Revised   Comprehension of a Paragraph   80%

Assesses ability to listen to a short paragraph and provide coherent statements about the content when asked literal comprehension questions. Christine's score demonstrates that her short-term memory for facts is adequate, particularly when she has visual support.

ECC–Revised   Comprehension of Story Inference   25%

Assesses ability to comprehend logical inferences in a short verbal presentation. Christine's ability in this area is weak. She will require support in understanding the process of inference and practice in applying this knowledge to all subject areas.

Tests and procedures assessing expressive language are listed below, including the possible impact of deficiencies on classroom performance.

CELF–4   Recalling Sentences   11

Assesses ability to process and recall spoken sentences of increasing length and complexity. Christine demonstrated a solidly average ability to store sentence-length information temporarily for later recall. This ability is particularly helpful when students take notes during lectures. It should be noted, however, that this ability has not generalized into Christine's being able to create complex sentences on her own.

CELF–4   Formulated Sentences   6

Assesses the student's ability to formulate simple, compound, and complex sentences. Christine presented with low-average ability to formulate grammatical sentences, particularly those featuring complex relationships. The majority of her responses were simple in nature, lacking age-appropriate complexity. The complex concepts common at this grade level require complex structures to explain them. Formulating sentences is critical to the writing process, as well as the process of oral communication; if Christine cannot express her thoughts orally at a grade-appropriate level, it is likely that her writing will reflect similar, and perhaps even more, deficiencies.

CELF–4   Word Classes–Expressive   7

Assesses the student's ability to explain relationships between associated words. Christine's ability falls in the low-average range. This skill is necessary in order to understand and use language, particularly within the school environment, where students are expected to explain connections between curriculum-based vocabulary, e.g., substituting appropriate synonyms to reduce redundancy or using antonyms to contrast meaning. Failing to use correct terms to describe synonymous, opposite, spatial, temporal, or whole–part relationships will make communicating concepts orally or in writing difficult.

CELF–4   Sentence Assembly   9

Assesses the student's ability to apply grammar and transformations to given content. Christine's ability to assemble words and phrases into logical, grammatically correct sentences fell in the average range. The ability to change statements to questions and vice versa allows a student to pose possible examination questions given notes containing facts.

CELF–4   Word Definitions   6

Assesses the student's ability to analyze and define words by referring to class relationships and shared meaning. Christine's ability to define terms fell in the moderately low range. Accurately defining new terms is an integral part of every subject at the high school level and is necessary to acquire new vocabulary and connect new information to previously learned concepts. Defining new terms concisely and with precision is a requirement of most writing assignments. Teaching Christine strategies to learn and retain definitions is a logical first step.

CELF–4   Expressive Language Score   88

Indicates this instrument's evaluation of an overall ability to translate thoughts into spoken language. Christine's score suggests that she has a slightly below-average ability in this area but represents an overall strength, although the difference between the two areas is not statistcally significant.

Evaluating Communicative Competence (Expressive Language Subtests)

Note: *ECC* is a criterion-based instrument.

ECC–Revised   Semantically Appropriate Use of   20%
                Clausal Connectors

Assesses ability to use a given clausal connector in a semantically appropriate manner to formulate a complex sentence. Christine's extreme difficulty in this area may be reflective of her problems in interpreting how ideas are related. The ability to make such judgments and express them in grammatically, semantically correct sentences is crucial in all subjects at her grade level. Teaching the meaning of these connectors may be necessary.

ECC–Revised   Expression and Justification of Opinion   50%

Assesses ability to express and defend a personal opinion on an issue. This ability is essential in those subjects where opinions must be specifically supported by facts, e.g., language arts, social studies. Christine's score reflected that she was able to state an opinion, but she did not marshall facts to state why she felt as she did.

ECC–Revised   Twenty Questions   50%

Assesses ability to gather information through systematic questioning. Understanding what you don't know and formulating a query that will allow you to gather specific information is a necessary part of gaining knowledge in any subject and is an integral part of studying for exams. Christine's ability in this critical area is deficient.

CELF–4	Composite Language Scores in Addition to Previously Reported Receptive and Expressive Language Scores	(82 and 89, respectively)
	Core Language	85
	Language Content	82
	Language Memory	88
	Working Memory	94
	Word Classes subtests—Total	7 (scaled score)

Overall, the CELF–4 indicates that Christine's combined receptive and expressive language as measured by this instrument is slightly below average, with strengths and weaknesses in specific linguistic tasks, as noted. The difference between the two scores, although not statistically significant, indicates that Christine's overall ability to comprehend language, particularly if it is complex or requires inference, is weaker than her ability to put her thoughts into words. It should be noted, however, that creating complex language structures and explaining her thought processes are lower than her other expressive abilities. Her working memory for information that does not require interpretation is age appropriate and represents a potential strength.

Presenting Problem: Receptive and expressive language deficits in organization and specific areas of semantics and syntax. These deficits occur in both oral and written discourse, particularly those involving complexity of thought or form.

Summary and Impressions: Christine Mason, a 15-1-year-old student was referred for an initial speech–language assessment secondary to parent–teacher concern regarding increasingly poor academic performance. Her mother expressed concern that Christine was increasingly discouraged as she tried but failed to keep up with classroom demands. Christine presents as a concerned, cooperative, friendly adolescent. Overall, she presented with scattered receptive and expressive language abilities. Evaluation data point to her limitations in understanding complex language, as well as expressing herself cogently and cohesively in verbal and written forms. Based on observation, analysis of written work, and the results of standardized and criterion-based testing, Christine appears to have adequate working memory and understanding of single-word vocabulary, can repeat syntactically correct sentences, and can even manipulate them if the words are present. Although not a strength, her grasp of semantic concepts appears marginally sufficient. When she is confronted with clausal connectors in syntactically complex sentences, however, she struggles, missing 8 out of 10 on the ECC and scoring poorly on the Formulated Sentences and Word Definition subtests of the CELF–4. This deficit directly affects her ability to understand and use logical connections (*because*), disjunctions (*but, although, except*), temporal relationships (*before, after, when, while*), and the conditional (*if … then*). Unfortunately, there is scarcely a high school subject that does not routinely use these connectors. In the ECC, she displayed acceptable skill in comprehending and remembering single facts and directions, but her ability to use inference was strikingly lower; that is, when she had to use the information and apply it, she faltered. She stated an opinion but provided no elaboration; similarly, there was no logical progression to her questions when she tried to identify an object that had been removed. Her classroom difficulties reflect these deficits. On the basis of her language profile, it would seem prudent to evaluate a longer writing sample from English class by identifying the types and number of clauses per T-unit, calculating the Subordination Index, and comparing these to spoken samples. Christine's ability to understand and use figurative language routinely present in grade-level material should be checked. Discovering what level of visual support leads to improvement would be helpful also (e.g., using partial outlines, semantic webs).

Classroom and Home Recommendations:

1. Allow extended time to process oral and written information and produce a response.
2. Provide a visual demonstration in addition to verbal directions or use other multiple modalities to present new information.
3. Provide a partially completed organizational outline or other scaffolding for lecture material.
4. Ask open-ended questions and provide verbal cues to facilitate increased elaboration and organization of oral and written language tasks.
5. Provide multiple-choice questions for a segment of examinations.
6. Encourage use of compensatory strategies to facilitate organization, e.g., diagrams, forms, templates, computer software to organize information and elaborate on her ideas.
7. Encourage Christine to recognize and ask for repetitions as needed to confirm information and increase understanding.
8. Where practical, provide experiences for hands-on learning.

Other recommendations, e.g., the possiblity of including Christine in a small reading comprehension support group, will be discussed at her upcoming TEAM meeting. It was a pleasure to evaluate her. If you have questions regarding any aspect of this report, please feel free to contact me at Anytown High School (123) 555-4321.

Jacqueline Meyer, MHS, CCC-SLP

Chapter 4

◆ ◆

Individualized Educational Programs

Eileen H. Gravani

I f you ask any speech–language pathologist (SLP) working in the public schools about roles or responsibilities, inevitably the term Individualized Educational Program or IEP will emerge. Because SLPs typically serve students with special needs, they are involved in the development and implementation of IEPs for these students. This chapter will cover information concerning the IEP and related topics such as due process and services for younger children.

THE IEP

An Individualized Educational Program (IEP) is essentially an outline of a child's special educational needs and the means to meet those needs. It is the basic building block for a specially designed program for a child with special education needs. Practically speaking, an IEP is a written planning tool for a child's special education that is developed by school personnel and parents together. This document is developed to meet the special needs of a child with disabilities that affect the child's education. Every student from 3 to 21 years of age who has a disability that significantly affects educational progress should have an IEP. It does not outline the regular education program unless there are classroom modifications or testing modifications. In other words, if a child is in a regular education classroom without any changes due to his or her special needs and receives only speech services, the classroom program and goals will not be outlined on the IEP, although the speech goals will be integrated into the regular education curriculum and state learning standards may be addressed.

A key phrase in the paragraph above is that the IEP outlines special needs that affect education, both in academic and functional performance. If a communication problem is mild in severity or does not affect the child's educational performance, then that child may not have an IEP. An example of this would be a first-grade child with a frontal production of /s/ and /z/ who is doing well academically and has appropriate social relations with his or her peers. This distortion of /s/ and /z/ is an example of a mild problem that is not educationally significant. So you might ask, "When is a problem educationally significant? And exactly what is 'educationally significant'?"

Typically, stating that a problem is educationally significant indicates that the problem affects the child's performance in the educational setting—the classroom. It might affect the child in academic subjects, social development, or self-esteem. Neither federal nor state legislation has specifically indicated what constitutes an educationally significant problem. This allows some flexibility in making decisions and allows for differences between children. For example, two children may have similar problems but different needs because of the way their classroom performance is affected.

In an effort to determine eligibility for special education and related services, some school districts have developed specific guidelines. These guidelines vary among school districts. Some require that diagnostic testing indicate a deficit of 1.5 standard deviations below the mean. This would place a child in the moderate range for severity. Refer to Chapter 3 for a full discussion of test score interpretation.

Children who do not qualify for an IEP may still receive speech–language services—for example, through speech improvement groups. This will be discussed later when we talk about the IEP meeting and eligibility for services.

Now that we have discussed very generally what an IEP is, we will cover what occurs before an IEP is developed, who develops it, and when it is developed. Later, we will talk about each of the parts or components of the IEP and work on some practice cases.

EVENTS THAT OCCUR PRIOR TO THE IEP

The typical sequence of events in developing an IEP is that the child is referred (by a teacher, a parent, a doctor, a school nurse, oneself, or another professional) or has demonstrated difficulty on a screening test. The 2004 Reauthorization of IDEA (PL 108-446) establishes a 60-day time line after a parental request for an initial evaluation or from the time parental consent is obtained from the school district. Eligibility and needs must be determined by the end of the 60 days. States may develop an alternative time frame. For example, if a child fails a screening test on September 10, the building administrator or principal is notified, and a letter is sent to the parents. This letter informs the parents that the child has demonstrated some difficulties and will require further testing. The letter also includes a consent form that the parents or guardians need to sign for the school district to begin testing. If the parents send this back by September 25, then the school district will arrange an IEP meeting.

To illustrate, we will follow a 5-year-old (5 years 2 months) boy, Martin Greene (Marty), through the IEP process. Unlike the students introduced in the chapter on assessment, Marty will have a phonological problem only. After reviewing his IEP, the other cases, which are more complex, will be presented.

Marty is a child in kindergarten who just moved into a new school district in Texas and demonstrated difficulty with the speech section of the screening test on October 1. His teacher reported that she has difficulty understanding him and often asks him to repeat comments or answers. She indicated to the speech–language pathologist that although she can usually understand children's speech patterns after they have been in her class for 2 weeks, she still has trouble understanding Marty and often relies heavily on the context of the situation. A letter was sent to the parents on October 7, indicating the need for testing and requesting permission. The parents returned the signed consent for testing on October 8, and the arrangements were made for diagnostic testing. The IEP meeting was set for November 7.

Evaluation Procedures

Federal regulations outline some considerations for testing children to determine if an IEP is needed and to identify the areas of strength and weakness. Tests and diagnostic materials must

- be validated for a specific purpose. This is true for tests in our field.
- be administered by trained personnel.
- reflect the student's actual ability rather than the influence of a sensory or motor disability. For example, you might want to be sure that the student has the motor ability to point to a choice of three or four pictures, as in some receptive vocabulary tests, or clearly see outline drawings.
- assess the child in all areas of disability.

PL 108-446 has modified the requirement regarding testing in a student's native language. The reauthorization of IDEA in 1997 provided that evaluation be "provided and administered in the child's native language or other mode of communication, unless it is clearly not feasible to do so." The 2004 Reauthorization states that evaluation must be "provided and administered in the language and form most likely to yield accurate information on what the child knows and can do academically, developmentally, and functionally unless it is not feasible to provide or administer." ASHA supports the development of clearer guidelines concerning testing of children who have Limited English Proficiency (LEP), also called English Language Learners (ELL). Clearer guidelines would help reduce the number of ELL students in special education (ASHA, 2005).

If a child had suspected problems in phonology and in receptive and expressive syntax and morphology, you would need to assess each of these areas. If during your testing you noted any other possible areas of difficulty, these would also need to be assessed.

A minimum of two measures of assessment per area of suspected disability is required. A single test is not sufficient to document a disability. This is to verify that a child actually does demonstrate a problem so that a diagnosis is not based on a single assessment measure. Additionally, the results need to be evaluated by a multidisciplinary team. This consists of a minimum of one teacher and one specialist in the area of the suspected disability.

Marty's testing was completed by October 15, and the IEP meeting was set for October 28. Next, we will discuss the people who need to be present at the IEP meeting.

Individuals Involved in the IEP Preparation

People typically at the IEP meeting include

- a representative of the public educational agency who is qualified to provide, administer, or supervise the specially designed instruction. This person needs to have the authority to ensure that services outlined in the IEP will actually be provided.

- the child's teacher, to provide information about the general education curriculum and performance in the classroom.
- The parents or guardians, and anyone they invite.
- the child (if appropriate).
- a member of the evaluation team or a person who is knowledgeable about the evaluation procedures used and the instructional implications of the results.
- at least one special education teacher or special education provider.
- other appropriate individuals.

The parents or guardians must be invited to the meeting in enough time to make arrangements for attendance. Efforts should be made to schedule the meeting at a convenient time and place for all invited. Parents may *choose* not to attend. Any attempts to reach the parents or to reschedule the meeting need to be documented. Additionally, the 2004 Reauthorization of IDEA provides for video conferencing and conference calls.

The preceding list reflects requirements under IDEA. Additional individuals may be required to attend in different states, depending upon state law or policy; however, states are responsible for compliance with federal IEP requirements.

A typical IEP meeting for a child receiving only speech–language services might include only

- a district administrator (the principal or director of student services)
- the speech–language pathologist
- the parent or guardian
- the child (particularly if the student is an adolescent or young adult)
- the classroom teacher

A child who has more special needs, has had an initial evaluation, or is changing placements might have more people in attendance. In addition to the individuals listed above, these might include

- a psychologist
- an occupational or physical therapist
- the school nurse
- a social worker
- evaluation team members
- the classroom teacher
- a vocational counselor
- other appropriate individuals, such as representatives from community agencies

The Reauthorization of IDEA in both 1997 and 2004 contains provisions related to parent involvement in the IEP process. Smith (2001) notes that having parents involved in the IEP process can be beneficial, because it

- provides information for teachers about the home environment,
- increases the parents' knowledge of the child's educational setting,

- fosters better communication and discussion between parents and school, and
- increases the chances that IEP goals will be achieved.

Note that parents may invite a friend, relative, representative from an outside agency, or another advocate to the meeting.

Educational agencies (typically school districts) need to document who is present at these meetings. This is done by listing the people attending or having individuals sign the IEP form. This type of documentation is important if later questions arise about a decision made at the meeting. The 2004 Reauthorization of IDEA also states that members of the IEP team can be excused from an IEP meeting if the parent and local educational agency (e.g., school district) agree and the agreement is in writing. The excused person must provide written input to the parent and the IEP team. Additionally, the 2004 Reauthorization of IDEA allows for a child's IEP to be modified or amended without having an additional IEP meeting.

In Marty's case, a school district administrator, his parents, the classroom teacher, the speech–language pathologist, and a psychologist planned to attend the IEP meeting.

DEVELOPMENT OF THE IEP

The IEP is developed at a meeting with the participants listed above (agency representative, teacher, parent, and possibly the child) before special education and related services are provided. It makes sense that the most appropriate placement for a child with disabilities cannot be determined without first knowing what that child's needs are. Having this as law is actually a safeguard against placing a child in an inappropriate placement without knowledge of the child's abilities and needs. This does not mean that a child cannot be served to some extent by special education before the development of the IEP. It is possible for a child to be placed in a temporary placement as part of the evaluation process. This actually becomes part of the diagnostic information, and the child's performance in the program is considered at the IEP meeting.

A variety of Web sites present information on IEPs. Two examples are the Nebraska Department of Education and the Cooperative Educational Service Agency, Department of Special Education in Chilton, Wisconsin.

COMPONENTS OF THE IEP

Each IEP must include

- present levels of performance (including strengths and needs, evaluation and observation)
- disability

- annual goals that are measurable
- specific special education and related services to be provided, along with program modifications
- projected dates for initiation of services and modifications, and the anticipated frequency, location, and duration of services and modifications
- an explanation of the extent (if any) to which the child will not participate with nondisabled children in a regular class
- any individual modifications for state or district-wide assessment of student achievement
- a statement of how the child's progress toward the annual goals will be measured
- information concerning how and when the parents will be regularly informed of the progress
- information related to transition services, if appropriate
- benchmarks or short-term instructional objectives (needed for students who participate in alternate assessments aligned to alternate standards)

We will discuss each one of these components and also some recommended items that should be included in a good IEP. Note that school districts will have developed IEP forms that meet federal and state regulations and include all the necessary components. These components will include all of the following topics.

Present Levels of Performance

This section may include a variety of information, depending upon the child and her needs, such as academic or educational achievement (i.e., pre-academic or academic levels), intellectual functioning, functioning in other areas such as speech and language, and possibly level or type of pacing for the effective acquisition of a skill (e.g., reinforcement, repetition, and learning style).

This section needs to address the strengths and needs of the student and reflect "how the child's disability affects the child's involvement and progress in the general education curriculum." This information needs to be instructionally relevant, address parents' concerns, deal with functional performance, and provide data that will later be used to measure progress. It should refer to assessments in such a way that the information can be easily understood, including information from state or district-wide assessments.

For a child who demonstrates a specific problem in phonology, as Marty does, this information might include

- IQ score (performance and verbal).
- classroom performance: information on how a child performs in the classroom, in terms of academics, attention, and interactions, particularly focusing on intelligibility and phonological awareness; any scores on standardized tests (e.g., Stanford Achievement Test) or district-wide

assessment (since Marty is a new kindergarten student, that information will be limited).

- information on the child's speech and language abilities, stimulability, etc.
- information on any other areas of suspected deficits.

Information concerning social development—interactions with peers and adults, self-perception, adjustment to the environment—is also included. In an effort to verify the accuracy of this type of information, Gelzeiser et al. (1998) studied the IEPs of two school districts and found that peer interactions were accurately described under "Present Levels of Performance" when compared to the data collected by the researchers.

Information regarding physical health and development is also included, in the amount of detail that is appropriate. This would cover general health: vision and hearing abilities, medications, injuries, motor development, and so forth.

Information regarding the amount of adult supervision or support needed might also be included. Obviously, this would be related to the academic, social, and physical areas.

For Marty, all this information is contained in Figure 4.1. (Citations for tests have been added to these IEP exhibits for your reference only.)

Disability

IDEA (2004) provides definitions of the disabilities covered under the law. The definition of specific learning disability has changed from IDEA (1997), but the other definitions have remained the same. They can be found in Section 300.8 of the proposed regulations and include autism, deaf-blindness, deafness, emotional disturbance, hearing impairment, mental retardation, multiple disabilities, orthopedic impairment, other health impaired, specific learning disabilities, speech or language impairment, traumatic brain injury, and visual impairment including blindness (U.S. Department of Education, 2005).

Annual Goals

Annual goals are measurable statements that include behaviors in specific areas that reflect the child's needs and can reasonably be achieved within an academic year. There must be a direct link between the annual goals and the information contained in "Present Levels of Performance." Annual goals may include both academic and functional goals. The annual goals relate to how the child can make progress in the general education curriculum. Many states now require that annual goals clearly relate to state learning standards.

Typically, there is an annual goal for each priority educational need. Therefore, a child with a very specific speech–language need may have only one or two annual goals on his IEP. However, a child with multiple needs will have more goals. These annual goals provide a framework or guidelines for the educational plan designed for a specific child.

Name:	Martin Greene	**Birthdate:**	8/1/2000
Age:	5–2	**School:**	Johns School
Address:	987 Summers Drive	**Grade:**	Kindergarten
	Littletown, TX	**Teacher:**	Mrs. Kerrins
Parents:	Barbara and William Greene	**Student/Teacher Ratio:**	20/1
Dominant Language:	English	**Date:**	10/28/05
Medications:	☐ Yes ☒ No	**Status:**	Referral

I. Present Level of Performance

A. Academic

Reading: Prereading and readiness level; recognizes upper- and lower-case letters; reads one-syllable words from the following word families: *at* (*cat, bat,* etc.); *an* (*man, fan,* etc.), and *en* (*hen, ten,* etc.).

Math: Counts to 100 by 1s and 10s (with articulation errors); matches pictures of items to the appropriate numbers for 1–12; does well with sequences and patterns.

Written language: Writes the appropriate letter (for initial sound) when sounding out a word 75% of the time.

Other: Interested and attentive during science activities.

Speech–language articulation: Marty's spoken language is difficult to understand. Intelligibility when context is not known is approximately 60%. When the context is known, intelligibility increases to 70%. Marty's teacher indicates that usually after a few weeks, she can understand children but she still has some difficulty with Marty. Teachers who see him less frequently do not understand him. At times, the other children in the class do not understand him, especially when he is excited and talking fast. Marty was recently moved to the school district and was recommended for testing based on the results of his screening. Testing, using the *Weiss Comprehensive Articulation Test* (Weiss, 1980), indicates that intelligibility is 70%; stimulability is 80%; errors with fricatives becoming stops (stopping) and palatals becoming alveolars (depalatization) were noted. An analysis of a spontaneous speech sample indicated stopping, depalatalization, and some weak syllable deletion. Fricatives in the final position were sometimes deleted rather than stopped.

Language: Classroom observation indicated that Marty understands and follows directions given in class. He appears to have appropriate vocabulary for the classroom. His teacher indicates that he has an extensive knowledge of animals and plants, beyond his classmates. Language testing, including *The Peabody Picture Vocabulary Test* and the *Test of Language Development–Primary* indicated scores in the typical range.

Intellectual functioning: Wechsler Preschool and Primary Scale of Intelligence (WIPPSI) indicates above average intelligence, with verbal and performance abilities similar.

Curricular needs: From Texas Essential Knowledge & Skills (TEKS):

- Make announcements, give directions, and make introductions. (Marty needs to do this so others will easily understand him.) (Listening/Speaking)
- Act out plays, poems, and stories. (Listening/Speaking)
- Clearly request, retell, or describe stories and experiences. (Listening/Speaking)
- Retell or act out important events in a story. (Reading)
- Express ideas orally and visually. (Social Studies)
- Use words and numbers to describe relative sizes of objects. (Mathematics–Number, Operation, and Quantitative–Reasoning)
- Describe position in a sequence of events. (Mathematics–Number, Operation, and Quantitative–Reasoning)
- Describe and identify objects. (Mathematics–Geometry and Spatial Reasoning)
- Describe, identify, and compare shapes. (Mathematics–Geometry and Spatial Reasoning)
- Compare and order objects by length, capacity, or weight. (Mathematics–Measurement)

(continues)

Figure 4.1. IEP for Marty.

B. Social development

Self: Takes pride in his work; comments to peers and adults, "I don't talk very good."

Peers: Liked by classmates; aware of others' feelings; frustrated when others do not understand him; and sometimes has ignored children when they do not understand him.

Adults: Does not initiate conversation but does answer questions; angry when not understood after second attempt; has kicked the wall and table when not understood; refused to talk in gym and music because the teachers have difficulty understanding him; cried and wanted to go home when there was a substitute teacher and she did not understand him.

Family/community: Parents report that Marty is a helpful child. They understand him but realize that he rarely talks with neighbors or relatives because "They don't know my words."

C. Physical development

Health information: History of middle ear infections; PE tubes inserted in August. Otherwise health history is unremarkable.

Vision: Normal

Hearing: Normal

Gross Motor: Good

Fine Motor: Right-handed; can copy detailed designs; printing typical for age.

D. Management needs

No significant management needs.

II. Disability

Speech or language impairment.

III. Annual Goals

Improve intelligibility of spontaneous speech in the classroom to approximately 80%, focusing on decreasing stopping, depalatization, and weak syllable deletion. This annual goal relates to the speaking components of TEKS, in addition to selected math and social studies components that emphasize describing, explaining, and comparing.

IV. Recommended and Related Services

Speech therapy for 90 minutes per week. Some sessions will take place in the classroom to ensure generalization.

V. Date for Related Services

November 12, 2005.

VI. Participation in Regular Education

Regular kindergarten classroom.

Program modifications: A "speech buddy" system will be established when there is a substitute teacher. This child will help Marty if he is not understood by the substitute.

(continues)

Figure 4.1. *Continued.*

VII. Assessment

Marty will participate in any district-wide assessment and state assessment.

VIII. Measurement of Progress and Report on Progress

Data will be kept on intelligibility in the classroom and on accuracy for individual speech sounds. Reports on progress in speech will be made with report cards and at parent conferences.

Figure 4.1. *Continued.*

Some children have special needs that on a severity scale would be termed severe. These children might also demonstrate regression over summer vacation and not retain what had been learned during the academic year. These children have IEPs that extend for 12 months and will be labeled accordingly.

Some states or school districts have annual goals available on computer. These may be specific to certain states since they relate to those states' learning standards. This does make IEP preparation easier. However, as a speech–language pathologist, you should be certain that you are not choosing goals simply because they are printed and missing a goal that an individual child might need. This would be a disservice to the child and would miss the point of the word *individualized* in an IEP. A source that may be helpful is *Linking IEPs to State Learning Standards: A Step-by-Step Guide* by Miller and Hoffman (2002).

For goals related to peer interaction, settings and situations may include

- classroom (collaborative or partner activities, peer instruction, social opportunities in class)
- cafeteria (where the student eats lunch and with whom, peer interactions)
- hallway (walking with and greeting friends)
- peer interactions (conversations with peers, number of peers in contact with student)
- extracurricular activities (Gelzeiser et al., 1998).

For Marty, there is only one area of need, so there is only one annual goal: Improve intelligibility of spontaneous speech in the classroom to approximately 80%, focusing on decreasing stopping, depalatalization (palatal fronting), and weak syllable deletion. This goal relates to the speaking component of learning standards in Texas, called the Texas Essential Knowledge and Skills (TEKS) and would relate to any part of the curriculum or state standards dealing with oral language. Components of the standards might include sharing ideas; comparing, analyzing, and explaining information; and social interaction. As noted previously, Marty lives in Texas, so his annual goal will relate to the learning standard for TEKS.

Specific Special Education, Related Services, and Modifications To Be Provided

Each educational agency or school district is required to offer a variety of educational programs and services to meet the needs of students with disabilities. These services need to support the attainment of annual goals and the child's progress in the general curriculum. Obviously, children with different strengths and needs are going to require different types of services. This variety is often referred to as a continuum of services. The educational agencies are required to provide the least restrictive environment (LRE) to the maximum extent that is appropriate. This means that children with disabilities should be educated with children without disabilities as much as possible. IDEA (2004) states that educational programs and related services should be based on peer-reviewed research.

Educational programs can include classroom services and related services such as speech–language therapy, audiology, psychological services, physical therapy, occupational therapy, counseling, and assistive technology devices and services. These services may be necessary for the student to benefit from classroom instruction, but the goals and objectives for these services may not directly relate to the classroom curriculum. An example of this might be a physical therapy goal for increasing trunk control. Although this goal does not directly relate to specific classroom curricula, it does relate to the student's daily life and will relate generally to the student's educational performance.

This continuum of services can include the following:

- *Regular education classroom with consultant teacher services.* This type of placement provides either direct or indirect services to students with disabilities in full-time regular education. Indirect consultant services provide consultation to the classroom teacher to assist in modifying materials or presentation to meet the needs of students with disabilities. The times for these consultant services need to be arranged so that as the curriculum changes throughout the year and the child's needs change, there is continued assistance. With direct service, the specialist works with individual students or provides group instruction. This may be done within the classroom so that the student can benefit from the regular education program. Students may also be taken out of the regular education classroom for services.
- *Resource room.* This provides specialized supplemental instruction in an individual or small-group setting. Resource room programs typically supplement classroom instruction. Resource room teachers work in cooperation with the classroom teachers to maintain or improve academic performance. Groups are often composed of students with similar academic, social, physical, and management needs.
- *Special classroom.* The guidelines for these classrooms vary from state to state and typically are concerned with teacher–student ratio and

student instructional needs. Students in these classrooms may spend a part of their day with peers in regular education, but their primary placement is in a special education classroom. This placement may be necessary to provide the adult attention and direction that the student needs to learn.

- *Special schools.* Special schools, in separate buildings, are also used in order to supply intensive services for students with severe or multiple problems. School districts and states vary in the use of these special school placements. A survey by Hasazi, Johnston, Liggett, and Schattman (1994) compared programs that use a high percentage of separate classrooms or schools for special education placements with programs that use separate placements less frequently. Factors that were cited as important were finances, organization of special education, parent advocacy, implementers (e.g., at the state level), and knowledge and values of the site implementers.

- *Private schools.* Students whose needs cannot be appropriately met in public school programs may be served in programs provided by private schools. These schools may have day school or residential components and may be in state or out of state.

- *State schools.* These schools have a specialized focus and are available for students who have specific educational needs. These programs may have day school or residential components. An example would be a school for students who are deaf or severely hearing impaired.

- *Home or hospital instruction.* At times, students require temporary instruction at home due to severe illness or special circumstances. These students are still entitled to services. State laws indicate guidelines for serving these students. Because these are very restrictive placements and allow limited social interaction, they should be reevaluated frequently.

All special education and related services necessary to meet the child's special education needs must be listed on the IEP.

Classroom Modifications

For the student to be successful in the classroom and the general education curriculum, there must often be modifications in the classroom program. These modifications should reflect input from the family and the teachers, and need to be documented so that they can be implemented appropriately. Modifications may include

- specialized equipment such as a computer or word processor, communication board, braille writer and books, large-print books, auditory training equipment, or, for students with physical disabilities, a prone board or a transfer board for moving from a wheelchair

- assistive technology devices and services
- modified directions
- increased time to respond verbally
- taped texts
- highlighted texts
- note-taking assistance (from another student or in the form of a partial outline)
- notes keyed to the pages in the text
- an outline for the text
- a parallel text (similar material but at an appropriate reading level)
- assistance with the organization of materials
- shortened or alternate assignments
- peer tutoring or "buddies"
- study sheets
- reduced paper-and-pencil tasks
- use of a calculator
- preferential seating
- an interpreter
- frequent breaks
- a behavior management system
- a modified response mode
- modified input (e.g., visual aids, concrete examples, hands-on activities)

Keep in mind that this list, though fairly thorough, is not all-inclusive; you may see an IEP with other classroom modifications noted.

Testing Modifications

Modifications in testing or assessment also need to be noted. This will allow their use throughout the school year and in state- and district-wide assessment. This is specified by P.L. 108-446. Some of the frequent modifications include

- time limits, extended or waived
- location of exams
- method of recording answers
- type of questions asked or omitted
- presentation of questions (signed, read aloud, use of braille, large type)
- breaks during testing
- writing directly on the test (rather than on the answer sheet)
- rewording directions
- explaining or rewording test questions
- use of a calculator
- use of a spell-checking device

Thus a student with a severe hearing loss who signs might have parts of an exam signed rather than given orally, or a student who has difficulty with written expression might be allowed to give test answers orally or in written phrases.

A special location might be a quiet nondistracting environment. It might also allow the student the opportunity to read the information aloud. Fuchs et al. (2000) found that students with learning disabilities benefited from reading material aloud during large-scale assessments.

Projected Dates and Anticipated Frequency, Location, and Duration of Services and Modifications

This section of the IEP includes the date that the recommended program is to begin and the duration of the services. Typically, the services and modifications are provided as soon as possible after the IEP is finalized. Some exceptions can occur, particularly when the meeting occurs over the summer or during other vacation time or if transportation needs to be arranged. This section also needs to include whether the IEP is to be in effect for 12 months or the academic year.

The amount of time also needs to be listed and clearly stated for the development of the IEP and its implementation. The total amount of service typically is changed without another IEP meeting. A sample statement would be "Speech–language services 90 minutes per week with time in the classroom. Services to begin September 15 and continue until annual review."

Explanation of the Extent to Which the Child Will Not Participate with Nondisabled Children in a Regular Classroom

This section needs to be specific and may give the percentage of the time *not* spent in regular education or list specific regular education classes that the child will *not* attend. The rationale needs to be included. This is a change from IDEA (1990), which required listing contact with nonhandicapped students and reflects a philosophy that children should be educated in the general education curriculum within the regular classroom if possible.

An example might be "Regular education classroom, second grade, excepting reading and social studies" or "Regular education classroom, speech–language sessions that establish use of sounds are not part of the classroom curriculum and will be taught outside of the classroom."

Students with severe disabilities may be in special classes most of the academic day, and their IEPs would reflect this. They may have contact with nondisabled peers during noncurricular activities such as lunch, school assemblies, and club activities.

Modifications for Assessment of Student Achievement

Information on modification for testing is included in the section above, "Specific Special Education, Related Services, and Modifications To Be Provided." Students with severe disabilities may require an alternate assessment. The IDEA amendment of 1997 requires states to develop guidelines for participation of children with disabilities in an alternate assessment if they will not be able to participate in state and district-wide assessment. The individuals at the IEP meeting must decide on an individual basis whether the child will participate in the state assessment measures or in an alternate assessment. If it is determined that it is not appropriate for a student to participate in regular state or district assessments but instead to participate in an alternate assessment, that needs to be stated on the IEP. IDEA (2004) requires an explanation of why the alternative assessment is needed. In New York State, three criteria are used to determine a child's participation: (a) the student has a severe cognitive disability and significant deficits in communication or language and adaptive behavior; (b) the student requires a highly specialized educational program that facilitates the acquisition, application, and transfer of skills across natural environments; and (c) the student requires educational support systems, such as assistive technology, personal care services, health or medical services, or behavioral intervention. Although states may have different guidelines, some clear guidelines or criteria should be used for deciding if a student will have an alternate assessment. A statement needs to be included with the IEP stating why the student is not taking part in the state assessment. The No Child Left Behind Act of 2001 (the Reauthorization of the Elementary and Secondary Education Act) specifies that students with the most significant cognitive disabilities may take an alternate assessment that is aligned with the state learning standards (Rebhorn, 2002).

Out-of-level testing may be considered. This means that a student would not participate in grade-level assessment but would take the assessment at a different grade level. For example, a sixth grader might take the fourth-grade language arts exam. However, difficulties with this include the fact that Section 300.137 of the 1997 IDEA regulations states that the performance goals for students with disabilities should be consistent with the standards and goals established by the state for all children to the maximum extent appropriate. In addition, out-of-level testing may not address the same standards at different grade levels and may lower expectations for students with disabilities (for more information, refer to http://www.wrightslaw.com).

Student performance may be documented using a variety of methods. These include student written work or other student "products," videotapes, audiotapes, observation of student performance in real-life situations, and so forth. Typically, multiple pieces of work would be collected in a portfolio or datafolio and then reviewed. Salvia and Ysseldyke (1998) suggest gathering data from multiple sources, including observation, recollections through interviews (of the student, peers, teachers, therapists, employers, family), a review of records, and any testing. States may have different mechanisms for review. They may include a rating scale, checklist, or rubric. Some states, like New York and Kentucky, which are using rubrics for assessment of students in the general education curriculum, are also using rubrics for alternate assessment.

Kleinert, Haig, Kearns, and Kennedy (2000) suggest aligning aspects of the alternate assessment with regular assessment in terms of the language used for scoring, the scoring categories or dimensions, and the educational outcomes. This helps to ensure that the alternate assessment is seen as a part of the school's assessment. This is important because under Title I, state assessment systems must explain how alternate assessment systems are integrated into their accountability systems. The No Child Left Behind Act of 2001 also has requirements for alternate assessments.

Progress Toward Annual Goals and Reporting

On the IEP, there must be clear ways to document whether a student has achieved or made progress toward annual goals and short-term instructional objectives or benchmarks if appropriate. These may be standardized testing or less formal means of assessment, such as pre- or posttesting, classroom observation, and class assignments. A new requirement of IDEA is parent notification of the child's progress. Parents of children with IEPs must receive information concerning their child's progress as frequently as parents of nondisabled children receive progress reports. What this means is that progress reports have to be sent to the parents as frequently as report cards are sent. There is no set format for the reporting of this information. Some school districts make copies of the annual goals. Progress is then noted during that marking period. Typically, for children receiving only speech or language services, a one-page assessment is enclosed with the report card. If it has been noted on the IEP, a phone call may be made to update the parents on progress. The call will then need to be documented (Karr, 1999).

Reports often indicate progress on short-term objectives linked to the annual goals, but short-term objectives are no longer a required component of the IEP for children who participate in statewide and districtwide assessment. Although short-term objectives and benchmarks are no longer required, they will be used in this chapter to reflect task sequencing and a means of reporting progress toward an annual goal. They will also be linked to the general education curriculum. They would be useful in reporting to parents on a child's progress.

For Marty, the annual goal of improving intelligibility would be addressed by

- increasing use of /f,v,s,z/ in single words to 80% for common and classroom vocabulary, e.g., counting numbers.
- increasing use of /f,v,s,z/ in short sentences to 80% when responding in class, particularly during class meeting time.

- increasing use of /ʃ/ in words to 80% for common and classroom vocabulary. (Note: Marty was highly stimulable for this sound.)
- decreasing weak syllable deletion to 20% in sentences when responding in class.
- decreasing weak syllable deletion in conversational speech in the classroom to 20%.
- increasing use of /f,v,s,z/ to 70% in appropriate words during a class play.

For a science unit on habitats in the general education curriculum, some suggested goals will be given for students with language disorders. Some ways to achieve the annual goal "Increase semantic skills" might be

1. After listening to a description, ___ will point to the correct habitat 90% of the time.
2. ___ will verbally label four types of habitats and list two characteristics of each.
3. ___ will compare and contrast two habitats, listing two similarities and two differences.
4. When given a habitat, ___ will list three animals living in that habitat.

For the annual goal "Increase syntactic skills" a goal related to the habitat unit might be that the student "will use conjoined sentences using disjunctive and causal conjunctions when discussing habitats, for one fourth of his sentences."

For annual goals in a language arts unit on folktales in the general education curriculum, more specific curricular goals are listed:

- Improve pragmatics (organization of information and clarity):
  1. ___ will retell a folktale with a clear beginning, middle, and end.
  2. When retelling a folktale, ___ will include a clear statement of the problem and the resolution.
  3. When retelling a folktale, ___ will stay on topic without reminders, three out of four times.
- Improve syntactic skills: ___ will retell a folktale with complete sentences, using a visual prompt.
- Improve semantics, using specific vocabulary: ___ will retell a folktale, using a minimum of eight adjectives.
- Improve phonology:
  1. ___ will retell a folktale with 90% intelligibility.
  2. When retelling a folktale, ___ will use velars in all positions of words, 80% of the time.
- Improve morphology:
  1. When retelling a folktale, ___ will use regular past tense 90% of the time.
  2. When retelling a folktale, ___ will use the third-person pronouns "he" and "she" appropriately 80% of the time.

Short-Term Instructional Objectives

The Appendix to the March 12, 1999, IDEA Final Regulations states that "once the IEP team has developed measurable annual goals for a student, the team must develop either measurable intermediate steps [short-term objectives] or major milestones [benchmarks] that will enable parents, students and educators to monitor progress during the year." However, there was a change with the 2004 Reauthorization of IDEA (P.L. 108-446). Short-term objectives and benchmarks are now required only for children who take alternate assessments, with alternate achievement standards.

Short-term instructional objectives are intermediate measurable steps between the present levels of performance and the annual goals. *Benchmark* is a term relating to local and state standards and used in general education to refer to a milestone documenting achievement toward standards. Benchmarks in special education are typically more specific than those used in general education. Short-term instructional objectives cover a period of several weeks to months. These short-term instructional objectives should reflect the sequence necessary for learning the targeted skills and should build upon each other.

Both short-term objectives and benchmarks need to relate to the student's needs and enable the child to progress in the curriculum. They must be measurable or able to be documented. Documenting objectives can be accomplished by a variety of means, including structured observation of the target behavior both in and outside of the classroom, a portfolio of assignments, teacher checklist or other behavioral charting, student self-monitoring checklist, audiovisual recordings, and so forth.

Examples of verbs and verb phrases that can be used to describe and specify a student's behavior include *verbally label, respond, verbally express, point to, look at, follow directions, select, calculate, read, spell, answer questions, write, sequence,* and *describe*. Conditions might include the following: *within a 5-minute period; three out of four times; three times daily;* or *for three consecutive days.* Conditions might also include the following phrases: *during class activities; when asked a question; when reading a story;* or *in small work groups*.

Information on Transition Services

IDEA (1997) required a statement of need for transition services to be included on a student's IEP at age 14 years, with transition services implemented typically at age 16 years. However, the 2004 Reauthorization of IDEA states that transitions services begin no later than 16 years. The goal for such services is a successful transition from school to adult life in the community, specifically "for further education, employment, and independent living" (§602(d)(1)(A)). An example of a transition goal might be taking a public bus independently.

Sample transition goals that might involve speech–language services include the following:

- investigate and select an assistive technology (AAC) device that will increase the student's communication and enhance community involvement

- train the student to use the AAC device in a variety of settings
- develop self-advocacy skills and the communication skills necessary for the student's success in employment or life in the community
- increase the student's use of appropriate interpersonal communication and social skills for different settings—for example, school, recreation, peer outing, workplace.

A sample transition goal related to further education might be for a student with a moderate learning disability. This student might have instructional needs related to organization and developing sentences and paragraphs. He has an interest in computers and would like to work with them after graduating from a technical college.

   ◀▶ **IEP Transition: _____ will complete courses in computer technology in preparation for studying computer programming at a technical college.**

Other IEP goals would address organization and writing skills (Bar-Lev, 2000).
     Hasazi, Furney, and Destefano (1999) studied nine sites across the United States for transition services. They found six themes that related to successful implementation:

- incorporating system-wide strategies that are student and family centered, with attention toward encouraging their participation and the student's skills in self-determination;
- fostering effective and significant interagency collaboration involving written agreements and meetings with schools and community agencies;
- facilitating systematic professional development related to the development and evaluation of transition practices;
- leading at the administrative level to encourage innovative ideas and develop leadership;
- coordinating reform efforts with an interest in the impact on all students—for example, for community-based learning; and
- making connections between local and federal transition initiatives (e.g., the School-to-Work Opportunities Act).

REVIEWING IEPS

Some general questions that may be helpful to ask in reviewing IEPs include the following:

- Does the information concerning the student's present level of performance clearly describe the impact of the disability on the student's educational performance?
- Does the IEP reflect the student's needs? Does it reflect the student's needs to progress in the general education curriculum?

- Is there a clear relationship between the present level of performance, recommended program, annual goals, and short-term objectives or benchmarks (if needed)?
- Do the goals and objectives focus on the special education needs of the student?
- Do the current goals relate to goals from previous IEPs?
- Does the IEP list all the services that the child needs, and are the frequency and duration of services clearly documented?
- Are the individuals who will provide the services clearly specified in the IEP?
- Is contact with nondisabled peers documented?
- Are the IEP goals functional? Will they assist the child in his present environment or an anticipated environment?

IEPs are sometimes challenged on the basis of procedural violations. An example might be the time line or the people in attendance at the IEP meeting. A meeting between a parent and a teacher or speech–language pathologist is not a legal IEP meeting. Another reason that an IEP might be challenged is a possible violation of parental rights, such as lack of notification concerning the meeting, insufficient time allowed for notification, or a notification that was not in the parents' native language.

ANNUAL REVIEW

IEPs must be reviewed at least every 12 months. Students age 18 years and older with IEPs emphasizing the coordination of multiple agencies with adult programs may have a 3-year IEP. The purpose of the annual review is to evaluate whether the program described in the IEP is still appropriate and meeting the student's needs. Progress made throughout the time that the IEP has been in effect is reviewed, and recommendations are made. Progress cannot be simply standardized test scores but must relate to classroom curriculum. If appropriate, information from district and state assessments should be considered. Information provided by the parents and anticipated needs should also be in consideration. The individuals involved in this process are essentially the same as those present at the initial meeting:

- a representative of the school district
- the parents
- the classroom teacher
- speech–language pathologist (if the student is on the caseload)
- other professionals who are responsible for implementing goals on the student's IEP
- the student (if appropriate)
- other individuals or representatives (e.g., of community agencies)

The LRE is considered, and a recommendation is made to continue, modify, or discontinue the student's special education program. This may mean a change in classification, placement, contact with nondisabled students, or the way that the services are delivered. If the student will continue to have an IEP, new annual goals and short-term instructional objectives (if needed) are written.

REEVALUATION

The IDEA 1997 Amendments eliminated the required triennial assessment. Now the IEP team meets and decides if a full assessment is necessary. This is based upon collected data and information from the parents, teachers, and other service providers. A decision is made as to whether a disability continues to be present, and whether special education services and modifications are necessary. The parents are involved in this decision process.

A child's parent or teacher may also request a reevaluation. Or one may occur if the school district determines that the child's performance warrants a reevaluation (possibly the child's school performance is improving significantly, or, conversely, the child is not making progress toward IEP goals). If the school district has requested the reevaluation, the parents' consent is needed. If the parents do not consent, and the school district has "taken reasonable measures to obtain such consent," the district may conduct a reevaluation.

IF A STUDENT IS NOT ELIGIBLE FOR AN IEP

We have discussed the scenario of a child who is referred, is evaluated, and receives an IEP—in other words, the student who is found to have a problem that is educationally significant. But at times, testing indicates that a child's problem is mild or mild to moderate in severity and there appears to be no impact on classroom activities. In such a case, there would be an IEP meeting, and after the findings were reviewed, the student would be ruled ineligible to have an IEP. However, the student might still receive some services. Many school districts have speech improvement programs and would enroll a child who has misarticulations that are not affecting her education. Additionally, the speech–language pathologist might consult with the classroom teacher and set up a classroom program for that child. Another possibility might be to place that child on a watch list and monitor her progress.

If a student is found to be ineligible for an IEP, after the IEP meeting the parents receive a letter from the school district. The letter outlines reasons for the decision, citing specific testing and information about performance in the classroom. The letter also outlines the parents' rights to appeal and the due process procedure.

An alternative for a student who does not qualify for services or modifications under IDEA is to evaluate whether the student might qualify for services or modifications under Section 504. Section 504 of the Rehabilitation Act of

1973 requires that schools (or any recipient of federal funding for any programs of the agency) do not discriminate, but unlike IDEA it provides no funding. Its definition of *disability* is broader than IDEA's, with both academic and nonacademic needs considered. The differences between IDEA and Section 504 are outlined in an article by deBettencourt (2002).

DUE PROCESS

At times in the IEP process, the school district and the parents or guardians of the child are not in agreement. Typically, differences are discussed informally. IDEA (1997) encourages mediation and requires that states offer mediation as a means to resolve disputes between parents and the school district when there is a disagreement. The 2004 Reauthorization of IDEA retained much of the same language. If mediation is used and a resolution is reached, a legally binding written agreement is signed by both the parents and the educational agency. Parents may refuse the mediation and request a due process hearing.

The set of procedures called due process is designed to protect the rights of students with special needs, the parents of those students, and school districts. These rights are ensured by federal and state law.

Typically, informal resolution is attempted first. If that is not successful, formal procedures may be requested by the parents or guardians or the school district. Parents may request due process procedures for a variety of reasons:

- failure to follow the appropriate time line for evaluation
- an inadequate IEP
- lack of education in the least restrictive environment (LRE)
- failure of the school district to implement the IEP recommendations
- failure of the school district to consider an independent evaluation when making IEP recommendations
- disagreement with the IEP recommendations
- failure of the school district to review the student's program on an annual basis
- failure of the school district to reevaluate the student every 3 years

Due process procedures may also be initiated by the school district. The local educational agency (typically a school district) is responsible for ensuring that students with special needs receive a free appropriate public education. One reason that a school district might initiate due process is the school district wants to establish that its evaluation is appropriate and avoid paying for an independent evaluation.

IDEA (2004) requires that before the due process hearing, the school district must arrange a meeting or resolution session with the parents and relevant members of the IEP team. This occurs within 15 days of receiving the parent's due process complaint. The school district has a total of 30 days from when the complaint was filed to resolve the complaint to the parent's satisfaction.

The due process hearing is conducted by an impartial hearing officer. This individual may not be an employee of the school district and should not have a personal or professional interest in the case that would interfere with making impartial decisions. Hearing officers need to have familiarity with special populations, education, and legal issues. IDEA (2004) provides clear qualification requirements for hearing officers.

Parental rights prior to the hearing include the parents or someone they delegate having access to the student's educational records relating to the identification, evaluation, educational placement, and provision of a free appropriate public education (FAPE). Copies of records must be supplied at a reasonable cost. A right of both the parents and school district is that information to be presented at the hearing be available at least 5 days before the hearing. This is to allow both parties access to the same information. Remember, the goal of hearings is not "to win" but to supply the student with the most appropriate educational program to meet his needs.

A notice is sent to both parties giving the date, time, and place of the hearing. A list of the rights of both parties at the hearing is supplied. These rights include the following:

- Counsel (a lawyer) may be present to give advice.
- Experts in the field may be present to give advice.
- Evidence may be presented by both parties.
- Cross-examination of witnesses is allowed.
- Witnesses (e.g., school district employees) may be required to attend.
- Issues raised in the hearing must have been included in the due process complaint.
- Written or taped recordings of the hearing must be made available.

Rights of the parents also include deciding whether the hearing will be open to the public and whether the child may be present. An interpreter for the deaf or a translator must be available to the parents at the hearing if needed.

The time line for these hearings is fairly quick. This is to ensure that the student receives the most appropriate services. Federal law requires that the final decision from the hearing must be reached and copies mailed to each party within 45 days from the request for the hearing. In the interim, the student remains in his or her original placement.

If either the parents or the school district wishes to appeal the decision of the hearing officer, they may appeal to the state educational agency. A designated official will review the entire set of records related to the hearing, ensure that the procedures followed federal and state laws, and request additional evidence if necessary. Both parties are given the opportunity to present written or oral arguments. The state educational agency official makes the decision concerning the arguments. A final decision is made within 30 days of the request, and copies of the decision are mailed to both parties.

If either party is dissatisfied with the decision, that party may bring civil action in either a state court or a federal district court. Issues that deal with federal law and may affect decisions in other states are typically brought to federal district courts.

The 2004 Reauthorization of IDEA includes statutes of limitations. There is a 2-year statute of limitation for requesting a hearing. The 2 years begins on the date that the parent(s) either knew or should have known about the alleged action or situation. The limitation does not apply if the local educational agency (e.g., school district) either misrepresented information (e.g., falsely indicated that it had resolved the problem) or withheld information from the parents. The interpretation of "should have known" is critical and may be the potential source of litigation.

Common Issues in Due Process

Some recent due process decisions have dealt with integration into regular education, the LRE, and testing modifications. Summaries of these cases are included below.

Need for Integration

Parents of a 6-year-old student with autism wanted their child to be placed in regular education on a full-time basis. The school district initially recommended placement in a special education classroom for 21 to 24 hours per week and 1 to 4 hours in regular education. This was in early May and only for the May and June time period. Information would be reviewed and a longer-term placement would be determined. The parents then requested homebound placement with supportive services. A due process hearing was requested.

One conclusion of the hearing was that the student did not have an absolute right to be placed in a regular education classroom but did have a right to be placed in regular education to the greatest extent possible, with appropriate support. The hearing officer noted that on the IEP the Present Levels of Performance section was lacking strengths and weakness. The hearing officer agreed with the school district's intent but indicated that the steps to be taken for evaluating placement were not clearly outlined. Placement for September and October would include both special education and general education classrooms. The hearing officer ordered that a new IEP be developed in November that would consider the student's need for integration into a regular education class. The officer ordered the parents and school district to work together to develop a plan that would establish ways for keeping data on the student's performance and would include involvement in regular and special education classrooms (Detroit Public Schools, 1993).

Least Restrictive Environment

A case outlined in the *Individuals with Disabilities Education Law Report* (IDELR; 1994) concerned parents of an 8-year-old with a hearing impairment. The parents were not in agreement with the school district regarding placement.

The school district had placed the student at a regional day school for the deaf, 17 miles from her home. At the school, the student was mainstreamed into a regular education classroom with an interpreter. She received instruction in total communication from the speech–language therapist and auditory training, language reinforcement, and tutoring from the deaf-education teacher. The parents wanted their child placed at her local school. The parents argued that the educational placement was 30 minutes from their home and limited their daughter's interaction with friends outside of school. It also prevented them from participating in programs at the school and presented difficulties to the family because they had children at the local school with different vacations than their 8-year-old daughter. They requested a due process hearing.

The hearing officer found that the district's placement on the IEP was appropriate for that student and that the IEP was being implemented in the LRE. The hearing officer based this on the fact that the student's academic abilities were significantly behind grade level and that she needed the comprehensive services offered at the regional school. There was no evidence that the program offered at the student's local school would be appropriate for her educational needs. In addition, services for students with hearing impairments were centralized at the regional school, and the availability of services at other locations was limited.

A recent Supreme Court decision, *Schaffer v. Weast*, concerned a due process challenge about the adequacy of an IEP. Parents of a middle school student with learning and speech–language disabilities challenged a proposed IEP and requested tuition compensation for a private school (Boswell, 2005). The Supreme Court ruled that the burden of persuasion should fall "upon the party seeking relief" [in this case, the parents] (*Schaffer v. Weast*). This case affects about half of the states, which do not have state statutes or regulations regarding burden of proof. Nine states, along with Washington, D.C., assign the burden of proof to the school district, while 17 states have regulations or statutes that put the burden of proof upon the moving party (Wright, 2005).

Classroom and Testing Modifications

IDELR (Child with Disabilities, 1993) reported on a case concerning parents who requested a due process hearing to change their child's IEP. The school district used a special education aide to record the student's oral responses to essay questions. The parents wanted to limit the personnel who could record the oral answers and maintained that the district's use of the aide violated federal law, specifically IDEA. The parents argued that the teacher would be able to include prompting or interpretation of classroom material while giving the exam.

The hearing officer noted that accommodations listed oral responses, not teacher prompting, and concluded that a trained special education aide was an appropriate person to record answers, and that the IEP should not be changed. The hearing officer also concluded that IDEA requires that IEPs be developed to provide educational benefit for the student, including special instruction and related services. However, federal law does not require IEPs to include every service or modification that might possibly be of some value.

The number of due process hearings is rising (Getty & Summy, 2004). After reviewing the results of 414 published cases, Newcomer and Zirkel (1999) noted the amount of time, effort, and resources involved in litigation and encouraged the use of mediation. (See Chapter 1 for a discussion of their findings.)

Preparing Yourself for Due Process Challenges

These are only a few of the cases that deal with common issues in due process. Although due process hearings are not common, and many disputes between parents and school districts are resolved informally, you should be prepared. If you conduct yourself professionally and are accountable, you can protect yourself in case of due process. Things you can do include the following:

- Administer the test according to the way it has been standardized.
- Note any modifications you make.
- Use the most current version of the tests.
- Be aware of the population used for standardization of the tests you use—sample size, whether it is representative of the U.S. population, and whether it is representative of your client's linguistic and cultural background.
- Be aware that all testing must follow the federal guidelines stated earlier in the chapter (e.g., tests administered in the child's native language).
- Make sure there are two measures for each area of disability.
- Be sure that the annual goals and short-term instructional objectives (if needed) clearly relate to the identified needs.
- Keep attendance, noting the reason for any absences.
- Keep brief notes on each session, including the goal, general activity, and performance of the student.
- Document any conversations or correspondence with parents.
- Keep in contact with the classroom teacher to learn about communication behaviors and generalization in the classroom.

SERVICES FOR YOUNGER CHILDREN

Services are available for children who are younger than school age. These services are divided into two categories: services for children from birth to 3 years of age, and services for children 3–5 years of age. Since the procedures for children ages 3–5 are similar to those for school-age children, these will be discussed first.

Services for Children Ages 3 to 5 Years

Many children entering elementary school may have been identified as having a disability and received special services prior to entry into kindergarten.

As you are reviewing children's folders and reading reports, this will become increasingly evident. The procedure for evaluating and providing services to preschool children with special needs is strikingly similar to that for children in public schools.

A referral for evaluation is made to the appropriate agency. In many states, services for preschool children are administered through the school districts. When a district receives a referral, a letter is sent to the parents. This letter includes a list of evaluators and requests the parents' consent for the evaluation. The letter also informs the parents of their due process rights. After the parents give written consent for the evaluation, it is scheduled. The evaluation includes a physical examination, psychological examination, social history, parent interview, observation of the child, and assessment in all areas related to the possible disability. While the evaluation process is occurring, the meeting to determine recommendations (IEP meeting) is arranged. This meeting needs to occur within 30 days of the referral.

At the meeting, the evaluation results and other information are reviewed. The child will be found either eligible or ineligible for special education services. If the child is found to be ineligible, there needs to be clear documentation of the reasons. The explanation should include specific tests or reports that led to the recommendation and the rationale for the decision. Also included are a list of due process rights in case the parents wish to appeal. If the child is determined to be eligible for special education services, an IEP is developed. The IEP for a preschool child is similar to an IEP for a school-age child. It includes a statement of the recommended program, a list of present levels of functioning, annual goals, short-term instructional goals (if needed), criteria, and whether the placement is the least restrictive alternative. Also included are descriptions of the program and placement options and the rationale for rejection of any option not selected. The program or related service provider is notified, and arrangements for services are made. The parents need to give written consent for the placement. Transportation may be arranged unless the child is to receive the services at home or in a day care setting. The IEP must be implemented within 30 days of the IEP meeting. As with school-age children, the IEP must be reviewed after 12 months. At that time, the child's progress and present levels of functioning are reevaluated, and if the child continues to be eligible for services, a new IEP is developed. Before the child begins kindergarten, a meeting is arranged to discuss the types of services for which he or she may be eligible. This meeting will help plan the transition from preschool to a school-age program and will ensure that the child continues to receive services during the transition.

Early Intervention

Federal laws support states' efforts to provide services to infants and toddlers with disabilities. In many states, services for children from birth to their third birthday are overseen by the state department of health. In other states, the managing agency is the state department of education, and a few states use other state agencies. For a list of coordinating agencies and contact information for each state, check the Web site maintained by the National Early Childhood Technical Assistance Center (NECTAC), www.nectac.org.

The law requires states that accept funds for services for infants and toddlers (early intervention services) to provide those services to children who demonstrate delays that can be measured in at least one of the following areas:

- cognitive development
- physical development
- communication development
- social or emotional development
- adaptive behavior

Services must also be provided to children who have a diagnosed mental or physical condition with a high probability that a developmental delay will result.

The NECTAC Web site provides a summary of the guidelines for each state and includes the states' policies.

The general procedure is similar to the development of the IEP for school-age children. The time line follows:

- Identification (by any of a variety of people, such as health care providers, hospitals, child care providers, local school districts, qualified personnel) occurs.
- Referral is made (within 2 days of identification).
- Family is informed of rights.
- Parents give consent for testing.
- Evaluation is completed.
- An Individualized Family Service Plan (IFSP) meeting is held within 45 days of referral.
- The IFSP is developed.
- The family must be provided with a review of the IFSP every 6 months.

The IFSP is a written plan for services and includes

- the child's present level of functioning
- information concerning the family's resources, priorities, and concerns (some of this information is included only with parental consent)
- major expected outcomes (also criteria, procedures, and time line to measure progress)
- specific early intervention services to be provided
- dates, duration, and frequency of services
- location of services (environment) and justification if not in a natural environment, e.g., home or day care

- identification of the service coordinator who will be responsible for implementing and coordinating the plan (from the profession most immediately relevant to the needs of the child)
- transition plan for preschool (upon reaching the age of 3 years).

The transition plan should involve both the sending provider (early intervention provider) and the receiving provider (school district or other provider). Family participation in this transition process and in plans should provide opportunities for both the family and the child to visit the new program. Transition planning should begin early enough to allow for adequate planning, possibly 6–9 months before the child's third birthday.

The primary difference between the IEP and the IFSP is the emphasis on family involvement, both in the IFSP and in the delivery of services. The plan may include not only services directly to the child but also family training and counseling (Bruder, 2000).

Suggestions for improving IFSPs include discussing with the parents what they would like their child to be able to do (as a result of intervention); reviewing the child and family outcomes on the IFSP with the parents; discussing the need for consistency; discussing the types of communication environments that the child is in; and including the family's information about the child's skills (Polmanteer & Turbiville, 2000). If parents have concerns about the IFSP, procedures are available that are similar to the due process procedures for school-age children and their parents.

A change in P.L. 108-446 allows states to combine early intervention and preschool programs. If the state participates in this change, when their child reaches the age of 3 years the parents may choose to have the child remain in the same program (Part C of the law) rather than a program provided by the local school district (Part B of the law). This is contingent upon the early intervention program providing a program that includes school readiness, preliteracy, language, and numeracy skills.

It is evident that when services to children with special needs are provided, there should be a strong commitment toward meeting the child's needs and dealing with family concerns, as well as a strong emphasis on accountability and documentation. As you can see in the IFSPs and IEPs for younger children and IEPs for older students, there also is an emphasis on assisting these individuals as they make transitions from early intervention programs to preschool services to school and later to the community.

CASE STUDIES

Figures 4.2, 4.3, and 4.4 give IEPs for the first three cases whose assessment you followed in Chapter 3: Zachary, James, and Christine. Figure 4.5 gives an example of the Report of Progress to Parents.

Name:	Zachary Johnson	Birthdate:	8/28/97
Age:	6 years, 6 months	School:	Smallville School
Address:	24 Winget Road	Grade:	First
	Anytown, IL	Teacher:	Ms. Cato
Parents:	Susan and Samuel Johnson	Student/Teacher Ratio:	20/1
Dominant Language:	English	Date:	April 27, 2004
Medications:	☐ Yes ☒ No	Status:	Referral

I. Present Level of Performance

Language:

Classroom observations: When summarizing language arts or science activities, Zachary omits past tense endings (e.g., *mixed, pasted, counted*). In longer sentences, he omitted small words such as articles and prepositions, particularly the article *a*. This pattern also occurred during sentence imitation tasks.

Strengths: Zachary showed appropriate sequencing and explanation for narrative after sequencing the pictures. Testing indicates that vocabulary is a strength.

Peabody Picture Vocabulary Test–3:	Standard score—111
Expressive One Word Picture Vocabulary Test–R:	Standard score—92

Other testing from *Clinical Evaluation of Language Functions Preschool–2* indicating language strengths:

Subtest	Standard Score
Concepts and Following Directions	9
Basic Concepts	12
Sentence Structure	8
Recalling Sentences	4
Expressive Vocabulary	9
Word Structure	7
Word Classes—Receptive	10
Total	9
Core Language Score	88
Receptive Language Index	93
Expressive Language Index	81
Language Content Index	93
Language Structure Index	79
SPELT–II	% Correct: 76

Articulation: In spontaneous speech, he omits syllables (words of three syllables or longer). Classroom examples include *triceratops* ("ceratops"), *Inuit* ("Init"), and *chrysalis* ("chrislis"). He also had difficulty with /l/ and /r/. However, this is a typical error for his age.

Phonological Awareness: During small group activities in the classroom, Zachary demonstrated the following:

Segmentation: 3 syllable words by clapping; unable to do longer words
Rhyme: 50% with pictures and slow rate; no independent production
Onset (Alliteration): 10% with pictures; no independent production

(*continues*)

Figure 4.2. IEP for Zachary.

Standardized Testing using the *Phonological Awareness Test* indicates strengths for segmenting sentences and syllables and separating the initial phoneme in a word. Scores follow:

		Raw Score	Standard Score
Rhyme	Discrimination	6/10	65
	Production	1/10	66
	Overall Rhyme		61
Segmenting	Sentence	9/10	105
	Syllables	8/10	107
	Phoneme	0/10	
	Overall Segmenting		NA
Isolation	Initial	9/10	94
	Final	0/10	<69
	Medial	0/10	<81
	Overall Isolation		NA
Deletion	Compound Words and Syllables	5/10	78
	Phonemes	2/10	77
	Overall Deletion		75
Substitution	With Manipulation	0/10	Discontinued
Blending	Syllables	8/10	78
	Phonemes	2/10	74
	Overall Blending		71
Graphing	Consonants	15/20	84
	Vowels	0	No Total
Decoding	VC	5/10	101
	CVC	1/10	87
Spelling	Nonsense words	Only initial sounds	Discontinued

Comprehensive Test of Phonological Processing (CTOPP; ages 5 and 6)
  Note: Only subtests dealing with phonological memory were administered.

Subtest	Standard Score
Memory for Digits	7
Nonword Repetition	6
Phonological Memory Composite Score	79

Reading decoding: Teacher reports that Zachary has difficulty decoding unfamiliar words. He seems to struggle with decoding words. Standardized testing indicates performance at the 10th percentile. Title I reading teacher, Mrs. Ruiz, notes difficulty with sound–symbol relationships and has seen slow progress.

Reading comprehension: Teacher reports that comprehension is a relative strength. Zachary appears to use pictures and the context of the sentence to aid comprehension. Standardized testing indicates performance in the low-average range.

Spelling: Uses one sound (initial position) to spell unfamiliar words; does not retain correct spelling of words on spelling lists.

Writing: Writes very short sentences with subjects and verbs (often difficult to understand due to spelling). Zachary appears frustrated when people have difficulty reading his writing.

Math: Can count to 100; adds and subtracts to 10. Math concepts appear to be strong; however, computational skills are relatively weaker.

Intellectual functioning: Wechsler Preschool and Primary Scale of Intelligence (WIPPSI) Verbal IQ = 98; Performance IQ = 127; Full Scale = 112. Overall score is within high average range. Performance is significantly higher than verbal scores.

(*continues*)

Figure 4.2. *Continued.*

Curricular needs:

- *Phonological awareness:* Needs to count syllables, recognize rhyme and onset in words.
- *Phonemic awareness:* Blend or segment phonemes in one-syllable words.
- *Reading:* Use phonics to decode simple words (age-appropriate); recognize 100 high frequency sight words; use appropriate strategies to decode a word (pictures, context, phonics, word patterns); use letter–sound correspondence; recognize miscues and self-correct.
- *Spelling:* Use phonemic cues and developmental spelling patterns.

Social development: Zachary interacts and cooperates with the children and teacher. He follows classroom rules. He appears to rely on classmates for some work. He appears anxious during reading activities and shows frustration when attempting to decode words or write. He seems embarrassed if classmates notice him struggling.

Physical development: Small for age. No health issues, normal level of activity, normal vision and hearing. Gross motor skills are adequate.

Management needs: There are no needs. He follows classroom rules.

II. Disability

Speech or language impairment.

III. Annual Goals

1. Improve phonological awareness skills and apply these to reading (decoding of short words). *Note:* This corresponds to Illinois State Goal 1 for English Language Arts (Read with understanding and fluency) and Learning Standard 1A (Apply word analysis and vocabulary skills to comprehend selections).
2. Improve morphological skills, using endings in spontaneous speech and writing. *Note:* This corresponds to Illinois State Goal 3 (Write to communicate for a variety of purposes) and Learning Standard 3A (Use correct grammar, spelling, punctuation, capitalization, and structure). The spontaneous speech segment of the Annual Goal corresponds to Illinois State Goal 4 (Listen and speak effectively in a variety of situations) and Learning Standard 4B (Speak effectively using language appropriate to the situation and audience).

IV. Recommended and Related Services

Ninety minutes per week, including small group work on phonological awareness both within and outside of the classroom.

V. Date for Related Services

May 12, 2004

(continues)

Figure 4.2. *Continued.*

VI. Participation in Regular Education

Regular first grade classroom. Some work on phonological awareness and morphology will be completed outside the classroom because activities need to be highly structured and intensive. Additionally, Zachary is aware of his difficulties and would work better in a small group.

Program Modifications

Reading: Program to emphasize phonological awareness and symbol sound awareness, such as the Wilson Program or Sound Reading.

VII. Assessment

Zachary will participate in district-wide assessment and state assessment with no modifications.

VIII. Measurement of Progress and Report on Progress

A report on Zachary's progress will be sent to his parents with each report card. This will include documentation on his progress in phonological awareness during small groups tasks, spelling of CVC words, and reading using strategies based on phonological awareness skills. Information concerning spontaneous speech in the classroom and in speech–language therapy will address morphology.

Figure 4.2. *Continued.*

Name:	James Jones	**Birthdate:**	9/1/94
Age:	8	**School:**	Anytown School
Address:	1234 Stream Drive	**Grade:**	Third
	Anytown, FL	**Teacher:**	Mrs. Dwyer
Parents:	Mary and Robert Jones	**Student/Teacher Ratio:**	24/1
Dominant Language:	English (AAE)	**Date:**	10/1/02
Medications:	☐ Yes ☒ No	**Status:**	Referral (Transfer Screening)

I. Present Levels of Performance

Language: During a classroom observation, James demonstrated word retrieval (word finding) problems indicated by hesitations and use of nonspecific words such as *place* for *habitat* and empty words (e g., *thing, one, stuff, this,* and *that*) during an oral report for his cooperative learning group. His teacher reported this occurs at other times and it was noted during spontaneous conversation. His performance on the *Test of Word Finding* (2nd ed.), Oral Vocabulary subtest of the *Test of Language Development* (3rd ed.; TOLD–3), and expressive portion of the *Comprehensive Receptive and Expressive Vocabulary Test* (CREVT) indicated word retrieval problems. Difficulties with automatic recall of common sequences were indicated by his performance on the Rapid Automatic Naming subtest of the *Clinical Evaluation of Language Fundamentals* (4th ed.; CELF–4).

James displayed difficulties with spatial concepts on a map task in social studies, and on the *Test of Relational Concepts* (Rev.; TRC–R), he showed difficulty with spatial concepts, ordinal numbers, and temporal concepts. He has demonstrated confusion concerning due dates for long-term assignments.

Language strengths: Receptive vocabulary is a strength. Scores on the TOLD–3 Picture Vocabulary and the receptive portion of the CREVT indicate scores in the average range. Also on the TOLD–3, Grammatic Understanding was in the average range, indicating appropriate comprehension of morphological markers and syntactic structures. The two subtests requiring expressive use of grammatic markers, Sentence Imitation and Grammatic Completion, were in the borderline range with a standard score of 7.

Reading: Oral reading skills are within the average range for his class (as indicated by his teacher). Reading comprehension is within normal limits as indicated by testing at the end of second grade. Reading decoding is within the average range.

Spelling: Grade appropriate.

Math: Computation is grade appropriate. He can add and subtract using three places. He knows multiplication through the "eights" and can do simple division. He has occasional difficulty with word problems.

Social studies: James demonstrates difficulty understanding and using directional and spatial words (e.g., *left, right, between, north*) necessary for completing map skills assignments and comprehending directions. He is interested and attentive and has done well in cooperative learning groups.

Science: James understands concepts presented but has difficulty with temporal concepts and ordinal numbers necessary to explain sequences.

Intellectual functioning: WISC–IV indicates normal intelligence, with performance subtests higher than verbal.

(continues)

Figure 4.3. IEP for James.

Curricular needs:

- *Language Arts–Reading:* James has knowledge of antonyms and synonyms; knowledge of root words and prefixes and suffixes. (ELA Standard 1)
- *Language Arts–Writing:* James demonstrates precise word choices. (Writing Standard 1)
- *Social Studies:* James uses maps, globes, charts, map key, and symbols to gather and interpret data. (Social Studies Standard 1)
- *Science:* James knows that materials such as water can be changed from one state to another; knows ways that living things interact. (Science Standard 1)

Social development: James is quiet and rarely asks for help. Instead, he will sit until the teacher or a peer approaches him. His requests for assistance are frequently vague. He relates well to the other children in his class although he does not have any close friends yet.

Physical development: Appropriate.

Management needs: There are no management needs for the classroom.

II. Disability

Speech or language impairment.

III. Annual Goals

1. During a spontaneous conversation, James will use word retrieval strategies to reduce the number of nonspecific or empty words from 10 to 3 in a 3-minute conversation. (Florida Sunshine State Standards in the subject area of Language Arts—Reading Standard [LA.A.1.2.3] and Listening, Viewing, and Speaking Standard 3 [LA.C.3.2.3])
2. James will use spatial and temporal concepts to construct and explain science processes, maps, and graphs, using five specific spatial or temporal terms for two different science activities and two different social studies activities. (Florida Sunshine State Standards in the following subject areas: Mathematics—Geometry and Spatial Sense Standard 2 [MA.C.2.2.1] and Data Analysis and Probability Standard 1 [MA.E.1.2.1]; Social Studies People, Places, and Environments Standard 1 [SS.B.1.2.1]. Science—How Living Things Interact with Their Environment Standard 1 [SC.G.1.2], The Nature of Science Standard 1 [SC.H.1.2])
3. When information presented in class has not been understood, James will ask the teacher to clarify specific parts instead of sitting quietly or saying, "Huh?" or "I don't know what to do," with no more than one prompt on three out of four opportunities. (Florida Sunshine State Standard in the subject area of Language Arts—Listening, Viewing, and Speaking Standard 3 [LA.C.3.2.2])

IV. Recommended and Related Services

Language therapy will be provided for 90 minutes per week.

V. Date for Related Services

October 16, 2002

VI. Participation in Regular Education

Regular third-grade classroom. Language services may be provided outside of the classroom in order to initially teach strategies to James.

(continues)

Figure 4.3. *Continued.*

Program Modifications: Visual cues such as timelines, calendar, and picture cue cards will be used. Visualization will be encouraged. Classroom teacher will use word finding cueing techniques such as use of the initial sound, category name, visualization, and similar word. Teacher will also allow sufficient pause time to allow for retrieval.

VII. Assessment

James will participate in district-wide assessment and state assessment, without modification.

VIII. Measurement of Progress and Report on Progress

Checklists and classroom observations will be used to indicate progress on goals. Report on progress in speech will be made with report cards and at parent conferences.

Figure 4.3. *Continued.*

Name:	Christine Mason	**Birthdate:**	2/11/89
Age:	15 years, 1 month	**School:**	Southtown High School
Address:	567 Stream Drive	**Grade:**	Tenth
	Anytown, CA	**Program:**	General
Parents:	Mary and Robert Mason	**Date:**	4/20/2004
Dominant Language:	English	**Status:**	Referral from Team
Medications:	☐ Yes ☒ No	**Teachers:**	Mrs. Able (English)
			Mr. Dunn (Social Studies)
			Ms. Smith (Science)
			Mr. Lee (Math)

I. Present Level of Performance

General: Christine's academic performance has been declining. Her average in several courses is just above the minimum for passing. She has switched from precollege to a more general high school program. At that time, she was also transferred to a science class with a lower class ratio and hands-on activities. She has been encouraged by the fact that her grades in science have clearly improved. Her science teacher reports that she seems to understand material after demonstrations and lab activities. Recently, Christine has begun to receive private tutoring for reading. Christine's parents have expressed their desire to work on curriculum-related vocabulary and concepts in a nonreading context.

Teacher report and observation (during social studies): Although Christine works hard, she has difficulty understanding complex material from lectures or texts. The use of material from primary sources is particularly difficult for her. She is quiet and does not ask questions. When called upon, she gives responses that are disorganized and comments that are irrelevant to the specific class topic. She appears to do better in small group activities. Her notes are disorganized, and she appears to have difficulty taking them.

Both her social studies and science teachers note that oral reports are sometimes allowed because written reports take extensive time for Christine. They indicate that these oral reports are disorganized with lack of support for statements, lack of main ideas or central thesis, and limited description of detail. This is also seen in written essay questions on tests. Written work typically includes correct spelling and grammar with simple vocabulary and grammatical structures and generally correct punctuation.

Her math teacher indicated that at times Christine will identify the correct answer for a math problem but is unable to explain the process that she used or why she chose it.

Intellectual Functioning: Christine's overall score on the WISC–IV is within the average range. There is a 12-point discrepancy between verbal score (84) and performance score (96), indicating that language is a relative weakness. Language testing was recommended.

Reading: Christine's reading comprehension is between −1 and −1.5 standard deviations below the mean, according to testing. She reports having difficulty with reading longer sentences. Reading decoding is relatively strong. Informal assessment tasks indicate Christine has difficulty with interpreting conjunctions and inferring information. Use of strategies to aid comprehension of logical conjunctions (e.g., *because, so, since, therefore*) increased comprehension of five selected paragraphs from her textbook.

A review of previous testing indicates that Christine has consistently scored between −1 and −1.5 standard deviations below the mean for reading comprehension. She received Title I services for reading in second grade through fifth grade and again in seventh grade and made improvements.

(continues)

Figure 4.4. IEP for Christine.

Language strengths: Receptive understanding of single word vocabulary is a relative strength. Christine scored in the low average range on the *Peabody Picture Vocabulary Test* (3rd ed.). On the *Clinical Evaluation of Language Fundamentals* (4th ed.; CELF–4), Christine did well on sentence imitation (Recalling Sentences subtest) and was able to apply grammatical rules when given the words (Sentence Assembly subtest). She also demonstrated a strength on the Word Classes receptive subtest of the CELF–4, which indicates understanding of word relationships (synonyms, antonyms, and other associations). Performance in the borderline range occurred on the Semantic Relations (receptive) and Word Classes (expressive) subtests involving explaining relationships.

Receptive language: Teacher reports indicate that Christine seems to have difficulty following lectures. She sometimes answers questions with irrelevant material and has difficulty inferring information.

Subtest	Scale Score	Implications for the Classroom
CELF–4 Understanding Spoken Paragraphs	6	difficulty understanding and recalling the main idea; probable difficulty with lectures
ECC Comprehension of Story Inference	(25% correct)	difficulty comprehending logical inferences

Expressive language: Teacher reports indicate that Christine's explanations are grammatically correct although simple. However, they are highly unorganized and difficult to understand.

Subtest	Scale Score	Implications for the Classroom
CELF–4 Formulated Sentences	6	lack age-appropriate complexity of sentences; effects on oral reports
CELF–4 Word Definitions	6	difficulty explaining word meanings
ECC Semantically Appropriate Use of Causal Connectors	(20% correct)	difficulty using causal connectors to explain how ideas are related
ECC Expression and Justification of Opinion	(50 % correct)	could state opinion but unable to support or state reasons
ECC 20 Questions	(50% correct)	unable to evaluate what doesn't know and unable to form questions; related to lack of questions in class

Parent report: The parents report that Christine was a late talker and received language therapy for a year when she was a preschooler. They indicated that they have tutored Christine throughout elementary and middle school. She has always spent a long time on homework, and they report that Christine spends so much time on homework that it is often a choice between sleep and finishing homework. School has become increasingly challenging for her in the higher grades. Her mother feels that this is because her textbooks have become more complex and the language level is more abstract. The parents feel that reading comprehension is difficult and have recently employed a tutor to assist Christine in this area. They stated that Christine had received help from Title I for reading; however, they wondered if there was "a problem beyond reading" because she had difficulty sometimes with other classroom activities, such as understanding lectures. They noted that Christine babysits during the summer and enjoys it. She reads to the children and does art and baking projects with them. She has not been able to continue with this during the school year due to the time demands of her academic classes.

(continues)

Figure 4.4. *Continued.*

Student report: Christine reported experiencing difficulty with both reading and writing. She indicated frequent re-reading of material. She pays attention to words that are bold or in italics and pictures or diagrams in the text but did not indicate using any other strategies with texts. She reported all subjects and assignments as "hard." She likes science more than other subjects because it involves "hands-on" activities and some lab experiments provide information in lists with the steps clearly outlined. Christine indicated that she pays attention in class, but sometimes cannot answer the teacher's questions, and that is frustrating and embarrassing. She indicated that she enjoys babysitting and often plays with the children, reads to them, or does art or baking projects. When asked about reading new recipes, she indicated that was not difficult because she knows the vocabulary and the steps are "in a list that makes sense."

Curricular needs: In order to succeed in 10th grade, Christine needs the following skills:

- The ability to form judgments and to support them with evidence. (Listening 1.1, Speaking 2.2)
- To support thesis. (Listening and Speaking 1.6)
- To compare and contrast. (Listening and Speaking 1.2—Ways Media Cover an Event; Social Studies 10.2—Philosophers and Effects on Revolutions)
- Describe and analyze patterns. (Social Studies 10.3—Industrial Revolution, 10.4—Global Change: New Imperialism)
- Recognize and use logical patterns of organization. (Sequencing, cause–effect, and topic; Listening and Speaking 1.3; Writing 2.4a)
- Generate relevant questions. (Reading 2.3)
- Synthesize information from different sources. (Reading 2.4)
- Evaluate argument. (Reading 2.8)

Social development: Christine is quiet. She appears to relate well to other students in class.

Physical development: Appropriate.

Management needs: There are no management needs for behavior in the classroom.

II. Disability

Speech or language disability.

III. Annual Goals

1. Develop oral and written position with a central thesis and a minimum of three pieces of supporting evidence with explanations. The supporting evidence will be clearly related to the main idea, with an organized presentation of the information. This will be demonstrated on a written and an oral assignment. (State Standards: Listening and Speaking 1.3, Speaking 2.2a and 2.5; Writing 1.1, 1.4, 2.3a; Social Studies 10.3, 10.5, 10.6, 10.7, 10.8, 10.9)
2. Provide an explanation when asked a question when involved in a project or working in small groups in class, three times in a given week. The explanation will consist of a response (main idea) and two pieces of supporting information. Notes may be used for reference. (State Standards: Listening and Speaking 1.3)
3. Read information and integrate with material presented in class (including primary source material). Accurately paraphrase the information three out of four times. (State Standard: Reading Comprehension 2.4)

Figure 4.4. *Continued.*

IV. Recommended or Related Services

Language therapy will be provided 90 minutes per week. Services will include small group and
work in the classroom.

Reading support will be provided with an emphasis on reading comprehension strategies, 60 minutes per week. Services will be in small groups and in the classroom.

V. Dates for Related Services

May 5, 2004

VI. Participation in Regular Education

Regular 10th-grade classroom. Language therapy will occur outside the classroom when initially
learning strategies.

Program Modifications

- Classroom
    1. Visual demonstration of material presented in class.
    2. Prepared outline or semantic map to organize material for lecture and text.
    3. Extended time for assignments.
    4. Use of parallel text, with similar content but easier reading level.
    5. Hands-on activities if possible.

- Testing
    1. Extended time for testing.
    2. Part of test as multiple-choice questions or a word bank provided.
    3. Topics grouped together on test (or sequenced).
    4. Essay questions may be answered orally after Christine prepares an outline.

Media specialist from library will suggest resources that provide visual support to curriculum (e.g.,
movies, videos such as those from Discovery and History channels, and computer programs).

VII. Assessment

Christine will participate in district-wide assessment and state assessment, with extended time.
She will be encouraged to use detailed outlines to formulate answers to essay questions.

VIII. Measurement of Progress and Report on Progress

Rubrics and checklists will be used to document progress. Report on progress will be made with
report cards and at parent conferences.

IX. Transition Service Needs (Optional at Age 15 Years)

Christine will have regular meetings with her guidance counselor to discuss her interests and plans
beyond high school. High school courses will be selected that emphasize hands-on activities (like
her science course) and use of sequenced steps that are clearly related (as in baking, which she
enjoys). Based on her interest in children, Christine and the counselor will identify possible programs in the community that have counselor-in-training programs for summer camp. They will also
identify courses that relate to child care and child development for her high school program.

Figure 4.4. *Continued.*

To: Mr. and Mrs. Greene   Re: Martin Greene   Speech and Language Therapy
From: Classroom Teacher: Mrs. Kerrins   Date:

These areas relate to the Annual Goals listed on Martin's IEP. This reflects the progress since the development of the IEP. (*Note:* If this were later in the school year, it might state "since the November Progress Report.")

Goal	Progress
Intelligibility of speech in the classroom	Approximately 70% for short utterances; 65% for longer utterances (e.g., stories)
Use of f, v, s, z	/f/ and /s/ are used 60% in the beginning of words.
Use of /ʃ/	Not begun yet.
Use of words with three syllables	Marty is using three syllables for common vocabulary in the classroom.

To: Mr. and Mrs. Johnson   Re: Zachary Johnson   Speech and Language Therapy
From: Classroom Teacher: Ms. Cato   Date:

These areas relate to the Annual Goals listed on Zachary's IEP. This reflects the progress since the development of the IEP.

Improve phonological awareness	a. Zachary segments words with 3–4 syllables by clapping for each syllable. b. Zachary can identify words that rhyme for 8 out of 10 words. c. Zachary can match short words based on similar beginning sounds for 8 out of 10 words. d. Zachary uses 2 correct sounds when spelling CVC words.
Improve use of morphological markers	Zachary uses morphological markers such as the past tense marker in short sentences 8 out of 10 times.

(*continues*)

Figure 4.5. Possible statements for Report of Progress to Parents.

To: Mr. and Mrs. Jones Re: James Jones	Speech and Language Therapy
From: Classroom Teacher: Mrs. Dwyer	Date:

These areas relate to the Annual Goals listed on James's IEP. This reflects the progress since the development of the IEP (*Note:* If this were later in the school year, it might state "since the grading period.").

James will use strategies for word retrieval and decrease use of empty words.	a. For words from science and social studies, James retrieved the correct word 80% of the time using semantic and phonological cueing. b. James used semantic and phonological cueing to answer questions using a maximum of 1 empty word for 5 questions. c. James used a concept map for an oral presentation and included 10 words from the curriculum unit.
James will use spatial and temporal concepts in explanations.	a. James completed directions containing directional and location terms using graphs and maps with 80% accuracy. b. James used at least three directional and spatial concepts when constructing graphs and science experiments with 80% accuracy. c. James followed directions containing at least three ordinal numbers or temporal terms for social studies and science (in three different activities). d. James used four ordinal numbers or temporal terms correctly when explaining a scientific process or experiment three times.
James will ask questions in class for clarification.	a. James asked the teacher to repeat information during two activities. b. James asked the teacher question when he was confused about the meaning of a phrase.

Figure 4.5. *Continued.*

To: Mr. and Mrs. Mason From:	Re: Christine Mason Homeroom Teacher: Ms. Smith— 10th grade	Speech and Language Therapy Date:

These areas relate to the Annual Goals listed on Christine's IEP. This reflects the progress since the development of the IEP.

Christine will have a thesis and three pieces of supporting information for oral and written work.	a. Christine completed a concept map relating eight events and ideas. She used the map to write an essay that outlined three pieces of information. The essay was judged acceptable on a rubric used for class. b. Christine completed an outline with assistance and used it for an oral presentation. It had an introduction, thesis, and three pieces of information.
When asked a question, Christine will provide an explanation.	Christine can explain how she arrived at a math answer using a checklist as a cue sheet, 2 out of 3 times.
Christine will read information and paraphrase it.	Christine differentiated between sections of a reading passage that she can understand and cannot understand three times. She underlined words or phrases not understood and answered questions correctly 80% of the time.

Figure 4.5. *Continued.*

CONCLUSION

IEPs are an integral part of providing services for children with communicative disorders when those disorders have an impact on their education. IEPs outline the services that need to be provided, accommodations to be provided, and goals for students. Goals are typically linked to the curriculum and to state standards. IFSPs outline services for infants and young children with disabilities. Those services are provided to the child and the family, as the name indicates.

REFERENCES

American Speech-Language-Hearing Association. (2005). *2005 IDEA proposed rules on Part B and Part D*. Retrieved on September 5, 2005 from http://www.asha.org/about/legislation-advocacy/federal/idea/prelim-ideaB-D.htm?print=1

Bar-Lev, N. B. (2000). *Writing transition statements on the IEP.* Retrieved on September 9, 2005 from http://www.cesa7.k12.wi.us/sped/issues-IEPissues/writingiep/transitionat14.html

Boswell, S. (2005). U.S. Supreme Court upholds school districts in special education case. *ASHA Leader, 10*(17), 2 & 10.

Bruder, M. B. (2000). *The individual family service plan.* Retrieved September 9, 2005 from http://www.ericec.org/digests/e605.html

Child with Disabilities. (1993). *Individuals with Disabilities Education Law Report, 20,* 314–315.

China Springs Independent School District. (1994). *Individuals with Disabilities Education Law Report, 21,* 468–472.

Cooperative Educational Service Agency No 7, Department of Special Education, Chilton, WI. (2005). *IEP issues/Writing IEP goals.* Retrieved on September 1, 2005 from http://www.cesa7.k12.wi.us/sped/issues-IEPissues/writingiep/writingindex.htm

deBettencourt, L. U. (2002). Understanding the differences between IDEA and Section 504. *Teaching Exceptional Children, 34,* 16–23.

Detroit Public Schools. (1993). *Individuals with Disabilities Education Law Report, 20,* 406–414.

Fuchs, L. S., Fuchs, D., Eaton, S. B., Hamlett, C., Binkley, E., & Crouch, R. (2000). Using objective data sources to enhance teacher judgements about test accommodations. *Exceptional Children, 67,* 67–81.

Gelzheizer, L. M., McLane, M., Meyers, J., & Pruzek, R. M. (1998). IEP-specified peer interaction needs: Accurate but ignored. *Exceptional Children, 65,* 51–65.

Getty, L. A., & Summy, S. E. (2004). The course of due process. *Teaching Exceptional Children, 36,* 40–44.

Hasazi, S. B., Furney, K. S., & Destefano, L. (1999). Implementing the IDEA Transition Mandates. *Exceptional Children, 65,* 555–566.

Hasazi, S. B., Johnston, A. P., Liggett, A. M., & Schattman, R. A. (1994). A qualitative policy study of the least restrictive environment provisions of the Individuals with Disabilities Education Act. *Exceptional Children, 61,* 491–507.

Individuals with Disabilities Education Act. (1990). Public Law 101-407.

Individuals with Disabilities Education Act Amendments of 1990. (1990). Public Law 102-119.

Individuals with Disabilities Education Act. (1997). Public Law 105-17.

Individuals with Disabilities Education Improvement Act. (2004). Public Law 108-446.

Karr, S. (1999). Action: School services. *Language, Speech and Hearing Services in Schools, 30,* 212–222.

Kleinert, H. L., Haig, J., Kearns, J. F., & Kennedy, S. (2000). Alternative assessments: Lessons learned and roads to be taken. *Exceptional Children, 67,* 51–66.

Miller, L., & Hoffman, L. (2002). *Linking IEPs to state learning standards: A step-by-step guide.* Austin, TX: PRO-ED.

Nebraska Department of Education. (1998). *Developing the IEP—Putting the pieces together.* Retrieved on Sept 1, 2005 from www.nde.state.ne.us/SPED/iepproj/develop/dindex.htm

Newcomer, J. R., & Zirkel, P. A. (1999). An analysis of outcomes of special education cases. *Exceptional Children, 65,* 469–480.

No Child Left Behind Act. (2001). Public Law 107-110. Retrieved July 19, 2005, from the U.S. Department of Education Web site: http://www.ed.gov/nclb/landing.jhtml

Peters-Johnson, C. (1994). School services. *Language, Speech, and Hearing Services in the Schools, 25,* 275.

Polmanteer, K., & Turbiville, V. (2000). Family-responsive Individualized Family Service Plans for speech–language pathologists. *Language, Speech, and Hearing Services in Schools, 31,* 4–14.

Questions & Answers About IDEA, Students with Disabilities and State and District-wide Assessments. Retrieved July 19, 2005, from the Wrightslaw Web site: http://www.wrightslaw.com/law/osep/faqs.idea.assessment.htm

Rebhorn, T. (2002). *Developing your child's IEP.* Retrieved July 19, 2005, from the National Dissemination Center for Children with Disabilities Web site: http://www.nichcy.org/resources/iep1.asp

Rehabilitation Act of 1973. (1973). Public Law 93-112.

Salvia, J., & Ysseldyke, J. (1998). *Assessment* (7th ed.). Boston: Houghton Mifflin.

Smith S. W. (2001). Involving parents in the IEP process. *ERIC Clearinghouse on Disabilities and Gifted Education.* (Eric EC Digest #E611). Retrieved on September 5, 2005 from http://ericec.org/digests/e611.htm

U.S. Department of Education. (2005). 34 CFR Parts 300, 301, 304: Assistance to States for the Education of Children with Disabilities: Preschool Grants for Children with Disabilities; and Service Obligations under Special Education–Personnel Development to Improve Services and Results for Children with Disabilities; Proposed Rule. *Federal Register.* Vol. 70, No. 118, June 21, 2005, pp. 35862–35892.

Weiss, C. E. (1980). *Weiss Comprehensive Articulation Test.* Austin, TX: PRO-ED.

Wright, P. W. (2005). *Schaffer v. Weast: How will the decision affect you?* Retrieved on January 4, 2006, from http://www.wrightslaw.com/law/art/schaffer.impact.pwright.htm

Chapter 5

♦ ♦

Intervention and Models of Service Delivery

Jacqueline Meyer,
with Tracy Crouch
and Nanette Clapper

present three quotations as an introduction to this chapter on intervention. The first is a seminal concept from Stark and Wallach reported in Butler over a quarter of a century ago (1980): "The single most significant deterrent to educational growth [of students] remains the inability to use oral and written language, to speak and to read" (p. 6).

The second quote comes from critic Jack Beatty (1985) in an *Atlantic Monthly* review of a work by author Studs Terkel. Beatty describes Terkel this way:

> His social perceptions flow from his literary and musical culture ... Style, language, story, rhythm, voice, tone, laughter: these aesthetic qualities, these properties of language and music, have made him feel more. Feeling more, he sees more. Seeing more, he cares more. The arts and humanities, his example suggests, are the proper stuff of character education. (p. 100)

The third one occurred during a class discussion in a course that included both speech pathology and education majors. The second day of class, a social studies teacher looked at several speech path students and said, "What is it that you people do?"

The long answer to that question is the subject of this chapter; the short one is that SLPs attempt to decrease speech and language deficits so that the students who have been placed in our care can access the glorious stuff of oral and written language, the foundation of character and lifelong education.

You may remember that in the very early days of our field, "speech correctionists" trained teachers how to help students in their classrooms who had "speech problems," most commonly either articulation or fluency deficits. Gradually, however, school speech–language specialists removed students from their classrooms, and the years of our providing itinerant service and pull-out intervention became decades. Since the 1980s, however, new and markedly different ways to deliver intervention have been introduced under a bewildering variety of names, such as collaboration, team teaching, consultation, push-in, pull-aside, inclusion, multiskilling, response to intervention, and curriculum-based instruction. Professionals in our field have been hard pressed to understand the changes inherent in these service delivery models, let alone keep up with them.

My personal experience has led me to adopt two premises regarding service delivery: (a) flexibility is one of the most powerful clinical attributes in providing effective intervention, and (b) the appropriate delivery system is the one that most benefits the student at a specific time. No longer do most school clinicians say that they "consult" or "use pull-out" exclusively. This means that although the pull-out model can be the most efficient type for a student at a particular juncture, a combination of two or even three others may best serve another pupil. To understand the strengths and weaknesses of individual models, we will look at each type in Section 1 of this chapter, with occasional descriptions of specific examples. Section 2 will recount the work of two SLPs, Tracy Crouch and Nanette Clapper, who currently work in the school environment.

Tracy Crouch has been a speech–language professional in the schools for 12 years and is known for her motivating and creative intervention materials and methods. She is an example of the caliber of professionals in our field who have chosen the school as their special place to provide services. Tracy will describe her successful intervention activities with students in the early elementary grades and the philosophical and legal foundations on which they are based. Some examples of her work offer alternatives to intervention suggestions in Figures 5.3 to 5.6 in Section 1. This apparent redundancy is deliberate, a further example that there is no one single way to accomplish a therapeutic goal.

Nanette Clapper, who wrote about authentic assessment in Chapter 3, will discuss motivating and effective procedures she and her colleagues have used with students in Grades 6 through high school. She describes her transition from providing therapy exclusively within the pull-out model to engaging in therapy within the classroom. In addition, she reports the experiences of several other speech–language pathologists who work with students in the upper grades, a quite different teaching environment compared with elementary school. I agree with Kamhi (1999) that the way to justify using an approach is the seemingly simplistic "because it worked" (p. 93). In an article describing the factors that influence the selection of new treatment approaches, Kamhi stated that this reasoning is consistent with research that indicated that teachers (and SLPs) did not generally base their choices on theoretical grounds but adopted a new idea (or service delivery model) when they "saw changes in their students' learning abilities [particularly] when it enhanced performance in difficult-to-teach students" (p. 93).

This chapter will conclude with Section 3, a description of the types of intervention chosen for Zachary, James, and Christine, the cases begun in Chapter 3 and continued in Chapter 4. By the end of this chapter, we will have determined alternate ways to address the Individualized Educational Program (IEP) goals of the first three students. What will be missing, however, are lengthy descriptions of general intervention techniques, such as how to use minimal pairs in articulation intervention or semantic maps to meet language goals, because I am assuming that you have already completed course work in clinical treatment. The specific techniques that are listed were chosen only to illustrate how different service models can affect your choice of approach and materials and vice versa. The ASHA Committee on the Roles and Responsibilities of the School-Based Speech–Language Pathologist underscored this point when it described our field as "dynamic and evolving" and said, "Additional emerging roles or responsibilities should not be precluded from consideration *if* they are based on sound clinical and scientific research, technological developments, and treatment outcomes data" (ASHA, 1999, p. 4).

SECTION 1: TYPES OF SERVICE DELIVERY MODELS

The list that follows is not exhaustive, nor do all professionals agree on the definitions; I have narrowed the number of categories to make the differentiation between them clearer than they probably are in actual practice. My intent is to encourage you to understand and consider the choices you make when you implement IEP goals. You should be aware that in addition to our field, many of these models are used in the schools by occupational and physical therapists, school psychologists, and learning disability and reading specialists. Further, there are different perspectives concerning not only the most appropriate model in a given situation, but also the role of the speech–language professional within that model (Prelock, 2000). Types of service delivery models include the following.

- Pull-out intervention provides intermittent direct services. Speech and language services are provided as supplementary services to regular or special education programs. Intervention may be aimed at an individual student or a group of students. Typically, the students scheduled into a group session exhibit similar communication disorders (e.g., language, articulation, fluency, and voice; Neidecker & Blosser, 1993, p. 187). ASHA's 2000 Schools Survey, an update to a similar survey undertaken in 1995, reports that this traditional service delivery model "continues to be the most commonly used model … in the school setting … an average of 23 hours providing services [out of 26] per week" (ASHA, 2000, p. 1).
- Consultative (indirect) intervention provides information to regular education teachers to assist in adjusting the learning environment and modifying their instructional methods to meet the individual needs of a pupil with a handicapping condition who attends their classes (New York Board of Regents, 1988). Several disorders discussed in Chapter 6 reflect the extension of our intervention activities into the classroom. This model is most closely associated with the therapeutic approach adopted by Ehren, who differentiates between the teacher's role of instruction, "the activity that occurs in the normal course of the school day," and the role of the SLP, who provides intervention or, in the role of consultant, makes specific suggestions for the teacher "when typical instruction is insufficient for a particular student to achieve mastery in language that is required in the curriculum" (Ehren, 2000, pp. 220–221).
- Collaboration: The definition most widely accepted is from Idol, Paolucci-Whitcomb, and Nevin (1986): "Collaboration is an interactive process that enables people with diverse expertise to generate creative solutions to mutually defined problems. It enhances the outcome and produces solutions that are different from those that the individual team members would produce independently. It provides effective programs for students with needs within the most appropriate context, thereby enabling them to achieve maximum constructive interaction with their non handicapped peers" (p. 1).
- Team teaching can be defined as a synonym for collaboration, but it can also refer to a system in which two teachers share students. They prepare lessons independently, often divided along subject lines. For example, one instructor teaches math and the other language arts. In the case in which a speech–language pathologist team-teaches with a classroom

teacher, one may "take over" the whole class for an assignment, or they may teach a single lesson at the same time. In either case, team teaching "emphasizes the use of naturalistic environments and meaningful contexts" (Miller, 1989, p. 155).

• Self-contained language class: In this case, the speech–language pathologist or special education teacher is the primary teacher and offers intense intervention on a continual basis within the context of the curricula. At the younger level, the classrooms are often developmentally based, as in a pre-first transitional class. Other students may be served in a special language course for students who are hearing impaired at the high school level. Self-contained classes may also include cross-categorical groups, such as a mixture of students whose conditions (e.g., autism or a cognitive impairment) all require language intervention.

• Multiskilling: This term, more commonly applied to the health care field, refers to a single professional who is cross trained to "provide more than one function, often in more than one discipline" (Pietranton & Lynch, 1995, p. 38). What is different about this model compared with others we have discussed is that a person so designated could replace another professional. For example, a "'rehab specialist' could practice across multiple scopes of practice, [including] speech–language pathology, occupational therapy and physical therapy" (Pietranton & Lynch, 1995, p. 40). Multiskilling is often suggested as a means of saving money.

• Inclusion represents a philosophy of valuing diversity by educating students who have disabilities within the regular education program; this includes their having access not only to the classroom but to other facilities and extracurricular activities, as well. Buschbacher and Fox (2003) state that "the inclusion movement in education, work, and community living is based on the notion that individuals with disabilities have a fundamental right to access normal patterns of learning, working, and living that should not be compromised because of the disability" (p. 218). The disabilities may be severe, and the children who are included under this model may be challenged in ways that heretofore have rarely been seen in the typical classroom. Chapter 8, "Augmentative and Alternative Communication in School Settings," contains related information on the topic of inclusion, as does the section of Chapter 12 dealing with physical and occupational therapy. Remember that intervention is also an integral part of the concept of authentic assessment discussed in Chapter 3. Many of the service delivery models described above can include authentic assessment and intervention, although it may not be mentioned specifically in the examples.

• Prevention: Although it is not a service delivery model, the role of the school-based SLP has extended beyond diagnosis and intervention to include disseminating information that will "avoid or minimize the onset or development of communication disorders and their causes" (ASHA, 1999, p. 16). The IDEA revisions of 2004 specifically include authority for local educational agencies to use some of their local IDEA moneys to provide early intervention services, the intent of which is to reduce or eliminate the future need for special education. Under the rubrics of primary, secondary, and tertiary prevention, emphasis in the schools includes, but is not limited to, disseminating information to parents, educational personnel, and policy-making bodies in settings that can range from individual conferences to school- or district-wide in-service presentations. Ways to foster early literacy or prevent vocal abuse are typical examples. Prevention also includes early detection and treatment, even if the disorder of the student in question is not considered severe enough to warrant a label—for example, providing fluency-enhancing strategies for a suspected developing stutterer.

Rationales for New Intervention Types

Why have all of these service delivery models appeared? Has something changed to make the pull-out mode not as desirable? In a word, yes. Pressure for change has come from a number of sources and for a number of reasons. Let us look first at some general reasons for altering the ways intervention is being provided in the school environment (Eger, 1992; Farber & Klein, 1999; Huffman, 1992):

- Changing school populations have resulted in a far more varied caseload. Consider first just the number and variety of cultures in the schools compared with 25 years ago. In addition to the likelihood that more students will be at risk, ponder the other stresses on family life that changing demographics and a volatile economy can produce. Think about the possible speech and language implications of autism or cerebral palsy for students who are now part of the regular classroom for the first time. Be careful, however, that you do not ascribe results to reasons without research to substantiate your conclusions. Often it is not easy to sort out cause and effect in language disorders. Let us suppose that Jason watches TV nonstop and rarely engages in conversation. Does he not talk because he was so entranced by television that he did not practice enough, or did he turn to TV because he had language deficits? Both? Neither?

- Diminishing or limited economic resources serving many sectors of our society have had one sure effect: less funding. Taxpayers are demanding results, and specialists' services have become suspect. The people who pay the bills, and their school board member representatives, are demanding a person who can wear more than one hat or at the very least can engage in cooperative endeavors with a variety of other professionals.

- As the general field of education has undergone changes, new buzz words have appeared in a climate of out with the old, in with the new. How members of our profession deal with such trends as site-based, total-quality, or outcome-based management; the whole-language and "no child left behind" movements; charter schools; curriculum-based learning; the National Outcomes Measurement System (NOMS); and increased use of high-tech equipment will determine whether we will have a real role in the larger educational community.

• Almost all states have instituted standards-based reform (Silliman, Bahr, Beasman, & Wilkinson, 2000). At the time this edition was written, the federal government had also weighed into the standards issue, demanding that all schools be held accountable for their students' performance, including those with special needs. Many schools will look to professionals in our field to help formulate remediation plans for students who are "low" but not labeled.

Pressure for changes has also specifically affected our profession:

• The knowledge base that speech–language pathologists are expected to have has exploded. The contents of Chapters 3 and 4 barely scrape the surface. Our field remains one that educates our newest members as generalists, but clearly there is too much to absorb and remember. Consequently, we must learn to rely on other professionals to share some of our load, and that usually means working in teams of one sort or another.

• We are required to prove the connection between language deficits and problems in school, plus demonstrate how intervention can both improve academic performance and enhance our students' ability to function productively in society (i.e., outcomes-based assessment and intervention).

• As we work with other professionals, we must be willing either to translate our terms into ones used in the educational world or to adopt theirs. Syntax may have precise meaning for us but not necessarily for the art teacher. Formal in-service presentations and informal sharing of information will be an increasing, regular part of our academic year, because there is a critical need for shared understanding of instructional purposes.

• The ability to work effectively with colleagues from different professional backgrounds is no longer just desirable, it is absolutely necessary. This means understanding curriculum as well as instructional and therapeutic techniques aimed at larger and more varied groups of students. In Chapter 12, representatives from those fields allow us to gain new perspectives.

• We must acknowledge and accept the responsibility that continual postgraduate education is a necessity in cutting-edge areas like assistive technology. ASHA's new rules for continuing certification presented in Chapter 2, enacted since the first edition of the text, are a formal acknowledgment of this fact. Many states also now require a minimum number of continuing education hours before renewing an SLP's educational certification or professional licensure.

• Because the law requires that students with handicapping conditions must receive services in the least restrictive environment, we must be prepared to develop and justify alternate modes of service delivery rather than to rely routinely on the pull-out model. If the pull-out model *is* the best choice, we have to prove why using it is in the best interests of the student.

• Research within our field has sensitized us to the needs of children who may not appear obviously at risk for a speech–language disorder. These include children who do not seem to have language problems but who score poorly on reading tasks (Hill & Haynes, 1992), as well as some students Launer (quoted in Paul, 1995, p. 478) refers to as "porpoise kids": children who can compensate in earlier grades, but whose language deficits come to the surface when the amount and complexity of work markedly increase in upper-level classes.

• Increasing numbers of students qualify for speech–language services, and there is a chronic shortage of speech–language pathologists in many areas.

• Research has shown that early language problems, translated into later learning problems, follow students through adolescence and into adulthood (Hall & Tomblin, 1978). As discussed in Chapter 7, this is particularly apparent in reading, writing, and spelling tasks.

Factors Affecting the Choice of Specific Service Delivery Models

Deciding which service delivery model best addresses the needs of a specific student is a complex task. The following descriptions of how various models work in the classroom will give added insight into factors that will govern your choice. The models include consultation, collaboration, team teaching, pull-out therapy, self-contained class intervention, multiskilling, and inclusion. The theme approach, which can be applied to many of the models, will be examined also.

Consultation

I have listed this category first, because I think that all models include consultation to some degree. I concur with Zins et al. (quoted in Curtis & Meyers, 1985, p. 35), who stated, "Consultation represents the foundation on which alternative services delivery systems are based. It is the problem solving process through which students' needs are clarified and appropriate strategies for intervention are developed and implemented." Although the authors of that article are school psychologists, all specialists now concur that consultation enhances the effectiveness of any type of intervention in the schools. It does so by improving classroom teachers' understanding of the serious educational implications of different conditions, as well as increasing their skills in addressing them within the regular class. In our particular field, generalization of consultation benefits to nonlabeled students has led to improved long-term academic performance (Roller, Rodriquez, Warner, & Lindahl, 1992).

The term *consultation* is used so loosely, however, that you should always look carefully at what authors mean when they are encouraging its use in our field. It can include everything from giving information to a teacher while providing no direct intervention, to the fully collaborative model explained under the heading "Collaboration" in this book. It can also vary from a situation in which one specialist assumes the role of expert (i.e., the advice giver) to one in which consultant and consultee roles shift back and forth depending on the situation.

In one of my earliest attempts at consulting, I assumed that I was the "expert." With a number of children on my caseload in her first-grade class, I planned to give Karen, their teacher, the benefit of my training in language diagnosis and intervention, and often I did. One day, however, I was presenting a language enrichment lesson to the entire class using an "art" component that required scissors, glue sticks, and so on. I carefully handed out the materials and began giving directions, but because the children were horsing around with all the neat stuff I had given them, they barely heard my instructions. In the most tactful of tones, Karen commented later, "Jackie, with first graders it's usually better to give directions before you hand out materials." As the months passed, I learned from Karen and Marie and Ann (first grade) and Cindy and Michelle (second grade) how to handle groups of 25 or more children with vastly varying abilities; what first-, second-, and third-grade children were expected to learn during those critical years; and the importance of providing seat work so that class members not involved in my group could continue learning. And I had to do this without losing sight of the goals I had set for "my" students. In short, I learned what Montgomery (1992) meant when she said, "The practice setting for a school based speech language specialist is the world of education" (p. 364).

Based on this insight, here is but one example of information from our professional background that I shared with those same elementary school teachers: The reason some students were not completing spelling assignments correctly was that the directions in their spelling books were too syntactically complex. How to deal with it? By explaining to the teacher what constitutes syntactic complexity and then demonstrating how to simplify unintentionally difficult classroom material.

I have included this example because if I had not been present in her classroom, I would never have considered addressing this issue, nor would the teacher have thought to ask me. Nelson and Kinnucan-Welsch (1992) presented verbatim comments transcribed from audiotaped interviews with school speech–language pathologists that detail their experiences and personal reactions to collaboration. The entire issue of *Language, Speech, and Hearing Services in the Schools* (Volume 31, No. 3) in July 2000 is devoted to rationales and descriptions of six different types of in-class collaboration. Tracy Crouch and Nanette Clapper contribute detailed descriptions of the collaborative process in the real world you are entering in Section 2 of this chapter.

With IDEA's continuing emphasis on curriculum-based intervention, collaboration in some form has become a given. In my personal experience, it opened exciting opportunities to expand my professional expertise. In addition to learning specific information about the classroom, I discovered that effective consulting was based on certain suppositions. Those that follow are not listed in order of importance because they are equally valuable:

- The consultee must feel free to accept, reject, or adjust any of the consultant's ideas. With shifting roles, this is particularly important; for consultation to work, coercion cannot be part of the mix.

- The consultant's and the consultee's ideas should receive equal consideration.

- Partners (or team members) must really listen to each other, not just wait for a pause in the dialogue to insert their own ideas. If the members of a team are from different sociocultural backgrounds, potential differences in interpersonal style may complicate interchanges. Because you are the professional who has had training in the effect of cultural differences on communication, expect to take the lead in dealing with this issue.

- Confidentiality must be an accepted part of any planning meeting. The teachers' lunchroom is no place to air the details of a conference. All team members must feel free to throw out ideas spontaneously without worrying about being quoted in an unflattering light later.

- Consider both short- and long-term goals. Although the primary intent of collaboration is an agreement on goals and techniques to address a specific student's deficits, a secondary consideration is to improve the ability of both colleagues to respond more effectively to a similar situation at some future time—our old friend generalization, or in the new parlance, dynamic assessment and intervention.

- Schedule *regular* meetings to review progress and to adjust goals and techniques as necessary. The two school-based co-authors of this chapter stress this point. According to Curtis and Zins (1981), initially a specialist's role is often determined more by what others expect than by what they desire. This is very important when you consider the third quotation at the beginning of this chapter: "What is it that you people do?" Many teachers and administrators have a very fuzzy idea indeed of our job as SLPs, often equating our field exclusively with articulation deficits. Finding the time to do this in busy schedules is a major hurdle to overcome.

- Implementing the results of consultation implies that administrators have agreed to abide by them. It is usually the case that the "specialist" bears the brunt of explaining the concept of consultation to people in charge, so be prepared to do so, particularly if this service delivery model is a new program in your school. Tactfully reviewing the legal requirements of IDEA may be necessary.

- If consultation is a relatively new concept in your school, do not emphasize how dissimilar it is from the present program; comparing its similarities to familiar procedures will help speed acceptance. Change is more likely to occur if manageable objectives are chosen that allow participants to blend new ideas with existing practices (Crais, 1992).

- As goals are discussed, but before they are implemented, you should clarify the problem and the objectives, explore the resources available, and evaluate and choose among alternatives (Curtis & Meyers, 1985).

- After implementation, evaluating approach effectiveness is necessary. Regardless of the delivery system, accountability still means proving that intervention using these new procedures leads to superior results.

Figure 5.1 is based on the work of Nancy Huffman: Duplicating this as a handout can be a good introduction to the within-the-classroom collaborative model for teachers and administrators.

In addition, the following adaptation from Christensen and Luckett (1990) can serve as a checklist of 10 steps for presenting an oral language lesson to a class:

1. careful planning;
2. classroom discipline;
3. teacher involvement;
4. a good lesson plan;
5. effective follow-up activities;
6. keeping good records of your IEP targeted student performance;
7. being on time for class; most classroom teachers keep very tight schedules;
8. providing the classroom teacher with several backup activities in case an emergency causes you to miss the class;
9. involving the classroom teacher in active participation during your presentation; and
10. asking the classroom teacher to critique your presentation, particularly if lessons involving the whole class are new to you; consultation can also include roles that do not stress the collaboration described above.

---

1. SLP co-teaches a subject area with a classroom teacher. This engages both in curriculum analysis, facilitating an increased awareness that all areas have language components.
2. SLP accompanies student or class to physical education, music, or art to work on following directions, positional concepts, and basic concept development.
3. SLP accompanies a student to a work-study site to reinforce communication abilities with less familiar people or strangers.
4. SLP becomes involved with a long-term language arts project, such as a class newspaper, pen-pal relationship with another classroom, poll taking, or letter writing for persuasion or information.
5. SLP is in classroom during free play to foster or manage peer communication, turn taking, and social skills for targeted children.
6. SLP can teach or practice wh concepts with classroom teacher. Students can interview each other, practicing wh questions and publish a "Who's Who" book as a classroom project.
7. SLP can co-teach a telephone communication unit, including rules for use, behavior, sequencing, taking messages, appropriate conversation, and so forth.
8. SLP can work with teacher to develop materials to augment classroom instruction, such as experience stories, game boards, picture stories, augmentative communication books and boards.
9. SLP preteaches social communication skills that would be appropriate at a restaurant, store, or museum where a field trip is planned.

Note. From N. P. Huffman, 1992, *ASHA, 34*(11). Copyright 1992 by the American Speech-Language-Hearing Association. Reprinted with permission.

Figure 5.1. Mediating speech–language–hearing competence: arenas of action for the speech–language pathologist.

Be aware that not all SLPs agree on what role they should assume in the classroom. Ehren (2000) makes a clear distinction between the role of the teacher and the role of a therapist. She sees the therapist at one end of a continuum in which "therapy is a very specific, more intensive type of intervention, requiring focused expertise of the provider in the area of language and language disorders" (p. 221). The teacher, on the other hand, provides instruction or "teaching that occurs in the normal course of events in a school curriculum" (p. 220). This does not necessarily mean that all instruction of either type is provided within the classroom setting. Wherever the intervention occurs, however, it should be built around or supplement the information being taught in the classroom. Therefore, although SLPs must know curricular content, they teach learning strategies that apply to the language deficits in any content area, rather than reviewing content-specific information. In short, curricula becomes the context for acquiring language strategies, not an end in itself.

Figure 5.2 features an example of a letter written by Tracy Crouch that can introduce the collaborative model to teachers in your school. Providing a written outline can allow your colleagues some time to consider the possibilities of the approach without having to respond immediately to your request.

Service delivery models can also include roles that do not stress the collaboration described above. The following represent only a few of the many hats you may wear:

- If you are a part of a district's diagnostic team, your results may be presented in a report, and although you may meet with teachers, most probably it will not be on a continuing basis; you, personally, may never work directly with the student.

Dear _____ ,

Greetings from your speech–language pathologist. I am looking forward to working together this year. As you may know, I am in the process of developing an intervention program to meet the needs of the students in your classroom who need speech and language services. In order to do this most effectively, I am asking for your help. Attached is a copy of the classroom planning sheet I have developed as a guideline for planning curriculum-based activities for the students. One of the ways we will implement the plan is to use a "push-in" model. Unfortunately, because of our busy schedules, I am not able to sit down and plan with each of the teachers of my students, but I am very interested in your ideas. Therefore, I am asking you to fill out the attached form. This is not meant to be a time-consuming task for you. Although I will be placing one in your box each week, if you choose to fill it out on a monthly or biweekly basis, that is fine. Please do whatever is easiest for you. Once you have filled it out, you can drop it in my mailbox or stop by my room. I always welcome your visit. If you have any questions, please do not hesitate to ask. I am looking forward to another wonderful year of working with you doing what we do best: putting children first and foremost so that great things happen!

Fondly,
Tracy Crouch

Figure 5.2. Introductory letter to teachers.

- As a school speech–language pathologist, you may apply your general expertise to adapting mainstream materials so they are appropriate for a labeled student or adapting intervention materials for classroom use, as in making changes in level, curricular area, material, equipment, input–output mode, or skill–sequence rules (Schuh, Tashie, & Jorgensen, 1981).
- After observing the interaction between student and teacher in the classroom environment, you may make suggestions addressing a mismatch of teaching and learning styles.
- As an "expert" in a specific area, you may educate parents about preschool language development and the importance of developing preliteracy skills or teach organizational strategies to middle school students with language impairments.
- You may provide information about a specific disability (e.g., Asperger's syndrome) to teachers and administrators either individually or through in-service presentations.
- You may present in-service training to teachers or other speech–language professionals on augmentative communication (Haney, 1992; Light & McNaughton, 1993), developing listening skills (Dollaghan & Kaston, 1986; Edwards, 1991), or dysphagia.
- You may demonstrate how computers can be used to implement IEP goals (Cochran & Masterson, 1995; Masterson, 1995; McGuire, 1995).

Conversely, another professional may acquaint you with information concerning a new reading series or teach you the basic curricular content of second-grade mathematics and science. It is time again for the reminder that when you begin intervention, you have not left assessment behind. Each time you evaluate the effect of intervention on a student's skills, you make a decision what to do next: continue without change, move "up" or "down," or embark on another goal. These decisions should be reflected in daily notes as part of your accountability procedures.

In sum, then, what are the advantages of language intervention provided within the regular classroom environment? Most commonly cited are cost effectiveness; extended opportunity for labeled students to practice pragmatic objectives; increased relevance of speech and language goals to the curriculum; enhanced generalization; and heightened teacher understanding of student language goals, the techniques and procedures used by speech–language professionals, and the overall impact of language on learning (Eger, 1992; Masterson, 1993; Nelson & Kinnucan-Welsch, 1992; Silliman et al., 2000). Goodman (1986) stated that language intervention presented in the classroom is easier to learn because it has a discernible purpose and is inherently more interesting, relevant, "whole," and part of a real event. In a series of articles on collaboration by school speech–language professionals, the practitioners all point to the presence of language learning throughout the day; unexpected, increased gains in student language skills; and the chance to use a writing process approach as an integrated part of a student's literature, science, and social studies course material (Borsch & Oaks, 1992; Brandel, 1992; Ferguson, 1992; Montgomery, 1992; Roller et al., 1992).

Other authors (Hoskins, 1990a, 1990b; Marvin, 1987; Simon, 1987; Simon & Myrold-Gunyuz, 1990) have cited additional advantages of collaboration: enabling the speech–language specialist and the classroom teacher to identify and teach speech and language skills critical for academic success; preventing future speech and language problems by serving whole classrooms of students; and addressing all students' cognitive and linguistic disabilities, developmental language problems, and social communication skills. ASHA (1991) has also provided helpful guidelines for the school-based collaborative service delivery model. Being familiar with these advantages gives you the means to counter automatic "knee-jerk" arguments against collaboration.

Are there disadvantages to consultation and collaboration? Elksnin and Capilouto (1994) reported that survey results of 31 school speech–language professionals listed these potential negatives: the need for additional hard-to-come-by planning time, increased paperwork, difficulty in scheduling, IEP goals that were hard to incorporate into these models, possible lack of individualization, possible boredom or lower expectation on the part of the "typical" students, addressing difficult behavior problems in large groups of students, and dealing with a different teaching philosophy or an uncooperative teacher. You should be aware that some of these factors were reported by speech–language pathologists who had never actually adopted the new models.

Disadvantages noted by classroom teachers may affect your ability to convince them of the advantages and efficacy of new modes of delivery: perceived lack of planning time, decreased instructional time, "invasion" of territory, and the fear that higher-level students would become bored. Other sources have reported that parents may have difficulty accepting that individual pull-out sessions are not necessarily more valuable than sessions that take place in the classroom (Eger, 1992). According to Sanger, Hux, and Griess (1995), educational professionals questioned whether speech–language specialists were prepared to deal with problems like behavior management, reading and writing issues, and English as a second language. Other authors have warned that teachers may become uneasy because "good oral language interaction can often be very noisy" (Christensen & Luckett, 1990, p. 111). They have also stressed that if the regular education teacher is not directly involved in "your" language lesson, your presence can serve as an excuse to run an errand or use the Xerox machine.

Some administrators may also prefer to stay with the way things have been done before, particularly when state and federal laws dictate conditions under which intervention should be provided. On the other hand, Guilford (1993), a supervisor of a speech–language–hearing program, stated, "In my experience staff know that there is a need for change [in service delivery models] spurred on by the increasing number of students who qualify for speech language services and the chronic shortage of SLPs. However, they want the changes to occur for other people—not them" (p. 63). Change is harder for some people than others, but it is a fact of life in our field. If you are just beginning your career as a speech–language specialist, try to accept "Thou shalt not become rigid" as the Eleventh Commandment. Nelson and Kinnucan-Welsch (1992) stated, "The cycles of unlearning and relearning are uncomfortable, but the discomfort is essential" (p. 47). In a sense, your status as a novice in the field is an advantage; you do not have as much to unlearn as some of the rest of us.

Conoley and Conoley (1982) also have some words of assurance: You do not have to consult in every single classroom. If this concept is unfamiliar or scares you, pick only one or two teachers at first, preferably those with whom you have the best rapport. Encourage them to be honest about what they feel the two of you can realistically accomplish in a collaborative endeavor. At first, be willing to serve in a capacity in which you will be least disruptive to the classroom routine, such as assisting your students during a classroom writing lesson. Be flexible about scheduling; perhaps you could start by being in the classroom only once a week. Here is an editorial comment from an issue of *Word of Mouth* that you may want to hang on your wall: "We ... need to be kinder with ourselves for not being an expert on everything. That's the reason team intervention exists. There is too much to know these days for everybody to be good at everything. We can rely on others for knowledge that we have not yet obtained. And regardless of the criticism that others may have when we don't know something, it makes people feel good to believe they can teach somebody something" (Editorial Comments, 1995, p. 10). Amen and amen.

Collaboration

As you have probably deduced by now, collaboration relies heavily on the consultation model described above. In fact, some authors use the term *collaborative consultation* (Russell & Kaderavek, 1993). I have separated the two terms because while consultation does not necessarily require at least two professionals working closely over an extended period of time, collaboration always does. Russell and Kaderavek stressed that although cooperation is the goal of coordinated service delivery in the schools, in practice this theoretical construct is "not necessarily evident in the actual practice of the model" (p. 76). They suggested that peer coaching and co-teaching are possible solutions to the barriers of the hierarchical relationship that often exist between consultants and classroom teachers and the consequent negative attitude that develops because of it. As noted previously, it is not uncommon for teachers to consider their classrooms their kingdoms and resent any interference with their right and obligation to teach as they see fit. Not infrequently, teachers want you to take children, "fix" them, and then return them to their tutelage. Collaborative models are designed to diminish that desire.

In the peer coaching model, the speech–language professional and the classroom teacher both model techniques for each other; neither is superior. This model involves (a) a preobservation conference, (b) the actual intervention, and finally (c) the postobservation conference (Schmidt & Rodgers-Rhyme, 1988, cited in Russell & Kaderavek, 1993, p. 76). I hope this reminds you of some of the assessment steps described in Chapter 3. The peer teaching model fits particularly well if the teacher has been the source of the referral because in that case the observation part of the peer coaching process has been started, and a working relationship has already been established. Discussion may focus on possible adaptations of curricular material by the classroom teacher, or, as Ehren (2000) suggests, teaching curriculum vocabulary by focusing on affixes, metaphors, or idioms. After therapeutic intervention has taken place, its effectiveness is evaluated, and, based on that, further plans are developed. Co-teaching differs from team teaching (see below) in that the classroom teacher plans activities that address curriculum goals, and the SLP incorporates communication objectives into those goals. Therefore, the two professionals together develop both curricular and language intervention goals, plan the activities, implement them, and then evaluate their students' progress.

Team Teaching

The name of this model can be used as a synonym for collaboration, but it can also refer to a system in regular education in which two teachers share students. They prepare lessons independently, usually divided along subject lines: For example, one sixth-grade teacher instructs all math lessons, and the other sixth-grade teacher instructs all language arts activities. In the case in which a speech–language pathologist team teaches with a classroom teacher, the SLP may take over the whole class for a period or they may both be involved in teaching a single lesson at the same time. In either case, team teaching "emphasizes the use of naturalistic environments and meaningful contexts" (Miller, 1989, p. 155). A speech–language pathologist can also team-teach with a special educator or a learning disabilities specialist to help increase awareness that all subjects have a language component (Eger, 1992). He or she can accompany students to classes in physical education, art, music, computers, or industrial arts to work on following directions, positional concepts, and basic concept development within the context of the subject. An example of this is described in articles by Ellis, Schlaudecker, and Griess (1995a, 1995b). Physical education teachers, the classroom instructor, and the SLP incorporated the teaching of basic concepts into a kindergarten PE class that emphasized the 28 most missed concepts on the *Boehm Test of Basic Concepts* (3rd ed.; Boehm, 2000). The program ran for 8 weeks, and the students received 30 minutes of concept instruction each week by the classroom teacher or a speech–language pathologist. The activities were often suggested by the speech–language pathologist. An additional 30-minute physical education period integrated the concept into the regular P.E. curriculum (e.g., throwing a ball to the "first person in line").

I team-taught a class one period a week with Marty, a seventh- and eighth-grade social studies teacher. Our experience illustrates the many, often unanticipated, ways that a single program can address a variety of goals and the needs of a group of students. Marty was concerned that "my kids" never expressed any opinions during class discussions. (Note that teachers will often bestow on you ownership for students you see, sometimes giving you credit for their improvement but also holding you at least partly responsible for any behavioral lapses.) When I considered the three students who were in Marty's class, I was not surprised that they did not venture an opinion. First, their language deficits and limited cultural literacy precluded their being aware of current events. One of Marty's questions concerned the demolition of the Berlin wall. None of my students had any idea where Berlin was, let alone the historical significance of the wall that had divided the east and west portions of the city. Typically, students with language learning disabilities do not, or cannot, read *Time* magazine or a newspaper, and they avoid watching national news on television altogether.

Marty and I planned a year-long program designed to teach students how to state, substantiate, and defend opinions. Students with limited language skills are usually asked lower-level questions, which, as classified in Bloom's taxonomy (Bloom, Engelhart, Furst, Hill, & Krathwohl, 1956), test only knowledge or comprehension. Consequently, labeled students frequently have little opportunity to answer the type of questions that will be increasingly required in middle and high school and found on statewide tests. The program, called What's Your Opinion?, helped students develop and practice the language of evaluation as a natural part of successful communication in the classroom. Several opinion questions were presented weekly, one as a basis for oral discussion and the other requiring a written response. At first, the questions were general, and students did not need to have read widely or "be smart" to answer them—for example, whether school should be in session year-round, or what the best bad-for-you junk food was. Later questions, however, related directly to the seventh-grade social studies syllabus, such as whether we should return land to Native Americans that had been unfairly taken from them in the past. Written answers were graded and counted as a completed assignment, and detailed comments were included with every assignment handed back. As the students' skill increased, they were required to use textbooks, the newspaper, *Junior Scholastic*, and similar sources to gather background and supporting arguments. Cooperative learning groups were frequently used, with labeled students placed in heterogeneous, not homogeneous, teams. Class sessions were regularly videotaped. I will discuss how this program related to other modes of delivery in the "Pull-Out Intervention" section later in this chapter.

One of the most motivating features of What's Your Opinion? was the role of the camera. Each week after written opinions were completed, six students were chosen by lot. Copies of their opinions were typed, individually framed, and placed on a bulletin board in the front hall of the school next to their photographs. The camera work was done by three other students who were credited for their photographic talent. During the second semester, the students also created opinion questions for second graders, an opportunity to practice the metalinguistic skill of adjusting language for students younger than themselves.

The program was originally instituted as a way to assist the labeled, mainstreamed student. Almost immediately, however, it became clear that every class member was a beneficiary. This was particularly true for the students who usually "slip through the cracks"—those who were not severely impaired enough to be labeled but whose limited language skills made classroom interchanges difficult for them. Last, the program represented a structured, natural way for an SLP to introduce IEP goals to the middle school teachers.

It is instructive to read the following guidelines that Marty and I created for the program because they speak so clearly to the shared nature of our collaborative endeavor. They also reflect the careful planning that is always at the heart of effective teaching and intervention:

- Regardless of ability, all students will contribute opinions during discussions as well as through written assignments.
- Both the SLP and the classroom teacher will be supportive and encouraging, even when neither agrees with the students' responses.
- Teachers will restate or clarify opinions as necessary, so that all group members can follow the direction of the discussion.
- Conversations should be as free-flowing as possible; strict adherence to "raise your hand before speaking" will not be required.
- All groups will be heterogeneous, and only rarely will cooperative learning groups be formed other than by random selection.
- When background information is to be given by one of the teachers, written outlines will be used to limit "lecture" time.
- Even when the topic is serious, the tone of the classroom will be as light as possible within the parameters of appropriate classroom behavior.
- Before each completed written assignment is returned, detailed written reactions by the teacher or specialist will be added to it.
- As much as possible, the opinion questions will feature the current week's curriculum topic.
- Each student will be encouraged to use the word-processing program on the classroom computer, a Polaroid or digital camera, and video-taping equipment.

As a result of this program, students gained skill in thinking of, formulating, and answering questions that required evaluation, the highest level of thought in Bloom's taxonomy. Students also learned to support their opinions with cogent reasons and to appreciate the ideas of others, even if they did not agree with them. They learned skills in interviewing and use of the word processor and camera as tools. They also discovered ways to find and record facts as they listened to or read background information, and they gained increased awareness of the larger world around them. Finally, they applied these new skills directly to the seventh-grade social studies curriculum in the presence of their typical classmates, thereby addressing both the New York State English Language Arts Standard for the social use of language and one section of the Social Studies Standard. In a pull-out program, they would have had little opportunity to do this.

From my point of view as an SLP, I found myself entering into a new phase of my career. I helped develop a list entitled "14 Steps to Nurture Independent Research" and practiced using "anticipatory set" to gain student attention at the beginning of a lesson. I relearned the Bill of Rights, who first circumnavigated the globe, and the constitutional powers of the governor of New York State. In addition, I discovered how to present this information in an interesting fashion to 28 seventh graders at 8:30 A.M., first period in the morning, something Marty had been doing that period plus six periods more a day for years.

One of the criticisms of the team-teaching model from speech–language pathologists is that they fear losing their sense of identity: They worry that they will become a tutor or a teacher's aide, not the specialist they have worked so hard and for so many years to be (Ehren, 2000). I think that is why the collaborative aspect of team teaching is so important. Each professional brings to the discussion the richness of his or her training and experience. We bring background, focus, and training in evaluating and instructing in the area of language development, including the specific effect of language difficulties on school performance and social behaviors. We have the ability to perform task analyses that will facilitate school performance and a keen understanding of the overlapping roles of listening, speaking, reading, and writing across all content areas. We have an acute awareness of how individual differences can affect learning and the role motivation plays in language learning (Wadle, 1991).

I would add that we also recognize the implication of such concepts as school "scripts" and the role of pragmatics on the nonacademic performance of the student, which, if deficient, can be utterly devastating. You may not consider yourself an expert on the effect of multicultural differences on the school population after you read Chapter 9, but you will probably know more than many educators do. What team teaching and collaboration are all about is how to apply this knowledge to the needs of a particular student, at the same time sharing the information with colleagues whose training is different from our own.

Let us consider these two oral sequencing goals: "By April 2004, Benjamin will sequence four items in a logical order without assistance, as measured by a 30% improvement on the _____ test" versus "By April 2004, Benjamin will be able to retell four events in correct order from a story in his fourth-grade literature book so that he can take part in his classroom oral book reports" (Montgomery, 1992, p. 363). Obviously, the second goal will assist Benjamin in the classroom in a way that the first one might not. I hope that it is equally clear that speech–language pathologists must understand the requirements of the classroom environment before they will be capable of writing pertinent goals.

Pull-Out Intervention

Usually speech–pathology students are familiar with this mode of service because it is the one used in the majority of university speech and hearing clinics, and, as stated previously, it is still the most common service delivery model in the school setting (ASHA, 2000). As part of your clinical courses, you have probably written lesson plans for individual clients or members of small groups. Secord (1989) listed these as advantages of the pull-out model: It allows for highly structured training, and you are free to use a variety of approaches to learning without being concerned whether they will fit in with a lesson or be appropriate for other students. You can preteach a topic or vocabulary well in advance of the time it will be used in the classroom. If you have discovered a basic weakness, you can address it immediately and directly without linking it to the curriculum. Thus, the pull-out model allows very focused, intense intervention and may be the mode of choice when your student requires much repetition or when the presence of other students would be detrimental.

Criticizing one's own performance is often difficult for a student who has a language-based learning disability, and therefore the privacy inherent in a pull-out session can be a distinct advantage. When I wrote down errors observed during classroom conversational exchanges and pointed them out to students later, they frequently argued, "I didn't say [or do] that!" During my discussion of team teaching in Marty's seventh-grade social studies class, you may remember that I referred to videotaping the cooperative learning groups. Later, in follow-up pull-out intervention sessions, my students and I reviewed those tapes to identify examples of good and poor topic maintenance, eye contact, body language, and sequencing during classroom discussions. In addition, we often examined how effectively the student used pragmatic "rules" to substantiate an opinion, defend his or her own point of view, and identify weakness in his or her own and others' opinion statements. Prior to this program, my students' typical response to a classmate's opinion was "That's [or you're] stupid!"—guaranteed to be fighting words in the seventh grade. It appeared easier for students to identify and criticize their own inappropriate responses when they could point to a videotaped image. In some way it created a necessary buffer: They were criticizing the image, not themselves.

Using pull-out intervention is also preferable when you must teach a student how to produce a phoneme for the first time by employing a mirror or an implement near a student's mouth. An older student may find this procedure humiliating if it is performed in the presence of a classmate. Being embarrassed is one of the chief reasons that older students do not like the pull-aside model in the regular classroom. Adolescence is a time when few students like to be seen as different. The disadvantages of this mode of service were covered under the earlier "Rationales" section as the advantages of models depending on classroom interactions.

Self-Contained Language Class

Some speech–language pathologists prefer this model over all others because they can spend hours a day with the same students, continually addressing their deficits as an integral part of every subject. Usually, the class is limited in size, so caseloads are often far smaller than average. If the class represents full-time placement, the speech–language pathologist in most states must also possess elementary (or secondary) classroom certification. In some schools, a speech–language specialist spends a half day in a kindergarten or pre-first class and the remainder of the day working with additional students, using other service delivery models.

Larson, McKinley, and Boley (1993) described a for-credit high school language course that is offered at the same time as other classes; it focuses on remediating deficits in thinking, listening, speaking, reading, and writing skills to enable the student to succeed not only in academic situations but in social and vocational ones, as well. The authors stated that assigning academic credit provides motivation and incentive for student participation. Another similar course addresses study and organizational skills; depending on the district, speech–language pathologists, special education teachers, or learning disabilities specialists may instruct these classes.

Frequently, inclusive preschool programs use the self-contained model—that is, the speech–language pathologist is one of several teachers in the classroom throughout the day. Planning is usually done by a team, and general as well as specific goals are set for the students in the class. In 1993, these goals hung on the walls of the preschool class in the Main Street School, North Syracuse, New York:

Play/cognitive:

categorization/grouping	colors
matching	counting, number concepts
spatial relations	role play/pretending
comparison/contrast	order
shapes	

Social:

problem solving	sharing
expressing feelings	cooperative play
routine self-help	

Sensory:

imitating designs	cutting
orientation/positioning	representation
pasting/gluing	grasp/hand dominance
colors	blocks
play/building/constructing	

Language:

awareness of auditory information	relaying simple messages
imitating communication	relating events out of context
making choices	phrases / word combinations
sequencing	answering simple questions in
imitating / producing words / sign	context

Given the age of the students, the necessity for integrating goals is exceptionally clear. With the possible exception of some small motor tasks, each of the other categories has strong language implications.

Multiskilling

As stated previously, how this service delivery model might be applied to the schools is far from clear. Pietranton and Lynch (1995) stated, "At best, [multiskilling is] viewed as a sincere, patient focused effort to improve efficiency and effectiveness of service delivery. At worst, it can sacrifice clinical standards in the name of lower costs" (p. 37). Questions of professional training, effect on the existing practitioners, quality of services, professional ethics, clinical liability, and risk management would all need to be addressed. Multiskilling as it is now defined is not the same as incorporating another discipline's goals into the provision of speech–language services.

Collaboration might include this scenario: After consultation with an SLP, an occupational therapist integrates exercises involving small-muscle control into a language activity—for example, having Sally Student color portions of a cartoon strip in a specific manner as she discusses the sequence of actions in the story. In multiskilling, the occupational therapist would make decisions regarding speech–language goals on her own; no speech–language pathologist would be required at any stage. ASHA's insistence on the highest-qualified provider is in direct conflict with this delivery model, "thus teaching other professionals *how to do* what SLPs do, rather than teaching them *about* what we do is contradictory to ASHA policy" (*Asha Leader,* 2003, p. 30).

Inclusion

Often specialists and teachers are comfortable having students who have mild to moderate disabilities in the classroom but resist the inclusion of those who are more severely impaired, such as those with serious behavioral problems, multiple handicaps, autism, or severe cognitive impairments. Those professionals who support their presence in the classroom to the greatest degree possible state that it is the civil right of these students to be assigned to the least restrictive environment, or to be placed, to the greatest extent possible, with their nondisabled peers. "The inclusion movement in education, work, and community living is based on the notion that individuals with disabilities have a fundamental right to access normal patterns of learning, working, and living that should not be compromised because of the disability (i.e., the concept of normalization)" (Buschbacher and Fox, 2003, p. 218). They assert that inclusion leads to improved learning outcomes in socialization, communication, adaptive behavior, and functional skills and a better quality of life marked by a broader range of choices, self-determination, and richer social connections (McSheehan & Jorgensen as presented by Sonnenmeier & McGuire, 1995).

Sonnenmeier and McGuire stress that it is our job as speech–language pathologists to create opportunities for all individuals to demonstrate their skills, using chronologically age-appropriate materials and under conditions of high expectations; our goal should be to support all efforts in this regard, not only to provide intervention. They argue that we should be prepared to explain and interpret to others that the sometimes negative behaviors are the only means of communication open to some children to let someone know that they want a change of activity or that they do not understand what is expected of them. Therefore, as part of our planning, we need to identify typical routines in the classroom and describe to what level we expect students to participate within each of them. We should identify the opportunities for communication within each routine and the length of time a specific student with special needs is likely to be able to participate. Aids to communication can include picture symbols, schedule books, and modified materials and supports. Examples of such adaptations are found in Chapters 3 and 9.

One of the most sensitive issues in the schools is the provision of a para-professional, often a one-to-one aide, to assist the classroom teacher in the day-to-day implementation of these laudatory goals. With tight budgets, teachers are sometimes expected to manage with part-time help and may resent the time taken away from the typical classroom pupils and their already crammed teaching schedule. There is no easy answer to these issues other than to try to keep the lines of communication open as we struggle to provide the best service we can to every student in our care. If you have students with severe handicaps on your caseload, be sure to check educational sources for additional information (Giangreco & Meyer, 1988; Schulz & Turnbull, 1984).

The Theme Approach

Integrating goals is also the intent of one of the most popular programs in the schools today, the theme approach. I have listed this topic separately because themes work equally well in collaborative or pull-out situations, and part of a curricular unit can be substituted for a theme topic. Themes can introduce concepts and vocabulary in a relevant, contextual manner, and they permit flexibility and creativity in meeting individual academic and language needs of students who may have very different academic deficits. Because language-learning deficits can profoundly affect students' ability to read and write (see Chapter 7), the same students may be seen not only by us but by a reading specialist and a special educator, as well. Consequently, it is easy for fragmentation to occur as each specialist treats his or her "part" of the student. Using themes as part of an interdisciplinary approach to remediation reduces this artificial separation, and for the SLP, units also offer many effective, time-efficient opportunities.

There are two basic ways to use a theme. SLPs can develop a curriculum-related topic that will be motivating to most of the students on their caseloads, or they can work within a preexisting school-wide or individual classroom unit. If you are choosing a theme, try to do it in concert with other specialists, so that fragmentation can be diminished as much as possible. Initially, examine the following list of language areas and match one or more to the IEP goals of a student or student group. Next, using the selected theme—be it space, animals, scarecrows, or world flags—plan an activity that meets IEP goals but also integrates the vocabulary and books required as part of the students' curricula. The authors of Section 2 in this chapter describe the process in detail.

Using thematic units has a number of advantages:

1. You are indirectly providing in-service training on the complexity of language when you review with teachers the linguistic areas that can be addressed through a thematic unit.

2. When you target one area repeatedly in various themes presented throughout the school year, students become aware that intervention techniques can generalize to new circumstances. For example, if a student has vocabulary limitations, you may choose to address adjectives, adverbs, synonyms, antonyms, associations, and categorization during each thematic unit. This tells the student that the strategies used in learning new vocabulary is a continuing process that crosses subject lines.

3. By becoming aware of curriculum content, speech–language pathologists can choose themes that have a clear relationship to classroom subjects. Jill, a special education colleague, and I chose space as a theme partly because she knew that the space race of the 1960s was covered in eighth-grade social studies and the planetary system in fourth-grade science. Similarly, when water was the theme, we covered ocean names because in the seventh-grade social studies unit on explorers, it is assumed that students already have this information. A communication theme was a natural subject to reinforce the names of inventions and their developers.

4. Literacy skills are usually an integral part of thematic units. Choosing interesting books, particularly in concert with the school librarian, can add to students' world knowledge as well as improve specific literacy skills (see Chapter 12).

5. There is often a parent component in thematic units. As part of a theme, students frequently build objects, complete artwork, write stories, or use computers or videotape to generate projects. Among other items, my students developed and illustrated cookbooks and built spaceships, sports arenas, Native American dwellings, miniatures of their own houses copied from a photograph, and mobiles of animals, fish, and characters in fairy tales. It is a rare parent who will not make a trip to school to see something concrete a son or daughter has created. This is particularly helpful with the family of a "labeled" student because parent meetings so frequently deal with problems, not celebrations.

How each language area is related to the educational environment is explained below. In many cases, a target language area can also be used to support work on a student's IEP goal, particularly if the IEP goal is directly related to classroom curriculum. Part of this list of language areas had its origins in the work of Catherine Bush in 1980. The innumerable books and materials featuring themes that have been published since then can serve as ready resources.

Developing your own, however, allows you to target topics of interest to your particular students. In addition, the interaction between colleagues as you plan units usually leads to more activities than you could ever use, as well as creating energy and wonderful rapport.

- *Adjectives and adverbs:* Most students with language disabilities overuse a few adjectives, such as *neat* and *gross*. Practice not only teaches new vocabulary, it encourages precision. Example: Provide two adjectives that go with the noun *blimp* and two adverbs that go with the word *drive*. Apply this linguistic area directly to written class work.
- *Analogy:* Before students can do proportions or solve many word problems in math, they have to learn to complete analogies, which commonly appear on standardized tests and are often used as a teaching technique. Having students explain concepts presented during class by using an analogy is good practice (e.g., moving troops across the ocean to Iraq is like packing for a long trip when you don't know if any stores will be available).
- *Antonyms and synonyms:* Both forms appear on most school-wide standardized tests. Learning antonyms (*enormous–minuscule*) and synonyms (*enormous–gigantic*) as a pair is a vocabulary-expanding shortcut. Students who overuse a few adjectives need practice in supplying alternatives and in choosing adjectives with a specific shade of meaning. Example: Give three synonyms for *walk*. Write a paragraph about walking, using your synonyms. What word is the opposite (antonym) of *horizontal*?
- *Association:* The ability to associate is necessary for storing information in short- and long-term memory, as well as for recalling related subjects. This is particularly important in writing tasks that require organization within a paper. Brainstorming ideas for a project or paper is good practice for this skill. Example: Say all the words you can think of as fast as you can that could go with the word *wheelchair* (*motor, ill, sit, strong, disability, hands, basketball, person, ramp, injury, illness, roll, fast, smooth, access,* etc.). Word retrieval practice is helpful for word-finding problems.
- *Categorization:* Placing items or facts into correct categories is a necessary first step in ordering information so that it can be retained and recalled. This is exceptionally useful for a student with word-finding problems, as well as a good topic for a study skills course.
- *Cloze:* Cloze involves the semantic and syntactic knowledge of what word would make sense if inserted in a blank space in a sentence. Fill-in-the-blank questions are commonly found on examinations. It is important that students be aware of the differences between convergent types (only one correct answer) and divergent ones (many correct answers). This concept can be taught in a unit on study skills. You can practice cloze orally and then in written form, using sentences from grade-level texts.
- *Fiction and nonfiction stories:* Being able to distinguish between fantasy and reality is not always easy for the student with language problems. Telling and writing stories of both types on a single-theme topic is a means

of internalizing the rules that govern each. Reading examples of both in the classroom can also serve as a basis for discussion.

• *Following verbal directions:* Of all the language skills most commonly used in the classroom, this is the one that can cause the most trouble if the student is deficient. It is typical of students with a language-learning disability (LLD) that they absorb only a portion of the directions and consequently complete only part of the assignment. In a unit on communication, my older, mostly male, students built radios from kits. The more skillful readers read the directions aloud, and then the members of the small groups took turns completing the action. There was no need to impose "penalties" if they did it incorrectly; they all knew that if every single connection was not finished as it should be, the radio was not going to work. Troubleshooting in the event that the radio did not work on the first try was a valuable life lesson as well.

• *Idioms, proverbs, metaphors, similes:* Most students with language deficits have profound difficulty understanding idioms and proverbs, partly because these students tend to interpret language in concrete terms and partly because it requires metalinguistic skill. This is the same reason they have difficulty "getting the joke." Understanding figurative language is also necessary for higher-level comprehension. Example: Older students can locate metaphors and similes in their literature texts, or, if that is too difficult, explain the meaning of ones you find.

• *Part and whole relationships:* The ability to "see the forest for the trees" is a difficult concept for many students. Often, students remember a small piece of information but fail to see how it relates to the whole. Discriminating between the entirety and its components is a first step and is closely related to differentiating between the main idea and supporting details. Example: Name the parts of a ring (stone, setting, prongs, band, diamond, etc.). Now name something a ring can be part of (the planet Saturn, an engine, a jewelry collection, etc.).

• *Question forms:* Being able to ask a specific question and resolve confusion over something the teacher said is a skill many students with LLD do not have. Playing *Jeopardy* using the classroom curriculum is a fun way to practice formulating questions, but applying the skill to classroom subjects will also require teaching students how to know *when* to ask them.

• *Riddles:* Solving a riddle involves inferential reasoning, common in literature, social studies, and mathematics. Riddles are another good topic to include in a unit on study skills for the older student and are a way to increase the complexity of comprehension questions for younger readers.

• *Rhyme:* Current research has indicated that the ability to rhyme— that is, to create a pattern—is a necessary prerequisite for spelling (encoding) as well as reading (decoding). Example: Find five different words in Chapter 4 of your science book that rhyme with *near* (hint: they may not all look alike).

• *Scrambled sentences:* Proper word order is necessary for coherent communication; practicing unscrambling also encourages a student to break out of the "article + noun + verb" sentence structure common in less complex syntactical forms. Use topics from the theme or curriculum. Example: Using the four words *hogan, abandoned, the, is* from the vocabulary list of your current social studies unit, create two different sentences.

• *Sentence construction:* Using specific words in a sentence requires a knowledge of both semantics and syntactic relationships. It is a metalinguistic skill. Example: Take three vocabulary words from a theme (or any classroom subject) and put them into a single sentence. Recognizing the difference between a correct sentence, a sentence fragment, and a run-on sentence is necessary in editing tasks.

• *Sentence types:* This is another example of a metalinguistic skill: using language to explain, analyze, and manipulate language. Most students with LLD experience great difficulty in identifying and defining grammatical information. Once students can produce different kinds of sentences verbally, you can work on transferring them to written work. Example: Using the word *shark,* create declarative, interrogatory, exclamatory, and imperative sentences; now write a paragraph in which you have an example of each sentence type.

• *Sequence of actions:* Understanding a sequence of actions and placing them in proper order is a necessary skill in narratives, mathematics, history, and science. Using an activity that demonstrates a clear sequence is one of the easiest forms to use if a student must write a paper. Example: Using a map, draw Magellan's path around the world. Explain his journey to a class member. Write a book report that contains at least six sequential events.

• *Similarities and differences:* Although many students can see either differences or similarities, it is frequently difficult for them to see both. Another common problem is choosing an insignificant comparison while ignoring the most important. These abilities are the basis of all "compare-and-contrast" questions in many subjects. Use the curriculum as the subject here, as in the example. Example: Using a Venn diagram, list three ways the American Revolutionary and Vietnam Wars were alike and two ways they were different.

• *Vocabulary:* Preteaching some therapeutic aspect of vocabulary can be an effective means of making classroom information more relevant and understandable to a student with language deficiencies. Ask to borrow word lists from the teacher, or make a list from the books that are being featured as part of the unit. Be aware that there is no substitute for knowing the curriculum; when Jill, my special educator colleague, and I were planning an animal unit, she, not I, understood that students would not be asked, "Where does this animal live?" Instead, they would be expected to answer the question, "What is this animal's habitat and range?" Although both words *habitat* and *range* relate to where animals live, the terms are not synonymous. Example: Using your last three vocabulary lists, find a word that starts with each of the letters of your first and last names; define each.

- *Word definition:* Although this is a skill that is generally used in writing, using it verbally gives practice without worrying about spelling, handwriting, and so on. It also encourages precision. It is often difficult for the student with language deficits, and you will need to scaffold the steps carefully. For example, when the student is defining *orbit,* visualization may help the student to appreciate how the word *path* is a good word to use in the definition. Students should also be specifically taught how to use root words, prefixes, and suffixes to help discern or remember a word's meaning. Example: Using the root word *tract,* add different prefixes to make words, and define each (e.g., *protract*).

Although not linguistic areas, these additional categories of activities also lend themselves to collaboration:

- introductory letters to the families explaining the theme and asking them to complete specific home activities with their child (Figure 5.2 is an example of a similar one for teachers);
- written products, often in conjunction with the classroom, special education, or English teacher: spelling words, written vocabulary activities, a factual essay, or a sequential writing activity;
- reading, as an integral part of any thematic unit, using a variety of reading materials: fictional works, basal readers, magazines, the Internet, biographies, and newspaper articles, plus activities in decoding, comprehension, and library resource skills;
- mathematics applications, such as charting, graphing, and word problems; and
- computer applications, such as word processing, developing games, using e-mail, and using search engines on the Internet or creating a report using Powerpoint.

Figure 5.3 features a form that can be used to plan theme-related goals involving several subjects; Figures 5.4 and 5.5 can be used to plan daily activities that will also indicate the delivery model used to accomplish individual objectives.

One important warning in using thematic units: It is very easy to become so involved in the topic and its motivating activities that you neglect the goals on the student's IEP or the classroom curriculum. Make sure that all intervention procedures address the most crucial student weaknesses as well as their curricular implications.

In conclusion, the service delivery models you use to provide intervention will vary from student to student and year to year. As surely as I am typing this, someone in our field, or an allied one, is developing a new way. For example, the DeSoto County (Mississippi) schools are using specialization to provide "the most efficient services" to a large and diverse caseload of students. Under this model, speech–language specialists are divided into committees focusing on fluency, voice, language, and articulation; membership on the committees

---

Theme: Flags

Subjects: Art, Social Studies, Language Arts

Goals:
1. Use appropriate vocabulary to describe flags.
2. Explain how flags represent countries.
3. Draw a picture of the flag of a Middle Eastern country.
4. Demonstrate how to locate the country belonging to the flag on a map of the Middle East.
5. Plan a Flag Day celebration for June 14.
6. Using sequencing terms, describe the development of the American flag from Revolutionary times to the present.
7. Recite three rules for displaying the American flag.
8. Create a flag representing the class, a family, or an individual.

Vocabulary:
field, symbol, staff, halyard, hoist (noun; part nearest the staff), *hoist* (verb), *fly* (noun: outer part of the flag), *fly* (verb), *banner, etiquette, bar, stripe, fringe, pennant, canton*

Ongoing Concepts and Areas Related to IEP Goals and State Standards

___ Vocabulary	___ Sentence types	___ Word definitions
___ Rhyme	___ Scrambled sentences	___ Associations
___ Part/whole	___ Sequence of actions	___ Adjectives/adverbs
___ Idioms	___ Similarities/differences	___ Sentence formulation
___ Similes	___ Proverbs	___ Metaphors
___ Cloze	___ Riddles	___ Analogy
___ Categorization	___ Verbal directions	___ Question forms
___ Fiction/nonfiction stories	___ Other	___ Antonyms/synonyms

---

Figure 5.3. Theme unit overall planning sheet.

is based on the interest and expertise of the speech–language specialists who work in the district (Zarrella, 1995). Are you wondering how in the world you can master all of these models? In the past, most SLPs preferred to learn about the principles of collaboration by attending conferences or in-service sessions rather than formal university courses. As you work in the field and you find opportunities to learn new models, take advantage of them. Almost always, they feature "hands-on" practical suggestions; if you are fortunate enough to do your student teaching under an SLP who is engaged in other than pull-out intervention, ask questions, keep a notebook, observe, and learn, learn, learn. And don't forget to pass your good ideas along to others.

Caseload Size and Service Delivery Models

Part of the process in choosing service delivery models is deciding how many other students, if any, should be included as intervention takes place with a particular student. Because of new models of service delivery, group size has in some ways become irrelevant; if intervention takes place within the classroom,

Theme:	Flags	Day/Date:	Mon 5/22
Anticipatory set:	Show "Don't Tread on Me" flag from Revolutionary War period		
Teacher:	Meyer	Goal:	Flag vocabulary
Location:	Speech room	Individual Objective:	Students will demonstrate knowledge of 50% of flag vocabulary
Materials:	Pictures of old and new flags, "blank" flags	Activities:	Label different parts of flag using visualization as memory strategy; discuss as a group the importance of flags in history; introduce concept of symbolism; present blank flag for students to label parts.
Closure:	Set up meeting time to see flag raised in front of school	Special Considerations for:	Jenny: preprint parts names on stickers
Theme:	Flags	Day/Date:	Tues 5/23
Anticipatory Set:	Pledge of Allegiance		
Teacher:	Meyer/Smith	Goal:	Introduce Flag Day theme to class
Location:	Classroom	Individual Objective:	Students will learn flag vocabulary, brainstorm activities for celebration on June 14
Materials:	same as 5/22 plus larger blank flag	Activities:	Label different parts of flag; discuss the importance of flags in Middle Ages, modern times; discuss symbolism in heterogeneous cooperative groups; present large blank flag for students to label parts.
Closure:	List places where students have seen flags	Special Considerations for:	Be sure all students from 5/22 use memory strategies and encourage them to display their knowledge in their small groups.

Figure 5.4. Daily planner for introduction to theme activities (Day 1).

other children will be present, often in very fluid arrangements. During a portion of a class period, you may work next to the child at his or her desk for 5 or 10 minutes, then include the child in a small group for practice, and later observe the child as part of the entire class applying what he or she has learned. Clearly, however, there remain times when a student must be seen outside the classroom on an individual basis for any number of reasons—for example to provide intensive drill, to protect confidentiality, or to teach a difficult, highly individualized technique. Complications arise when you must describe group size on his or her IEP or in an end-of-the-year report that usually includes designations of group size only up to five members. Throughout the country,

Theme: Flags	**Day/Date:** Tues. 5/23	**Anticipatory Set:** Pledge of Allegiance
Teacher: Meyer/Smith	**Goal:** Introduce Flag Day theme to class	
Location: Classroom	**Individual Objective:** Students will learn flag vocabulary; they will brainstorm activities for celebration on June 14	

Materials: Same as 5/22 plus larger blank flag

Activities: Label different parts of flag; discuss the importance of flags in Middle Ages, modern times; discuss symbolism in heterogeneous cooperative groups; present large blank flag for students to label its parts.

Closure: List places where students have seen flags

Special Considerations: Be sure all students from 5/22 use memory strategies and encourage them to display their knowledge in their small groups.

Figure 5.5. Daily planner for continuation of theme activities (Day 2).

speech–language specialists are struggling to fit these new delivery models to an "old" law; I have every confidence that as long as we honor the spirit of the legislation, we will work through these difficulties.

The question of caseload size has been and continues to be one of the most emotionally charged subjects in speech–language pathology in the schools. Cassandra Peters-Johnson (1992), in a historical review of caseload size, wrote that in the 1960s, speech–language pathologists reported serving 111 students per week on the average, with about three quarters of them at second-grade level or below. Approximately 80% of the caseload involved articulation. More fluency cases were seen than those involving any other type of language disorder. After the passage of Public Law 94-142, a dramatic downward shift in numbers occurred. The average fell to 43, and language and articulation cases became equally represented. Numbers of older students on the caseload also increased. By 1992, the upward trend appeared to have stabilized at about 52, but the author cautioned that this is an average and that "some speech–language specialists have caseloads much higher and others much lower than the average … with some … caseloads of 70, 80, 90 and even 100" (p. 12).

In 2002, ASHA published a position statement describing a workload analysis approach for establishing speech–language caseloads in the schools to "insure that students receive the services they need, instead of the services SLPs have time to offer or services based on administrative convenience" (p. 89). This paper makes a clear distinction between caseload, typically the number of students who have IEPs, and workload, all the activities required and performed by SLPs as they comply with IDEA and other mandates. When you accept a position in the schools, you would be well advised to ask what the state and district guidelines are regarding maximum caseload—whether those numbers take into account relative severity and whether time is provided to complete evaluations, meet with teachers, attend conferences, and so forth. Meeting with 10 groups of children a day, 5 days a week, with no breaks other

Time	Monday	Tuesday	Wednesday	Thursday	Friday
7:45–8:00	Primary meeting	7th–8th-grade meeting	K meeting	Plan	Child study team
8:00–8:15	Jerry (& aide)	Bus duty	Jerry	Bus duty	Jerry (& aide)
8:30–9:10	Pat, Sally, Jamar	3rd-grade "s" group	*Pat, Sally, Jamar	3rd-grade "s" group	Pat, Sally, Jamar
9:15–9:55	K-garten—Smith	Kim	K-garten—O'Hara	Kim	Test
10:00–10:40	Mitch, Andy, Joe	Brad	Mitch, Andy, Joe, Brad	Brad	Test
10:45–11:25	7th-grade social studies	8th-grade English	Kristine, Chris, Joe L.	Kristine, Chris, Joe L.	Test
11:30–12:00	Lunch	Lunch	Lunch	Lunch	Lunch
12:00–12:40	Jake, Ben, Ann, Abel	Jason, Bill,	Jake, Ben, Ann, Abel	Jason, Bill	Jake, Ben, Ann, Abel
12:45–1:25	Lindsay, Beryl, Katie, Blake, Chou	6th-grade reading	Lindsay et al.	5th-grade reading	Lindsay et al.
1:30–2:10	Jamie, T'rique, Kristin, Corey	William, Mei, Rakia	*Jamie, T'rique, Kristin, Corey	William, Mei, Rakia	Jamie, T'rique, Kristin, Corey
2:15–2:55	Stephen, Beth, Gaby	2nd-grade lang arts	Stephen, Beth, Gaby Whitney, Bill	Patricia, Sue	Sue, Patty, Whitney, Bill
3:00–3:30	CSE premeeting	Planning	Planning	CSE meeting	Planning

*Meets in classroom.

Figure 5.6. Planning a schedule for elementary grades.

than a 30-minute lunch is burnout waiting to happen. An exhausted, overworked SLP puts the children he or she serves at risk. Figure 5.6 illustrates a typical schedule in an elementary school. Note the inclusion of bus duty and other nonacademic activities.

Scheduling groups and choosing a mode of delivery can be complicated and frustrating. Deciding whether to group by disorder, age, grade, degree of severity, personality compatibility, availability at a specific time, or teacher preference requires the wisdom of Solomon and the patience of a saint. One fact is certain; as soon as you arrive at an acceptable schedule, something will happen that will necessitate change. Regardless of the circumstances of the workplace, after their first year, all SLPs write their schedules in pencil—and have a large eraser at the ready.

Another area of trial and error involves choosing the format for weekly lesson plans and daily logs. In an attempt to decrease paperwork, IDEA's 2004 revision and reauthorization eliminate the requirement for "benchmarks and short-term objectives" on IEPs for all children with disabilities except those who are the most severely cognitively disabled (IDEA, 2004). Because SLPs must be accountable for their results, however, it is necessary that objectives or benchmarks focusing on student performance continue to exist in some form, whether or not they appear on an IEP. There is no one correct way to accomplish this task. Some professionals prefer quite detailed plans, a slightly streamlined version of the ones most of you used in your college programs. Others employ a highly abbreviated single page for the week but keep individual or group logs in more detail. Almost none take detailed data every session for every student. Most school districts distribute lesson plan books, but these are not always applicable to intervention in speech and language. I suggest that you use your master teacher's system as a starting place and gradually develop your own. Figure 5.11, created by Tracy Crouch, illustrates one way lesson plans can appear on the same sheet with data from a session, regardless of service delivery mode. Completed plans are kept in the student or group folder and filed every month or so. Because the sheet also lists the activity's IEP objective and applicable state learning standard for each student, it is easy to make sure that all goals are being addressed on a regular basis. It also facilitates gathering information for quarterly report cards or end-of-the-year reports.

SECTION 2: PULLING IT ALL TOGETHER IN THE REAL WORLD

In this section of the chapter, school-based SLPs Tracy Crouch and Nanette Clapper describe the rationale and details of their daily work. As you read this section carefully, you will recognize many of the concepts discussed in Section 1 and discover additional, exciting ways theory can be applied to the classroom environment.

A Successful Intervention Program: Tracy Crouch

I came to a school setting after having been clinic based, which was a difficult transition—knowing how and where to start was my greatest challenge. My intention in this chapter is to help others who are starting out in school programs become aware of some of the problems they are likely to face and discuss ways they can develop and provide effective intervention for their school-aged students.

To me, the key to developing a successful intervention program is identifying and addressing three component parts:

- *The first component is creating goals and objectives that target the individualized learning needs of the students on your caseload.* Sometimes you formulate these goals based on your own diagnostic assessment, or, as a new clinician, the goals may reflect assessments performed by the therapist who preceded you in your position. Most important, however, is that the goals can be easily measured and attained within the framework of the primary-level curriculum and your state's learning standards.

- *The second essential component is having a clear understanding of the primary-level (K–2) curriculum that is being covered in the school district in which you are employed.* As a school speech–language professional, I find it crucial to learn what is expected of all students in the specific curricular areas of reading, writing, science, social studies, and math. This is because students with deficits in language functioning typically struggle in these academic areas and need to be taught strategies and methods to help them compensate or overcome their weaknesses. If we do not have a clear understanding of what is being taught in our students' classrooms, it is difficult to know the most effective way to help them function successfully among their peers.

- *The third component is collaborating with regular education teachers, administration, and your student's primary caregivers.* Regardless of the type of service delivery model you provide at your particular school, it is extremely beneficial to have a good working relationship with your students' regular education teachers, because your students spend the majority of their day with that person. In addition, if classroom teachers have a good understanding of their students' specific individualized needs and goals that you identified, they are better able to support your intervention program. Similarly, it is necessary to have guidance and support from your administrators in order for effective program results to take place. Although it may be more difficult with school-aged students, parental involvement and follow-through at home are additional elements important to a student's academic success and lifelong learning.

In Chapter 4, you learned how to develop an Individualized Educational Plan (IEP). For your students who receive mandated services, that document is the foundation on which you build your intervention program. As you are likely aware, not all students who receive speech and language services have an IEP. Students may also qualify for services under Section 504 of the Rehabilitation Act of 1973. In that case, they will have a 504 plan. Other students who don't qualify for an IEP may be seen as a part of a speech improvement group. Because this is considered a service offered through regular education, many school districts require that specific guidelines and goals be put in place to demonstrate progress. Consequently, it is necessary to outline goals and objectives specific to the students' individualized learning needs, whether they have a label or not. This too will serve as a building block for establishing a proper intervention program. Since IDEA requires that students at risk be the recipient of modifications within the regular classroom, your speech improvement goals can serve this function, as well.

Once student goals and objectives have been set and, when possible, you have grouped the students on your caseload according to similar needs, the planning process for your intervention program begins. The beauty of planning lessons and activities for your school-aged students is that there exists no one, foolproof way of doing it. This allows practitioners in our field the freedom to be creative. As with any task, however, there must be a starting point, and I have found that the easiest place to begin is by establishing a long-range plan. This entails outlining what skills need to be addressed and then assigning those skills to the appropriate month and weeks of the school year (refer to Figure 5.7). In conjunction with this schedule, you can construct other ones that address the content or curriculum units (Figures 5.8 through 5.10). As you can see, this outline indicates what units are being taught each month in the different subject areas across the primary grade levels. Once this has been established, it is much easier to incorporate the specific skill areas or objectives that you have set into the classroom curriculum.

Stated simply, the rationale behind this method of intervention is that students can make greater sense of what is being taught to them when it is functional, meaningful, and has an obvious purpose. For example, if a group of second graders is having significant difficulty understanding and explaining similarities and differences among items, it makes greater sense to use curriculum vocabulary to teach strategies rather than to use random or arbitrary material to overcome this weakness. So if this group of second graders is learning about butterflies in science, I might choose to teach vocabulary related to the development of an adult butterfly. I would help the students develop the life cycle of the butterfly and then compare and contrast the differences between butterflies and moths using a Venn diagram as a visual aid to show how the two insects are related. After making a plan like this, it is always wise to ask yourself if you are, in fact, targeting the goals you set out to address in the lesson. In this case, because you know that the students have already spent some time learning about the life cycle of the moth, they are able to bring their prior knowledge about moths into the lesson. Remember also that this group of second graders' language weaknesses involves problems in understanding how two objects can be both alike and different at the same time. The butterfly–moth activity clearly provides the students with an opportunity to practice their developing

For Group #7
Josh, Sam, Mike, Brenda

September
• categorization, similarities, differences
• sequencing, retelling, verbal directions, sentence building
• sound skills, discrimination, imitation

October
• categorization, associations, classification
• sequencing, retelling, problem solving
• sound skills, discrimination, imitation

November
• prepositions, associations, classification
• question forms, retelling, problem solving
• sound skills, discrimination, production

December
• attributes, antonyms, synonyms
• question forms, verbal directions, sentence building
• sound skills, production, rhyming

January
• riddles, classification, description
• auditory memory, sentence building, grammatical structures
• sound skills, production, rhyming

February
• prepositions, associations, classifying,
• sequencing, visual memory, problem solving
• sound skills, production

March
• antonyms, synonyms, auditory memory
• sequencing, retelling, sentence building
• sound skills, production

April
• vocabulary—categorizing, superlatives, prepositions
• sequencing, retelling, sentence building
• sound skills, production

May
• part/whole relationships, similarities, differences
• sequencing, cloze, sentence building
• sound skills, production, rhyming

June
• analogies, part/whole relationships, cloze
• sequencing, retelling, sentence building
• sound skills, production

Figure 5.7. Long-range skills plan.

skills in comprehending and using both similarities and differences, the intended outcome of the lesson. More important, the skill was taught within the framework of the second-grade science curriculum.

Although my example may be a somewhat simplistic one, it does illustrate the importance and relevance of curriculum-based instruction for the students who have language delays or learning disabilities. Figures 5.8 through 5.10, the sample unit plans, were developed in collaboration with a kindergarten, first-, and second-grade teacher with whom I work. It is a piece of the sometimes elaborate planning that goes into developing lessons that target the diverse needs of the students on my caseload, as well as their typically developing classmates. It was designed to provide clinicians in the school setting a way to understand and appreciate this type of service delivery model.

Figure 5.11 is a sample of the document that I developed to use during planning meetings with classroom teachers. As you can see, it provides a simple framework to help design activities that target specific objectives. The most valuable aspect of this form has proven to be its simplicity. It can easily be

Grade	Month	Theme/concepts	Activity	Objectives/skills
K	September	• colors	• prism experiment with overhead projector	• identify & label 4–6 colors
K	October	• autumn leaves	• collect a variety of leaves in bags, sort by different characteristics of size, color, shape, etc.	• identify & label 6–8 colors • identify and use superlatives in context • classify objects into 2 categories
1st	September	• apples	• examine apple, identify parts • design life cycle with construction paper, label parts • read *Arnold's Apple Tree* (1984) by Gail Gibbons	• describe objects using 3–5 attributes • respond to a variety of question forms • follow 2–3-step directions • identify & label pictures
1st	October	• pumpkins	• carve pumpkin, examine seeds, plant a seed • read *Pumpkin Pumpkin* (1990) by Jeanne Titherington	• answer questions related and unrelated to a story • complete a 6-step sequence • recall 3–4 story events • describe objects using 3–6 attributes
2nd	September	• butterflies	• identify and discuss life cycle of butterfly using a Venn diagram • compare and contrast a butterfly with a moth	• identify & describe 3–4 similarities & differences between 2 objects • respond to a variety of questions orally & in writing
2nd	October	• light	• shadow experiments • when given a variety of objects, determine which will refract or reflect light • present to class	• orally define words • identify & describe how items are similar & different using a complete sentence • increase vocal projection in large group speaking situations

Figure 5.8. Science unit.

completed during an actual planning session with a teacher, or by a classroom teacher, or it can be finished at another time. Although it would be wonderful to assume that you will have time to sit down and plan with every teacher of every student on your caseload, depending on your caseload size, you might have to plan with 15 or more teachers a week. Clearly, this is an impossible task. The form shown as Figure 5.7 is an especially useful tool when I decide to

Grade	Month	Theme/concepts	Activity	Objectives/skills
K	September	• friendship	• read *Land of Many Colors* by Conde (1999) • trace & cut paper person in color of choice • act out story • brainstorm how to be a friend	• identify & label 4–6 colors • retell 2–3 events from the story • follow simple 1–2-part commands • respond to wh questions using a complete sentence
1st	October	• family	• read *Families Are Different* by Nina Pellegrini (1991) & discuss how families are similar and different • pair students & illustrate one another's family • circle what is the same • orally share observations with the class	• identify 2–4 similarities & differences between 2 objects • increase turn-taking skills • maintain topic for 3–4 interchanges
2nd	November	• Thanksgiving	• read *Oh, What a Thanksgiving* by Steven Kroll (1988); using a Venn diagram compare and contrast the first Thanksgiving to Thanksgiving today	• identify 3–6 similarities & differences among events or situations • respond to a variety of questions orally and in writing.

Figure 5.9. Social studies unit.

pull students out of a classroom. It becomes a resource guide that I can choose to use when I plan specific skill work or activities for the students working in the smaller group setting.

Figure 5.2, presented previously, is a sample of the letter sent to classroom teachers with the planning sheet. I have found that teachers appreciate it when you ask for their input. In the beginning of the school year, I provide all of my students' teachers with a summary of each student's needs and classroom accommodations. I place them in individualized folders for confidentiality; this method also makes it easy for teachers to find it in a busy classroom. Teachers have said that the information contained in it increases their understanding of the specific learning requirements of the special needs student in their classroom. It also allows the teacher to have easy access to the student information and facilitates their making necessary adaptations for that child.

Figure 5.12 provides you with an example of information distributed to teachers to help ease the transition of the student with special needs into the regular education classroom.

Grade	Month	Theme/concepts *From regular education classroom curriculum*	Activity	Objectives/skills *From students' IEPs*
K	September	• letter recognition • sound awareness • name recognition	• read *Chicka Chicka Boom Boom* (Martin & Archambault, 1989) • each student traces 2–3 letters of the alphabet & puts it on class alphabet tree when his letter or sound is called	• identify letter names • discriminate initial sounds • follow 1–2-step directions
1st	September	• rhyming	• read *Green Eggs & Ham* (1973) to begin Dr. Seuss author study • each student will be given a picture–word stimulus card & must find the corresponding rhyme pair • student partners will brainstorm additional rhyming words	• identify & label pictures • identify ending sounds • maintain attention & focus for 5–10 minutes • utilize turn-taking skills for 3–4 exchanges • follow a 2-part related command
2nd	September	• sequencing	• read *Frog & Toad, The Kite* (1979) by A. Lobel • together fill in story map • have students sequence events of story • all students design their own kite with construction paper	• orally respond to a variety of question forms using a complete sentence • sequence 3–6 events • name 3–5 attributes to describe an object

Figure 5.10. Language arts (reading, writing, speaking, listening) unit.

In their entirety, Figures 5.2, 5.11, and 5.12 are particularly helpful when a classroom teacher is new to the district; they serve as an introduction to the services that I am prepared to provide and assures her that she is not alone in working with students who have special needs.

At the beginning of this chapter, Jacqueline Meyer described several different intervention models to consider as you decide on the individual learning requirements and learning styles of students in a typical caseload. In my experience, curriculum-based intervention, including the thematic approach, has proven to be the most successful way for students to master the goals and objectives on their IEP. The way I provide this type of intervention, however, generally depends on what works best for the individual student at a

---

What's Happening in Mrs. Kelly's Second-Grade Classroom
For the week of September 18–22

UNIT—Language Arts

Literature Being Used
Frog and Toad Are Friends by Arthur Lobel (1970)
I Need a Friend by Sherry Kafka (1990)
Frog and Toad, The Kite by Arthur Lobel (1979)

Concepts/Skills Being Taught
compare/contrast   sequencing skills
story elements retelling

UNIT—Science (2-week unit)

Concepts/Skills Being Taught
Understanding the life cycle of the butterfly

Vocabulary to reinforce:

- life cycle   • stages   • caterpillar   _____
- pupa   • metamorphosis • milkweed   _____
- chrysalis   • larva   • life span   _____

UNIT—Social Studies

Concepts/Skills Being Taught
Citizenship: The students will brainstorm two ways to be a good citizen. A poster contest will be held on September 29.

Other Need-to-Know Information
Reading assessments will be on Thursday.
Pull-out speech–language students complete writing piece for portfolios.
Science vocabulary test September 25.

Figure 5.11. Planning document.

particular time. I have found combining a push-in and team-teaching approach with a pull-out model has been a successful mix for meeting the needs of my students. In my experience, working within your students' classroom presents many wonderful opportunities. It allows you to see how your students cope within the regular education setting and also provides you with an occasion to see how typical students are performing. Being in the classroom has also served as a means to identify additional at-risk students. By working directly in the classroom setting, you become acutely aware of the need for—and consequently develop—accommodation plans for your students. The presence of the speech–language pathologist in the classroom gives classroom teachers the opportunity to observe their students as they work with another trained adult. It also provides them with a colleague who can serve as a brainstorming partner, particularly when they are discussing a student who represents a real challenge.

To: Mrs. Kelly
From: Mrs. Crouch, speech–language pathologist
Date: Fall, 2005
Re: Classroom Accommodation Plan

For: Josh W.

Listed below are the accommodations that have been included in Josh's IEP so that he may experience greater success in the classroom. Thank you for taking the time to become familiar with
this accommodation plan. Your continued support is what ensures that good things can happen!
Please remember that this is a confidential document that must be locked up and examined for
your review only. Complete information regarding this student can be reviewed in his school file in
the office. Thank you for your consideration.

Classroom/program accommodations:
1. Provide student with additional wait time to process verbal information.
2. Have student repeat or rephrase instructions to ensure his understanding.
3. Provide student with multiple repetitions and visual cues to learn new concepts.
4. Allow student frequent breaks or opportunities for movement to decrease frustration.
5. Provide preferential seating to assist with attending behaviors.
6. Have school nurse monitor hearing on a monthly basis.

Test modifications:
1. Provide a separate location.
2. Allow extended time for tests (2×).
3. Read directions and test items aloud to student.
4. Allow student to answer orally.

Figure 5.12. Letter to teachers re classroom accommodations.

I think it is fair to say that it takes a great deal of time and trust to build
this kind of relationship between two professionals. True collaboration between individuals may not be easy and rarely takes place overnight. From a
speech–language pathologist's perspective you must have the confidence in
yourself to accept new challenges, to learn curriculum, and to understand and
appreciate that your students are not your only priority—the entire class becomes your priority. Furthermore, you have to view yourself as your colleague's
equal. This can be especially difficult when you or your teammate has strong
opinions on how something should be taught or on a particular student issue.
Likewise, the classroom teacher must be open minded and willing to accept
you as a joint partner.

There are also some challenges to working directly in the classroom.
Often the students on our caseload are easily distracted by their surroundings
and have difficulty concentrating within a large group setting. It is frequently
necessary, therefore, to pull them out to provide an environment that is safe,
comfortable, and has minimal distractions. Also, students with learning problems often feel that they cannot "measure up" to their peers. They may become
withdrawn or unwilling to participate within a large group. When brought into
a smaller setting the same students may be successful at answering questions
they previously felt were too difficult. Another advantage of pull-out programs

is that they provide students with the opportunity to practice the skills or compensatory strategies you have taught prior to actually using them in the classroom. Some of my students have said to me that they like how we go over a topic, story, or skill before doing it in the classroom. Preteaching can help increase students' success in the classroom, as well as be instrumental in building a skill base they need for later learning. As you can see, then, there is no one correct way of providing intervention. You must determine what works best for you and your students at any point. In the 13 years I have been employed in the public school setting, besides not using one approach exclusively, I have changed my methods from year to year.

As we know, the activities that you develop for students on your caseload must target the goals stated on the students' IEPs. Thinking of activities becomes easier when you have themes or specific skill areas to work on. At the end of the chapter, I have included a list of materials I have found to be very helpful as I plan lessons and activities. What can be difficult, however, is making sure that you are addressing all the goals and objectives on the IEP and that you document student progress and performance. One way I do this is by developing a monthly code bank of goals and objectives.

Figure 5.13 provides an example of how I organize my students' IEP goals so they are easily accessible. As you can see, the goals and objectives are coded, which I have done for several reasons. It is much quicker to write codes in my plan book than very long and frequently repetitive goals and objectives. Furthermore, it is easy to see at a glance if I am including a variety of objectives in my plans or if I am concentrating on only one or two areas of deficit. Moreover, this system allows me to see immediately when a child is demonstrating success or struggling in an area. If a goal has been met, it is no longer necessary to incorporate it into my plans. Other goals, however, may require me to target them over and over or develop different criteria levels before the student can completely master them.

In addition to a goals and objectives code bank, I have included a New York State Learning Standards code bank on my lesson plan sheet. Figure 5.14 provides you with a brief overview of the New York State Learning Standards, typical of those developed in many other states. These standards are directly correlated to the curriculum being taught in the primary classrooms in my state. School districts have made it a policy to incorporate these standards in our daily planning; therefore, it is important to understand what each standard represents. Many states are developing new standards, and speech–language professionals should have a thorough knowledge of their content.

Figure 5.15 provides you with a sample lesson plan for a group of language-impaired kindergarten students. This method of planning has proven successful for me, but only you can know what method of planning is best for you. It is an ongoing process and inevitably involves a period of trial and error.

Much of this chapter has addressed planning for the student with a language impairment. Keep in mind that the same process of planning can also be pertinent for the student with articulation problems. Although the majority of my school-aged caseload consists of students with language-based deficits, I do have some primary students who exhibit articulation problems or a phono-

---

Student Goals and Objectives for September

Student Goals
Group #7 (Josh, Sam, Mike, Brenda)

1. To increase student's understanding and use of vocabulary and concepts (J,S,M,B).
2. To improve student's sound production skills (J,B).
3. To improve student's understanding and use of language (J,S,M,B).

Student Objectives
SWBAT (Students will be able to):

1. a. describe words using 3–4 specific attributes (J,S,M).
   b. understand and use directional prepositional concepts with 75% accuracy (S,M).
   c. identify/name items within a specific category with 75% accuracy (J,S,M,B).
   d. describe how items are similar and different with 70% accuracy (J,S,M,B).
   e. use critical listening skills to recall specific details with 75% accuracy (J,S,M,B).
   f. use words in a complete sentence with 80% accuracy (J,S,B).
2. a. discriminate target sounds (*k, g* blends, *f, v*) in isolation in 6/10 trials (J,B).
   b. understand the components necessary for good speech production (J,B).
   c. identify and demonstrate proper tongue placement for target sounds (*k, g, f, v*) (J,B).
   d. produce target sounds in words in all positions with 70% accuracy (J,B).
   e. produce target sounds in phrases with 70% accuracy (J,B).
   f. produce final consonants in words following a model with 80% accuracy (J,B).
3. a. follow novel one- and two-step commands with 70% accuracy (S,M,B).
   b. respond to wh questions related and unrelated to a story with 80% accuracy (J,S,M,B).
   c. identify letters of the alphabet with 80% accuracy (J,S).
   d. sequence a four-part event with 80% accuracy (M,B).
   e. identify and label colors with 80% accuracy (J,S,M).

Note. The above goals were taken directly from the IEPs of the four kindergarten students who make up group #7 on my caseload. The goals are a combination of each of the four IEPs included on one primary goal sheet for the month of September. Next to each of the goals and objectives is the initial letter of the name of the student to whom the goal pertains.

Figure 5.13. Student goals and objectives.

logical delay. I have found it more successful to work on their errors within the framework of a language-based activity, since many of them have weaknesses in that area, as well. Even if their language is age and grade appropriate, teaching them strategies to compensate for their errors is much easier when it is in a context that makes sense to them. Helping these students learn how to slow their rate, achieve appropriate placement, and demonstrate an awareness of good sound production often takes a great deal of time and practice.

I have included the following because most new clinicians benefit from several shelves of good materials to use as they plan effective intervention activities for the students on their caseload. Here are some of my favorite published materials:

Ausberger-Weiner, C. (1991). *Cut-n-color language development activity book.* Youngstown, AZ: ECL Publications.

English Language Arts (ELA)
1. Reading, writing, listening, and speaking for information and understanding
2. Reading, writing, listening, and speaking for literary response and expression
3. Reading, writing, listening, and speaking for critical analysis and evaluation
4. Reading, writing, listening, and speaking for social interaction

Mathematics, Science, Technology (MST)
1. Using mathematical analysis, scientific inquiry, and engineering design
2. Managing information systems
3. Understanding and applying mathematical concepts and principles
4. Understanding and applying scientific concepts and principles
5. Understanding and applying technological concepts and principles
6. Understanding and applying common themes across mathematics, science, and technology
7. Interdisciplinary problem solving

Social Studies (SS)
1. Understanding the history of the United States and New York State
2. Understanding world history
3. Understanding the geography of the world
4. Understanding economics
5. Understanding civics, citizenship, and government

Figure 5.14. Examples of New York State Learning Standards.

Bryer, J. (1993). *Rap-n-rock musical activities for language and literacy.* Oceanside, CA: Academic Communication Associates.

Cardoza-Griffith, S. (1999). *Multiple intelligences: Teaching the way kids learn in Grade 1.* Grand Rapids, MI: Frank Schaffer.

Diamond, S. (1993). *Language lessons in the classroom.* Youngstown, AZ: ECL Publications.

Lyle, M. (2000). *The LD teacher's IDEA companion, grades K–5.* East Moline, IL: LinguiSystems.

Paredes-Barnett, I. (1999). *Multiple intelligences: Teaching the way kids learn in kindergarten.* Grand Rapids, MI: Frank Schaffer.

Toomey, M. (1997). *Teaching the language of time.* Marblehead, MA: Circuit Publications.

The Collaborative Model in the Upper Grades: Nanette Clapper

Growing up, I often heard this message from my elders, identifying the difference between wisdom and knowledge: Knowledge is acquiring important information, having the facts. Wisdom is knowing how to apply that knowledge to everyday situations.

I was reminded of that saying when I initiated therapy within the classroom setting at my school. Unlike many therapists facing a new type of service delivery model, I had an advantage, a big advantage. I was not asked to participate in this approach or forced into it. I suggested my participation in it. After 20 years, I felt quite confident in my understanding of the speech and language

Week of: September 11–15   **Classroom:** AM Kindergarten   **Theme/Unit:** Friendship

Week Day: Monday   **Number Day:** 3

Activity Description

Read to whole group *The Land of Many Colors*. While reading, highlight the elements of the story, including characters, setting, problem, solution, and events. Engage the class in a discussion of what it means to be a friend. Brainstorm ways to be a friend. Chart on paper. Have students illustrate their favorite part of the story. Have student dictate in their own words their favorite part of the story. Write it down as part of their reader response.

Standards: ELA 1, ELA 2, ELA 4, SS 5   **Objectives:** 1e, 3b, 3e

Week Day: Tuesday   **Number Day:** 4

Activity Description

Divide class into 4 small groups. Rotate every 15 minutes. Provide students with a 4-picture story sequence sheet. Have the students color the pictures, cut them apart, and sequence them in the correct order from beginning to end to retell the events from the story that they heard earlier, *The Land of Many Colors*.

Standards: ELA 1, ELA 2, SS 5   **Objectives:** 1b, 1f, 2b, 2c, 2d, 3a, 3b, 3d

Week Day: Thursday   **Number Day:** 6

Activity Description

Model for the whole group the steps for making a "friendship flower." Have the students trace and cut out 5 petals in 5 different colors of paper. Have the students write their names on each of the petals and give them each to a different friend in the classroom. Have them verbally share with one another why they are friends with that person (e.g., "You are my friend because you like to swing with me on the playground"). Encourage the students to use complete sentences when orally sharing. Then have each student glue the petals of the flower onto a sheet of paper.

Standards: ELA 1, ELA 4, SS 5   **Objectives:** 1f, 3a, 3e

Figure 5.15. Speech and language push-in plans.

domains. I was also comfortable that I was using that knowledge to create interesting and challenging lessons. Therefore, it was difficult for me to come to the conclusion that the way I was providing services might not be the best way for my students to learn. Seriously contemplating in-the-classroom speech and language therapy was fueled by multiple considerations.

I had become concerned that in their classroom setting some of my students were not carrying over the strategies, language skills, and so forth that they had focused on in my therapeutic, pull-out environment. It appeared that these students had neither internalized nor organized the strategies learned in their pull-out sessions, nor had they applied them to their everyday communicative exchanges. I also saw that the classroom teachers were perplexed by a student's response or lack thereof. Teachers were very skilled in instructional techniques, but when a student's performance or response did not reflect comprehension, or did not meet the criterion for a correct response, they were often unfamiliar with specific strategies to facilitate a student's understanding.

My suggestion for a change in the service delivery model came after long deliberation on how I could improve therapy in a different setting. I met with an administrative committee headed by the director of pupil personnel services, Ms. Gisele Fox, and shared with the committee, the Least Restrictive Environment Committee, what I thought could be an ideal service delivery model. Once the program was accepted by the committee as a pilot project, I was allowed input into the selection of teachers and teacher's assistants with whom I would be working.

Delivering lessons in the classroom setting, however, posed new challenges. To begin with, before using this new service model approach, I was a solo act. With this new model, I found myself working beside other professionals—others who had their own agenda, their own goals and objectives, and their own way of doing things! When I had participated in the traditional service model, my planning time was flexible, based on my own schedule and availability. Becoming a member of a team meant working around other members' schedules, seeking times that were convenient for all those involved. As a pilot project, we were given the opportunity to arrange our schedules to reflect shared planning time at least one period a week. The school also afforded us the opportunity to have planning time before the start of the school year to integrate curriculum goals with the IEP goals of their students.

I also took into consideration the potential problems in scheduling students' therapy sessions as part of the collaborative service model. There was a particular class moving up that had a disproportionately large number of students who required speech and language therapy services. With that in mind, I sought to establish a collaborative classroom that would include several of those students. Focusing on those students, I was able to ensure that the goals and objectives I tailored for their personal learning profiles were relevant to their classroom instruction and performance.

The students receiving these services were not placed in a special education class. They were in a traditional classroom with their typically achieving peers, who, without a conscious effort on their part, served as excellent models. The classroom became enriched in the sense that the speech pathologist was a part of the classroom for at least one period a day, and the teacher and the SLP worked as a team, making every effort to weave relevant therapy approaches into the traditional curriculum.

Perhaps the greatest affirmation of this program, outside of the students' success, was the teacher's appreciation for the techniques, strategies, and diagnostic observations she acquired while being a part of the collaborative team. She felt that the strategies she observed and then carried over into the daily presentation of the curriculum were strategies she could use with all future students, whether they were students with special needs or not. By working with me, the classroom teacher recognized that the best way to facilitate language and auditory processing was not necessarily through auditory stimuli alone. From my perspective, I learned from her an abundance of information concerning reading and writing strategies that I was able to incorporate into my language strategies.

Parents also served as important team members in this collaborative service model. They were invited to meet with the school team before the school year started and share in the process of developing goals for the class. About 6 weeks into the school year, the parents were invited to meet with the rest of the team to learn strategies we had found particularly helpful. We shared observations about the students' learning profiles, and the parents were encouraged to share with us strategies and observations of their own. They were also asked to give us feedback regarding the work that went home with the student and to reflect and report on whether the student was carrying skills taught in class to the home environment. The parents also met with the school team on an individual basis to share specific strategies, concerns, and issues unique to their son or daughter. The classroom had an open-door policy in which each parent was invited to volunteer or observe at any time.

I attributed the success of the pilot program to many things. The school administration allowed us preparatory time before the school year began, and it supported consistent scheduling for planning time. The team was selected because of the proven skills of the teacher, Joan Sharkey; assistant, Sue Scerbo; and the other therapists involved. They were also willing to try something new. We learned that team compatibility is essential for a successful program. The team members recognized each others' contributions to the class and worked diligently at complementing each others' areas of expertise rather than duplicating them.

As the program's success was shared with the administration and faculty, requests for this service model approach increased. The quality of subsequent programs would be determined by the planning and cooperation of the team members involved. Planning with one team is time consuming; planning to the same degree with multiple teams can yield a program that is compromised. The implementation of multiple collaborative classes is a challenge faced by many school therapists. Balancing the benefits and pitfalls of this service delivery should be considered carefully when a therapist participates in more than one or two classes of this type.

When working collaboratively, it is essential that your plans reflect the means by which the student's goals and objectives (created on his Individualized Education Plan) can be facilitated within the classroom curriculum. It is imperative that the therapist be familiar with the grade-level curriculum for the students with whom he is working. Once acquainted with curriculum expectations and the proposed sequence of presentation, the therapist can integrate the student's individual needs with curriculum instruction.

In the following paragraphs I have divided specific examples of how this has been accomplished into activities appropriate to different grade levels across the upper primary, junior high school, and high school grades. In the upper elementary grades, I worked collaboratively within a special education class. This setup was unique and complex. Most of the students participated in other classes, making the collaboration team even larger and planning more difficult. The "homeroom" teacher (the special education teacher), however, eased the burden of my meeting with all of the other teachers by seeing the other teachers on at least a weekly basis and then sharing information, notes, goals, objectives, and plans with me when she met with me once a week.

There were two science units that proved to be particularly challenging for our students: the study of the solar system, and a unit on nutrition that included teaching the food pyramid. The teachers reviewed the units' curriculum contents, goals, and objectives. I examined my individual students' needs and developed a plan to incorporate their therapeutic needs within the contents of the curriculum.

Amber, a student in the class, had speech–language goals that included (but were not limited to) those of the New York Education Standard: English Language Arts #3: Language for Critical Analysis and Evaluation (New York State Board of Regents, 1998–2000). Amber's goal was "Improve use of morphological markers and syntactic structures in oral and written expression; 90% of sentences used in in-class samples will be without syntactic or morphological errors. 30% will be two-clause sentences." A second goal related to the New York State Standard: English Language Arts #1: "Improve comprehension and use of curriculum vocabulary. Amber will complete three end-of-unit assignments, answering questions and using new vocabulary correctly at an accuracy level of 80%."

Using these individualized goals and the contents of the curriculum, Amber (in concert with the other students) made a list of new words to learn, gleaned from the introductory unit. She chose a target word from her new curriculum vocabulary list and placed it in the center of a semantic word web. From that word in the web's center, she drew extensions that included the word's meaning, synonyms, antonyms, associations, and descriptives including size, color, shape, and quality. Using this web and other similar ones, Amber was able to compare and contrast the planets, as well as other aspects of the solar system. Hung around the room, under a student-drawn picture of the planet, were lists of the characteristics for each planet. The pictures reflected the students' understanding of what they had learned about that planet. The lists included facts about the planet and comparisons of that planet to others in the solar system. In order to obtain the facts listed, Amber had to use the critical thinking strategies identified in her IEP, specifically answering question types what, where, how, why, and "Is … ?"

Amber then used the target words to complete phrases and sentences that reflected her comprehension of curriculum content, including vocabulary. The sentences also enabled her to work on another objective, applying sequencing skills to organize information as she prepared an outline for a written composition. To include another of her goals, developing appropriate grammar and sentence structure, she and other students made entries in a daily journal. The journal was a piece of creative writing, pure fiction. They wrote about either their journey on a spaceship or what their lives were like visiting a new planet. They described in detail what this previously undiscovered planet looked like. They were encouraged to use comparatives, superlatives, transition words, and so forth.

The study of the solar system could have been challenging for our students who required support services. By using multiple modalities and strategies (e.g., word webs, lists, descriptions, comparisons, visual displays, written work) within the course of content instruction, the students were successful in attaining their curriculum goals, as well as working on their individualized goals and objectives. They had been given practice in using strategies to facilitate their learning, rather than drill, repetition, and short-term memorization.

A similar approach was used when the students studied nutrition. The teachers and therapists examined what the goals and objectives were for the curriculum in the unit, and I reviewed the students' IEPs and worked with the teacher to construct plans and activities that would meet the needs and learning profiles of the students.

In this unit, the students worked on categorizing by determining which food items belonged in a specific group. They studied labels for fat content, calories, vitamin and mineral content. They used comparatives and superlatives to describe foods within the same food group and foods in different food groups. This activity required them to use regular and irregular plurals, an objective from their grammar and syntax goal sheet. Auditory memory skills and strategies were taught, practiced, and encouraged as they discussed grocery items. The students listened to the items, listed them in written form, organized them by category, and then charted them on the food pyramid to see if the list reflected a balanced diet. They used critical thinking and reasoning abilities to plan menus and create corresponding grocery lists. They read flyers and compared prices of different brands, price per pound of bulk items, and the availability of coupons. Making choices required critical analysis and evaluation as they made inferences and drew conclusions from the relevant written information.

The students' enthusiasm and understanding of unit content affirmed that the integrated teaching approaches and specific strategy instruction worked. Perhaps the most significant sign of progress and success came when students working in a small group spontaneously suggested on their own, "Hey, let's make a list to help us remember, and then we can do a word web and come up with as many facts and associations as we can think of." Seeing students internalize new strategies and skills and then apply them to daily life skills or at least to the classroom curriculum is an affirmation of true learning.

One of the most creative efforts I had the pleasure of observing was that of a team working with upper-level students in the Phoenix Central School District in Phoenix, New York. The speech therapist, Mary Beth Calogero, worked closely with a team of classroom teachers. Together, the team created units that included the language arts, science, and social studies curriculum at the same time it met the students' therapeutic needs. The specialists made a concentrated effort to ensure that their therapy goals were educationally relevant for their students.

Among many successful collaborative lessons was one on the *Titanic*. At the time, the movie *Titanic* was making its debut. Young teens were captivated by the movie, the music, and the movie stars. Using another study guide as a model, the team took advantage of the students' excitement about a popular media event to teach them about a specific period of history (social studies), oceanography and weather (science), and communication (language arts).

Although that particular movie has passed into history, current movies and television shows continue to reflect a major teen passion. Consequently, they also represent a potential source of motivating topics, provided you can relate them to curriculum.

For the *Titanic* unit, the classroom was transformed into an event. Students began with basic vocabulary comprehension. Next, they prepared themselves to write journal entries and newspaper articles by expanding the vocabulary to include related synonyms, antonyms, and associations. Students chose characters from the story as the subject of a biography and studied words that described characteristics of the characters' personalities (e.g., ambitious, curious). Students sequenced events and recalled details (auditory memory) as they heard them. They worked on their critical thinking goal and objectives by analyzing and synthesizing information they had encountered in their research. In addition, they distinguished fact from fiction—that is, they differentiated between the events of the real disaster and its glamorized movie version. The integration of therapeutic goals and objectives within the core instruction was seamless and reflected thoughtful consideration by the special education and classroom teachers and the SLP.

Ms. Calogero also provided speech–language services to high school students using a different collaborative effort. She knew that the key to providing successful therapy for the teenage population was making their goals and objectives applicable to, and integrated into, their daily lives. The problem was that as students move into high school, their future plans begin to diverge. For example, all SLPs recognize how important it is for students to develop adequate written language skills. In high school, however, learning to write well may be a means to different goals. Some of Ms. Calogero's upper-class students were scheduled to take challenging year-end New York State Regents examinations, and they wanted to pass them at a high enough level to get into a college. Ms. Calogero also recognized the need for daily life skills, including writing, for those who were not planning to pursue a college career. She targeted the requirements of both types of students by creating individualized therapeutic goals and objectives to meet those needs. For example, some of her students learned how to write a résumé and complete a job application. Other students focused on expressive language skills and language for social interaction by enacting job interviews, phone calls to perspective employers or college interviewers. Hard-to-motivate students were more apt to show interest in activities that they viewed as purposeful and valuable.

In summary, collaborative teaching, also known as push-in therapy, is an approach encouraged by many school districts across the nation as they attempt to meet the demands of IDEA. The impetus is supported by the recognition that therapeutic needs for many students are best met when they are presented within the least restrictive environment and are related to the student's curriculum. From my own experience, and the reflections of the other therapists with whom I have worked, the collaborative approach is successful given certain parameters. The team must be given ample time to plan as a group. Our experience has been that when this does not happen, therapeutic goals and objectives are not clearly addressed and our therapeutic intentions are compromised. It is important that team members are compatible and recognize the contributions of each other's area of expertise. This recognition is a very important component and when properly addressed avoids the pitfall of a therapist's becoming an assistant or just an extra set of hands in the classroom.

Perhaps the greatest challenge of being a therapist participating in the collaborative approach, however, is the question "How do I do it all?" While I consider the collaborative approach as possibly the most successful approach I have been part of, I also recognize how time consuming the planning for this service delivery model is. Until caseloads and workloads are decreased, or the number of therapists increased, within a school, I do not think this approach is feasible for an entire caseload. SLPs need to meet with team members weekly. Multiple teams translate to multiple meetings, and these place more time constraints on the therapist's already tight schedule. At this point, time and resources can negatively affect a student's opportunities to receive therapeutic intervention within the least restrictive environment.

SECTION 3: CASE STUDIES

Returning now to the case studies, we discuss the SLP's next step in meeting student needs: intervention. Previously, you planned and interpreted an evaluation (Chapter 3), and then chose appropriate goals (Chapter 4) for each of the cases. Now, given this information, what are some ways you could address the students' deficits? As before, we will take the cases in order from youngest to oldest.

 ## Zachary

Considering Zachary's age, his grade, his teachers' styles, and his specific IEP, what service delivery model(s) and short-term objectives would you employ? I hope you recognize that most of Zachary's annual goals could be addressed through a variety of single- or multiple-service delivery models, such as collaborative, team teaching, and pull-out. Before reading on, list and defend your choice of service delivery model as you consider each of his goals.

Here are some of my suggestions. It is essential to identify an underlying goal first and then choose different means to implement it; the goals and objectives listed in Chapter 4 (no longer required on an IEP but necessary nonetheless) reflect the beginning of this process. As stated in one of his goals, Zachary is to develop basic phonological awareness skills at a conscious level. He must recognize that words are composed of syllables and phonemes and that they begin and end with different (or the same) sounds (Hodson, 1994). Once he has accomplished these goals, he must learn how to manipulate phonological information with increasing speed, that is, rapidly perform mental operations on sounds. He must also transfer this auditory knowledge into written form—that is, spelling and reading (decoding). Combining these modalities is in keeping with research that indicates that reading and writing develop concurrently and relatedly, not sequentially (Montgomery, 1995).

We should list our target phonological awareness skills and determine Zachary's present level in each: segmentation (sentences into words, words into syllables, and words into phonemes), rhyme (detection and production), alliteration (detection and production of initial, final, and medial sounds), and spelling. This is, in effect, the baseline, or the initial stage in a rubric. Next, we should decide how to integrate some of the skills with others, teaching more than one of them at a time. For example, we could link alliteration and segmentation, or segmentation and rhyme. In each case, however, we should start from a point where Zachary is confident—for example, because he recognizes what a "word" is, he could place Legos in a pattern with one Lego for each word (*he* + *is* + *sad*). Building on that skill, he could progress to Legos standing for syllables in compound words (*bird* + *house*), non-compound two-syllable words (*lum* + *ber*), or a sound plus a "word family" (*p* + *at*, or *p* + *in*). Gradually Zachary will move into those areas that represent new learning (e.g., four- and five-syllable words or separating a word into phonemes).

Using Legos takes advantage of the fact that Zachary finds learning easier when he has visual cues. If these actitivies are too elementary for the whole class, it might be accomplished only by the "low" group in an extended reading lesson, or in an individual pull-out or pull-aside session. Either you or Ms. Ruiz, his Title One reading teacher, could direct this while the other person teaches another group (collaboration and team teaching). You may suggest that picture card representations of "popping" or "windy" sounds from the Lindamood program (2000) be posted on a bulletin board, or that any teacher involved in the reading process with Zachary adopt the use of hand signals to cue a particular sound in the final position, thus employing different kinds of visual cues to assist his growing auditory awareness (Masterson, 1993).

Assessing Zachary's spelling level can determine what phonological skills he is bringing to the task—that is, what stage of spelling he is in, probably early phonemic, and then moving him into the next stage, even though it may not be age appropriate. To bring his attention to the sound at the end of a word, you could use Legos again (e.g., for the "t" sound in *pat, sit,* and *cut,* "t" could be a red Lego). This approach lends itself to teaching spelling, as well (e.g., putting a *t* on the Lego and gradually using the letter only). We can use sound families (*an, at, ot,* etc.) to help Zachary understand that what makes words rhyme is the presence of the same sounds at the end of words. As a speech–language pathologist, you realize that initially presenting continuant phonemes before noncontinuant ones enables Zachary to hear the sound longer.

Within the regular first-grade curriculum, we, or the teacher, can read poems and stories containing rhyme, and create alliteration or nonsense-sound activities ("deanut dutter danwich," "beanut butter banwich"). Ask the music teacher if the choral curriculum could include selections with alliteration ("The Sneaky Snake") or rhythmic and rhymed repetitions. Music is a natural for segmentation because the musical beat can bring attention to words and syllable boundaries in an unforced way.

You may also wish to discuss with the reading specialist the possibility of a reading method for Zachary that will emphasize phonology (Haskell, Foorman, & Swank, 1992). One of the possibilities suggested by Bradley and Bryant (1983) is using onset-rime. In an onset-rime approach to reading, Zachary would learn to segment and blend single-syllable words. For example, the initial consonant *f* (the onset) is combined with the vowel and remaining consonants *-in* (the rime) to make *fin*. Be careful, however, that you do not appear to dictate any one approach as the only possibility. Remember, Ms. Rose and the reading specialist have many years of experience. Your role is to point out how Zachary's apparent deficits in metaphonology may make certain reading approaches more appropriate. In the meantime, you will share with them how your goals in intervention are designed to address these underlying problems. You may wish to refer to some of the references that target metaphonology: those by Swank (1994), Catts (1991), Masterson (1993), Temple and Gillett (1984), Hoffman (1990), Hodson (1994), and Haskell et al. (1992). The International Dyslexia Association is a source of reading programs that feature the Orton-Gillingham approach. Before you can suggest any of these, or the surfeit of new materials available in catalogues, you need to become aware of the underlying philosophy of various reading programs.

Zachary must be able to match a "new" reading word to one previously stored in his memory; therefore, it is important that his new vocabulary words exist in proper phonological form. When you or Ms. Rose preteach vocabulary, try to choose words from class science lessons or reading books or those commonly used when teachers give directions (*top, bottom, circle, underline,* etc.). Using them and employing the techniques discussed previously, practice identifying initial and final sounds or segmenting words by syllables or phonemes (Catts, 1991). If Zachary needs more practice than others in his group, again you could provide it in pull-out (or pull-aside) intervention. A whole-class activity could feature printing signs for each major object in the first-grade classroom (*door, computer, desk, sink,* etc.), with Zachary deciding what the final sound should be or identifying the number of syllables in the word. Old articulation materials are easily adapted to sound identification in all word positions, including blends. Better yet, use the games as templates, but substitute words that Zachary is learning in any subject area, including spelling.

Other authors suggest these ways to establish and practice applied metaphonological principles: incorporate sound play into the classroom curriculum or theme; create nonsense words for common objects; suggest structured activities like choosing the word in a three-out-of-four series that does not rhyme or has a different initial or final sound; use additional visuals (boxes = sounds) or key terms, for example, "noisy nose" for a nasal sound. Catalogues are now full of new phonologically based materials and reading programs. Van Kleeck (1990) presented another sequence of acquisition that could serve as a springboard for dialogue between the reading specialist, the classroom teacher, and the speech–language pathologist.

Because Zachary's listening comprehension, including sequencing, also appears to be strongly affected by whether visual cues are present, the presence of pictures and manipulatives should help him become more successful in following directions. In addition to improving the coding of new words into Zachary's memory, it will help him to retain vocabulary if there is increased relevance of linguistic targets—that is, if the teacher makes sure he knows how and why he should learn them. Small-group or whole-class activities could include using predictable books to teach morphology (past tense, plurals, etc.), as well as more sophisticated syntax based on curricular needs ("Someone has been sleeping in my bed"). The techniques described to target final sounds and onset-rhyme can be adapted to teach morphological endings by substituting root word–plus–ending for initial sound-plus-rime. This is also a good way to introduce the fact that, although regular past tense ends in *ed,* it can be pronounced "t," "ed," or "d." Similarly, regular plurals can sound like "s," "z," or "ez." A typical first-grade science experiment addressing state can be used to bring attention to morphological endings ("Here the ice cube is solid; here it is melt*ing* [or it *melts*]; here it is melt*ed*").

Using Zachary's strengths to compensate for his weaknesses should be another goal of your intervention—for example, providing more opportunities to use his growing social skills to increase his ability to ask clarifying questions. If motoric sequencing is part of the problem in /r/ production, it may be advisable to use pull-out intervention, perhaps as part of an existing articulation group. Because his only articulation errors occurred in liquids, these will be incidentally addressed within the context of other goals. Certainly, in the initial stages of intervention, a large part of your job is translating your diagnostic findings into activities that will improve classroom competence by exposing all of Zachary's teachers to both his language goals and your procedures.

 James

We have now determined that James has pervasive word-finding deficits that directly affect expressive tasks; a receptive and expressive semantic problem involving concepts; and deficits in articulation, morphology, and syntax that can be attributed to a language difference. Let us tackle the language difference issue first. How will you handle this? Will you develop ways to change his language to reflect standard American English pronunciation and forms? Think about this before reading on.

First, is this difference affecting his overall classroom performance? Often, you need to share with teachers and administrators what the concept of a language difference entails, as well as describing the specific African American English forms James is using. After I gave this information to his teacher, Ms. Dwyer, she stated that the differences in question were not affecting James either academically or socially. Please note this last comment. It is a fact of life in schools that pragmatics are often ignored in an evaluation unless there is a clear indication of serious deficits. Ms. Dwyer recognized the value that children place on being accepted at school and acknowledged that James, even though shy and new in the school, interacted well and was liked by his classmates.

In a case like this, in which dialect is not negatively affecting academic subjects, SLPs can simply mention its presence during a regular conference with the parents and explain that the ability to switch code from the language students use at home to the standard forms valued at school can serve them well both academically and later in the workplace. At no time, however, should SLPs disparage the richness inherent in AAE. Sadly, many districts will not allow their specialists to work with students who are not on their caseload. Even if this is the case, however, SLPs can present in-service training to administrators and faculty or develop a unit on dialect that could be team-taught at various grade levels.

Both annual goals listed as part of James's IEP in Chapter 4 reflect nondialectical deficits that were identified during testing: James requires help in acquiring and using specific types of vocabulary (temporal and spatial terms); in addition, he needs to increase his ability to ask his teacher for help when he is confused or needs assistance. A primary barrier to meeting either goal is James's anomia. Word-finding problems can originate from either inefficient word storage or inefficient retrieval strategies. Storage strength is an indication of how well learned words are, that is, how available they are in memory. Retrieval strength reflects the accessibility of that information (Nippold, 1992). It is important to identify which one (or both) of these is implicated because intervention strategies will be different. For discussion purposes, let us assume that you have already determined through extension testing that James needs help in both areas. What type of intervention and what service delivery models could you use?

Here are some ways I might address meeting James's goals. The more often a student studies and uses an item of information, the more storage and retrieval strength increase. Nippold (1992) stated that retrieval practice is more powerful for increasing the ability to store and retrieve. Therefore, we need to prioritize the specific vocabulary James needs to succeed in different subjects, particularly those in which the terms are brand new, such as scientific concepts. One of the most efficient ways to address this need is by preteaching vocabulary, done individually in pull-aside or pull-out intervention, in a small group within the class, or by engaging parents or aides as partners. It is important to note the difference here between teaching the meaning of new words (the teacher's, aide's, or parent's role) and the SLPs therapeutic role, teaching James strategies to remember the words (e.g., visualization).

German's work (1992, 1994) provides detailed information on word-finding problems. Finding sources like this provides a solid foundation on which you can build. The author suggests teaching different attribute and associate cueing strategies as a way to help students call up a specific word. Under attribute cues, she lists the following: providing students with an initial sound or syllable; providing the category name or function of the word; telling the student to visualize the referent; and drawing a sketch or using a gesture associated with the word. Associate cues refer to an intermediate word that can help cue the target word (e.g., *crayon* for *pencil*). She also suggests that students be taught to consciously circumlocute (i.e., to use a synonym, a description, or a category name until the word is retrieved). Students should be taught to deliberately pause to give themselves time to think of the word, and to reduce their use of proforms, nonspecific words like *thing*. Finally, she suggests that students must learn to self-monitor, self-evaluate, and self-correct. As we have noted in earlier chapters, for any strategy to work, students must feel that it is worth the effort—that is, James must be confident that if he uses one of the strategies, he will be able to retrieve the word he wants.

To increase retrieval strength, it is especially important that James be able to pronounce each word easily. It is difficult to retrieve a word you cannot pronounce. When he reads a new vocabulary word for the first time, encourage him to say it out loud. Specific phonemic cues can be used when the terms are taught, and those same cues can be employed again when retrieval is practiced: for example, "Ants have antennae." You will also want to use categorization, grouping items that have something in common (insects that fly) and associative clues to help aid memory (the sound some insects make, or visualizing six legs). As part of your consulting you could teach Ms. Dwyer some of German's cueing techniques to use throughout the class day. She could also use word boxes or matching questions to test vocabulary, at least initially.

To the greatest extent possible, the first words addressed by these techniques should have concrete referents. Because James will need many, many repetitions to put these words into storage and access them easily, you should plan with the teacher or librarian (collaboration, consultation) to have available books, pictures, computer programs, film strips, and posters that can provide many opportunities for continued discussion. Spelling words can also be used. Remember, you are teaching the process of how to store and retrieve words, as well as the actual vocabulary. Be very explicit about what you are doing so that in later months and years, James can use these methods to learn new material. Note that learning new vocabulary is required of every student in school and that the means of memorizing effectively is a valuable skill. Others may not need the number of repetitions or the cues that James will, but they would certainly benefit from learning such techniques as visualization, word webs, semantic maps, and Venn diagrams presented as part of whole-class instruction.

Decreasing proforms can be done partly within the context of teaching the processes just described. It could also be addressed directly by teaching how to define or describe objects, sequences, or events. Consider collaboration with the art or physical education teacher in teaching spatial and temporal terms. Unfortunately, most teachers assume that students have mastered calendar facts by second grade at the latest. For students like James, it can be both confusing and embarrassing not to know in what months holidays come, whether spring is a season or a month, whether today is Monday the 27th, or what the day and date of the day before yesterday was. Consequently, part of your job will be to help him review this information until it becomes automatic, using classroom routines as much as possible, such as counting down days on a calendar on his desk until assignments are due. A time line can serve as a visual cue to help him understand temporal concepts, as well as review concept vocabulary.

As we did with Zachary, think of ways you could combine some of James's short-term objectives both in and out of the classroom. Assume the class is studying different climates in diverse geographical areas. Use visualization and drawing to help James "see" a desert and a swamp. Help him learn and list specific adjectives to describe each: *dry, sandy, hot, arid, quiet, bright* versus *humid, green, dripping, wet, dank, shaded, noisy.* The adjective lists could be part of a compare and contrast diagram. Have James locate deserts and swamps on a real map and plot how to get from one place to the other using map words and other spatial terms. He could write a journal, à la Lewis and Clark, about his adventures along the way using sequential terms. He could plan the journey, listing what he should do before he leaves home, while he is on the trip, and after he returns home. (Note that the entire class could take part in some or all of the activities.) Since James is part of a military family, perhaps his father and mother could discuss the places family members have lived (in sequence) and describe how they traveled from one to the next. As he is completing these activities, cue him as neccessary as you help him start using his own word-finding strategies. Encourage him to recognize the need for asking questions as his plans unfold.

As you develop these programs with James's teacher, be sure to plan how you will maintain records verifying the effectiveness of intervention; remember, accountability is required for all service models, not just pull-out.

Christine

You have moved from first to third and now tenth grade. How will you adapt your intervention procedures to reflect this change in age and situation? List at least two activities for each of the goals developed in Chapter 4 using three different service delivery models.

One of the imperatives at the high school level is using curriculum materials and assignments exclusively when you plan intervention. A second consideration should be to teach a process that can be applied to as many different subjects as possible and that addresses more than one goal. You want to help Christine learn to recognize the underlying organizational structure of material she is reading. At the same time, she can practice applying those organizational schemas to her written assignments. This could be done collaboratively with her reading or classroom teachers. An example is teaching the concepts behind and use of verbal organizers. Westby (1994) presents a list of text structures (sequence, comparison–contrast, cause–effect, etc.), including the function of each, key words for recognizing them, and comprehension questions that Christine could use to create study guides. Using Figure 7.2, "Linking Expressions That Signal Cohesion and Organization," in Chapter 7 could be a starting place, as well. Paul (2001) has compiled a number of visual organizers that could assist Christine in learning the meaning of various clausal connectors.

Be aware that Christine may need to start at a basic level—for example, differentiating between a main idea and supporting detail. One of the ways to practice this concept is by teaching her how to paraphrase content area materials. Donahue and Pidek (1993) recommend this holistic skill because it requires a knowledge of syntax and vocabulary to rephrase information. It allows the SLP to check recall, comprehension, and ability to discern the organizational pattern of the text at the same time the skill is being taught and practiced. Depending on Christine's ability, the authors suggest that paraphrasing can involve simple retelling (easiest for a narrative), a summary of main ideas (good for expository discourse), or an elaboration of the original message (useful in persuasive essays). Paraphrasing is also useful because if Chris gets lost, she can be encouraged and taught how to ask for repetition or clarification, two quite different prompts.

Another way to approach Christine's reading comprehension is to teach her how to summarize expository text by beginning at the paragraph level (Swanson & De La Paz, 1998). Swanson and De La Paz suggest that teachers require students to use a single sentence to summarize information found in a paragraph. They use three steps to accomplish this end: They begin by having students retell the main idea in a single expository sentence. Next, they teach students how to retell two sentences of text in 15 words or less. Finally, they gradually lengthen the material to an entire paragraph until students can summarize it in 15 words or less.

Teaching Chris how to use her textbook's headings, subheadings, boldfaced key words, chapter summaries, and review sections will also aid in her understanding of organization. You could accomplish this by co-teaching with a special education colleague during a resource room period. Since Christine is in class with a number of other low-average students, teaching these ways to understand a given material's organization schema will be helpful to most of them.

Ms. Williams, Christine's English teacher, could provide you with a list of future writing assignments or oral presentations that would allow you to review the appropriate structures and clausal connectors for a specific assignment type. Push-in, collaborative, team teaching, and pull-out modes could all be used, depending on the situation at the time. Working on the actual assignment could also give you an opportunity to discuss such topics as transitions between paragraphs, topic sentences, and supporting statements. Graham and Harris (1987) discuss how to teach students self-prompts when they are rereading or editing their own work. Turpie and Paratore's (1995) pilot program featuring assessment and intervention could prove useful in diminishing Christine's discouragement. It features parent involvement and would allow Christine a voice in setting academic goals.

At the same time, Christine will need instruction and practice in how to improve her note-taking skills in lecture. She will need assistance not only in organization but also in decoding the meaning when it is not directly stated. Adapting Christine's textbook could include, at least initially, the SLP's simplifying some of the syntactic complexity of certain very difficult sections so that the meaning can be deciphered. At a later date, the reverse procedure could take place—for example, taking the two simple sentences you extracted and reforming them into a longer one. Giving Christine a textbook for her permanent and exclusive use would let her highlight topic sentences or section titles. It would also prove useful to her reading tutor. You could highlight clausal connectors in some sections so Christine could see how they are used in actual grade-appropriate materials. The highlighted text, perhaps with a few margin notes, could also serve as a study guide.

Teachers could initially offer lecture outlines for Christine to follow that would teach her various ways information is organized. These could gradually be faded to include only the main outline with numbers and letters to indicate that information should be filled in. Fry, Polk, and Fountoukidis (2000) provide a useful list of "signal words," words that authors and lecturers use to tell the reader or class members how to read and listen. These include "continuation signals" (meaning there are more ideas to come: *moreover, furthermore, in addition*) and "change-of-direction signals" (meaning we're doubling back: *despite, rather, conversely, even though*). Finding these terms in different textbooks could provide additional practice.

Finally, it is important to consider how to support Christine's transitional goals. Her guidance counselor will help her select elective courses that build on her academic strengths (her preference to learn by doing, particularly when information is presented in clear sequences, e.g., in science experiments, cooking) and personal interests (working with children). As her SLP, you can suggest to teachers curriculum-related assignments that reflect her interests. For instance, if the class is studying colonial history, Christine could report on games children played or books they read during that period.

Megan

Consider the goals you developed for Megan at the close of Chapter 3 and discuss how they might be implemented. If you have not used each service delivery model, try the remaining ones for at least some of the goals.

CONCLUSION

As you conclude this fourth case, I hope you are feeling more confident in your ability to assess strengths and deficits; interpret your findings; and plan appropriate, motivating intervention for students like Zachary, James, Christine, and Megan. These students may not exist, but every fact about them is based on the experiences of real students with real needs who are counting on all of us to put forth our best effort. Finally, I trust that if someone asks, "What is it that you speech–language people do?" you will be able to tell them more than they want to know. Enjoy.

STUDY QUESTIONS

1. Define the term *service delivery model*.
2. What factors have led to so many different kinds of service delivery models?
3. Compare and contrast six different service delivery models, giving at least one positive and one negative aspect of each.
4. List six different speech–language roles that do *not* use the collaborative approach—that is, ways that you may serve the school other than direct intervention.
5. According to Ehren, what is the difference between teaching and therapy?
6. Create a language lesson plan that could engage an entire class but would also provide an opportunity for a therapeutic focus for two students on your caseload who have vocabulary deficits.

7. Define *learning strategy*. What is the advantage of using one when providing intervention?
8. Why might a classroom teacher resent your intrusion into his or her classroom? What are some positive steps you can take to blunt this feeling?
9. Compare and contrast the intervention strategies used by Tracy Crouch and Nanette Clapper.
10. Create a week-long thematic unit that will address both curricular and language goals. Explain how your unit can do both.
11. Reread the cases describing Zachary, James, and Christine. Create an appropriate activity for each student, employing a different service delivery model for each one; provide a lesson plan to share with classmates.
12. List additional ways in which you could address Christine's transitional goals.

REFERENCES

American Speech-Language-Hearing Association. (1991, March). Guidelines for the collaborative service delivery for students with language-learning disorders in the public schools. *Asha, 33*(5), 44–50.

American Speech-Language-Hearing Association. (1999). *Guidelines for the roles and responsibilities of the school-based speech–language pathologist.* Rockville, MD: Author.

American Speech-Language-Hearing Association. (2000). Special report: Service delivery. *2000 Schools Survey,* 1–2.

American Speech-Language-Hearing Association. (2002). A workload analysis approach for establishing speech–language caseload standards in the schools: Position statement. *ASHA Desk Reference, 3,* 89–90.

Bashir, A., Conte, B., & Heerde, S. (1998). Language and school success: Collaborative challenges and choices. In D. D. Merritt & B. Culatta (Eds.), *Language intervention in the classroom* (pp. 1–36). San Diego, CA: Singular.

Beatty, J. (1985, February). A voice for the underdog. *Atlantic Monthly,* p. 100.

Bloom, B., Engelhart, M., Furst, E., Hill, W., & Krathwohl, D. (Eds.). (1956). *Taxonomy of educational objectives: The classification of educational goals. Handbook I: Cognitive domain.* New York: David McKay.

Boehm, A. (2000). *Boehm test of basic concepts* (3rd ed.). San Antonio, TX: Psychological Corp.

Borsch, J., & Oaks, R. (1992). Clinical forum: Implementing collaborative consultation. Effective collaboration at Central Elementary School. *Language, Speech, and Hearing Services in Schools, 23,* 367–368.

Bradley, L., & Bryant, P. (1983). Categorizing sounds and learning to read: A causal connection. *Nature, 30,* 419–421.

Brandel, D. (1992). Clinical forum: Implementing collaborative consultation. Collaboration: Full steam ahead with no prior experience! *Language, Speech, and Hearing Services in Schools, 23,* 369–370.

Buchoff, R. (1990, Winter). Attention deficit disorder: Help for the classroom teacher. *Childhood Education,* 86–90.

Buschbacher, P., & Fox, L. (2003) Understanding and intervening with the challenging behavior of young children with autism spectrum disorder. *Language, Speech, and Hearing Services in Schools, 34,* 217–227.

Bush, C. (1980a). *Language remediation and expansion: 100 skill-building reference lists.* Tucson, AZ: Communication Skill Builders.

Bush, C. (1980b). *Language remediation and expansion: School and home program.* Tucson, AZ: Communication Skill Builders.

Butler, K. (1980). The path to a concept of language-learning disabilities. *Topics in Language Disorders, 1*, 6.

Catts, H. (1991). Facilitating phonological awareness: Role of speech–language specialists. *Language, Speech, and Hearing Services in Schools, 22*, 196–203.

Christensen, S., & Luckett, C. (1990). Getting into the classroom and making it work. *Language, Speech, and Hearing Services in Schools, 21*, 110–113.

Cochran, P. S., & Masterson, J. J. (1995). NOT using a computer in language assessment/intervention: In defense of the reluctant clinicians. *Language, Speech, and Hearing Services in Schools, 26*, 213–222.

Conde, M. (1999). *Land of many colors and Nanna-Ya.* Lincoln: University of Nebraska Press.

Conoley, J., & Conoley, C. (1982). How to enter: When to stay. In J. Conoley & C. Conoley (Eds.), *School consultation: A guide to practice and training* (pp. 106–133). New York: Pergamon.

Crais, E. (1992). *Family-centered assessment and collaborative goal-setting.* New York State Speech-Language-Hearing Association Annual Conference, Kiamesha Lake, New York.

Curtis, M., & Meyers, J. (1985). Consultation: A foundation for alternative services. In A. Thomas & J. Grimes (Eds.), *Best practices in school-based consultation: Guidelines for effective practice* (pp. 35–38). Washington, DC: National Association of School Psychologists.

Curtis, M., & Zins, J. (Eds.). (1981). *The theory and practice of school consultation.* Springfield, IL: Thomas.

Dollaghan, C., & Kaston, N. (1986). A comprehension monitoring program for language-impaired children. *Journal of Speech and Hearing Disorders, 51*, 263–271.

Donahue, M., & Pidek, C. (1993). Listening comprehension and paraphrasing in content-area classrooms. *Journal of Childhood Communication Disorders, 15*(2), 35–42.

Edwards, C. (1991). Assessment and management of listening skills in school aged children. *Seminars in Hearing, 12*, 389–401.

Eger, D. (1992). Why now? Changing school speech–language service delivery. *Asha, 34*(11), 40–41.

Ehren, B. (2000). Maintaining a therapeutic focus and sharing responsibility for student success: Keys to in-classroom speech–language services. *Language, Speech, and Hearing Services in Schools, 31*, 219–229.

Elksnin, L., & Capilouto, G. (1994). Speech–language specialists' perceptions of integrated service delivery in school settings. *Language, Speech, and Hearing Services in Schools, 25*, 248–267.

Ellis, L., Schlaudecker, C., & Griess, K. (1995a). Effectiveness of a collaborative consultation approach to basic concept instruction. *Language, Speech, and Hearing Services in Schools, 26*, 69–74.

Ellis, L., Schlaudecker, C., & Griess, K. (1995b). Effectiveness of a collaborative consultation approach to basic concept instruction with kindergarten children. *Language, Speech, and Hearing Services in Schools, 26*, 63–69.

Farber, J., & Klein, E. (1999). Classroom-based assessment of a collaborative intervention program with kindergarten and first grade children. *Language, Speech, and Hearing Services in Schools, 30*, 83–91.

Ferguson, M. (1992). Clinical forum: Implementing collaborative consultation. An introduction. *Language, Speech, and Hearing Services in Schools, 23*, 371–372.

Fry, E., Polk, J., & Fountoukidis, D. (2000). *The reading teacher's book of lists* (4th ed.). San Francisco: Jossey-Bass.

German, D. (1992). Word-finding intervention for children and adolescents. *Topics in Language Disorders, 13*, 33–50.

German, D. (1994). Word finding difficulties in children and adolescents. In G. Wallach & K. Butler (Eds.), *Language learning difficulties in school-age children* (pp. 323–347). New York: Merrill.

German, D. (2000). *Test of word finding* (2nd ed.). Austin, TX: PRO-ED.

Giangreco, M., & Meyer, L. (1988). Expanding service delivery options in regular school and classrooms for students with severe disabilities. In J. Graden & M. Curtis (Eds.), *Alternative educational delivery: Enhancing instructional options for all students* (p. 257). Washington, DC: National Association of School Psychologists.

Gibbons, G. (1984). *Arnold's apple tree.* Orlando, FL: Harcourt Brace.

Goodman, K. (1986). *What's whole in whole language?* Portsmouth, NH: Heinemann.

Graham, S., & Harris, K. (1987). Improving composition skills of inefficient learners with self-instructional strategy training. *Topics in Language Disorders, 7,* 68–77.

Guilford, L. (1993). Letter to the editor. *Language, Speech, and Hearing Services in Schools, 24,* 63.

Hall, P., & Tomblin, J. (1978). A follow-up study of children with articulation and language disorders. *Journal of Speech and Hearing Disorders, 43,* 227–241.

Haney, C. (1992). The place for assistive technology. *Asha, 39*(11), 47–49.

Haskell, D., Foorman, B., & Swank, P. (1992). Effects of three orthographic/phonological units on first grade reading. *Remedial and Special Education, 13*(2), 40–49.

Hill, S., & Haynes, W. (1992). Language performance in low-achieving elementary school students. *Language, Speech, and Hearing Services in Schools, 23,* 169–175.

Hodson, B. (1994). Helping individuals become intelligible, literate and articulate: The role of phonology. *Topics in Language Disorders, 14*(2), 1–16.

Hoffman, P. (1990). Spelling, phonology, and the speech–language specialist: A whole language perspective. *Language, Speech, and Hearing Services in Schools, 21,* 238–243.

Hoskins, B. (1990a). Collaborative consultation: Designing the role of the speech–language specialist in a new educational context. In W. A. Secord (Ed.), *Best practices in school speech–language pathology* (pp. 29–36). San Antonio, TX: Psychological Corp.

Hoskins, B. (1990b). Language and literacy: Participating in the conversation. *Topics in Language Disorders, 10*(2), 46–62.

Huffman, N. (1992). Challenges of education reform. *Asha, 34*(11), 41–44.

Idol, L., Paolucci-Whitcomb, P., & Nevin, A. (1986). *Collaborative consultation.* Austin, TX: PRO-ED.

Individuals with Disabilities Education Improvement Act. (2004). Public Law 108-446.

Kafka, S. (1990). *I need a friend.* San Antonio, TX: Harcourt Brace.

Kamhi, A. (1999). Research to practice. To use or not to use: Factors that influence the selection of new treatment approaches. *Language, Speech, and Hearing Services in Schools, 30,* 92–98.

Kroll, S. (1988). *Oh, what a Thanksgiving.* New York: Scholastic.

Larson, V., McKinley, N., & Boley, D. (1993). Clinical forum: Adolescent language. Service delivery models for adolescents with language disorders. *Language, Speech, and Hearing Services in Schools, 24,* 36–42.

Light, J., & McNaughton, D. (1993). Literacy and augmentative and alternative communication (AAC): The expectations and priorities of parents and teachers. *Topics in Language Disorders, 13*(2), 33–46.

Lindamood, P., & Lindamood, P. (2000). *The Lindamood phoneme sequencing program for reading, spelling, and speech.* Austin, TX: PRO-ED.

Lobel, A. (1970). *Frog and toad are friends.* New York: HarperCollins.

Lobel, A. (1979). *Frog and toad—The kite.* New York: HarperCollins.

Martin, B., & Archambault, J. (1989). *Chika chika boom boom.* New York: Simon & Schuster.

Marvin, C. (1987). Consultation services: Changing roles for speech–language specialists. *Journal of Childhood Communication Disorders, 11,* 1–16.

Masterson, J. (1993). Classroom-based phonological intervention. *American Journal of Speech–Language Pathology, 2,* 5–9.

Masterson, J. J. (1995). Computer application in the schools: What we can do—What we should do. *Language, Speech, and Hearing Services in Schools, 26,* 211–212.

McGuire, R. A. (1995). Computer-based instrumentation: Issues in clinical application. *Language, Speech, and Hearing Services in Schools, 26,* 223–231.

Miller, L. (1989). Classroom-based language intervention. *Language, Speech, and Hearing Services in Schools, 20,* 153–170.

Montgomery, J. (1992). Clinical forum: Implementing collaborative consultation. Perspectives from the field: Language, speech and hearing services in schools. *Language, Speech, and Hearing Services in Schools, 23,* 363–364.

Montgomery, J. (April, 1995). *Language, literacy and learning.* Presentation to Long Island Speech Language Hearing Association.

Multiskilling. (2003). *Asha Leader,* 8(10), 30.

Neidecker, E., & Blosser, J. (1993). *School programs in speech–language: Organization and management.* Englewood Cliffs, NJ: Prentice Hall.

Nelson, N., & Kinnucan-Welsch, K. (1992). Curriculum-based collaboration: What is changing? *Asha,* 34(11), 45–47, 50.

New York Board of Regents. (1988). *Amendment to Part 200 Regulations of the Commission.* Available from the University of the State of New York, State Education Department, Office for Special Education Services, Division of Program Development and Support Services, Room 1069, Education Building Annex, Albany, NY 12234.

New York Board of Regents. (1998–2000). *Learning standards.* Albany: University of the State of New York State Education Department.

Nippold, M. A. (1992). The nature of normal and disordered word finding in children and adolescents. *Topics in Language Disorders, 13,* 1–14.

Paul, R. (1995). *Language disorders from infancy through adolescence: Assessment and intervention.* St. Louis, MO: Mosby.

Paul, R. (2001). *Language disorders from infancy through adolescence: Assessment and intervention* (2nd ed.). St. Louis, MO: Mosby.

Pellegrini, N. (1991). *Families are different.* New York: Holiday House.

Perry, T. (1990). Cooperative learning = Effective intervention. *Language, Speech, and Hearing Services in Schools, 21,* 120.

Peters-Johnson, C. (1992). Professional practices perspective on caseloads in schools. *Asha, 34,* 12.

Pietranton, A., & Lynch, C. (1995). Multiskilling: A renaissance or a dark age? *Asha,* 37(6, 7), 37–40.

Prelock, P. (2000). Prologue. Multiple perspectives for determining the roles of speech–language pathologists in inclusionary classrooms. *Language, Speech, and Hearing Services in Schools, 31,* 213–218.

Riley, A. M. (1991). *Evaluating acquired skills in communication–Revised.* Austin, TX: PRO-ED.

Roller, E., Rodriquez, T., Warner, J., & Lindahl, P. (1992). Clinical forum: Implementing collaborative consultation. Integration of self-contained children with severe speech–language needs into the regular education classroom. *Language, Speech, and Hearing Services in Schools, 23,* 365–366.

Russell, S., & Kaderavek, J. (1993). Alternative models for collaboration. *Language, Speech, and Hearing Services in Schools, 24,* 76–78.

Sanger, D., Hux, I., & Griess, K. (1995). Educators' opinions about speech–language pathology services in schools. *Language, Speech, and Hearing Services in Schools, 26,* 75–86.

Schmidt, H., & Rodgers-Rhyme, A. (1988). *Strategies: Effective practices for teaching all children (participant guide).* Madison, WI: Wisconsin State Department of Public Instruction, Bureau of Exceptional Children. (ERIC Document Reproduction Service No. ED 304 231)

Schuh, M., Tashie, C., & Jorgensen, C. (1981). *Strategies for modifying and expanding curriculum for students with disabilities.* Concord: University of New Hampshire, Institute on Disability.

Schulz, J., & Turnbull, A. (1984). *Mainstreaming handicapped students.* Newton, MA: Allyn & Bacon.

Secord, W. (1989, November). *Developing a collaborative language program.* Paper presented to to Central New York Speech, Language and Hearing Association, Oneida, NY.

Seuss, D. (1973). *Green eggs and ham.* New York: Random House.

Silliman, E. R., Bahr, R., Beasman, J., & Wilkinson, L. C. (2000). Scaffolds for learning to read in an inclusion classroom. *Language, Speech, and Hearing Services in Schools, 31*(3), 265–279.

Simon, C. (1987). Out of the broom closet and into the classroom: The emerging speech–language specialist. *Journal of Childhood Communication Disorders, 11,* 41–66.

Simon, C., & Myrold-Gunyuz, P. (1990). *Into the classroom: The speech–language specialist in the collaborative role.* Tucson, AZ: Communication Skill Builders.

Sonnenmeier, R., & McGuire, K. (1995, March). *Supporting the communication skills of children's language learning needs in inclusive settings.* Paper presented at the Central New York Speech Language and Hearing Association Spring Conference, Syracuse, NY.

Swank, L. (1994). Phonological coding ability: Identification of impairments related to phonologically based reading problems. *Topics in Language Disorders, 14*(2), 56–71.

Swanson, P., & De La Paz, S. (1998). Teaching effective comprehension strategies to students with learning and reading disabilities. *Intervention in School and Clinic, 33*(4), 209–218.

Temple, C., & Gillett, J. W. (1984). *Language arts learning processes and teaching practices.* Boston: Little, Brown.

Titherington, J. (1990). *Pumpkin, pumpkin.* New York: Harper.

Turpie, J., & Paratore, J. (1995). Using repeated reading to promote reading success in a heterogeneously group first grade. In K. A. Hinchman, D. J. Leu, & C. K. Kinzer (Eds.), *Perspectives on literacy research and practice: Forty fourth yearbook of the national reading conference* (pp. 255–264). Chicago, IL: National Reading Conference.

van Kleeck, A. (1990). Emergent literacy: Learning about print before learning to read. *Topics in Language Disorders, 10,* 25–45.

Wadle, S. (1991). Clinical exchange: Why speech–language clinicians should be in the classroom. *Language, Speech, and Hearing Services in Schools, 22,* 277.

Westby, C. (1994). Advanced communication development. In W. Haynes & B. Shulman (Eds.), *Communication development: Foundations, processes and clinical applications* (pp. 341–384). Englewood Cliffs, NJ: Prentice Hall.

Word of mouth. (1995). Editorial Comment, 6, p. 10. New York: Harper.

Zarrella, S. (1995). Specialization facilitates service delivery in schools. *Advance, 5*(29), 3, 15.

Expanding Roles of School-Based Speech–Language Pathology: Educationally Relevant Intervention

Chapters 6–10 make up this section of the text. Building on the information in Section II, assessment, goal setting, and intervention issues are examined in the light of the who, the what, and the how of application. Each chapter addresses a way in which clinical speech–language pathology skill requirements have expanded in recent years to meet the demands of different groups of individuals, different disorders, and the ways assessment and intervention take place in today's schools.

Chapter 6 has two main sections. The first section describes the challenges inherent in assessment and intervention for students with three disorders or conditions that have gained new prominence in school-based practice. These include autism spectrum disorders (ASD), traumatic brain injury (TBI), and medical fragility. Swallowing problems (dysphagia) related to the last two conditions are also discussed. The second section of Chapter 6 discusses the ramifications of undertaking assessment and intervention within the context of the school curriculum.

Chapter 7 follows naturally from the second section of Chapter 6. It addresses a specific curricular area new to many speech–language pathologists: their role in helping students who are experiencing problems in reading, writing, and spelling that are language based. Typical developmental progressions and assessment and intervention issues are discussed for each of the three literacy areas.

Chapter 8 describes the role of augmentative and alternative communication in school-based practice. It includes the large range of AAC options and employs case histories to acquaint readers with the ways choices are made in this rapidly changing field.

Chapter 9 has been expanded to include the issues involved in assessment and intervention for students who are culturally and linguistically diverse. General principles are presented, plus specific information about groups whose members have gained new prominence in school populations.

Chapter 10 addresses the complexity of third-party payments and the important topics of supervision and support personnel. These issues are not often encountered in undergraduate or graduate courses, but school administrators assume that SLPs know about them, particularly when it comes to monetary reporting requirements.

Chapter 6

◆ ◆

Serving Students with Challenging Disorders and Conditions

Eileen H. Gravani
and Jacqueline Meyer

As noted in Chapter 1, the history of speech–language pathology has been one of continuing growth. In school-based practice, the expansion has been particularly apparent in the additional types of disorders SLPs are now expected to evaluate and treat. Although a number of low-incidence populations are increasingly encountered, including students with conditions stemming from maternal substance abuse, specific syndromes, behavioral disorders, psychiatric disorders, and physical abuse and neglect (Sparks, 1984, 2001), the first part of this chapter will provide a brief overview of three disorders that have gained gained new prominence on SLPs' caseloads in the last 10 years: pervasive developmental disorder (PDD)—or the term more frequently encountered in schools, autism spectrum disorder (ASD)—traumatic brain injury (TBI), and medical fragility. The latter two conditions can be complicated by swallowing problems (dysphagia). This chapter should not be read in isolation. The general principles of evaluation, goal writing, and intervention outlined in Chapters 3–5 should be applied with children who have the disorders and conditions discussed in this chapter. It is also important to note that each of these three areas requires a multidisciplinary team for identification and treatment. Chapter 8, which addresses augmentative and alternative communication, and the portion of Chapter 12 that discusses the roles of occupational and physical therapists will be particularly instructive.

In addition to the above disorders and conditions, SLPs have been encouraged to extend their assessment and intervention into educational areas once considered to be the exclusive domain of elementary and secondary classroom or special education teachers. Implicit in this expanded role is the irrefutable effect of language limitations and disorders on a student's acquisition of curriculum. The rationale and intervention implications of this increased role for speech–language pathology will be the topic of the second part of the chapter. This section of Chapter 6 will serve as both a summary of the educationally relevant intervention information in Chapters 3–5 and an introduction to our profession's role in literacy, detailed in Chapter 7.

DISORDERS AND CONDITIONS INCREASINGLY FOUND IN SCHOOL-BASED PRACTICE

In common with other disorders, the educational and communicative implications of ASD, TBI, medical fragility, and dysphagia extend along a continuum from impairments that are relatively mild to those that are severe. Detailed descriptions of assessment and intervention for subdivisions within the disorders are beyond the scope of this text but are available in articles and textbooks devoted to the subject and should be consulted if you require specific information. Regardless of the severity of the condition, however, speech and language therapy goals for students with these conditions must be aligned with classroom curriculum and to state learning standards in the same way disorders that have previously been present on a "typical" caseload.

Pervasive Developmental Disorders

First, a word about terminology. Physicians employ the term *pervasive developmental disorder* (PDD) because the *Diagnostic and Statistical Manual of Mental Disorders–Fourth Edition–Text Revision* (DSM-IV-TR; American Psychiatric Association, 2000) uses this designation; consequently, doctors use PDD when an individual is diagnosed with one of many subtypes of the disorder. However, according to Patricia Prelock, our "literature is using [the term] Autism Spectrum Disorders because it is more descriptive of the range and severity of symptoms that are often associated with children who have autism, Asperger's and PDD-NOS" (personal communication, May, 2003). Prevalence estimates range from 1 in 500 children (Prelock, 2001) to 1 in 160 individuals of all ages (Cowley, 2003). Individuals with this disorder exhibit deficits in the ability to use communicative functions to engage in typical social behaviors. Subtypes of this family of disorders (PDD or ASD) are characterized as psychiatric afflictions because of their more clearly established neurological base compared with those disorders classified as behavioral conditions (e.g., elective mutism). This categorization was not always the case; when autism was first identified in the 1940s, a prominent researcher suggested that the condition was caused by "cold" mothers (Kanner, 1943).

In recent years, researchers using imaging techniques have clearly established the biological roots of ASD, including indications that in some cases there is a genetic connection (Rutter, Bailey, Simonoff, & Pickles, 1997; Volkmar, Carter, Grossman, & Klin, 1997). Two medical researchers, Walsh and Usman (2001), are investigating a possible defect in metal metabolism as a causative factor in autism. Other researchers are working hard to determine the underlying causes of the disorder with a hope of prevention. As implied above, the subdivisions of PDD (or ASD) also represent a spectrum range of relatively mild to severe communicative difficulty. Contrary to its previous appellation, "infantile autism," the symptoms of 95% of the individuals who are diagnosed with PDD will persist throughout the life span (Volkmar et al., 1997).

According to the *Diagnostic and Statistical Manual of Mental Disorders– Fourth Edition* (DSM-IV; American Psychiatric Association, 1994), the major categories of Pervasive Developmental Disorders include Asperger's Syndrome, Autism, Childhood Disintegrative Disorder, Pervasive Developmental Disorder-Not Otherwise Specified (PDD-NOS), and Rett's Disorder. Paul, Parent, Klin, and Volkmar (1999) state that PDD-NOS is the most common form, diagnosed five times as often as autism. Regardless of type, according to the National Research Council, children with autism spectrum disorders constitute "the fastest growing category of children in special education" (Westby, 2001a, p. 10). There may be differences in age of onset, relative delays in specific areas of language development, cognitive involvement (degree of coexisting mental retardation), physical complications (loss of bowel or bladder control, difference in motor skills), but all PDDs (or ASDs) have certain characteristics in common (Paul et al., 1998). The "mix," however, may vary.

For simplicity's sake, we will use the term autism spectrum disorder from this point forward. A word of caution: If you suspect that a student has autism, describe his behaviors to parents and teachers, but do not label him as "autistic" until a doctor has made the diagnosis. General characteristics of the disorder include the following; not every child will display all of them:

- withdrawal from interpersonal contact
- intense tantrums
- use of ritualistic behavior
- cognitive limitations, particularly in the ability to transfer information across multiple domains
- lack of understanding and use of the principles of pragmatics
- lack of intentional communication and reciprocal speech
- abnormal stimulus selectivity and sensitivity, including obsessive focus on a narrow interest
- problems with abrupt transitions; preference for routine
- concreteness
- language impairment in specific areas, e.g., presence of echolalia; mechanical, robotic-like speech patterns; lack of imaginative play; and difficulty using deixis, figurative language, verbally based humor, and multiple-meaning words

Regardless of the presence of "splinter skills"—rapid, accurate math calculation; hyperlexia, exceptional musical ability—SLPs should remember that autism commonly cooccurs with mental retardation. This is important information because higher overall IQ scores are a good prognostic indicator for relative independence in adulthood (Paul, 2001). Therefore, consultation with a school psychologist experienced in evaluating the cognitive development of students with ASD is essential. Similarly, for those students with cooccurring physical or behavioral limitations, the expertise of behavioral, physical, and occupational therapists is a necessary part of evaluation and intervention.

In recent years, a number of assessment tools that diagnose autism have been published; some use parent interviews, some employ checklists, and others provide tasks for children to complete. Several instruments are included in Table 6.1 (Lord, Rutter, & DiLavore, 1998, cited in Paul, 2001; Lord, Rutter, & LeCouteur, 1994; Schopler, Reichler, & Renner, 1988). Although SLPs as individual practitioners do not diagnose autism, they are often part of interdisciplinary teams that do. Prelock (2001) suggests that SLPs can assist doctors in diagnosing autism by encouraging pediatricians to monitor language and social skill development at all well-child visits, to support early referral for audiological and speech–language evaluations for patients with a suspected language delay, and to encourage parents to enroll children at risk in early intervention programs as soon as possible. Prelock's focus on the school environment as a determining factor in evaluation is a welcome one, as "ultimately the goal of assessment is to devise an educational program that addresses a child's needs in the areas of social interaction, communication, play, behavior, and overall learning" (p. 6).

Another important part of assessment and intervention for children with ASD is the role of the family. Most clinicians routinely involve parents

Table 6.1 Sample of Evaluation Instruments To Help Identify Autism Spectrum Disorders

Test Name	Authors	Ages	Description	Date
Asperger's Syndrome Diagnostic Scale (ASDS)	Myles, B., Jones-Bock, S., & Simpson, R.	5–18	Quick rating scale that identifies children; provides AS quotient; 50 items.	2000
Autism Screening Instrument for Educational Planning–Second Edition (ASIEP–2)	Krug, D., Arick, J., & Almond, P.	18 mos–adult	Uses 5 components to measure 5 behavior areas; interaction; communication; learning rate; vocal behavior. Can be used to monitor progress.	1993
Childhood Autism Rating Scale (CARS)	Schopler, E., Reichler, R., & Renner, B.	2–adult	15-minute behavior scale.	1988
Gilliam Asperger's Disorder Scale (GADS)	Gilliam, J.	3–22	Norm referenced; 32 items divided into 4 subscales; can be used by parents & teachers.	2001
Gilliam Autism Rating Scale (GARS)	Gilliam, J.	3–22	Items on scale based on definitions of autism adopted by *DSM–IV* & Autism Society of America; norm referenced.	1995
Krug Asperger's Disorder Index (KADI)	Arick, J., & Krug, D.	6–21	Distinguishes students with Asperger from other forms of high-functioning autism.	2003

in therapy when their clients are under age 5, but often include them less once the children are in school. According to Buschbacher and Fox (2003), this is a mistake because "the importance of parent involvement in children's individualized education plan (IEP) assessment and implementation has been well articulated [in the research] and is mandated through IDEA. In most cases the family is and will remain the most essential, enduring and knowledgeable resource for the child with autism throughout his development" (p. 220). In the same journal issue, which is dedicated to ASD, Prelock states, "Families have expert knowledge about their children that is essential for the team to know and understand" (Prelock, Beatson, Bitner, Brode, & Ducker, 2003, p. 200). This includes understanding the family's culture.

Mirenda (2003) reports that "one third to one half of children and adults with autism do not use speech functionally" (p. 203). Many articles and materials targeting deficits associated with ASD are either formally or informally divided into two categories: those addressing the needs of essentially nonspeaking students and those more suitable for students who exhibit communicative function at a more advanced level. Because students' skills in expressive language exist on a continuum, this is clearly an artificial designation; however, we have adopted the division to simplify our discussion of intervention.

Addressing Needs of the Severely Affected Student with ASD

Recently one of the authors of this chapter listened to a lecture given by an English professor discussing setting and point of view in early 20th-century short stories. As she held aloft an antique stereopticon, an early version of a *Viewfinder,* the speaker explained that to make it work you needed a photograph with two identical pictures printed side by side. When a person places the card in a holder a short distance from the eye pieces, the photograph appears to have three dimensions. The professor explained that when students encounter a short story written in another time, they should perform a similar act. With one "eye," they should view the story from their own perspective of the 21st century, but with the other, they must try to see it through the eyes of the author and the readers of the time in which it was written. When the two views merge, true perspective is achieved.

This is a useful analogy when SLPs address the educational and communicative needs of a student with ASD, particularly one who is nonspeaking. With one eye, we SLPs must use all our knowledge and insight into the hows and whys of language and this specific disorder, but with the other eye, we must seek to understand what is happening from the point of view of the student with ASD. From his perspective, head banging may be the only way to communicate anger, want, or frustration. Our job is to take what we know and try to help the student use other means to convey his message. Buschbacher and Fox (2003) remind us that the amendments to IDEA "have mandated that components of the process of functional behavioral assessment and PBS [positive behavior support] be provided to students with disabilities whose placements in the least restrictive setting are in jeopardy because of challenging behavior" (p. 217). The following intervention suggestions are adapted from Koegel, Koegel, Frea, and Green-Hopkins (2003); Paul (2000); Prizant, Schuler, Wetherby, and Rydall (1997); and Schuler, Prizant, and Wetherby (1997):

- Create the most motivating activities you can to engage the student (talk to his parents and teachers to discover what appeals to him).
- Use communication temptations to expand socially based intents—for example, place a wanted item out of reach.
- Respond to the student's behavior as if it were acceptably communicative (head banging) while you work toward a more acceptable alternative (slapping the table, a nonlinguistic vocalization).
- Be flexible in allowing, encouraging, and modeling different ways for the student to communicate his intent. These can include using ritualized phrases, gestures, single words, buzzers, and so forth to indicate that he approves (or disapproves) or agrees (or disagrees) with what you said or asked of him.
- Create an environment that supports better communication by providing pictured schedules, using the same words and intonation every session to express required behaviors, employing a set routine during

intervention, limiting your language both in length and complexity, using yes/no boxes.

- Use routine to shape behavior. After you have established a routine, begin it and then wait for some sign of anticipation from the student and encourage some gesture, word, or sign that he wants you to proceed. Reinforce any acceptable response and gradually shape it to a more appropriate one.

Addressing Needs of the Less Severely Affected Student with ASD

Reading about autism as described by a person who is affected by the disorder is another way for SLPs to gain new perspective. Temple Grandin, an assistant professor of animal science at Colorado State University, who was diagnosed with autism when she was 2, wrote *Thinking in Pictures* (1996), in which she relates her struggles with the disorder. Although much of the book is personal history, she includes some practical suggestions for students with autism and their instructors. One of these is teaching vocabulary to older students by writing the word and a corresponding picture on the same side of a 3×5 card. She does not advise any specific intervention program but recommends that regardless of the type, it should feature 20 hours a week of "active involvement" (Uffen, 2001, p. 1). An article from a strengths perspective point of view is Sean Barron's "A Personal Story" (2001), in which he states that his "purpose is to show … how the world looks through the eyes of a child with autism." His description of his school years should be required reading for any SLP in an educational setting—for example, this excerpt: "My most terrifying moments as a … high school student occurred not in class, but between classes. My self-esteem was so low that when the halls exploded with 2,000 students, I felt on display. At times, I clung precariously to the wall's edge, holding on for dear life as I made my way to the next class" (p. 7). Finally, thumbing through *Artism: A Book of Autism Art* (Simmons, 2003) by children with various ASD disorders, is both fascinating and enlightening.

It is important to note that youngsters like Barron, who function at a higher level linguistically, often perform well on intelligence tests and commonly administered speech–language instruments like the CELF–3 and the TOLD–3 (Westby, 2001a). Westby notes that SLPs can help identify autism spectrum disorders by making sure we investigate the students' ability to initiate joint attention and communicative interactions, rather than focusing solely on their responses to requests. Evaluating the higher-functioning students' pragmatic skills in conversational and narrative discourse can be useful in documenting their major area of communicative deficit. She suggests the *Test of Pragmatic Language* (Phelps-Terasaki & Phelps-Gunn, 1995) and the *Test of Problem Solving* (Bowers, Huisingh, Barrett, Orman, & LoGiudice, 1994) as two possible instruments to use. The newly revised CELF–4 (Semel, Wiig, & Secord, 2003) now includes an optional pragmatics profile subtest, the results of which could be revealing and consequently useful in identifying an area of weakness not represented in the instrument's other subtests.

Treatment goals should focus on appropriate pragmatic interactions within the classroom as the student engages in the activities required by grade-level curriculum. Goals should also reflect those state standards dealing with the social uses of language. Prizant et al. (1997) offer these practical, general suggestions for higher-functioning students: Make use of reading and writing assignments that contain a socially communicative purpose (e.g., requests, thank-you notes); model and use scripts for commonly occurring events, including typical phrases and gestures to initiate and repair conversations; use visual organizational supports to discuss routine events, gradually expanding into those not currently occurring.

To decrease behavioral outbursts, prime students by exposing them to school assignments before their presentation in class (Koegel et al., 2003). A study conducted by Silliman et al. (2003) suggests also that clinicians use a hierarchy of prompts to increase inferencing ability in theory-of-mind tasks. These are defined as "the kind of social reasoning that allows them to understand that people's beliefs and desires, including their plans, feelings, emotions, and attitudes are causally related to the intentionality of their actions ... necessary because successful communication depends on how adequately conversational partners are able to infer the motivations underlying each other's mental states.... In addition a well integrated theory-of-mind is also essential for educational success ... across the domains of oral language and literacy" (p. 237).

Regardless of where on the spectrum of severity a student falls, Prelock (2001) provides a concise description of ways various researchers have characterized different treatment approaches. These include Heflin and Simpson's (1998) identification of three basic approaches (relationship based, skill based, and physiologically oriented interventions), and Prizant and Wetherby's (1998) continuum of traditional behavioral to social–pragmatic developmental approaches. The latter describes a middle ground that "offers children choices, shares control of teaching opportunities, and uses child-preferred activities and materials" (p. 6). With so many different ways to approach intervention, what then is "preferred best practice"? Prizant and Rubin (1999) and Freeman (1997) suggest the following as guidelines for SLPs as they choose among different approaches:

- be aware of your own biases;
- consider typical developmental patterns and choose an approach that matches the needs of the individual child and her developmental level;
- make sure the approach addresses the core deficits found in autism;
- understand the basis of the intervention approach you are using (the articles noted above would be helpful);
- select approaches that support quality of life, do no harm, and reflect the cultural values and priorities of the family; and
- select approaches that provide methods to determine efficacy.

Because we still have so much to learn about this disorder, it is wise to follow the advice of Prelock (2001), who states, "It is our responsibility as providers to this population to pursue the knowledge we need, remain current in our understanding of the issues, and share the ideas we have" (p. 7).

Medical Fragility

The term *medically fragile* refers to students who are in constant need of medical supervision to prevent life-threatening situations. More children with serious health issues are now surviving and subsequently request services within the public school. Murdoch (1999) presents a comprehensive review of the current treatment and outcome status of childhood cancers. Westby (2001b), in her review of that work, states that most SLPs accept the probability of speech–language involvement when a student has been diagnosed with cancer within the central nervous system. She continues, however, that as the survival rate for leukemia and other tumors increases, "treatments are saving lives, but they are also inducing structural and functional changes that can have adverse effects on speech, language and cognition ... not only as a result of the direct effect of cancer ... but also indirectly as a result of the combinations of drugs in chemotherapy and radiation therapy that may be used to prevent metathesis or recurrence.... These very treatments ... can cause CNS changes ... that impede academic achievement, social interactions, and vocational opportunities [and] can occur as acute reactions, early-delayed reactions, and late-delayed reactions" (p. 11). Change as a result of treatment is called iatrogenesis. As SLPs we need to know that approximately 30% of children who have survived pediatric cancers will develop language and academic difficulties, making a review of the medical history mandatory for any child referred for services.

The school-based SLP may now provide services for students with medical conditions that only hospital-based SLPs had previously encountered. Lubker, Bernier, and Vizoso (1999) state that children "classified as *chronically ill* (CI) are [also] at increased risk for psychoeducational and language-learning disorders" (p. 59). The authors state that there is comorbid evidence of language-learning disorders with the following diseases: leukemia, hemophilia, sickle cell anemia, juvenile onset diabetes, cystic fibrosis, and severe asthma. Because relatively little research has taken place on the prevalence of comorbidity, they suggest that SLPs keep careful records of the children on their caseloads who are suffering from these illnesses. IDEA assures a free appropriate public education (FAPE) in the least restrictive environment (LRE), with the FAPE consisting of special education and related services designed to meet individual needs and confer educational benefits regardless of the origin or severity of problems.

Related services are defined in IDEA (1997) as "transportation and other such developmental, corrective, and other supportive services (including speech pathology and audiology, psychological services, physical and occupational therapy, recreation, including therapeutic recreation, social work services, counseling services, including rehabilitative counseling, and medical services, except that such medical services shall be for diagnostic or evaluation purposes only) as may be required to assist a child with a disability to benefit from special education, and includes the early identification and assessment of disabling conditions in children." School health services are defined broadly and according to IDEA are "provided by a qualified school nurse or other qualified personnel."

A case concerned with the definition of related services and school health services was *Cedar Rapids Community School District v. Garret F.* (1999). Garret was a 12-year-old student who required continuous nursing care. He could only breathe with an electric ventilator or manual pumping. He had been paralyzed since he was 4, and his parents initially used funds from the insurance settlement to pay for a licensed practical nurse during school hours. When Garret reached middle school, his mother requested that the school district supply the services. The school district refused, and the parents requested a due process hearing. The hearing officer decided in favor of the parents, and the school district appealed. The U.S. District Court and the U.S. Eighth Circuit Court of Appeals' decision supported the parents, as did the Supreme Court (Katsiyannis & Yell, 2000).

The issue of special education funding may pressure Congress to act in the future. One possibility is that Congress may clarify language in IDEA on school health issues, including the nature and level of health services. Another possibility is that Congress may consider increasing funds for IDEA. (IDEA currently funds approximately 17% of related expenses for the education of students who are eligible for services; however, the initial intent was approximately 40%.)

Dysphagia (Swallowing Problems)

In the context of health-related problems, it is noteworthy that the January 2000 issue of *Language, Speech, and Hearing Services in the Schools* was primarily devoted to dysphagia in the public school population. In the prologue to the "Clinical Forum" section of the issue, Logemann and O'Toole (2000b) note that "changes in health care have dramatically influenced the types of children who are requiring, requesting, and receiving services for communication and swallowing problems in the public schools. Medically based communication and swallowing problems have dramatically increased in the public schools in the last 5 years and are likely to increase over the next few years" (p. 26).

Dysphagia is not defined or listed in IDEA (1997). ASHA submitted a recommendation in response to requests for input on the proposed regulations for IDEA, but it was not adopted. Some children may be classified as "other health impaired," and dysphagia services can then be provided. Decisions for dysphagia should be made at an IEP meeting and cannot begin simply with a physician's order (O'Toole, 2000). If the IEP team does not decide that services for dysphagia should be provided, the parents may file for a due process hearing. (See Chapter 7 for a discussion of the procedure.) They may also file for services under Section 504 of the Rehabilitation Act of 1973.

School districts and SLPs may be concerned about liability issues relating to dysphagia. O'Toole (2000) comments that claims and litigation may occur from "misdiagnosis, incorrect or inadequate treatment, injuries from equipment, failure to refer, and failure to obtain informed consent" (p. 59). IDEA does not allow parents to recover monetary damages. However, parents may utilize civil rights laws, coupled with IDEA. These include Section 504 of the Rehabilitation Act of 1973, the Americans with Disabilities Act, and Section 1983 of the Civil Rights Act (O'Toole, 2000).

According to the 1997 Omnibus Survey of ASHA (ASHA, 1997), approximately 19% of certified SLPs employed in schools work with children who have dysphagia. Guidelines addressing the knowledge base and the skills needed by speech–language pathologists who work with clients with dysphagia have been outlined by the ASHA Task Force on Dysphagia (ASHA, 1990). The guidelines note that the proficiencies will depend upon the population to be served and that the speech–language pathologist will not be required to be proficient in all areas.

Power-deFur (2000) notes that before speech–language pathologists either assess the problem or provide therapy they must be confident that they

- know anatomy and physiology relating to dysphagia;
- are familiar with the principles and practices of assessment and intervention for dysphagia;
- have observed an experienced speech–language pathologist working with a client with dysphagia; and
- can provide services under the supervision of an experienced SLP.

Power-deFur (2000) stresses the importance of this, because "inadequate preparation in dysphagia assessment and treatment may result in choking, pneumonia, or even death, of the patient" (p. 78). School districts should ensure that at least one speech–language pathologist has the background to provide services to students with dysphagia.

Some of the basic requirements for dysphagia programs in the schools include

- an emphasis on a team approach,
- interactions with the medical team that has provided services to the child,
- completion of imaging procedures to identify swallowing physiology because silent aspiration is a concern,
- knowledge of and adherence to both ASHA and state guidelines,
- malpractice insurance, and
- continuing education (Logemann & O'Toole, 2000a).

Because many school districts do not currently have programs in dysphagia already in place, the article by Homer, Bickerton, Hill, Parham, and Taylor (2000) is invaluable. The authors outline the procedures they took in developing a dysphagia program for their school system. Their primary concerns in setting up the program were to provide adequate nutrition and hydration for children and for safety during oral feeding. They developed seven goals for the program, concerned with identification, medical referrals, implementing emergency plans for "at-risk" children, evaluation, participating in modified barium swallow (MBS) studies when recommended, developing and implementing treatment plans, and developing compensatory strategies for safe swallowing if appropriate (p. 63).

The article describes the development of the team and initial concerns and procedures. A survey of the 92 speech–language pathologists and 11 occupational therapists in the system was used to identify students at risk. The survey employed is reprinted as one of the appendices to the article. The processes of referral and an observation of feeding, along with a sequence of events, including an IEP meeting, are outlined. For the feeding observation, a list of additional questions will provide important information (Arvedson, 2000; Arvedson & Rogers, 1993, 1997). Sample forms relating to medical services, as well as sample letters to physicians, are included in the Homer et al. (2000) article. This information is helpful as a prototype for other school systems that may be considering developing programs for children with dysphagia.

An overview of treatment procedures for children with dysphagia is provided in an article by Logemann (2000). She highlights compensatory treatment strategies, including postural changes, sensory enhancement procedures, and changes in the feeding pattern. Direct therapy strategies that require following directions for the purpose of changing swallow physiology are also outlined.

Many speech–language pathologists have limited hands-on experience with dysphagia, and many do not have experience with children. Some ways to improve your knowledge of dysphagia that are necessary for developing a program include

- regional workshops sponsored by school systems,
- continuing education workshops on dysphagia, and
- a graduate course.

CPR training should also be taken (Homer et al., 2000).

SLPs who are involved in treating children with dysphagia should

- follow ASHA's scope of practice, preferred practice patterns, and position statements;
- adhere to state licensure laws; and
- be concerned with confidentiality of clients' records.

O'Toole (2000) recommends that speech–language pathologists who work with students with dysphagia

- work within their acceptable standards for delivery of care;
- obtain information on the precise nature of the students' oropharyngeal swallowing disorders;

- keep proper clearances on file for sharing of information, following laws related to confidentiality of information; and
- refer children for medical follow-ups.

Traumatic Brain Injury

Another group served in the public schools who may present a challenge to SLPs are children and adolescents with traumatic brain injury (TBI). This category was added to IDEA in the 1990 reauthorization. The definition from IDEA (1997) states, "Traumatic brain injury means an acquired injury to the brain caused by an external physical force, resulting in total or partial functional disability or psychosocial impairments, or both, that adversely affects a child's educational performance. The term applies to open or closed head injuries resulting in impairments in one or more areas, such as cognition; language; memory; attention; reasoning; abstract thinking; judgment; problem solving; sensory, perceptual, and motor abilities; psychosocial behavior; physical functions; information processing; and speech. The term does not apply to brain injuries that are congenital or degenerative, or to brain injuries induced by birth trauma." DePompei (1999) cautions that a student with TBI may be able to state what an appropriate response should be in a specific situation, or speak in an acceptable manner for a limited period of time, but when he finds himself in an actual situation, he may be unable to formulate an appropriate response either verbally or using gestures. When assessing the impact of TBI, one of the factors for accurate assessment is the student's preinjury status, including information on previous classroom performance, social abilities, behavior, intelligence, family relations, and community involvement.

IDEA services are available to students with TBI, provided the problems related to TBI are educationally significant. However, sometimes schools are not notified of a head injury, or families assume that there will be little academic impact once the child has been released from direct medical care. If services are not available under IDEA, modifications may be obtained under Section 504 of the Rehabilitation Act of 1973. Some of these modifications might include changes in

- the schedule—length of classes, length of a school day, consistency of daily schedule;
- work expectations—length of assignments, speed of work;
- instruction—using best input and output modalities, multiple repetitions, graphic organizer, tape recorder;
- material—amount of print, size, modality, rate;
- cueing—print or pictured "cues" for tasks on desk, organizer, buddy system;
- flexibility—routines, shifting from class to class, shifting from task to task;
- test modifications—additional time, use of computer or calculator, enlarged print, breaks during tests, completion over several days, take-home tests;

- motivation and behavioral variables—self-selected tasks;
- social—use of social cues, social groups (Paradise, 2000).

Besides repeating some of the above, DePompei (1999) adds the following suggestions:

- Simplify communication by using shorter, clearer words or sentences, or restating information in a different way.
- Use slow rate of presentation.
- Give clear, step-by-step directions.
- Use a quiet voice and limit gestures and amount of information given at one time.
- Avoid an environment that is too loud, stimulating, or confusing.

In addition, SLPs can demonstrate to teachers and peers how they can assist the student's efforts to communicate by discussing his strengths and weaknesses, identifying the most supportive learning environments (e.g., a small group), and helping all communication partners appreciate the need to coach communication skills during actual events, not just during therapy. Finally, since communication skills can change over time, SLPs should monitor students with TBI for language changes. A checklist is available for this purpose (DePompei, 1999).

Ylvisaker and DeBonis (2000) strongly suggest teaching executive function skills to students with TBI to avoid the typical scenario of a student's chronic failure to generalize and maintain skills. Without such instruction, frustrated older students often turn to acts of aggression. Using the suggestions in the preceding two paragraphs as basic intervention procedures, the authors suggest that SLPs

- identify goals and create graphic organizers for complex tasks, beginning with a series of actual photographs that illustrate the task;
- monitor performance, noting the quality and quantity of completed work, but including a record of any behavioral relapses;
- assign high-success tasks before asking students to attempt more challenging ones;
- avoid verbal cues that students perceive as nagging;
- provide an acceptable escape phrase ("I need a break now") if a student feels that her anger or frustration has reached a dangerously high-level.

The *Clinical Evaluation of Language Fundamentals–3* (CELF–3; Semel, Wiig, & Secord, 1995) has been used to assess children and adolescents with TBI (Turkstra, 1999). Although it is not designed for TBI clients, it has a large sample size of adolescents, and its purpose of identification and diagnosis of individuals with language impairments is relevant for many students with TBI. Turkstra conducted a study of 11 adolescents with TBI. The CELF–3 identified the students who had diagnosed language problems. The CELF–3 results, however, did not indicate strengths and weaknesses for within-subject analysis. Turkstra noted that of the 6 children neither diagnosed as having language disorders according to the CELF–3 nor identified as having language problems, "… all of these students experienced difficulty with the listening, reading, writing and speaking demands of school, and required academic modifications and assistance. Thus a score within the normal range on the CELF–3 does not eliminate the potential for handicap in aspects of communication" (p. 139)

A test developed particularly for clients with TBI is the *Measure of Cognitive–Linguistic Abilities* (MCLA), for individuals 16–55 years of age (Ellmo, Graser, Krchnavek, Hauck, & Calabrese, 1995). It evaluates clients with mild to moderate impairments and includes a family questionnaire, a communication functioning interview, and an information processing checklist in addition to the test. Subtests include Paragraph Comprehension, Story Recall, Verbal Abstract Reasoning, Discourse Rating Scale, Narrative Discourse Analysis, Visual Confrontational Naming, Pragmatic Rating Scale, Reading, Written Narrative, and Oral Mechanism Screening.

When reviewing test results, it is important to consider when the test was given relative to the time of injury; a test given 1 month after the injury may not be a reflection of the student's abilities 6 months postinjury. Also, students with TBI may have more difficulty with tests that are timed or given in groups. Another factor to consider is whether the student was allowed to take breaks during the testing. When a student enters school following a TBI, educational services may need to be adapted according to IDEA or Section 504. See Chapter 1 for a review of those laws.

EDUCATIONALLY RELEVANT INTERVENTION

At the same time the areas discussed above achieved increased significance in school-based practice, the new requirements of IDEA "altered the role of school-based speech–language pathologists … [in that] IEPs must [now] be designed in the context of the general education curriculum to support content learning" (Silliman, 2000, p. 211). Whitmire (2000) states, "Speech language pathologists must now engage in collaborative consultation, authentic assessments, curriculum based intervention programs and classroom based services" (p. 194). While this may be less difficult for English Language Arts (ELA) Learning Standards, some SLPs find themselves working for the first time in other subject areas, such as math or social studies, as well. In addition, SLPs may be directly involved in the reading and writing process at all grade levels. In short, SLPs must address the relationship of underlying speech and language weaknesses present in an increasing variety of disorders to the demands of all subject areas within the school environment. Whether working with children who have particularly challenging disorders or conditions or entering areas previously the exclusive purview of teachers, SLPs will encounter a new emphasis on developing close working relationships with other professionals.

IMPROVING LANGUAGE SKILLS IN THE CONTEXT OF ACADEMIC SUBJECTS

Components of the IEP, including present levels of performance and annual goals, and benchmarks or short-term objectives are required by IDEA (2004) to support the student's progress in the general education classroom. Ehren (2000) states that the concept of functional outcomes in the educational environment "translates … in part to providing therapy that facilitates school success in terms of academic, social, emotional, and vocational progress. Speech language pathologists are being urged to provide educationally relevant therapy, which includes therapy that impacts curriculum acquisition" (p. 220).

Students with language or learning difficulties often benefit from explicit instruction. This process includes teaching in small sequenced steps, using guided practice, and ensuring that the practice is successful (McCleary & Tindal, 1999). In a study with two classes of sixth graders, McCleary and Tindal found that using explicit instruction, teaching a series of rules to guide the students, and using an outline to structure the rules provided support to students who were at risk or who had learning disabilities. This type of scaffolding is particularly useful to students with language disorders.

One of the most powerful skills that SLPs can teach in the educational setting is the use of strategies. Strategies provide organizational support and are designed to foster generalization to related assignments across subject areas whether they are used to plan, systematize, create an initial attempt, increase word retrieval, self-monitor, evaluate, or revise. Palinscar, Collins, Marano, and Magnusson (2000) discuss in detail the engagement and learning of students with language disabilities as they used an approach called Guided Inquiry supporting Multiple Literacies (GIsML). The authors state that using the strategies in GIsML "points to ways in which the skills of general educators and educational specialists could be used synergistically to advance the learning of students with special needs when they are participating in rigorous curricula and instruction" (p. 251).

Seidenberg (1988) describes a seven-step sequence to teach students learning strategies: introduction, explanation, description, modeling, practice with easier materials, evaluation of student performance, and practice using curricular material. Stevens and Englert (1993) state that in addition to teaching strategies, students should be specifically taught to recognize when a strategy has worked well for them and to acknowledge that fact (attribution). It is our personal experience that students will not use strategies unless they actually think they are worth the effort, that is, unless their use translates into a consistently better performance in their "regular" classrooms. Examples of specific strategies are presented in the chapters devoted to intervention (Chapter 5) and literacy issues (Chapter 7).

Many states now require that speech–language goals relate not only to the curriculum but also to that state's learning standards. As stated previously, it may be relatively easy for the speech–language pathologist to link goals to the state learning standards for English Language Arts, but, for a variety of reasons, the speech–language pathologist may be asked to support the student using other curricular material. Lee and Fradd (1998) discuss the fact that teachers may not be aware of the differences between social and academic language. Social discourse in the classroom is typically concrete, with the context fairly well established. Students can learn by observing, imitating, and interacting with others. Academic language is much more abstract and decontextualized in school discourse, and students must work independently to interpret the language, both direct and implied, that is used to describe events and tasks to be completed. Two areas that lend themselves to language goals are social studies and science; even math, however, can clearly relate to both language and organizational goals.

Improving Language Skills in the Context of Science

Science lessons and texts pose a variety of linguistic challenges. Vocabulary terms in science often assume a knowledge of the relationships among ideas and a variety of concepts. For example, the term *buoyancy* requires not only the definition but also a sense of the meaning of the concept and how it relates to other concepts such as "mass." Language is used for new functions, or functions are used in ways that rely less upon personal experience. These include describing, explaining, reasoning, hypothesizing, predicting, reflecting, and imagining. Science also promotes inquiry. This may present a challenge to students from other cultures who may not have been encouraged to ask questions (Trueba, Cheng, & Ima, 1993; Walker-Moffat, 1995).

Westby and Torres-Valasquez (2000) discuss the components of science learning, which include

- knowing science (vocabulary, concepts, relationships, knowledge),
- doing science (inquiry, strategies, problem solving),
- talking science (discourse and communication, participating in discussions),
- understanding scientific attitudes and values, and
- using scientific worldview.

The authors note that science requires not only knowledge of vocabulary and concepts but also a firm grasp of the relationships between terms, such as *vapors, condensation,* and *precipitation* in a unit on the water cycle. Students also need to understand and use conjunctions such as *because, so, if,* and *then.* Both science and social studies texts are also more lexically dense; that is, they contain more content words. Often a phrase including a verb is later used as a noun; this is called *nominalization.* An example of this comes from a science text discussing refraction: "Light *travels more slowly* through glass or water than it does through air. If light hits glass or air at an angle *this slowing down* makes it *change directions.* This *bending of light* …" (Unsworth, 1999, p. 514).

Improving Language Skills in the Context of Social Studies and Mathematics

Social studies poses similar linguistic challenges. It includes new vocabulary and relationships, complex syntax in textbooks, conjunctions used to discuss remote events, nominalization, and texts that are almost entirely decontextualized. Since social studies is so rich in language, it provides a wonderful opportunity for SLPs to work on underlying language limitations. One of the case studies at the end of Chapters 3, 4, and 5, Christine, includes a series of language-based social studies intervention activities. (Chapter 7 contains a segment that discusses different types of expository discourse as they relate to reading comprehension and is directly applicable to developing language goals within the context of social studies.)

The National Council of Teachers of Mathematics (NCTM; 1991) lists four basic processes that should be emphasized to meet the needs of all learners. These include problem solving, connectedness, reasoning, and communication. Communication is the most basic of these and is defined as "the ability to interpret and describe mathematical phenomena through various written, oral and visual forms" (NCTM, 1991). With its own language and its own symbol system, mathematics poses a problem for students with language difficulties. Terms and symbols used in math class may not be encountered outside the class. Several terms may be related or refer to the same concept. Difficulty with the language of math may present problems in learning the material and also limit use of problem-solving skills.

Salend and Hofstetter (1996) suggest analyzing instructions and word problems to identify the vocabulary and syntax that may present challenges and then using the analogies to guide instruction. They also suggest having students make their own math dictionaries listing a definition, symbols used, and related terms. For example, the term *quotient* would include the definition, the symbol for division, and related terms such as *dividend* and *divisor*. Another strategy is to link new material with information that students already know. The experience of breaking apart a candy bar to share with other children relates nicely to units on division and fractions (Scheid, 1994). Mathematics affords the opportunity to address skills in advanced morphology, such as prefixes (e.g., *mili-*, *deci-*), and to teach how information can be obtained by paying attention to the presence of the same or related word roots (e.g., *divide, dividend, divisor, divergence*).

A method of teaching that supplies not only the framework for learning the material but also a strategy for later independent use is one that is schema based (Jitendra, Hoff, & Beck, 1999). A schema-based approach maps important information for various types of problems and highlights semantic relations within the problem. This helps in the problem-solving process and ultimately in finding the solution. Initially, students begin with "stories" that include all of the mathematical information required to solve the problem. They are shown how to map the problem, extracting the important information and noting how it is related. Later, other word problems or stories are used, and students must identify which information is missing. Students are supplied with diagrams when they first learn the material and later supply their own diagrams. They are taught appropriate rules for solving specific types of problems and are given sequenced guided practice with problems. This method is effective for children who find word problems a mystery and may use the "best guess" strategy to their detriment.

This type of sequenced approach with identifying and mapping important information may also help children think about math. Lucangeli, Coi, and Bosco (1997) identified metacognitive skills as important for success in math as proficiency is in problem solving and calculating. They found that fifth-grade students who were poor in solving math problems were also low in metacognitive awareness of math. Mapping problems using the approach described above assists children in thinking about math and may improve metacognition as it relates to math.

Specific strategies for instruction and the use of manipulative materials can also help students learn math concepts. Peer-mediated instruction that encourages communication about math and self-instruction guided by a set of questions may be effective. "Boxing" problems so that numbers remain in their correct columns may assist students who have difficulty organizing information neatly. Mnemonics, such as DRAW (*discover* the sign, *read* the problem, *answer* or answer/check, and *write* the solution) may provide a structure and reminder for children with organizational difficulties (Salend & Hofstetter, 1996). SLPs should also consider using different means of input and output or responses for students. Crawley and Reines (1996) list four means of input: manipulate, display, say, and write. The four means of output for the student are manipulate, identify, say, and write. This can allow students to represent mathematical meanings in the manner easiest for them.

We do not mean to imply that SLPs should be science, math or social studies teachers. The fear that SLPs will become classroom teachers and their intervention neither sufficiently prescriptive nor intensive enough to qualify as the therapy they were trained to do is a real one (Ehren, 2000). However, communication specialists are uniquely trained to understand the language challenges faced by students in these courses and can provide the structure for them to learn the content of the course by teaching and scaffolding the underlying language required and providing information on organizational strategies. Remember that related services such as speech pathology need to support the student's progress in the classroom and provide access to the general education curriculum if possible.

Improving Language Skills in the Context of Language Arts

Following the theme of expansion of our roles and their relationship to the classroom curriculum, SLPs in the schools have seen the definitions of aspects of language, like syntax and phonology, expanded. Receptive phonology now encompasses work in phonological awareness, linked to success in reading (decoding) and spelling. (See Chapter 7 on literacy for more information.) SLPs are working not only with children who show deficits in this area but also with kindergarten and primary grades in classroom intervention programs. Emphasis on syntax has progressed beyond the sentence level into paragraphs—that is, looking at the ways we link sentences in discourse. Semantics now emphasizes not only vocabulary but relationships of concepts (discussed above) and semantic mapping (e.g., Venn diagrams). Pragmatics is crucial in the organization of information, a vital piece of most academic tasks. Morphology, as mentioned in the section on math, clearly affects both semantics and spelling. An example of this is the bound morpheme *a* meaning "not" in the words *amoral, atypical,* and *amorphous.* Related to language as well are executive function and self-regulation. These abilities are crucial for success in academic environments and were discussed in several cases at the end of Chapters 3 and 5.

CONCLUSION

The profession of speech pathology has been one of continuing change. Given medical advances, shifts in the laws governing our procedures, new research in communication disorders, and changes in education requirements and methods, it is likely that the rate of change will accelerate in the coming decades. Future editions of this text will reflect new information and insights. From a legal point of view, the days of "permanent" certification are behind us. ASHA and most state accrediting agencies now wisely require professionals to complete continuing education hours to maintain licensure or certification. These requirements recognize the underlying imperative that SLPs must remain current in their specialty in order to provide appropriate services to *all* students on their caseload. In short, we should follow the admonition of Prelock (2001) quoted earlier in the chapter: "It is our responsibility ... to pursue the knowledge we need, remain current in our understanding of the issues and share the ideas we have" (p. 7). To do less would violate the letter and spirit of our Code of Ethics.

STUDY QUESTIONS

1. Why has the role of the speech–language pathologist in school-based practice continued to expand?
2. Comment on the relationship between language deficits and a student's success in the classroom.
3. Prepare a list of activities appropriate for fostering communication in a nonspeaking child with ASD. What activities could be added for a child with higher verbal skills?
4. Comment on the appropriateness of including parents in your treatment plan for a student with ASD.

5. In what ways might a student with TBI be similar to a student with a language-based learning disability who has problems with organization?

6. Your principal assumes that you will be in charge of feeding students on your caseload with swallowing problems, but you have had minimal training in dysphagia techniques. What will be your response?

7. Why is it important to check a student's medical history when she has been referred to you for a speech–language evaluation?

REFERENCES

American Psychiatric Association. (1994). *Diagnostic and statistical manual of mental disorders* (4th ed.). Washington, DC: Author.

American Psychiatric Association. (2000). *Diagnostic and statistical manual of mental disorders* (4th ed., text rev.). Washington, DC: Author.

American Speech-Language-Hearing Association. (1990, April). Knowledge and skills needed by speech–language pathologists providing services to dysphagic patients/clients. *Asha, 34*(7), 15–33.

American Speech-Language-Hearing Association. (1997). *1997 omnibus survey caseload report: SLP.* Rockville, MD: Author.

Arick, J., & Krug, D. (2003). *Krug Asperger's disorder index.* Austin, TX: PRO-ED.

Arvedson, J. (2000). Evaluation of children with feeding and swallowing problems. *Language, Speech, and Hearing Services in the Schools, 31*, 28–41.

Arvedson, J., & Rogers, B. (1993). Pediatric feeding and swallowing disorders. *Journal of Medical Speech Language Pathology, 1*, 203–221.

Arvedson, J., & Rogers, B. (1997). *Pediatric dysphagia: Management challenges for school based speech language pathologists.* Pittsburgh, PA: RTN.

Barron, S. (2001). A personal story. *ASHA Leader, 6*(17), 5, 7, 17.

Bowers, L., Huisingh, R., Barrett, M., Orman, J., & LoGiudice, C. (1994). *TOPS–R elementary: Test of problem solving.* East Moline, IL: LinguiSystems.

Buschbacher, P., & Fox, L. (2003). Understanding and intervening with the challenging behavior of young children with autism spectrum disorder. *Language, Speech, and Hearing Services in the Schools, 34*, 217–227.

Cedar Rapids Community School District v. Garret F., (96-1763) 526 U.S. 66 (1999) 106 F. 3d 822, affirmed.

Cowley, G. (2003, July 28). Predicting autism. *Newsweek,* 46–48.

Crawley, J. E., & Reines, R. (1996). Mathematics as communication. *Teaching Exceptional Children, 28*(2), 29–34.

DePompei, R. (1999). Run a reverse left: Communication disorders after brain injury. *Brain Injury Resource, 3*(3), 22–24, 51.

Educational Amendments of 1965. (1965). Public Law 89-313.

Ehren, B. J. (2000). Maintaining a therapeutic focus and sharing responsibility for student success: Keys to in-classroom speech language services. *Language, Speech, and Hearing Services in the Schools, 31*, 219–229.

Ellmo, W., Graser, J., Krchnavek, B., Hauck, K., & Calabrese, D. (1995). *Measure of cognitive-linguistic abilities.* Vero Beach, FL: Speech Bin.

Freeman, B. J. (1997). Guidelines for evaluating intervention programs for children with autism. *Journal of Autism and Developmental Disorders, 27*, 641–650.

Gilliam, J. (1995). *Gilliam autism rating scale.* Austin, TX: PRO-ED.

Gilliam, J. (2001). *Gilliam Asperger's disorder scale.* Austin, TX: PRO-ED.

Grandin, T. (1996). *Thinking in pictures and other reports from my life with autism.* New York: Random House.

Heflin, S., & Simpson, H. (1998). Intervention for children and youth with autism. *Focus on Autism and other Developmental Disabilities, 13,* 212–220.

Homer, E. M., Bickerton, C., Hill, S., Parham, L., & Taylor, D. (2000). Development of an interdisciplinary dysphagia team in the public schools. *Language, Speech, and Hearing Services in the Schools, 31,* 62–75.

Individuals with Disabilities Education Act of 1997. (1997). Public Law 101-336.

Individuals with Disabilities Education Improvement Act. (2004). Public Law 108-446.

Jitendra, A. K., Hoff, K., & Beck, M. M. (1999). Teaching middle school students with learning disabilities to solve word problems using a schema based approach. *Remedial and Special Education, 20,* 50–64.

Kanner, L. (1943). Autistic disturbances of affective contact. *Nervous Child, 2,* 416–426.

Katsiyannis, A., & Yell, M. L. (2000). The Supreme Court and school health services: Cedar Rapids v. Garret F. *Exceptional Children, 66,* 317–326.

Koegel, L., Koegel, R., Frea, W., & Green-Hopkins, I. (2003). Priming as a method of coordinating educational services for students with autism. *Language, Speech, and Hearing Services in Schools, 34,* 228–235.

Krug, D., Arick, J., & Almond, P. (1993). *Autism screening instrument for educational planning* (2nd ed.). Austin, TX: PRO-ED.

Lee, O., & Fradd, S. H. (1998). Science for all, including students from non–English language backgrounds. *Educational Researcher, 27,* 12–21.

Logemann, J. (2000). Therapy for children with swallowing disorders in the educational setting. *Language, Speech, and Hearing Services in the Schools, 31,* 50–55.

Logemann, J., & O'Toole, T. (2000a). Identification and management of dysphagia in the public schools: Epilogue. *Language, Speech, and Hearing Services in the Schools, 31,* 79–87.

Logemann, J., & O'Toole, T. (2000b). Identification and management of dysphagia in the public schools: Prologue. *Language, Speech, and Hearing Services in the Schools, 31,* 26–27.

Lord, C., Rutter, M., & DiLavore, P. C. (1998). Autism diagnostic observation schedule–generic. (Unpublished manuscript, University of Chicago, Chicago, IL). Reported in R. Paul (2001), *Language disorders from infancy through adolescence: Assessment and intervention* (2nd ed., p. 140). St. Louis, MO: Mosby.

Lord, C., Rutter, M., & LeCouteur, A. (1994). Autism diagnostic interview–revised: A revised version of a diagnostic interview for caregivers of individuals with possible pervasive developmental disorders. *Journal of Autism and Developmental Disorders, 24,* 659–685.

Lubker, B., Bernier, K., & Vizoso, A. (1999). Chronic illnesses of childhood and the changing epidemiology of language-learning disorders. *Topics in Language Disorders, 20*(1), 59–75.

Lucangeli, D., Coi, G., & Bosco, P. (1997). Metacognitive awareness in good and poor math problem solvers. *Learning Disabilities Research and Practice, 12,* 209–212.

McCleary, J., & Tindal, G. (1999). Teaching the scientific method to at-risk students and students with learning disabilities through concept anchoring and explicit instruction. *Remedial and Special Education, 20,* 7–18.

Mirenda, P. (2003). Toward functional augmentative and alternative communication for students with autism: Manual signs, graphic symbols, and voice output communication aids. *Language, Speech, and Hearing Services in the Schools, 34,* 203–216.

Murdoch, B. (1999). *Communication disorders in childhood cancer.* London: Whurr.

Myles, B., Jones-Bock, S., & Simpson, R. (2000). *Asperger's syndrome diagnostic scale.* Austin, TX: PRO-ED.

National Council of Teachers of Mathematics. (1991). *Professional standards for teaching mathematics.* Reston, VA: Author.

New research suggests cause of autism. (2001). *Advance, 11*(23), 4.

O'Toole, T. J. (2000). Legal, ethical and financial aspects of providing services to children with swallowing disorders in the public schools. *Language, Speech, and Hearing Services in the Schools, 31,* 56–61.

Palinscar, A. S., Collins, K. M., Marano, N. L., & Magnusson, S. J. (2000). Investigating the engagement and learning of students with learning disabilities in a guided inquiry science teaching. *Language, Speech, and Hearing Services in the Schools, 31,* 240–251.

Paradise, R. (2000, March). *School reentry following traumatic brain injury: A cognitive linguistic and educational perspective.* Paper presented at the meeting of the New York State Speech Language Hearing Association, Saratoga Springs, NY.

Paul, R. (2000). Disorders of communication. In M. Lewis (Ed.), *Child and adolescent psychiatry* (3rd ed., pp. 510–519). Baltimore: Williams & Wilkins.

Paul, R. (2001). *Language disorders from infancy through adolescence: Assessment and intervention* (2nd ed., p. 140). St. Louis, MO: Mosby.

Paul, R., Coken, E., Rubin, E., Romanik, L., Klin, A., Shriberg, L., et al. (1998, November). *Communication profiles in autism and Asperger's syndrome.* Poster presented at the National Convention of the American Speech-Language-Hearing Association, San Antonio, TX.

Paul, R., Parent, D., Klin, A., & Volkmar, F. (1999). Multiplex developmental disorders: The rate of communication in the construction of a self. In R. Paul (Ed.), *Child and adolescent psychiatric clinics of North America* (pp. 189–202). Philadelphia: W.B. Saunders.

Phelps-Terasaki, D., & Phelps-Gunn, T. (1995). *Test of pragmatic language.* Austin, TX: PRO-ED.

Power-deFur, L. (2000). Serving students with dysphagia in the schools? Educational preparation is essential! *Language, Speech, and Hearing Services in the Schools, 31,* 76–78.

Prelock, P. (2001). Understanding autism spectrum disorders: The role of speech language pathologists and audiologists in service delivery. *ASHA Leader, 6*(17), 4–7.

Prelock, P., Beatson, J., Bitner, B., Broder, C., & Ducker, A. (2003). Interdisciplinary assessment of young children with autism spectrum disorder. *Language, Speech, and Hearing in Schools, 34,* 194–202.

Prizant, B., & Rubin, E. (1999). Contemporary issues in interventions for autism spectrum disorders: A commentary. *Journal of the Association for Persons with Severe Handicaps, 24,* 199–208.

Prizant, B., Schuler, A., Wetherby, A., & Rydall, P. (1997). Enhancing language and communication development: Language approaches. In D. Cohen & F. Volkmar (Eds.), *Handbook of autism and pervasive developmental disorders* (pp. 572–605). New York: Wiley.

Prizant, B., & Wetherby, A. (1998). Enhancing communication: From theory to practice. In G. Dawson (Ed.), *Autism, new perspectives on diagnosis, nature and treatment.* New York: Guilford Press.

Rehabilitation Act of 1973. (1973). Public Law 93-112.

Rutter, M., Bailey, A., Simonoff, E., & Pickles, A. (1997). Genetic influences of autism. In D. Cohen and F. Volkmar (Eds.), *Handbook of autism and pervasive developmental disorders* (pp. 370–387). New York: Wiley.

Salend, S., & Hofstetter, E. (1996). Adapting a problem solving approach to teaching mathematics to students with mild disabilities. *Intervention in School and Clinic, 31,* 209–217.

Scheid, K. (1994). Cognitive-based methods for teaching mathematics. *Teaching Exceptional Children, 26*(3), 6–10.

Schopler, E., Reichler, R. J., & Renner, B. R. (1988). *The childhood autism rating scale.* Los Angeles: Western Psychological Services.

Schuler, A., Prizant, B., & Wetherby, A. (1997). Enhancing language and communication development: Prelinguistic approaches. In D. Cohan and F. Volkmer (Eds.), *Handbook of autism and pervasive developmental disorders* (pp. 539–571). New York: Wiley.

Seidenberg, P. (1988). Cognitive and academic instructional intervention for learning-disabled adolescents. *Topics in Language Disorders, 8,* 56–71.

Semel, E., Wiig, E. H., & Secord, W. A. (1995). *Clinical evaluations of language fundamentals* (3rd ed.). San Antonio, TX: Psychological Corp.

Semel, E., Wiig, E. H., & Secord, W. A. (2003). *Clinical evaluations of language fundamentals* (4th ed.). San Antonio, TX: Psychological Corp.

Silliman, E. (2000). Editorial introduction. *Language, Speech, and Hearing Services in the Schools, 31,* 211.

Silliman, E., Diehl, S., Bahr, R., Hnath-Chisolm, T., Zenko, C., & Friedman, S. (2003). A new look at theory-of-mind tasks by adolescents with autism spectrum disorder. *Language, Speech, and Hearing Services in the Schools, 34,* 236–252.

Simmons, K. (2003). *Artism: A book of autism art.* Edmonton, Canada: Autism Today Publishers.

Sparks, S. (1984). *Birth defects and speech language disorders.* Boston: College-Hill Press.

Sparks, S. (1993). *Children of prenatal substance abuse.* San Diego, CA: Singular.

Sparks, S. (2001). Prenatal substance use and its impact on young children. In T. Layton, E. Crais, & L. Watson (Eds.), *Handbook of early language impairments in children: Nature* (pp. 451–487). Albany, NY: Delmar.

Stevens, D., & Englert, C. (1993). Making writing strategies work. *Teaching Exceptional Children, 26*(1), 34–39.

Trueba, H., Cheng, L., & Ima, K. (1993). *Myth or reality: Adaptive strategies for Asian Americans in California.* Washington, DC: Falmer.

Trueba, H., & Wright, P. (1992). On ethnographic studies and multicultural education. In M.-Saravia-Shore & S. Arvizu (Eds.), *Cross-cultural literacy: Ethnographies of communication in multiethnic classrooms* (pp. 299–338). New York: Garland.

Turkstra, L. S. (1999). Language testing in adolescents with brain injury: A consideration of the CELF–3. *Language, Speech, and Hearing Services in the Schools, 30,* 132–140.

Uffen, E. (2001). Learning to act: Temple Grandin shares her personal insights on autism. *ASHA Leader, 6*(10), 1, 9.

Unsworth, L. (1999). Developing critical understanding of the specialized language of school science and history texts: A functional grammatical perspective. *Journal of Adolescent and Adult Literacy, 42,* 508–521.

Volkmar, F., Carter, A., Grossman, J., & Klin, A. (1997). Social development in autism. In D. Cohen & F. Volkmar (Eds.), *Handbook of autism and pervasive developmental* (pp. 173–194). New York: Wiley.

Walker-Moffat, W. (1995). *The other side of the Asian-American success story.* San Francisco: Jossey-Bass.

Walsh, W., & Usman, A. (May, 2001). *Autism subtypes for research and therapeutic directions in a large autism population.* Paper presented at 154th Annual Meeting of the American Psychiatric Association, New Orleans, LA.

Westby, C. (2001a). Another kid with autism. Review of *Education Week* article: Pressing need seen to catch autism earlier. *Word of Mouth, 13*(1), 10.

Westby, C. (2001b). Cancer and communication disorders. Review of B. Murdoch, Communication disorders of childhood cancer. *Word of Mouth, 13*(1), 11.

Westby, C., & Torres-Valasquez, D. (2000). Developing scientific literacy: A sociocultural approach. *Remedial and Special Education, 21,* 101–110.

Whitmire, K. (2000). Action: School services. *Language, Speech, and Hearing Services in the Schools, 31,* 194–199.

Ylvisaker, M., & DeBonis, D. (2000). Executive function impairment in adolescence: TBI and ADHD. *Topics in Language Disorders, 20*(2), 29–57.

Chapter 7

◆◆◆◆◆◆◆◆◆◆◆◆◆◆◆◆◆◆◆◆◆◆◆

Reading, Writing, and Spelling: The Speech–Pathology Connection

Jacqueline Meyer
and Eileen H. Gravani

T
he earliest educational literature identified reading and writing as two of the "three R's": the basics of education. As sophisticated as learning objectives have become since that time, reading remains one of the most valuable skills children master. Good readers, by virtue of the ease with which they approach the task, enjoy reading, improve their skills, and become better readers. When they read, they also increase their vocabulary and world knowledge. Student experiences with reading directly influence their academic success, particularly when they are in third grade and beyond and use reading to access curriculum content.

As children progress through the grades, writing and spelling become increasingly important as a measure of a student's thought processes and ability to communicate in nonverbal terms. In this chapter, we will trace the development of the skills of reading, writing, and spelling and explain the ways in which language deficits can interfere with their acquisition. Some general intervention techniques will also be discussed.

THE DEVELOPMENT OF READING

Most researchers and educators consider that reading develops along a continuum, with children possessing many preliteracy skills prior to entering school. A toddler or young preschool child who recognizes a logo, covers the print on the page when an adult is reading, or holds a book and turns the pages correctly is making progress on the continuum of literacy. Typically, by the time a child begins to read, he has a wealth of experience and has already acquired skills that will help him to decode printed words and comprehend their message. Ehri (1999) proposed a continuum with four phases.

Prealphabetic Phase

During the prealphabetic phase, children do not use knowledge of the alphabet to decode words. Typically, they remember sight words by relying on one or two distinctive visual cues about printed words. For example, *doll* might be remembered because of the two tall *l*s. Students at this stage are interested in books and "pretend read" by memorizing text and then reciting it with the support of pictures from the book.

Partial Alphabetic Phase

In progressing to the partial alphabetic phase, children learn the names and sounds of both upper- and lower-case letters. They improve in phonological awareness skills—for example, recognizing onset (alliteration). They rely on a few salient letters (e.g., first and last letters) and sounds. When using these salient cues, they often make errors when reading similarly spelled words. For example, *bag, big, bug,* and *bang* may be confused.

Full Alphabetic Phase

Children in the full alphabetic phase understand the relationship between letters (graphemes) and speech sounds (phonemes). This linking of letters (visual) and speech sounds (auditory) helps them to begin to remember "sight words." They are able to segment words into phonemes. This skill then helps them to decode unfamiliar words. They also begin to make analogies between known words and unknown words (e.g., *night* and *fight*). They can read familiar words quickly and accurately and comprehend texts with familiar or predictable words.

Consolidated Alphabetic Phase

Skills in the consolidated alphabetic phase may begin during the full alphabetic phase. As words with common letter patterns are retained in memory, morphemes, syllables, onset, and rimes are also stored in memory. These units become part of spelling and are valuable for sight reading. As children get older, they read words with familiar letter patterns (e.g., *-est*) more accurately than words with unfamiliar letter patterns (Treiman, Goswami, & Bruck, 1990). This skill becomes more noticeable in second grade (Bowey & Hansen, 1994; Ehri, 1991; Juel, 1983). Similar findings have been noted with fifth graders, when they read words that share letter patterns more rapidly than words that have less common letter patterns (Juel, 1983). This pattern continues through at least eighth grade (Juel, 1991; Venezky, 1976).

Recent research in brain mapping as children read has assigned a part of the brain to each of three phases: the left inferior frontal gyrus (*the phoneme producer*) helps an individual vocalize words, silently or out loud, and begins to analyze phonemes; the left parieto-temporal area (*the word analyzer*) does a more complete analysis of written words by pulling words apart; and the left occipito-temporal area (*the automatic detector*) makes word recognition automatic (Gorman, 2003). Gorman also states, "In addition to the proper neurological wiring, reading requires good instruction" (p. 56). Brain mapping of children who have had problems learning to decode indicates that these students access different parts of the brain compared with children who have learned to read with little difficulty.

PRELITERACY FACTORS

Long before they begin to learn to read, however, typically developing young children have acquired language without explicit instruction. Parents and others provide language models during conversations and give feedback to their children in the context of social interaction. Most children learn new words without effort and gradually combine them into sentences; however, children typically do not acquire reading skills without explicit instruction. "Unlike speech, which any developmentally intact child will eventually pick up by imitating others who speak, reading must be actively taught" (Gorman, 2003, p. 55).

Prior to this explicit instruction, there are a cluster of experiences and abilities that support young children as they progress along the continuum to develop literacy. Oral language provides the foundation for the development of literacy, and the relationship of one to the other is reciprocal (ASHA, 2001). The following paragraphs present an overview of the multiple areas that provide support for literacy. Scarborough (2001) uses the analogy of intertwined strands of rope or cord to explain these numerous abilities and their relationships. This analogy is fitting not only because it reflects the multiple abilities, but also because it emphasizes the interrelationships and need for all of the "strands" to be strong.

Vocabulary

It has long been understood that there is a strong relationship between oral vocabulary and reading. Stanovich (2000, p. 182) notes that "the correlation between reading ability and vocabulary knowledge is sizable throughout development" (see also Stanovich, Cunningham, & Freeman, 1984). As is the case in most areas of reading research, correlational evidence is much more plentiful than experimental evidence (Anderson & Freebody, 1979; Mezynski, 1983). However, a growing body of data indicates that variation in vocabulary knowledge is a causal determinant of differences in reading comprehension ability (Beck, Perfetti, & McKeown, 1982; McKeown, Beck, Omanson, & Perfetti, 1983; Stahl, 1983). It seems probable that, like phonological awareness, vocabulary knowledge is involved in a reciprocal relationship with reading ability, but, unlike the case of phonological awareness, the relationship is one that continues throughout reading development and remains in force for even the most fluent adult readers.

As Whitehurst and Lonigan (1998) explain, if a child is "sounding out" a written word like *cot*, even adult support will not compensate for the lack of semantic representation for the word. In other words, if the child doesn't recognize that *cot* has meaning, she may attempt to substitute another word, such as *cat*.

World Knowledge

World knowledge is based on both direct experiences and indirect ones (afforded through books, television, and other experiences). It provides not only vocabulary, but also information about relationships. For example, sequencing is learned in activities like baking or assembling and building tasks. Cause and effect may be learned from a trip to the doctor (medicine helps you feel better) but also from what happens when you jump in puddles (Gilovich, 1991; Kahneman, Slovic, & Tversky, 1982; Nisbitt & Ross, 1980). Reports by the National Reading Panel (2000) and the RAND Reading Study Group (2002) confirm the importance of direct and incidental vocabulary development across age groups as students activate prior knowledge and imagery. Therefore, world knowledge helps build vocabulary in part because it allows students to use imagery techniques to assist in remembering new words.

Direct or personal experiences may be limited and consequently restrict children's world knowledge. They may also lead children to incorrect assumptions due to the narrowness of their scope (Baron, 1985, 1988; Dawes, 1988).

Syntax

Knowledge of how sentences are constructed also assists children in comprehending what they read. Scarborough (2001) indicates that syntax, in the form of sentence imitation tasks, is predictive of later reading abilities. For older students, difficulty in understanding the following structures can result in comprehension problems: passives ("The cat was chased by the dog"); embedded clauses ("The girl who has red hair is my cousin"); complex sentences ("Although we didn't finish the assignment, we took a break anyway"); ambiguous pronoun reference ("The quarterback threw a good pass to Jack but he blew it"); and causal relationships ("Because I'm a speech–path major, I work all the time") (Klecan-Aker, 1985; Liles, 1985; Smith & Elkins, 1985).

Exposure to varying syntactic constructions is one of the advantages of reading aloud to children. Books often contain more complex syntactic constructions (Biber, 1986; Chafe & Danielwicz, 1987)—for example, the perfect verb form in *The Three Bears:* "Someone *has been* eating my porridge! Someone *has been* sitting in my chair!"

Narratives

Understanding and using narratives is linked to later reading skills. The structure of a story includes a beginning, characters, a setting, events in a sequence, a problem or problems, and a solution. Children who understand these components and can discuss or rearrange them are demonstrating skills in metalinguistics that will be important for later reading and comprehension of story narratives.

Within a given narrative, syntactic structures and vocabulary are included. These language abilities are intertwined within a story. Narratives from books or a story that is not a personal experience are important because they provide language that is decontextualized. Decontextualized language skills are linked to later literacy (Dickinson & Snow, 1987).

Phonological Awareness

Snowling, Hulme, Smith, and Thomas (1994) define phonological awareness as "the ability to reflect upon and manipulate components of spoken words" (p. 161). This is a metalinguistic task and requires that a child be able to separate the word or label from its meaning, and to listen and analyze the sounds in the word.

The majority of studies concerning phonological awareness have focused on children at the kindergarten level or above. However, in the past 10 years, there has been an increasing number of studies concerning younger children. From these studies we know that 3-year-olds are able to segment some simple sentences (Fox & Routh, 1975)—for example, the sentence "I like cake," which has three parts. Norms for segmentation of multisyllabic words in listening tasks are not available in published form. Most researchers indicate that children are first able to segment compound words like *snowball* and *cowboy*, later progress to other two-syllable words like *zebra*, and then to longer words such as *telephone*. Many preschoolers are unable to segment words into phonemes (Lonigan, Burgess, Anthony, & Barker, 1998).

There have been varying opinions concerning the number of phonological awareness skills, their developmental ordering, and whether they function independently. Whitehurst and Lonigan (1998) proposed that there is a developmental ordering, with children showing sensitivity to the syllable level first and to the phonemic level later. This would indicate that segmenting syllables and noticing rhyme would precede the tasks that involve the phonemic level.

Three and four-year-olds typically are able to recognize rhyme by either matching or "odd one out" tasks (MacLean, Bryant, & Bradley, 1987)—for example, matching *can* with *man* (not *ball*) or when given the words *cat, hat, peach,* and *rat*, selecting *peach* as the one that doesn't rhyme. There is both anecdotal and preliminary research evidence that some 3- and 4-year-olds can produce rhyme (Gravani & Meyer, 2001; van Kleek, 1990). Recognition of alliteration or onset is also a skill that many 4-year-olds begin to develop. Sounds that are easier for children to recognize for alliteration include initial sounds that are visible (e.g., labials), sounds that may be prolonged (such as nasals and fricatives), and the sound at the beginning of the child's name. Alliteration production begins to develop before entry into kindergarten (Gravani & Meyer, 2001).

As children enter kindergarten as 5-year-olds, they build on previously learned phonological awareness skills and develop new ones. Often these new skills deal with individual phonemes rather than syllables and are therefore termed *phonemic awareness*. For clarification then, phonemic awareness refers to changes at the sound (phoneme) level; *phonological awareness* is the broader term and can include sound changes.

Early phonological awareness skills are critical, not only because logically they appear to provide the foundation for later ability, but also because recent research indicates that early skills and later ones at the phoneme level are clearly related. Using factor analysis, Lonigan, Burgess, and Anthony (2000) and Anthony et al. (2002) hypothesized that early phonological awareness skills and later phonemic skills represent an underlying phonological ability. Children who were more successful with tasks at the syllable level, such as rhyme detection, tended to also be more successful with phonemic awareness tasks (Anthony et al., 2002). Anthony et al. and Lonigan et al. propose that at different ages, various phonological awareness skills appear to be independently related to reading and have different levels of significance in their relationship to reading because they are developmental and children are more sensitive to different tasks at different ages. Lonigan et al. note that phonological awareness skills are relatively stable in children. Skills in younger children (3-year-olds) are less stable than for older ones (4 through 5 years).

Metalinguistics

Metalinguistics may also relate to reading. Metalinguistics is the ability to think and talk about language. This overarching ability may be associated both with decoding words while learning to read and with reading comprehension. The ability to break words apart into speech sounds (phonemic awareness) related to decoding (Whitehurst & Lonigan, 1998) suggests that this metalinguistic skill may also include the knowledge that sentences have words and events are components of narratives.

Letter Knowledge and Identification

The most basic level of letter knowledge is simply knowing the names of letters. Stevenson and Newman (1986) note that alphabet (letter) knowledge is one of the strongest predictors for both early and later success with literacy. Catts, Fey, Shang, and Tomblin (2001) had similar findings, with letter identification scores in kindergarten predicting reading difficulties in second grade ($p > .0001$).

However, intervention focusing on teaching children alphabet letter names does not seem to significantly affect later reading success. Adams (1990) proposes that this may be because children who are successful in letter identification often were not explicitly taught letter names but learned them within a literacy context, from books and other print materials. Therefore, it seems that intervention also needs to focus on letter names within a broader literacy context. However, other research has found that letter knowledge does influence phonological awareness or phonological sensitivity development (Bowey, 1994; Johnston, Anderson, & Holligan, 1996; Stahl & Murray, 1994).

Book Reading

Storybook reading, with an adult and a child, provides opportunities for exposure to new vocabulary, different syntactic structures, and written words and letters (Mason & Allen, 1986). For children from middle-class homes, storybook exposure was significantly related to oral language skills (receptive vocabulary, listening comprehension, and phoneme awareness), ($p < .017$) (Senechal, LeFevre, Thomas, & Daley, 1998). This study did not find book reading to be related to knowledge of written language in kindergarten, but oral language was significantly related ($p < .0001$). It may be that parent–child book reading relates to children's later reading skills through oral language.

READING PROBLEMS IN SCHOOL-BASED PRACTICE

In the early days of speech–language pathology, our predecessors hypothesized theories to explain oral language development and described age norms of a typical progression. After these were established, they embarked on two related goals: describing the effect of delayed or disordered development on comprehension and expression, and developing effective intervention techniques. A similar sequence is now underway for the language basis of reading and writing. At the beginning of this chapter, you were introduced to the developmental progression of reading and writing skills in students without speech and language deficits. Our next task, mirroring our history in oral language, is to consider the different ways this progression can be compromised and to describe the role of a school-based SLP in assessing and treating deficits in reading and written expression.

First, a commercial. Our expertise in speech and language development allows us unusual insight into underlying deficits that can negatively affect reading ability. Researchers in the field base their findings on the fact that reading is not just a visual–perceptual skill. Seeing the words on the page is simply another entrance into the language processing system. Our profession's full involvement in this area, however, has not broken any speed records. Butler (1999) outlined our start-and-stop history in recognizing reading issues as part of our professional responsibilities and described how slowly the majority of SLPs came to realize what we have to offer a struggling reader.

Now, in the early years of the 21st century, there remains little doubt that "considerable evidence has emerged in support of the language basis of reading disabilities" (Catts & Kamhi, 1999, p. 68). ASHA's report, *Roles and Responsibilities of Speech–Language Pathologists with Respect to Reading and Writing in Children and Adolescents* (2001), summarizes the research that identifies our role. Catts and Kamhi (1999) state, "Speech language pathologists with their knowledge and training in language and language disorders have become increasingly involved in the identification, assessment and treatment of individuals with reading disabilities. The contribution a language specialist can make in serving individuals with reading disabilities is gradually becoming recognized by teachers, reading specialists, special educators and psychologists" (p. 54). The fact that we were so slow to recognize our role should make us patient with some members of the school community who still may not appreciate the inherent connection between oral and written language. In a number of school districts, reading also represents a "turf" issue and speech–language professionals are actively discouraged from providing direct reading instruction. Therefore, it may be necessary to emphasize that our intervention is designed not to teach reading per se, but to target underlying language weaknesses that are making the process difficult. Ehren's (2000) article on the role of SLPs in school-based practice offers two key principles in preserving an SLPs professional identity: maintaining a therapeutic focus and sharing the responsibility for school success. The article contains a helpful chart that gives specific examples of activities that are and are not recommended for in-classroom services, including a number that are directly related to reading.

We should understand, however, that not all reading problems are part of our professional "territory." Having said that, please note that the line of demarcation between what is and is not within our purview is often blurred. Figure 7.1 contains a list of factors that can impede progress in learning to read and write that are not specifically speech and language based. Common sense will tell you, however, that some of these factors may be combined with elements that we do identify as legitimate goals for our intervention.

Most failures in learning to read and write are language based. The problems reflect underlying deficits in comprehending and using oral language; comprehending what you read requires all the same abilities as understanding what someone says to you. Words seen on the page make a connection with language-based information already stored in the brain. As indicated earlier, this language material includes sufficiently developed skills in metalinguistics, vocabulary, syntax, pragmatics, and memory, plus world knowledge, book reading experience, letter knowledge and identification, and an understanding of narratives and the organization of expository text.

Lack of attention: Sanders (2001) excludes the "normally occurring event" when the mind simply drifts away to other thoughts as we read. Instead, she is identifying the process that occurs while the reader is making an active effort to attend. Lack of sustained attention can include physiologically based difficulties or a low threshold for distractibility.

Poor emotional control: The opposite of this occurs when a reader realizes that he is not attending and successfully forces his thoughts back to the reading process rather than the topic that has interfered.

Anxiety: A type of poor emotional control that often exacerbates other reading problems during stressful situations, e.g., during examinations or reading out loud in front of the class. Anxiety can include anxious thoughts about the process itself or can be triggered by the content of the written text.

Vision deficits: Serious acuity or perceptual problems that reduce the ability to identify similar letter shapes accurately or markedly slow the process.

"Matthew effect": Students who have difficulty learning to decode are likely to avoid reading. This compounds the problem, because the act of reading itself improves decoding and other advanced reading skills. In short, it is an application of "the rich get richer and the poor get poorer," and it can lead to learned helplessness (Stanovich, 1986).

Figure 7.1. Factors that can impede learning to read.

Well-trained SLPs recognize that, developmentally speaking, individual linguistic areas are, as stated previously, intertwined like a coil of rope. At more advanced levels, another useful analogy is a French braid, as opposed to a straight sequential process. "Like a braid, language consists of multiple strands—phonology, semantics, syntax, discourse, reading and writing—that are picked up at various times and woven in with other strands to create a beautiful whole" (Dickinson & McCabe, 1991, p. 1). Therefore, even though this chapter segment will discuss language-based information under separate categories, in assessment and intervention they are usually combined.

That said, differences do exist in the ways that hearing a message and reading it differ. In conversation, the context of the message is usually here and now, with links between the topic and the listener's experience. Vocabulary is often familiar, and intonation helps comprehension. If the listener appears confused, the alert speaker can repeat, restate, or ask directly if the message is understood. The listener can stop the speaker and ask for clarification. In conventional reading assignments encountered beyond third grade, the language is similar to that found in formal lectures and class presentations—for example, material featuring unfamiliar words, elaborated syntax, and cohesion based on linguistic markers. Content is more abstract and often relates to unfamiliar topics and situations. In written text, no immediate feedback is possible. Clearly, the more sophisticated language skills that advanced reading demands can severely stress a limited or deficient language base.

Two Main Areas of Reading Problems

Reading deficits commonly occur in both *comprehension,* the ability to understand the meaning of a word, sentence, paragraph, chapter, and so on; and *decoding,* the ways a reader attacks an unfamiliar word to figure out what it says. Apel and Swank (1999) make this key point for the speech–language pathologist: Although "the goal of reading is comprehension ... comprehension is also heavily influenced by ease and accuracy in decoding" (p. 232).

Decoding

Students learning to read in kindergarten through second grade primarily exhibit problems in decoding, characterized by an inability to pronounce a word encountered on the page accurately and, as they approach second or third grade, rapidly. For example, read and then say the word *syzygy* out loud. Most of you will have pronounced the first two *y*s as a short *i* but the last *y* as a long *e.* Your *g* was like the one in *George,* not *go,* and you probably put the accent on the first syllable. Even if you have no idea what the word means, you successfully applied decoding rules to figure out what it sounds like. Efficient decoding requires a well-developed internal sound system that can differentiate between phonemes, plus basic phonological awareness skills that include the ability to take words apart as you sound them out, letter by letter or syllable by syllable (analysis), and then blend them together to make a word you recognize or at least one that sounds like a word in English (synthesis). It also requires sound–letter awareness that can sort out the accommodations required by a system that has 40 phonemes but only 26 letters to represent them and whose rules to accomplish this draw on the pronunciation dictates of many different languages that have influenced English. English has 1,130 different ways to spell its 40 phonemes; by comparison, Italian needs only 33 letter combinations to spell its 25 phonemes (Kher, 2001). Finally, the new reader has begun to build up a store of visual orthographic images (VOIs), "syllables, morphemes or words that are developed in memory by repeated successful experiences in decoding words" (Apel & Swank, 1999, p. 233). The roles of rapid naming ability and phonological memory, the coding of information for temporary storage in short-term memory (and the basis of VOIs), have recently been the subject of renewed interest (Wagner, Torgesen, & Rashotte, 1999).

Researchers have consistently found a correlation between the phonological awareness skills that allow readers to complete these tasks and their later emergence as competent readers (Ball, 1993, 1997; Ball & Blachman, 1988, 1991; Blachman, 1994; Catts, 1991, 1993; Muter & Snowling, 1998; Swank, 1997; van Kleeck, 1990). It should be obvious that if these abilities are not in place, decoding will remain a struggle. It will continue to require a significant allocation of mental resources that should be available to the student as she attempts to understand the meaning of longer, more complex material. "Simply put, limitations in phonological awareness lead to slow, labored and inaccurate decoding of words, which, in turn, leads to poor reading comprehension" (Lyon & Chhabra, 1996, p. 4). The ability to decode text quickly and efficiently and read it aloud (or silently) with correct phrasing, prosody, and stress is called *fluency,* an area of reading ability that has attained new significance among researchers (Carreker, 2002).

A number of new assessment tools specifically addressing phonological awareness have been published in recent years. Several are included in Appendix 3.A in Chapter 3. *Qualitative Reading Inventory–3* (Leslie & Caldwell, 2000) is an example of an instrument used to evaluate comprehension of different types of texts that is probably unfamiliar to most SLPs. Reading problems present another example of our need to collaborate with professionals from related fields. The instruments administered by reading specialists can provide additional, valuable information to combine with your findings. As speech–language therapists, we must understand what areas these instruments address, even though we never administer them ourselves.

In addition, excellent new textbooks and journals that emphasize the reading–language connection can be consulted for detailed information concerning formal and informal assessment and resultant intervention (ASHA's *Roles and Responsibilities of Speech–Language Pathologists with Respect to Reading and Writing in Children and Adolescents,* 2001; Catts & Kamhi, 1999; Mattes, 1997; Moats, 2000; and *Topics in Language Disorders,* Vol. 20[1], 1999; Vol. 17[3], 1997). Many school districts are adopting phonological awareness activities as part of their prereading and reading programs. SLPs can serve as sources of information for teachers who are unfamiliar with phonological development either as a separate subject or as it relates to reading and spelling achievement. Since catalogues in our field now feature dozens of products targeting this area, appropriate for kindergarten through third grade, the days when clinicians were forced to create materials from scratch are behind us.

Given the recent proliferation of "phonologically based" materials, however, Strattman (2001) cautions that SLPs are well advised to check research-to-practice studies before recommending that a particular reading system be adopted by a school district to verify that the "published programs and materials are based on solid treatment research" (p. 3). The No Child Left Behind Act (NCLB) specifically requires that schools prove their reading programs are research based to receive funding under the Reading First grants (Westby, 2004). An example of a system described in such terms is the Gaskins' Early Literacy Program (1998). Silliman, Bahr, Beasman, and Wilkinson (2000) state that this instructional program integrates reading and spelling "as the means for developing awareness of individual phonemes in spoken words, gaining insight into how letters represent phonemes in printed words, promoting active learning strategies to encode sight words in memory in a fully analyzed way … that makes instruction about sounds, letters and words relevant and sensible" (p. 269). The newest revision of IDEA also requires that assessment be technically sound (IDEA, 2004).

Silliman et al. (2000) differentiate between the intervention procedures that focus on decoding *content* (direct, skills-based instruction: the knowledge transmission model) and those based on the work of Vygotsky, described in Chapter 6, that feature *graduated assistance*. The latter can include "instructional conversation," in which the SLP "mediates interactions through supportive scaffolding sequences, adjusting the types and levels of assistance to the comprehension needs of individual students. With experience students learn … the strategies to apply, and eventually … appropriate the tools of instructional conversation as their own for the purposes of self regulating their learning" (Silliman et al., p. 267). The authors' detailed comparison of these two not necessarily mutually exclusive models for improving reading skills can be very helpful to the new school-based clinician.

Another role that the SLP can play in addressing early reading problems is to alert teachers to the probability that specific students, given their language profiles, may be at risk for reading problems. This "heads-up" can lead to early intervention, particularly important in light of the findings of Shaywitz, Fletcher, and Shaywitz (1994), who report that of those whose reading disability is not identified and addressed during intervention before the age of 9, 74% of students will continue to have reading problems, even through high school. Catts (1997) presents a helpful checklist for the early identification of language-based reading disabilities that includes a section on speech–sound awareness. The research of Larrivee and Catts (1999) found that, although there was considerable variability among students who exhibited phonological disorders, in general, the more severe the phonological disorder as measured by multisyllabic word and nonword phonological awareness tasks combined with concomitant poor language skills, the more likely it was that the student would experience reading problems. These are also the students with whom SLPs probably have had contact in preschool or early in their elementary school careers. Snow, Scarborough, and Burns (1999) suggest that SLPs also serve as coordinators with parents who are not aware of the relationship between their child's language and his reading problems. Since any reading program benefits when parents are involved, this can serve "to expand intervention activities into the child's daily life" (p. 56). Finally, the 2004 revision of IDEA, in recognizing the value of addressing likely reading problems as early as possible, permits local educational agencies (LEAs) to use up to 15% of their IDEA Part B funding for early intervening services for children who have not been identified as children with disabilities "but who need additional academic and behavior support to succeed in a general education environment" (IDEA, 2004).

Although decoding issues are paramount in the early grades, it is quite likely that you will also encounter older students who are experiencing comprehension problems, partly because decoding has not become automatic. Even adults who received phonology intervention during their earlier years and are accepted as "normal" speakers appear to have greater difficulty on phonological awareness tasks administered during testing for reading weaknesses (Hodson, 1994). A case study reported by Apel and Swank (1999) outlines assessment and intervention techniques used for just such an individual, a 29-year-old college student. The authors' list of factors that contribute to problems faced by older students as they decode unfamiliar words can prove useful to the SLP who is working in a middle or high school. In one of ASHA's excellent School Division publications, Parton (2002) recounts how he applied the FAME program (Foundation of Reading, Adventures in Reading, Mastery of Reading, Explanation) developed by Curtis and Longo (1997, 1999) in a high school setting, and Tirolo-Zaleski (2002) describes an intervention model promoting adolescent literacy. These are but a few examples of the growing interest in reading-related intervention for students in the upper grades. Although the work by Silliman et al. (2000), noted above, describes reading instruction to two third-grade students, the scaffolding techniques they used are equally applicable to students in upper grades. The International Dyslexia Association is an excellent source for information regarding reading instruction for adults and older students. A recent issue of its journal, *Perspectives,* contains a number of articles that specifically address this issue (Knight, 2002).

Reading Comprehension

Let us now discuss areas that can affect reading comprehension that are directly related to skills in oral language development. First, reading comprehension of text extends beyond knowing what single words mean; that is, "problems can occur in the ... comprehension and awareness of language at the ... sentence and discourse levels" (ASHA, 2001, p. 1). The work of Adler and VanDoren (1972), described in Catts and Kamhi (1999), describes four levels of comprehension:

1. understanding the literal meaning of words and sentences;
2. inspectional reading or systematic skimming (obtaining as much information as possible within a limited period of time);

3. analytic reading (thorough, complete—the best the reader can do); and
4. comparative reading (generating a critical interpretation of the text based on solid intellectual judgments).

Clearly, these abilities extend well beyond the decoding process.

The Role of Metalinguistics

Both decoding and comprehension tasks assume metalinguistic ability—that is, the ability to think about, discuss, and consciously manipulate speech and language segments. To succeed at tasks requiring phonological awareness, for example, children are asked to view speech or language as an object. Even the simplest of phonological awareness tasks extends beyond simple auditory discrimination, because they work on a conscious level. Children must concentrate, often for the first time, on the form of communication rather than its content (Yopp, 1992). This, as van Kleeck (1994) states, "is not intended to ... de-emphasize ... the nature and development of the ability to use language as a pragmatic tool.... [It is] another aspect of the language development process ... how children learn to treat language as a focus of cognitive reflection.... It is important as the crux of early reading, writing and spelling skills ... [and is] crucial to success in our academic institutions and in our highly literate society in general" (p. 55). Being able to think about language apart from its meaning is necessary in word play; beginning reading; making syntactic and morphologic grammaticality judgments; editing; second-language development; and an understanding of ambiguity, cohesion, coherence, verbal analogies, idioms, and other types of figurative language, humor, and synonymy (i.e., meaning coded in different ways: "the car hit the dog" and "the dog was hit by the car" are equivalent).

In addition, metalinguistics includes recognizing and categorizing parts of speech (verb, participle), segments of narratives (setting, characters), genres (poetry, essay), and divisions of longer segments (chapter heading, summary). It is not surprising that tasks requiring this kind of analytical thinking are often very difficult for students with language-based learning and reading disabilities (Gregg, 1991). Clearly, if you identified that a student demonstrates weaknesses in comprehending metalinguistic elements in orally presented information, you would likely find that those elements present equal difficulty in written material. Metalinguistic skills become increasingly important when students confront spelling and written expression demands. Hennings (2000) notes that an underlying deficit in metalinguistic ability as it is applied to morphology can create particular difficulty because "by adolescence, students are more liable to encounter problems with morphemic units (affixes and bases) and derivational consistencies or inconsistencies as they try to use and spell polysyllabic words" (p. 269).

Another metalinguistic task is one that uses questions to promote reading from a critical stance. McLaughlin and DeVoogd (2004) state that students need to understand both the author's intent and the sociocultural influences in order to comprehend text fully. They present a list of questions helpful to students in this regard—for example, whose viewpoint is expressed? whose voices are missing, silenced, or discounted? Critical reading is particularly important when students are required to answer document-based questions (DBQs) that rely on original material centuries old or representing a different culture. Massey and Heafner (2004) note that social studies in particular requires students to read a wide variety of texts including primary sources "written in a variety of language styles by well-educated and less well-educated authors ... [and other secondary sources that can include] non-fiction, fiction, poetry, letters and other textbooks" (p. 28).

We are including executive function and self-regulation in this category because these two concepts are so closely related to metalinguistics and metacognition. They reflect ways in which students develop plans for future actions (including reading comprehension), "holding those plans and action sequences in working memory until they are executed and inhibiting irrelevant actions" (Pennington & Ozonoff, quoted in Singer & Bashir, 1999, p. 266). As the plans are executed, the student must employ self-monitoring skills to ensure the desired end product. These actions require skills in analysis and, depending on the classroom requirement, often involve an understanding of narrative sequence or expository type. "The student, whether communicating orally or in writing (or seeking to comprehend oral or written information), needs to know how, when, where, and why to apply various amounts and kinds of control processes across ... assignments" (Singer & Bashir, 1999, p. 266). Using reading comprehension strategies requires metalinguistic analysis skills as students learn to talk to themselves about what they want to discern from the text, what they are actually accomplishing during the act of reading, and, when they have finished reading the text, whether they have succeeded. Block and Pressley (2002) present a series of research-based strategies that SLPs can consider when planning intervention to increase a student's reading comprehension. Each requires metalinguistic ability.

The Role of Metacognition

Metacognition, an individual's knowledge and control of his ability to think, is closely related to metalinguistics and executive function. Brown (1987) includes in this category establishing a reader's ability to understand his purpose for reading, identify important ideas, activate prior knowledge, evaluate a text for clarity, compensate for failure to understand, and assess one's level of comprehension. Ehren (2002) notes that while educators expect students' vocabularies to expand over the years, they have not always acknowledged other aspects of continuing development, including metacognition. "Difficulties in cognition—or cognitive awareness—will interfere with the learning of strategies required for academic tasks, including monitoring and repair of language comprehension and production" (p. 67). A student's conscious use of strategies that he accepts as valid ways to learn is an example of a metacognitive process that represents a skill "essential for students to be able to meet the curriculum demands of secondary education" (Ehren, 2002, p. 63).

Perera (1984) described these features of written language, absent in oral expression, that can help a student understand content: chapter headings, color and type alterations, summaries, and footnotes. The presence of charts and figures, word banks, glossaries, and indices can also be helpful in increasing comprehension. However, most students with a language-based learning disability will probably need to be specifically taught how and when to use these aids. Massey and Heafner (2004) suggest that "asking students to read through the subtitles, captions, and bold print before reading and then discussing what the chapter appears to be about provides students with a simple scaffold to enhance their comprehension" (p. 27). Rosenshine and Meister (1992) also stress that the scaffolding commonly used in strategy instruction applied to the learning-to-read process must be used on a continuing basis for it to be effective, that is, until students themselves take responsibility for problem solving with the tools of literacy. When that point is reached, if comprehension breaks down, students can implement a specific strategy that will help restore meaning to the text.

The Role of Vocabulary

A limited vocabulary is probably the most obvious reason for a student's difficulty in comprehending text. Studies by Bird, Bishop, and Freeman (1995), Catts (1993), Catts and Kamhi (1999), and Scarborough (1990, 1998) indicate that measures of receptive vocabulary, expressive vocabulary, and grammatical comprehension and production are the most predictive of later reading achievement (Justice, Invernizzi, & Meier, 2002). In a longitudinal study of the number of words children heard at home between 7 months and 3 years of age, Hart and Risley (2003) found that the vocabulary use of a child at 3 "was equally predictive of measures of language skill at age 9–10 … [and] was strongly associated with reading comprehension scores on the *Comprehensive Test of Basic Skills*" (p. 8). The numbers are astounding: Given a 14-hour waking day in a 100-hour week, the average child in a professional family had 215,000 words of language experience, those in a working-class family had 125,000, and those in a welfare family were exposed to 62,000. Hirsh (2001) states the implications of this on reading: "Many a low income child entering kindergarten has heard only half the words and can understand only half the meanings and language conventions of a high income child.… The verbal gap is not effectively compensated for by programs … which bring children to fluency in decoding skills yet do not sufficiently and systematically enlarge their vocabularies.… Hence, instead of the term 'reading gap' clarity would be better served by using a more descriptive term like 'language' [or] 'verbal gap'" (pp. 6–7).

Suzannah Campbell, a Massachusetts-based SLP, related this enlightening experience that describes the lasting effect of limited vocabulary growth on reading. After one of her middle school students had read a paragraph aloud, she checked for understanding. She quickly realized that although the student appeared to decode the words with little difficulty, he did not have a clue about the paragraph's content. She encouraged him to read it a second time, silently, making a real effort to understand what the author was talking about. Sighing, the student replied that it wouldn't do any good because he didn't know what a lot of the words meant. Using a dictionary in this situation usually does not help. Supposing the student looks up the unfamiliar word *entour* and finds that it means "to surround with a halo." If the student does not understand either *surround* or *halo,* checking the definition only adds to his frustration because it means two more words to look up. So what do you do to help students whose vocabularies form an inadequate base? First, texts and articles that address deficits in oral vocabulary and related issues often contain intervention techniques that can be used to support vocabulary growth in written language, as well. In other words, using categorization (e.g., semantic mapping) is as applicable to the language of textbooks as it is for preparing an oral report.

Having students memorize lists of words, even when they put them into sentences, does not ensure that those words will remain in long-term memory. New words should repeatedly be used in context, linked with a synonym if possible. This is one of the prime reasons that curriculum-based intervention should always include a prioritized list of essential vocabulary. Most teachers will, albeit reluctantly at times, provide a "bare bones" list of words that a student must master in a new unit. At the middle school and high school levels, it is clear that this must be done within the class as part of the consultation process, since SLPs cannot teach the new vocabulary contained in six or seven different subjects. What the SLP can do may include focusing on the metaphors or idioms contained in the textbook, or encouraging the subject-area teacher to create a learning station with a language master and master cards for any student to review during specific seat work times (Ehren, 2000). Computer software programs can also be created collaboratively.

Be aware that vocabulary intervention can be integrated into morphology, syntax, and general semantic goals. For example, a root word (e.g., *tour:* going from place to place), even when it is combined with different prefixes and suffixes (e.g., *entour, detour, tournament, tourist, tourniquet*), can often provide a clue to the meaning of the word that contains it. Hennings (2000) presents seven principles that assist students in acquiring vocabulary across the curriculum. She provides a series of seven figures that SLPs will find very useful, including a list of common roots or bases of words derived from Latin and Greek with examples from different subjects, two tables that feature word elements that tell "how many" or indicate a negative message, and a list of Web sites that deal specifically with words.

For younger students, adjectives and adverbs can be taught in pairs of opposites. Because students' comprehension of complex sentences depends on an understanding of different kinds of conjunctions, conjunctions can be taught as words that signal a relationship between two or more parts of a sentence or paragraph (Nippold, 1998). Figure 7.2 contains conjunctions and other linking expressions that contain this information. As noted above, it is important to realize that much vocabulary growth in schools is based on written material; that is, when they read, students are introduced to new words that they use

Compare (show similarities) and contrast (show differences): and, but, or, either, though, different from, also, less than, analogous to, on the contrary, by comparison, similarly, even so, even though, on the other hand, counter to, conversely, as opposed to, in contrast to, same, opposite, however, in the same way, likewise, like, as, although

Making transition according to:

Time: when, next, lately, first, second, third (etc.), at the same time, then, earlier, following, meanwhile, soon, until, since, beginning, eventually, once, at once, immediately, already, finally, during, now, little by little, after a while, later, before, after, in the meantime, eventually, as soon as, yesterday, tomorrow, afterward, prior to, till, thereafter, at last, secondly, while

Space: between, below, across, above, here, amid, against, beyond, in front of, right, left, over, near, in, into, middle, next to, north, south, east, west, under, toward, on, there, this, that, about, out, opposite, inside, adjacent, close to, beside, in back of, behind, alongside, far, outside, throughout, beneath, among, tangential to

Conclusion: finally, in conclusion, as a result, consequently, in summary, at last, nevertheless, hence, last of all, from this we see, therefore, accordingly, in short, due to, to sum up, all in all, last of all, a final point

Cause and effect: as a result, thus, so, therefore, if, reason, affected, influenced by, hence, cause, effect, because, for, as, so that, yet, resulting from, consequently, in order that, due to, for this reason, then, affected by, influenced, resulted in

Examples, enumeration, adding information: for example, that is, to illustrate, another, an example of, finally, again, moreover, also, and, for instance, further, together with, and, additionally, likewise, in addition, besides, equally important, along with, such as, in the same way as, specifically, similar to

Problem and solution: one problem, the problem is, a solution is, the issue is, the answer is

Emphasize a point: again, for this reason, truly, to repeat, indeed, with this in mind, in fact, to emphasize, a significant factor, a central issue, above all, especially important, especially relevant, important to note, most noteworthy, more than anything else, the main value, the basic concept, the most substantial issue, it should be noted, most important

Define and clarify: defined as, called, labeled, refers to, is something that, can be interpreted as, describes, is someone who, that is, in other words, put another way, stated differently, to clarify, for instance, restated, to make clear, to simplify

(Adapted from Nottingham Writing Team (2000); Fry, Kress, & Fountoukidis, 2000; Nippold, 1998; Rorabacher, 1956; Brown 1862 and Meyer & Freedle, 1984, Halliday & Hasan, 1976, Irwin & Baker, 1989, Wesby, 1991 cited in Ward-Lonegan, 2002)

Figure 7.2. Linking words and expressions that signal cohesion and organization.

later in oral or written work: "Spoken and written language have a reciprocal relationship, such that each builds on the other to result in general language and literacy competence, starting early and continuing through childhood into adulthood" (ASHA, 2001, p. 1). This is an example of the positive aspect of the Matthew effect—that is, as vocabulary grows and this aspect of comprehension becomes easier, it is likely that students will begin to perceive reading as more pleasurable.

Remember that vocabulary deficits can extend beyond abstract or unfamiliar words. Students with semantic weaknesses often struggle with multiple-meaning words, pronoun referents, lexical ambiguity ("She wanted long *nails*": Is she in a beauty shop or a hardware store?), categorization, idiomatic phrases, and figurative language in general. DeVilliers, deVilliers, Peason, and Burns (2002) list linking meaning across referents as an illustration of a potential vocabulary deficit not related to single words (e.g., cohesion in extended conversational turns). Encountering any of the above in written form may compound other comprehension problems.

Ward-Lonergan (2002) suggests the following ways to build grade-appropriate vocabulary:

- Improve literate and content-area vocabulary, e.g., by creating a dictionary, making semantic webs.
- Improve use of word retrieval strategies, e.g., by using a mini thesaurus, cueing.
- Improve comprehension and production of figurative language.
- Improve use of a context clues strategy.
- Improve comprehension and production of multiple-meaning words.

The Role of World Knowledge

World knowledge is closely related to vocabulary. The child who has been introduced to animals other than cats and dogs; is familiar with a city environment as well as a rural one; has experienced the differences between bitter, tart, and sour; and knows what happens when you plant a seed has amassed a storehouse of information that will support new learning and new vocabulary. *Corduroy*, a favorite preschool book set in a large multistoried department store, features the adventures of a teddy bear named Corduroy who is waiting to be sold (Freeman, 1968). The story includes a description of Corduroy's scary journey up an escalator. No problem for a city child, the concept of "a moving stair" that goes to "another floor" could be mystifying to children in a rural Head Start classroom who have never seen either. Limited world knowledge that prevents a child from connecting new information to previously learned material can extend well beyond preschool years. Among other characteristics of low-achieving students, Ehren included a "lack [of] much of the prior knowledge necessary to benefit from the secondary curriculum" (2002, p. 66). A colleague recently recounted a conversation with her high school daughter Kristin in which Kristin complained that because all of her classmates had been to Europe, but she had not, they were making historical connections she didn't immediately see. Although her mother was not particularly sympathetic, Kristin had a point: Experience does assist new learning. Having children link new information to what they already know speeds vocabulary growth and is one reason field trips or other extension activities can be a powerful source of language learning.

The Role of Syntax

One of the ways written language differs from its oral counterpart is in syntactic complexity and density. Perera (1984) characterizes spoken language as having relatively high frequencies of coordination, repetition, and rephrasing; that is, it is low in lexical density and high in redundancy. Written text, on the other hand, is high in lexical density and low in redundancy. In mathematics and scientific texts, for example, clauses are often piled one on top of the other and students with a weakness in syntax experience comprehension problems, particularly if difficult vocabulary is also present.

Comprehension of the complexity inherent in multiple clauses, however, is not just a function of the number of clauses present. Clauses can be joined by words like *if, when,* and *although* that signal the relationship between one or more clauses. Students must understand those relationships to comprehend the meaning of the entire structure. Figure 7.2 lists conjunctions and other expressions as ways in which authors link thought and make transitions.

Here is a clear example of how reading comprehension can also inform writing ability. Jill deVilliers (2002) noted that syntax is in the service of a pragmatic function, for example, understanding the implications of "a book" versus "the book," or knowing what question to ask a teacher to clarify the meaning of a difficult passage (deVilliers, deVilliers, Peason, & Burns, 2002). In a reading strategy called ReQuest, students generate their own questions and the answers to those questions. In discussing this technique, Massey and Heafner (2004) comment that "student-centered questioning can be very powerful in helping students understand social studies texts" (p. 36). The metalinguistic ability to change a declarative statement into a question is clearly a prerequisite to this technique. The skill is also necessary when students try to create exam questions that teachers are likely to ask about a reading assignment. Coherence, at the sentence, intraparagraph, and interparagraph levels, and cohesion, in its use of grammatical, transitional, and lexical ties, are further examples of how an understanding of syntax is necessary in reading comprehension.

Twenty years ago, Chall (1983) suggested that once beginning readers have achieved some mastery of decoding operations, they learn to exploit this knowledge as they shift from learning to read to reading to learn. Scarborough's (1990) work indicates that preschool syntactic competence is highly predictive of later reading levels and that syntactic delays at 2½ years were characteristic of children identified as dyslexic in the second grade. A firm foundation in syntax appears particularly important in terms of fluent reading, in which "students use their knowledge of word order and its rules and constraints to predict upcoming information in a sentence. Knowledge of cases and word order appears to help readers anticipate future information" (Snyder & Downey, 1997, p. 34). Greenhalgh and Strong (2001) identified students' use of conjunctions and elaborated noun phrases in narratives as one way to determine if they had moved from everyday oral language to literate language forms, "a contributor to academic success" (p. 114). Kamhi (2003) states that fluent readers "see clauses and phrases as chunks of text and use these chunks to read and write more quickly" (p. 6).

A study of pertinent research at this point, however, does not indicate that all students who experience problems in learning to read have concomitant deficits in syntax (Aram & Hall, 1989). Snyder and Downey (1997) conjecture that there may be subtypes of reading disabilities, one of which involving syntax, just as there is a subtype reflecting difficulty with phonological processing that does not involve other linguistic areas. This supposition represents another reason our training as SLPs is applicable to reading intervention; as professional SLPs, we are comfortable with the concept of identifying individual differences. It's one of the things we do automatically.

Identifying which specific linguistic areas are involved in a reading deficit, syntax, or otherwise is not always an easy task. Many of the techniques described as part of dynamic or authentic assessment in Chapter 3 are good choices because the "test" material features aspects of the curriculum the student is expected to master. ASHA (2001, 2003) provides general information concerning our role in both reading and writing. Westby's (1999) writing on assessing and facilitating text comprehension problems gives explicit details helpful to the clinician inexperienced in reading problems. She describes the types of linguistic and cognitive knowledge students need to comprehend text, including information on schemata, text grammar, differences between narrative and expository texts, assessing literary style, and different ways content is organized. She also discusses how to use literature to teach syntactic forms.

Gillon and Dodd (1995) compared the effects of training oral language on reading ability. The first part of their program featured phonological awareness abilities; the second part focused on syntactic and semantic processing skills. The authors concluded that whereas students with a relatively severe reading disability benefited most from oral phonological awareness instruction, for some other students, those not as impaired, an improved knowledge of sentence structure and use of word meanings in various contexts appeared to be as important for reading comprehension as improving their phonological processing skills. The authors conjectured that the students at a more advanced stage in word recognition skills may have the capacity to integrate syntactic and semantic knowledge into comprehension strategies, but others may be too overloaded.

One advantage of written compared with oral communication is that the reader does not have to understand content the first time he sees text on the page. He can read and reread as he attempts to understand and make the connections implied by cohesive ties. Even though we are discussing reading comprehension, we cannot divorce syntax from decoding. According to van Kleeck (1994), students cannot remember or comprehend complex sentences without subvocalization, and that requires conscious awareness of the phonemes that make up words.

Rasinski (1994) notes that proficient (fluent) readers automatically segment the text they are reading into syntactically appropriate units to help them understand the information. Poor readers, however, often have difficulty realizing that words are grouped together in meaningful phrases that are signaled by intonation and expression in their oral reading. Rasinski suggests that SLPs create a phrase-cued text segment by lightly marking the phrase boundaries with a penciled vertical line. Students can then read aloud the phrase-cued text excerpts as a means of both practice (marked texts) and assessment (unmarked text). Ward-Lonergan (2002) suggests paraphrasing as a way to facilitate and check comprehension and improve summarizing skills, for example, using the RAP strategy: **R**ead a paragraph, **A**sk questions about the main idea if necessary, **P**ut into own words.

The Role of Pragmatics and Narrative Structure

Story grammars specify the structural organization of stories "in the same way that syntactic grammars specify the structural organization of sentences" (Just & Carpenter, quoted in Catts & Kamhi, 1999, p. 13). These subdivisions include comprehending (and later discussing) setting, episodes, characters, context, initiating event, attempt, consequences, and—most difficult for students with receptive pragmatic limitations—the internal response and reaction of the characters in the story. As part of a story grammar, interpreting narrative text often demands a student to infer, analyze, and compare motivation; identify feelings; and judge whether characters' actions are socially appropriate. Linking these requirements are examples of the last two levels of reading posited by Adler and Van Doren (1972): analytic reading (thorough, complete, the best the reader can do) and comparative reading (generating a critical interpretation of the text based on solid intellectual judgments). It is important to note that narratives encountered during the upper grades may not follow a linear structure. Anstey (2002) provides specific examples of authors employing unusual uses of the narrator's voice, deliberately omitting information needed to understand the story, mixing genres within a single work, and deliberately avoiding a logical sequential pattern.

Clearly, narratives, especially more sophisticated types, can present particular problems for students who have nonverbal as well as verbal pragmatic deficits. Often students with pragmatic deficits are quite concrete; that is, they have difficulty changing from one point of view to another and appreciating how different characters may have different perspectives of an event or situation. Compounding this problem are narratives within a typical language arts curriculum whose action occurs in a far distant time or a very different geographical or social setting. Sometimes narratives even involve fantasy. Think of the difficulty a student may have analyzing how a group of alien beings are likely to behave in a world that does not exist when the student does not fully comprehend the rules of social interaction in the school lunchroom.

McFadden (1997) combines narrative structure with phonemic awareness concepts, and Hoggan and Strong (1994) describe 20 narrative teaching strategies created by different authors. The types are categorized under the following categories: the suggested grade level (primary, late elementary, and middle secondary); optimal presentation stage (pre, post, and during story telling); language areas employed (content, form, use focus); appropriate group size. Typical strategies include story mapping, think alouds, extensions, and internal state.

Bristor (1993) provides an example of using technology to address language goals. The author suggests that SLPs and teachers use videos to introduce, discuss, and model story or other text elements. This is particularly desirable in the middle grades, when students encounter lengthier and more complex reading material. Videos may be one of the few available means to encourage a discussion of story, voice, and tone in age-appropriate materials. When students' reading skills are severely depressed, material they can read easily may be years below their interest level. Using a video (e.g., *To Kill a Mockingbird* or *Where the Red Fern Grows*) allows students to learn vocabulary and take part in a classroom discussion about setting and plot that would be denied them otherwise.

The Role of Organizational Patterns of Expository Text

Narratives represent the most frequent literary genre in kindergarten and first grade. By third grade, however, students are expected to read and understand expository discourse in social studies, science, mathematics, and history texts. Instead of a story grammar, children are exposed to different ways in which content can be organized—for example, cause and effect; explanation; sequence (procedural); problem and solution; descriptive; enumerative, including definition and examples; comparison and contrast; classification; analogy; whole and part. For students to comprehend content completely, they must understand how the subsets of the content relate to each other. Helping students recognize the organizational schemas helps them retain the subject matter and connect new information with old (Hyerle, 2004). The corollary to this process is that it helps students recognize which pattern to use when they outline information for a paper. Students who do not understand or use these organizational patterns are at a significant disadvantage in the upper elementary grades through high school.

The Role of Letter Knowledge/Identification

Until very recently, orthography, the written equivalent of sounds, was largely ignored by speech–language professionals. After all, we prefer phonetic symbols to transcribe speech! Studies by Catts et al. (2001); Blatchford, Burke, Farquhar, Plewis, and Tizard (1987); Johnston, Anderson, and Holligan (1986); and Adams (1990), however, have identified a child's knowledge of letter names and ability to accurately and rapidly identify letters as important predictors of later reading success. Justice et al. (2002) state, "Although the relationship between rapid naming and reading achievement is likely bidirectional, such findings suggest that the extent to which representations of individual alphabet letters have been internalized and automated is a particularly important component of early literacy achievement" (p. 89). Grapheme–phoneme correspondence is defined as a student's ability to use a symbol to represent the sound of a phoneme—that is, a letter (or letters, as in *ch* and *th*). This ability indicates that the child has already acquired some degree of phonological awareness and has been a recipient of direct instruction, by either parents or teachers. Justice et al. cite the work of Fox and Routh (1984) and Vellutino and Scanlon (1987) as revealing "that helping children to develop accurate representations of the systematic relationship between letters and sounds facilitates reading achievement" (p. 89). Therefore, SLPs would be well advised to include letter naming and grapheme–phoneme correspondence as they teach phonological awareness skills, as well as early spelling and writing, even though, as indicated in the discussion of developmental norms in this area, intervention focusing on teaching children alphabet letter names does not seem to significantly influence later reading success. It is obvious, however, that children's skills in this area are prerequisite to their learning how to spell, a subject to be addressed later in this chapter.

The Role of Book Reading Experience

Another aspect of reading readiness is "emergent literacy" (van Kleeck, 1990). This involves the ways children begin to develop ideas of how written language works long before they begin to decode words. When adults or older children read to them, they discover that the light has to be on to see the thing called a page (light is inconsequential if someone is telling a bedtime story or reciting a prayer), that the book has a right way up, that you start at the "front," that those squiggles on the page are read in a certain way (left to right), that books can serve different purposes (telling about trucks or how to make cookies), and that those marks make short and long words. Goldfield and Snow (1984), among many others, have shown that children who are read to when they are young have an easier time learning how to read themselves. Clearly, a child who has not had that experience will be at a disadvantage. SLPs can take an active role as they encourage parents of young children to fill their lives with books. Recently, Head Start classrooms have put a new emphasis on literacy issues.

The Role of Memory

We have listed memory last in this section because it represents an integral part of each of the previously listed categories. Wagner, Torgesen, and Rashotte (1999) include subtests measuring phonological memory and rapid naming skills in their *Comprehensive Test of Phonological Processing* (CTOPP). Regardless of other strengths and weaknesses, students with serious memory problems will struggle in school because learning new facts depends, to some degree, on being able to access previously acquired related facts. Since entire textbooks have been written on memory theory, particularly in the field of psychology, the why of memory deficits will not be addressed in this chapter. As practicing SLPs, however, we can incorporate into other intervention targets those techniques that aid recall—for example, teaching general mnemonic devices; visualization; semantic webs; and the meaning of root words, prefixes, and suffixes. When you realize that specific students have memory limitations, it is imperative that what you ask them to remember during your time with them represents the most important information. In other words, prioritize as a matter of course.

What then is the role of the SLP when it comes to reading? Specific answers depend on the language basis of the students' problems. The underlying speech–language deficit should be targeted, but if at all possible, it should be done so within the context of the reading demands of the curriculum. If, for example, meager vocabulary is an issue, intervention should not require the student to learn 10 new words a day using a deck of vocabulary cards. Targeting new terms found in students' texts while teaching them how to use a knowledge of root words and affixes is a method that uses our knowledge base as it relates to reading. Relating new vocabulary to previously learned information is also helpful.

Massey and Heafner (2004) recommend teaching students specific comprehension strategies, which they describe and divide into those used before, during, and after a reading test. In this context, a strategy is a plan that students are able to implement when reading. Teaching a student how and when to use comprehension strategies and then practicing their appropriate use allows her to organize her work and take greater charge of her own learning. The authors also suggest that teachers (or SLPs) limit the number of strategies they present. "By limiting the strategies and teaching techniques used, teachers gain increasing confidence in [their use] and students gain increasing competence and independence with the strategies" (Massey & Heafner, 2004, p. 27). Conley and Hinchman (2004) recommend that adolescents in particular learn comprehension strategies, but they caution that they must understand where, when, and how to apply different types.

Increasing language growth and increasing reading prowess can and should be done at the same time. Particularly in the schools, language growth is bidirectional: As language skills improve, they help reading ability; as reading skills increase, language gains are accomplished. If language blossoms and reading becomes more pleasurable, education benefits. In many cases, teaching strategies that cross subject lines is the most productive way to spend therapy time. ASHA's new emphasis on literacy has resulted in an explosion of articles, conference presentations, and special interest groups detailing how to accomplish growth in this area. Use them, and share the ones you find most helpful with others. You can use ASHA's publication *Knowledge and Skills Needed by Speech–Language Pathologists with Respect to Reading and Writing in Children and Adolescents* (2003) as you target areas of personal continuing education.

Remember that books can be used to teach language, and language can be used to teach literacy. Figure 7.3 lists suggestions of ways SLPs can encourage book use at the same time they enrich a student's language base.

Book-Based Activities

Using a book as a basis for oral language intervention goals can serve literacy targets as well. There is no single way to accomplish both goals. Keep in mind what deficits you are targeting, or, if you are working with children who are typically developing, what skills you can teach them that will increase their literacy skills.

Carefully choose a book based on your goals: If you want to target rhyme, obviously, you will pick a book that features rhyme. Other possible goals include those listed in Figure 7.3. Different stimuli can be used: a request for specific information, modeling, recast (changing a question into a statement and vice versa), a self-correction request, cloze, expansion, parallel talk, repetition, group cooperation, and others. Different modalities can be used: videotape, interview, associated activity (e.g., cooking), music, puppets, flannel board, drama, drawing, commercials, painting, or sculpture. Remember that the use of books is not limited to preschoolers and the early elementary grades. Stages of narrative development, from the simplest to the most complex, can obviously be a target.

THE DEVELOPMENT OF WRITING

Growing up in a literate society, young children are interested in "writing" at an early age. Scribbling at age 2 years provides practice using fingers and hands with a variety of writing utensils. Beyond scribbling, children attempt writing before they have any formal instruction (Clay, 1975). At age 3, children may begin to use scribble writing. This differs from scribbling because scribble writing is linear and also patterned. During the preschool years, children may insert

Alliteration	Compare–contrast	Similes
Emotions	Increasing MLU	Word order
Word segmentation	Word analysis	Discourse–narrative
Part–whole	Fiction and nonfiction	Association
Metaphors	Sequencing	Prediction
Specific sounds and letters	Irregular forms	Politeness
Answering questions	Cause and effect	Pretending
Making choices	Syntactic forms	Syllable segmentation
Spelling families	General world knowledge	Multicultural aspects
Synthesis (blending)	Giving examples	Proverbs
Opinion	Problem solving	
Rhyme	Past-tense question formation	

Literacy terms: title, author, etc.
Motivation: providing reasons for actions
Specific vocabulary: nouns, verbs, adjectives, prepositions, possessives, prefixes, suffixes, ordinal numbers, etc.
Recognizing organizational format of expository material

Figure 7.3. Addressing language and literacy targets through book activities.

letters within the scribble writing. Harste, Woodward, and Burke (1984) note that even at age 3, most children appear to distinguish writing from drawing, and when given a pen, will write and when given a crayon, will draw. One of the first words that a child writes (or more accurately, prints) is his name.

Some children in kindergarten may begin the year interested primarily in scribbling and drawing, while others may be labeling or making lists. Children in kindergarten often produce letter strings and may copy words, dictate sentences or a story to an adult, and make attempts to write independently (Farris, 2001). Their spelling will be unconventional and based on the sounds in the words. For more information on this, see the spelling section later in this chapter.

Like reading, writing progresses on a continuum. Children in first grade continue to use phonetic or invented spelling for many words, with some conventional spelling. They often use sentences (subject plus verb) to express an idea. Upper and lower case may not be used appropriately, and punctuation may be used but not necessarily correctly. Typically, there is a tremendous development in writing between early first grade and the end of the school year. Dahl and Freppon (1995) note that the urban first graders they observed often used topics from reading for their writing. Within a second-grade classroom, there is likely to be an array of abilities. Children begin to write sample stories and talk about writing. They often use simple sentences and may join ideas by the favorite phrase "and then."

During third grade, children write not only narratives and stories but also factual reports and poetry. They become more aware of the use of paragraphs. Spelling becomes more conventional. Sentences are often single clauses (one subject and verb). Typically, classrooms use some type of writing and editing process, and third graders can make simple corrections. Capitalization and basic punctuation are correct.

Students are able to write from different points of view and are aware of their audience. Frank (1992) and Kroll (1985) found that fifth graders were able to modify their writing for two different audiences, third graders and adults.

Fourth- through sixth-grade children demonstrate use of quotes, and mechanics have clearly improved. Sentence structure is more complex, with more clauses per sentence. Students are able to revise and edit, and, in fifth and sixth grades, may use different audiences for different drafts. Even in fifth and sixth grades, however, organizing thoughts and ideas may be difficult.

Seventh- and eighth-grade (middle school or junior high) students are able to use more abstract terms, like *justice*. They can research a topic, take notes, and organize the notes. They can integrate information in their notes with previous knowledge. Langer (1986) points out that when students in sixth to ninth grade produce reports, they link ideas and elaborate on basic information.

In comparing written and oral expression from Grades 1 through 7, Loban (1976) found that words per communication unit were slightly higher for oral expression. In Grades 7 through 9, they were roughly equivalent, and in Grades 9 through 12, written expression had more words per communication unit. Table 3.1 in Chapter 3 contains this information.

Writing Problems and Intervention with the School-Aged Student

It should come as no surprise that the same underlying deficits in language that make learning to read difficult can cause problems when a student is learning to write. Weaknesses in phonological awareness, metalinguistics, vocabulary, syntax, or pragmatics and limited world knowledge, early book reading experience, or knowledge of narrative and expository structures: Each of these alone or combined with others can negatively affect some aspect of writing.

We will discuss student problems you are likely to encounter under two conditions: (a) as learners approach typical assignments in writing as process, and (b) as you match their work to sections of rubrics used to evaluate student writing. In other words, what you might see as you work with students on a writing assignment or when you or their teachers grade their written product.

Writing as Process

Scott and Erwin (1992) identified the following as common writing assignments in middle and high school:

- personal experience narratives
- story retelling
- factual retelling
- creating a fictional story
- expositions on how to do something
- descriptions
- reporting
- persuasive essays
- business letters
- friendly letters

The most difficult assignment for most students is the lengthy research paper or report. Although writing, particularly of this type, is a problem for all students, adolescents with a language-based learning disability exhibit even more difficulty mastering this advanced skill (Englert & Raphael, 1988). Fortunately for SLPs, there are many sources available in the education literature detailing the process of teaching typical students how to write a lengthy paper. Common process stages include prewriting, sentence generation, and revision (Hayes & Flower, 1987). Your first job will be to discern what kind of problems your students, given their individual language profiles, are likely to encounter when sections of the writing process are assigned by their classroom teacher. Your second task will be to provide effective intervention strategies to overcome those difficulties. For clarity, organization is included as an additional stage. Recognize that these divisions in themselves constitute a strategy for completing an assignment.

Collecting Information, the Prewriting Phase

Students are expected to collect, record, and sort the resources they need to develop their subject. This can include research in books or online, day dreaming, brainstorming, looking through journals and magazines, jotting down ideas on note cards, talking with other people, and identifying and exploring key words. Students will be at a significant disadvantage during this initial step if they have limitations in any of these areas: decoding, vocabulary, world knowledge, or comprehending multiclause sentences or cohesive ties.

Instructing students to visualize and verbalize their thoughts (Romero, 2002) and teaching them how to distinguish a main idea from its supporting details are good first steps. Be sure to read the section in Chapter 12 written by a school librarian, for ways a librarian can help; a good technology instructor may also be of assistance.

Organizing Found Material

The second step in the writing process is organizing the information a student has discovered. Students who are writing a narrative are expected to use story grammar markers (setting, episodes, characters, context, initiating event, attempt, consequences, internal response, and reaction of the characters in the story). Teachers who have assigned some aspect of expository discourse assume students will likely use one of the schemas listed previously under the heading "The Role of Organizational Patterns of Expository Text." Students with poor executive function, little understanding of point of view, or limited experience in reading books that could serve as either organizational models or examples of specific genres will struggle with this important phase of the writing process. Singer (1995) contends that some children with language-based learning disabilities fail to advance beyond the stage in which writing is simply talking written down.

Teaching how and when to use story grammar markers, specific graphic organizers, or other charts that make organizational patterns clear can be beneficial, although it may take much practice for these to become automatic. Students can also be helped to consider their intended audience and the purpose of their writing. Developing a vocabulary list can help them understand content. Teaching students how to define words gives them a way to start a paragraph. One way to define a word is by giving its specific characteristics, plus a general class word, or vice versa:

- The constitution is a *document* (class word) that *provides rules in a written form* (specific characteristics).
- A spider monkey is *a small, long-tailed* (specific characteristics) *primate* (class word).

Other ways to define words can be found in the *Reading Teacher's Book of Lists* (Fry, Kress, & Fountoukidis, 2000), along with dozens of other useful lists. Teaching the underlying meaning of cohesive ties (words like *therefore, but*), and expressions like *on the other hand,* is an effective way to show students how parts of their writing assignment relate to each other (see Figure 7.2). Using the journalist's 5W model (who, what, when, where, why) can be helpful in some cases. At the middle and high school levels, helping a student create a power point presentation is a good way to teach the concepts of main idea and supporting points.

Drafting

The third step is writing the first draft. It is the student's task to take her organized resources and begin to write. This is a messy, stop-and-start process that many students, particularly those with language deficits, find frustrating if not downright painful. Students with spelling problems frequently get hung up on that part of the process. Those with limited vocabulary or word-finding problems often get stuck or use the wrong word. Not having a sense of what constitutes a complete thought (i.e., a proper sentence) can create another roadblock to writing a draft. Based on the work of Carlson and Alley, Ehren (2002) identifies deficits in syntax as another of the characteristics of low-achieving students, stating that as a group "they have significant difficulties producing well-structured and complete sentences, taking notes from lectures, or writing well-organized, error-free paragraphs and themes" (p. 66). Sentence fragments and run-ons, tense shifts, and word omissions or additions are common. Often, students demonstrate shortened T-units and a low subordination index (Scott & Erwin, 1992). (SLPs should check for these markers as one means of evaluating writing products.) At the paragraph level, students omit topic sentences, leave out the beginning or ending, or fail to develop the middle paragraphs. Gregg (1991) asserts that students with a language-based learning disability also often struggle with coherence—for example, logical sequencing, temporal organization, and cause-and-effect and other relationships. Not understanding the correct use of the following is also a significant barrier:

- reference words: *pronouns, demonstratives, definite articles, comparatives*
- substitutions for words previously used: *likewise, the same (is true)*; using *synonyms*.
- ellipses: deletions of a word, phrase, or longer structure already understood: *some* came running (some of these people came: "of these people" deleted)

Teaching and then having students practice these concepts may be a vital first step in the writing process. A lack of understanding of these structures makes it very difficult for a beginning writer to maintain cohesion.

Similarly, before students can use referents, substitution, or ellipses in their own work, they must recognize cohesion demonstrated by transitional ties that show relationships *between* sentences (e.g., *hence, in fact, finally*), as well as lexical ties—that is, repeating in a following sentence the same word or its synonym ("Black Beauty stumbled near the end of the lane. Clearly, *the horse* was nearing exhaustion"). SLPs should include these structures (and other similar ones) as part of a student's IEP, using curriculum-based materials to provide practice during intervention.

Some students can use an outline and think through each sentence before writing it down; other students just need to get enough words down on paper or a computer screen to enable them to edit later. Even if your students are writing longer assignments, as an SLP you may have to review with them how to write a single paragraph. Encouraging a student to use a word-processing program on a computer can be enormously helpful because the physical act of writing in longhand is eliminated and spell and grammar checks are useful if not perfect. However, Scott (1999) cautions that her research indicates that the work of students using a computer shows more errors than their handwritten products and does not reflect longer or better structure. But if students perceive using a computer as less painful and are more willing to write when using one, that in itself is a positive. Dictating a draft to an aide, teacher, SLP, or another student can help the student clear the handwriting hurdle, provided this is permitted. Whoever takes the dictation should take care, however, to use only the student's words. Often, your single most difficult task will be convincing the student to complete an assignment, a draft, that is to be discarded.

Editing and Revising

The fourth part of the writing process is editing the product, revising it to meet expectations. When typically developing students revise their work, they read it critically, a vital step because it gives them a final opportunity to elaborate on ideas and make general improvements. Reviewing, replanning, reexecuting, and final editing can make the difference between an acceptable and an unacceptable paper. Students with language deficits are at a real disadvantage because their deficits often result in limited metalinguistic abilities. These may include a lack of organization and metacognitive skills, a sparse knowledge of word usage at the single-word level and beyond, and, at the middle and high school levels, a lack of syntactic subtlety. Because of this, of all the areas of the writing process, this last task can be the most frustrating for students with a disability. Reading a sentence over to see if it "sounds right" may seem to be a logical starting place, but more frequently than not, students simply do not perceive errors.

Luckner and Isaacson (1990), among others, suggest that teachers model the editing strategy they are suggesting, but only one aspect at a time. It is also important that students do not see possible changes as evidence of failure—for example, if a teacher makes suggestions. Sometimes a series of questions can be helpful for a student to ask herself—for example, Are my paragraphs well developed, unified, and coherent? A warm, supportive atmosphere in which students can make mistakes as they take risks is imperative (Luckner & Isaacson, 1990).

In its entirety this section on editing also represents a learning strategy. Using it can be an effective means of teaching students how to write, provided the students themselves see the process as worth the effort. Acknowledging that a strategy is helpful is called attribution training (Stevens & Englert, 1993); it can lead students to attest to the efficacy of strategy use as well as enhance their sense of control. If students do not believe that a strategy helps, they will not use it independently. The following steps include several suggested by Stevens and Englert (1993) and Seidenberg (1988):

How to Teach a Learning Strategy

- Introduce the concept of strategies by explaining what they are and their general use—for example, that they represent an activity within the student's control.
- Give some examples of different strategies.
- Describe the strategy, including a written list of steps.
- Explain why the strategy in question fits the assigned task and provide examples of successful applications to actual assignments.
- Model the strategy several times, encouraging the student to repeat the steps out loud.
- Practice with easier tasks first, having students use self-talk as they work through the steps.
- Provide prompts or other scaffolds as necessary to prevent discouragement.
- Have students evaluate their use of the strategy.
- Practice using curricular material.

Evaluating the Writing Product

The second way that you can determine the weaknesses and strengths a student brings to the writing task employs rubrics. Writing rubrics are increasingly used to measure quality and progress at all grade levels. They are commonly found in writing texts or as part of assessment information provided by state boards of education or local school districts.

A typical high school rubric used by teachers at Nottingham High School in New York State contains the following subdivisions to measure writing quality (2001):

- *Meaning:* the extent to which the product exhibits sound understanding, interpretation, and analysis of the task and resources.
- *Development:* the extent to which ideas are elaborated using specific and relevant evidence from the sources.
- *Organization:* the extent to which the product exhibits direction, shape, and coherence.
- *Language use:* the extent to which the product reveals audience awareness and purpose through effective use of words, sentence structure, and sentence variety.
- *Convention:* the extent to which the product exhibits conventional spelling, punctuation, paragraphing, capitalization, grammar, and usage.

The authors of this rubric provide detailed descriptions of six different stages within each of the above areas. Each stage reflects quality on a continuum ranging from poor (garnering 1 point) through excellent (garnering 6 points). From the previous discussion on the writing process, it should be obvious how specific language deficits would likely result in student scores of 1–3 rather than 4–6 on any or all of the areas. Rubrics such as the one from New York State, however, are ideally suited for establishing IEP goals. They foster measurable, specific objectives and follow a sequence. Often reflecting curriculum and state standards, they promote the types of measurable IEP goals required by IDEA. Discovering the ones used by your state or district is well worth your time.

THE DEVELOPMENT OF SPELLING

Like reading and writing, the foundations of spelling begin with exposure to print. As noted above, 3-year olds are aware that print is linear and that it uses a variety of symbols (Lavine, 1977). In one study, 4-year-old Israeli children's "writing" was linear and arranged with groups of characters and spaces (Tolchinsky-Landsmann & Levin, 1977). It appears, then, that preschoolers already have some knowledge of print. There seems to be general agreement that like the development of reading, spelling occurs in stages. Researchers have proposed different stage theories for reading and spelling (Ehri, 2000b). There appear to be four broad stages. The first three—prealphabetic, partial alphabetic, and full alphabetic—are similar to their counterparts in reading.

Prealphabetic Stage

The first spelling stage is prealphabetic. As the name implies, children in this stage have little understanding about the alphabet and how it relates to speech. They may recognize familiar words or logos and try to reproduce them, relying on the salient or important visual features of a word such as the printing for a stop sign or the golden arches for McDonald's (Masonheimer, Drum, & Ehri, 1984).

Partial Alphabetic Stage

In the second stage of spelling, called either partial alphabetic or semiphonetic, children begin to link alphabet letters and speech sounds. These links are not complete, however, and vowels or consonant sounds that do not clearly correspond to the letter name present difficulty and are often omitted. Children may remember words based on only a few letters. This may cause misreadings of new words. Ehri and Robbins (1992) found misreadings of similar words, with *save* (new word) read as *cave* (old word). When attempting to spell a word, children in this stage may produce only the most salient consonants and vowels. For example, the word *rainbow* might be spelled *rb* or *rbo*. Children at this stage may be unable to segment words into phonemes, and they may have difficulty with letter–sound correspondence (Ehri, 2000b).

Full Alphabetic Stage

The third stage of spelling is called full alphabetic. Children in this stage have the ability to segment words into phonemes. They also understand letter–sound correspondence. Their spelling attempts are based on their ability to "sound out words," so that *cat* may be spelled *kat*. In sounding out words, they may add sounds, such as *balaosis* for *blouses* (Ehri, 1986). Because they understand the grapheme–phoneme correspondence, they can remember how to spell words, and their attempts can be understood by adults. They have also stored words in their memory, so that attempting to read new work by analogy or comparison is possible (Ehri, 2000b).

Final Stage: Knowledge of Units of Letter Sequences

The final general stage of spelling involves the knowledge of units of letter sequences that recur across different words (Ehri, 2000b, p. 29). For example, children know prefixes and affixes such as *un-, re-, -er,* and *-est* not only with sound–letter relationships but also as units, or morphemes. They also know letter patterns that reoccur, such as *-ound* (in *sound, hound*) (Ehri, 2000b).

Research by Treiman, Cassar, and Zukowski (1994), and Treiman and Cassar (1997) indicates that children may use both phonology (*adic* for *attic*) and morphology (e.g., sensitivity to the past tense *ed* ending) to spell words.

Spelling Problems and Intervention Strategies

As we did in reading, let us now look at what happens when students fail to follow this learning sequence. Because of our training in phonetics and phonology, SLPs are in a unique position to evaluate and provide early intervention for spelling problems. Moats (2000) states, "The instructional materials common in classrooms are often misinformed about the structure of orthography and fail to give teachers any insight into the sound–symbol representation system or how to present it logically and coherently.... The linguistic knowledge required to interpret ... errors and plan lessons from them is not available in teacher training" (p. 85). She gives this example: The spelling of words like *pitch* and *fudge* is erroneously listed in spelling books as "unpredictable" because the authors did not realize that the "three-letter graphemes follow a short vowel and represent one speech sound" (p. 86).

From our years in school-based practice comes another example: Michelle, a second-grade teacher, was baffled because some of her students were spelling the word *train* as *chrain*. To an SLP this made perfect sense: /ch/ is a combination of /t/ and /sh/; therefore, the two blends (*t* + *r* and *ch* + *r*) are actually quite close. How to deal with it? First, we taught her students that in English, *chr* is always pronounced *kr* as in *Christmas* and *chrysalis,* and then we had them practice by dividing a group of mixed *chr* and *tr* pictures into two separate piles.

In elementary school, good and poor spellers appear to follow different developmental paths. Good spellers begin to make use of analogies as a strategy and less use of phonology between second and fifth grades (Goswami, 1988; Marsh, Friedman, Welch, & Desberg, 1980). For example, students who are familiar with the word *panic* might use it to spell a new word like *manic.* Poor spellers tend to continue to show increases in phonological strategies even beyond the fifth grade. When they are younger, they appear to rely more on visual matching and phonological position rules for spelling. This may be due to difficulty with rules for sound–letter associations. Masterson and Apel (2000) warn that assigning a student to a single stage of spelling development can be misleading, since it assumes that all aspects of a previous stage have been mastered. In fact, they state, "Particular lower-level orthographic features ... may become problematic again in the context of multi syllabic words" (p. 90).

Similar to reasons for reading deficits, there are a variety of factors that influence spelling ability. One of these is knowledge of letter names. While they are not perfect matches, all letter names except *h, w,* and *y* contain relevant sounds. For example, the letter *b* contains the sound /b/, and the letter *j* contains /dʒ/. This allows children a cue for 23 letter–sound associations. But this is only part of spelling, as English has 1,130 different ways to spell its 40 phonemes, as stated previously (Kher, 2001). Knowledge of common rimes is also helpful. Thirty-seven rimes can generate about 500 primary-grade words (Stahl, Osborn, & Lehr, 1990; Wylie & Durrell, 1970).

Knowledge of morphology is also critical. The most common morphological markers are suffixes: *-ed, -ing, -y, -ate, -er, -ion,* and *-ly* (Becker, Dixon, & Anderson-Inman, 1980). Morphological knowledge (on judgment tasks) has a significant correlation with spelling (Derwing, Smith, & Wiebe, 1995; Fowler & Lieberman, 1995). Often, words are spelled differently depending on whether they represent one or more morphemes (e.g., *pinned* vs. *wind* and *list* vs. *kissed*). Rubin, Patterson, and Kantor (1991) provide information on the relationship between writing and spelling skills and basic morphological knowledge. Their article would be particularly useful at the middle and high school levels because it gives insight into vocabulary building as well as morphology and spelling. It also includes a brief test that clearly presents the concept of morphology use at the advanced level.

Word familiarity also plays a role in spelling. This is indicated in a variety of studies, such as Ehri (2000a), Reitsma (1983), and Ehri and Saltmarsh (1995). Word familiarity allows the construction of visual orthographic images (VOIs). These are "representations of images or templates for words, morphemes and syllables in memory" (Masterson & Apel, 2000, p. 50). VOIs are as helpful in spelling as they are in rapid decoding.

Phonological awareness is crucial for the development of spelling. Children's early attempts at spelling are often phonetically based, for example, spelling *coat* as *kot* or *of* as *av.* Longitudinal research highlights the importance of phonological awareness. MacDonald and Cornwall (1995) found that phonological awareness abilities in kindergarten children were a stronger predictor of spelling abilities 11 years later than vocabulary and word recognition. Cognitive abilities, such as use of analogies, may also influence the development of spelling (Goswami, 1988; Treiman, 1997).

What is the role of the speech–language pathologist in spelling? While SLPs have traditionally not focused on spelling at all, that is changing. Lombardino and Ahmed (2000) suggest four areas that SLPs should target:

- Promote early literacy and identify children who may be at risk for literacy learning. Also provide information to parents and preschool teachers on literacy activities that are language based.
- Include early literacy assessment in speech and language screenings. This could involve phonemic awareness in oral language and in print.
- "SLPs should be prepared to conduct a comprehensive assessment of written language" (Lombardino & Ahmed, 2000, p. 84). Intervention for poor spellers should include both direct instruction and the extension of new spelling skills into writing.
- Use assessment information to develop treatment goals. This should include both classroom activities and small group or individual sessions.

Given what we know about factors that contribute to the development of spelling and about language and metalinguistics, how should spelling be evaluated? Masterson and Apel (2000) list several standardized tests that include dictated word lists. These may be valuable if a standard score or quotient, grade equivalency, or age equivalency is needed. In addition to word lists, samples of connected writing should be taken. These samples are valuable because they more closely reflect the demands within the classroom.

Recognition tasks are also commonly used to assess spelling. These typically consists of selecting the correct spelling of a word from four possible spellings. This clearly assesses a different ability from creating word lists and spontaneous writing, which require recall rather than recognition. Their use in the assessment of spelling has been both questioned (Ehri, 2000b) and dismissed (Moats, 1995).

Following the collection of data, the child's spelling skills must be analyzed. Patterns of errors should be described. Frequency of error patterns and their complexity should be noted (Bear, Invernizzi, Templeton, & Johnston, 1999; Henderson, 1990). Masterson and Apel (2000) present different procedures to sample and evaluate a specific student's spelling ability. Their Spelling Analysis Flowchart provides a useful means to identify spelling patterns and suggests possible causes of errors. The article also describes intervention procedures for various patterns.

In addition to information on spelling, SLPs should also obtain related information on reading, phonological awareness, and morphological knowledge (Bear et al., 1999). Formal reading assessment information often may be obtained from the classroom teacher, reading teacher, or support teacher. Miscue analysis (looking at all oral reading errors for patterns) also should be completed. This may provide information about skills related to both reading and spelling. Phonological awareness skills can be assessed by several standardized tests. The tests vary in the ages on which they are normed and the specific abilities assessed (e.g., segmentation, phonemic blending). The ability to segment words into phonemes is a strong predictor of spelling abilities in early elementary school (Nation & Hulme, 1997), and results should be carefully considered. A software program called SPELL–Links to Literacy (2004) is one example of an assessment procedure that identifies which language knowledge deficits underlie specific spelling errors. A sampling of typical instruments is given in Appendix 3.A in Chapter 3.

Like phonological awareness, morphological awareness involves metalinguistics. It appears that, similar to that of phonological awareness and spelling, there is a reciprocal relationship between morphological awareness and spelling (Treiman & Bourassa, 2000). This means that while an understanding of morphology aids spelling, experience with spelling can increase understanding of some morphological forms. Treiman and Bourassa (2000) and Masterson and Apel (2000) give some possible strategies for assessment. One example is to ask the student to spell words that are different morphologically but similar phonetically, for example *tuned* (with two morphemes) and *brand* (with one morpheme but a consonant blend) (Masterson & Apel, 2000). This is a valuable means of identifying a student's morphological knowledge; besides its application to spelling, it illuminates a specific area of reading comprehension.

Intervention for poor spellers should include both direct instruction and the extension of new spelling skills into writing. Problem-solving strategies and self-discovery of patterns should be emphasized. Word sorts and word hunts can be used. These can begin with known words to illustrate spelling patterns and similarities. Sound–letter and sound–letter group correspondence should be emphasized. For example, in the words *sing, ring, rang,* the /ɔ/ sound is spelled as -*ng*. Differences in spelling patterns can also be highlighted. Scott (2000) and others suggest beginning with known words and then contrasting them with unknown words. Scott provides a list of sample word sort targets (p. 74) and examples of three different multisensory study techniques to help students memorize words. These include saying the word (and letters), visualizing, writing, checking, and tracing (Allal, 1997; Berninger et al., 1998; Graham & Freeman, 1986; Horn, 1954).

Montgomery (2003) describes her invention and use of "Spellish," a cross between English and spelling. She teaches her students to say words they are learning to spell by pronouncing the words the way they are spelled, e.g., saying *machine* with the second consonant sound "ch" not "sh." She gradually fades out saying the word in Spellish herself, which her students have to remember on their own as she pronounces the word correctly. This technique is similar to learning to spell *Wednesday* by saying "Wed-nez-day."

Spelling lists should be short (6 to 12 words) (Graham & Voth, 1990) or presented in groups. Moats (1995) notes that children with dyslexia may need to write a word correctly 40 times before they can remember how to spell it. Therefore, she suggests that spelling lists contain both old and new words. Computer programs may be helpful to provide additional practice if they permit the SLP or teacher to add word strategies for teaching spelling. Other strategies for teaching spelling include multisensory techniques.

Research by Moats (1995) indicated that older students who were poor spellers demonstrated phonologically based errors (with clusters, noninitial liquids and nasals, vowels and consonants substitutions with phonemes having similar place and manner of articulation, for example /p/ and /b/, which are both bilabial stops and differ only in voicing). She attributes this to underlying difficulties with phonemic segmentation. Some morphological errors, such as plurals and past tense, may also be due to difficulties with phonemic segmentation (Moats, 1995). Minimal pair words can be used to highlight both spelling and meaning differences. In addition, "spelling demons," words that the child consistently misspells, should be targeted. Spelling words may then be incorporated into writing. It may be more meaningful if some of the target words are incorporated into a story, a letter or note, or a short report. This allows both the teacher and the child to note the words that are spelled correctly and the continued patterns of errors.

Writing activities can also be used to teach proofreading and self-correction of spelling errors. How to use spell check, a dictionary, and peer editing effectively can also be emphasized. A study by MacArthur, Graham, Haynes, and De La Paz (1996), of students with learning disabilities, indicated that use of spell checkers increased both the percentages of detected errors and subsequent corrections. Templeton (2002) suggests that for students in the late elementary grades and beyond, spelling and vocabulary "can become two sides of the same instructional coin" (p. 4). He encourages teachers to point out that because *crumb* is related to *crumble*, it ends with the letter *b* even though the *b* is not pronounced. Similarly, pairing *sign* with *signal* may help students to remember the silent *g*; *compose* with *composition* explains why the word isn't spelled *compisition*; and pairing *pleasing* with *pleasure* helps teach why the middle vowel is spelled *ea* rather than short *e*. The author concludes with this reminder of the bidirectional nature of spelling: "Developmental spelling research is helping us understand how students' knowledge of the spelling of words—their orthographic structure—can support students' ability to *read* words." (p. 5.)

CONCLUSION

Given the interaction between oral language and literacy acquisition and the link between literacy and academic success, we have no doubt that this chapter reflects only the beginning of ways in which school-based SLPs will be involved in the diagnosis and treatment of language-based problems in reading, writing, and spelling. It is likely that training programs in speech–language pathology will increasingly offer coursework to support students' theoretical knowledge in the area. In the meantime, all school-based clinicians must seek ways—study groups, online and other short courses, conferences, journal articles—to keep abreast of new research findings in the literacy area. The role of informed speech–language pathologists is crucial to the development of more effective strategies in assessment, goal setting, and intervention.

STUDY QUESTIONS

1. List 10 specific ways that a deficit in oral language can negatively affect learning to read.
2. What is the difference between reading decoding and reading comprehension?
3. List 10 factors that positively affect learning how to read; explain why 3 of these are particularly important.
4. What is phonological awareness? What is its importance to reading and spelling?
5. Discuss ways SLPs can work collaboratively with the classroom teacher, the special education teacher, and the reading specialist.
6. Briefly describe typical stages in learning how to read.
7. Explain: "In Grades K–2, children learn how to read; after Grade 3, they read to learn."
8. What is reading fluency? What can it tell you?
9. Explain how writing develops along a continuum, using several specific examples.
10. Define *literacy*; create an outline for a 30-minute talk to parents of children birth through 7 on the importance of reading to and with their children.
11. Choose a book suitable for fourth graders, and using Figure 7.3, discuss three language goals you could address using your book.
12. Discuss how to use at least two different strategies in reading comprehension and writing. Why is strategy instruction important in intervention with the older student?
13. Describe the four stages of spelling development and the implications for a child attempting to spell a word such as *wave*.
14. List and explain three of the intervention strategies for spelling. Why do you think they are effective?
15. What are two differences between good and poor spellers? Good and poor readers? Good and poor writers?

REFERENCES

Adams, M. (1990). *Beginning to read: Thinking and learning about print*. Cambridge, MA: MIT Press.

Adler, M., & VanDoren, C. (1972). *How to read a book*. New York: Touchstone Press.

Allal, L. (1997). Learning to spell in the classroom. In C. Perfetti, L. Rieben, & M. Fayol (Eds.), *Learning to spell: Research, theory, and practice across languages* (pp. 129–150). Mahwah, NJ: Erlbaum.

American Speech-Language-Hearing Association. (2001). *Roles and responsibilities of speech–language pathologists with respect to reading and writing in children and adolescents.* Rockville, MD: Author.

American Speech-Language-Hearing Association. (2003). Knowledge and skills needed by speech–language pathologists with respect to reading and writing in children and adolescents. *Asha,* Suppl. 23, 93–102.

Anderson, R., & Freebody, P. (1979). Vocabulary knowledge. In J. Guthrie (Ed.), *Comprehension and teaching: Research reviews* (pp. 77–117). Newark, DE: International Reading Association.

Anstey, M. (2002). It's not all black and white: Postmodern picture books and new literacies. *Journal of Adolescent and Adult Literacy, 45,* 444–457.

Anthony, J., Lonigan, C., Burgess, S., Driscoll, K., Phillips, B., & Cantor, B. (2002). Structure of preschool phonological sensitivity: Overlapping sensitivity to rhyme, words, syllables, and phonemes. *Journal of Experimental Child Psychology, 82,* 65–92.

Apel, K., & Masterson, J. J. (2000). What is the role of the speech language pathologist in assessing and facilitating spelling skills? *Topics in Language Disorders, 20*(3), 83–93.

Apel, K., & Swank, L. (1999). Second chances: Improving decoding skills in the older student. *Language, Speech, and Hearing Services in Schools, 30*(3), 231–242.

Aram, D., & Hall, N. (1989). Longitudinal follow up of children with preschool communication disorders. *School Psychology Review, 18,* 487–501.

Ball, E. (1993). Assessing phonological awareness. *Language Speech and Hearing Services in Schools, 24,* 130–139.

Ball, E. (1997). Phonological awareness: Implications for whole language and emergent literacy programs. *Topics in Language Disorders, 17*(3), 14–26.

Ball, E., & Blachman, B. (1988). Phoneme segmentation training: Effect on reading readiness. *Annals of Dyslexia, 38,* 208–225.

Ball, E., & Blachman, B. (1991). Does phoneme awareness training in kindergarten make a difference in early word recognition and developmental spelling? *Reading Research Quarterly, 26,* 49–66.

Baron, J. (1985). *Rationality and intelligence.* New York: Cambridge University Press.

Baron, J. (1988). *Thinking and deciding.* New York: Cambridge University Press.

Bear, D., Invernizzi, M., Templeton, S., & Johnston, F. (1999). *Words their way: Word study for phonics, vocabulary, and spelling instruction* (2nd ed.). Upper Saddle River, NJ: Prentice Hall.

Beck, I., Perfetti, C., & McKeown, M. (1982). The effects of long-term vocabulary instruction on lexical access and reading comprehension. *Journal of Educational Psychology, 74,* 506–521.

Becker, W., Dixon, R., & Anderson-Inman, L. (1980). *Morphographic and root word analysis of 26,000 high frequency words.* Eugene: University of Oregon College of Education.

Berninger, V., Abbot, R., Rogan, L., Reed, E., Abbot, S., Brooks, A., et al. (1998). Teaching spelling to children with specific learning disabilities: The mind's ear and eye beat the computer or pencil. *Learning Disabilities Quarterly, 21,* 106–122.

Biber, D. (1986). Spoken and written textual dimensions in English: Resolving the contradictory findings. *Language, 62,* 384–414.

Bird, J., Bishop, D., & Freeman, N. (1995). Phonological awareness and literacy development in children with expressive phonological impairments. *Journal of Speech and Hearing Research, 38,* 446–462.

Blachman, B. (1994). Early literacy acquisition: The role of phonological awareness. In G. Wallach & K. Butler (Eds.), *Language learning disabilities in school-age children and adolescents: Some principles and applications* (pp. 253–274). New York: Macmillan.

Blatchford, P., Burke, J., Farquhar, C., Plewis, L., & Tizard, B. (1987). Associations between pre-school reading related skills and later reading achievement. *British Journal of Educational Psychology, 13,* 15–23.

Block, C. C., & Pressley, M. (2002). *Comprehension instruction—Research based best practices.* New York: Guilford Press.

Bowey, J. (1994). Phonological sensitivity in novice readers and nonreaders. *Journal of Experimental Child Psychology, 58,* 134–159.

Bowey, J., & Hansen, J. (1994). The development of orthographic rimes as units of word recognition. *Journal of Experimental Child Psychology, 58,* 465–488.

Bristor, V. (1993). Enhancing text structure instruction with video for improved reading comprehension. *Intervention in School and Clinic, 28,* 216–223.

Brown, A. (1987). Metacognition, executive control, self-regulation and other mysterious mechanisms. In F. Weinert & R. Kluwe (Eds.), *Metacognition, motivation, and understanding* (pp. 65–116). Hillsdale, NJ: Erlbaum.

Brown, G. (1862). *The first lines of English grammar.* New York: William Wood.

Butler, K. (1999). From oracy to literacy: Changing clinical perspectives. *Topics in Language Disorders, 20*(1), 14–32.

Carreker, S. (2002). Fluency: No longer a forgotten goal in reading instruction. *Perspectives of the International Dyslexia Association, 28*(1), 1–4.

Catts, H. (1991). Facilitating phonological awareness: Role of speech–language pathologists. *Language, Speech, and Hearing Services in Schools, 22,* 196–203.

Catts, H. (1993). The relationship between speech–language impairments and reading disabilities. *Journal of Speech and Hearing Research, 36,* 948–958.

Catts, H. (1997). The identification of language-based reading disabilities. *Language, Speech, and Hearing Services in Schools, 28,* 86–89.

Catts, H., Fey, M., Shang, X., & Tomblin, J. G. (2001). Estimating the risk of future reading difficulties in kindergarten children: A research based model and its clinical instrumentation. *Language, Speech, and Hearing Services in Schools, 33*(2), 84–101.

Catts, H., & Kamhi, A. (Eds.). (1999). *Language and reading disabilities.* Needham Heights, MA: Allyn & Bacon.

Chafe, W., & Danielwicz, J. (1987). Properties of spoken and written language. In R. Horowitz & S. Samuels (Eds.), *Comprehending oral and written language* (pp. 83–113). San Diego, CA: Academic Press.

Chall, J. (1983). *Stages of reading development.* New York: McGraw-Hill.

Clay, M. (1975). *What did I write?* London: Heinemann.

Conley, M. W., & Hinchman, K. A. (2004). No child left behind: What it means for U.S. adolescents and what we can do about it. *Journal of Adolescent & Adult Literacy, 48*(1), 42–50.

Curtis, M., & Longo, A. M. (1997). *Reversing reading failure in young adults.* Retrieved July 22, 2005, from the National Center for the Study of Adult Learning and Literacy Web site: http://www.gse.harvard.edu/~ncsall/fob/1997/curtis.htm

Curtis, M., & Longo, A. M. (1999). *When adolescents can't read: Methods and materials that work.* Cambridge, MA: Brookline Books.

Dahl, K., & Freppon, P. (1995). A comparison of inner city children's interpretations of reading and writing instruction in the early grades in skills-based and whole language classrooms. *Reading Research Quarterly, 31,* 50–75.

Dawes, R. (1988). *Rational choice in an uncertain world.* San Diego, CA: Harcourt Brace Jovanovich.

Derwing, B., Smith, M., & Wiebe, G. (1995). On the role of spelling in morpheme recognition: Experimental studies with children and adults. In L. B. Feldman (Ed.), *Morphological aspects of language processing* (pp. 189–209). Hillsdale, NJ: Erlbaum.

deVilliers, P., deVilliers, J., Peason, B., & Burns, F. (2002, November). *Assessing pragmatics and syntax between age 4 and 9—Elicited production.* Paper presented at the meeting of the American Speech-Language-Hearing Association, Atlanta, GA.

Dickinson, D., & McCabe, A. (1991). The acquisition and development of language: A social interactionist account of language and literacy development. In J. F. Kavanaugh (Ed.), *The language continuum: From infancy to literacy* (pp. 1–40). Parkton, MD: York Press.

Dickinson, D., & Snow, C. (1987). Interrelationships among pre reading and oral language skills in kindergartners from two social classes. *Early Childhood Research Quarterly, 2,* 1–25.

Ehren, B. (2000). Maintaining a therapeutic focus and sharing responsibility for student success: Keys to in-classroom speech language services. *Language, Speech, and Hearing Services in Schools, 25,* 248–267.

Ehren, B. J. (2002). Speech–language pathologists contributing significantly to the academic success of high school students: A vision for professional growth. *Topics in Language Disorders, 22*(2), 60–80.

Ehri, L. (1986). Sources of difficulty in learning to spell and read. In M. Wolraich & D. Routh (Eds.), *Advances in developmental and behavioral pediatrics* (pp. 121–195). Greenwich, CT: Jai Press.

Ehri, L. (1991). Development of the ability to read words. In R. Barr, M. Kamil, P. Mosenthal, & P. Pearson (Eds.), *Handbook of reading research* (Vol. 11, pp. 383–417). New York: Longman.

Ehri, L. (1999). Phases of development in learning to read words. In J. Oakhill & R. Beard (Eds.), *Reading development and the teaching of reading* (pp. 79–109). Malden, MA: Blackwell.

Ehri, L. (2000a). Keys to in-classroom speech language services. *Language, Speech, and Hearing Services in Schools, 31*(3), 219–229.

Ehri, L. (2000b). Learning to read and learning to spell: Two sides of a coin. *Topics in Language Disorders, 20,* 19–36.

Ehri, L., & Robbins, C. (1992). Beginners need some decoding skills to read words by analogy. *Reading Research Quarterly, 27,* 12–26.

Ehri, L., & Saltmarsh, J. (1995). Beginning readers outperform older disabled readers in learning to read words by sight. *Reading and Writing: An Interdisciplinary Journal, 7,* 295–326.

Englert, C., & Raphael, T. (1988). Constructing well formed prose: Process, structure, and metacognitive knowledge. *Exceptional Children, 54,* 513–527.

Farris, P. (2001). *Language arts—Process, product and assessment.* Boston: McGraw-Hill.

Fowler, A., & Lieberman, I. (1995). The role of phonology and orthography in morphological awareness. In L. B. Feldman (Ed.), *Morphological aspects of language processing* (pp. 189–209). Hillsdale, NJ: Erlbaum.

Fox, B., & Routh, D. (1975). Analyzing spoken language into words, syllables, and phonemes. *Journal of Psycholinguistic Research, 4,* 331–342.

Fox, B., & Routh, D. (1984). Phonemic analysis and synthesis as word attack skills: Revisited. *Journal of Educational Psychology, 76,* 1059–1064.

Frank, L. (1992). Writing to be read: Young writers' ability to demonstrate audience awareness when evaluated by their readers. *Research in the Teaching of English, 26,* 277–298.

Freeman, D. (1968). *Corduroy.* New York: Viking Penguin.

Fry, E., Kress, J., & Fountoukidis, D. (2000). *The reading teacher's book of lists* (4th ed.). San Francisco: Jossey-Bass and Wiley.

Gaskins, E. (1998). A beginning literacy program for at-risk and delayed readers. In J. L. Metsala & L. G. Ehri (Eds.), *Word recognition in beginning literacy* (pp. 209–232). Mahwah, NJ: Erlbaum.

Gillon, G., & Dodd, B. (1995). The effects of training phonological, semantic and syntactic processing skills in spoken language on reading ability. *Language, Speech, and Hearing Services in Schools, 26*(1), 58–68.

Gilovich, T. (1991). *How we know what isn't so: The fallibility of human reason in everyday life.* New York: Free Press.

Goldfield, B., & Snow, C. (1984). Reading books with children: The mechanics of parental influence on children's reading achievement. In J. Flood (Ed.), *Understanding reading comprehension* (pp. 204–218). Newark, DE: International Reading Association.

Gorman, C. (2003, July 28). The new science of dyslexia. *Time, 162(4),* 52–59.

Goswami, U. (1988). Children's use of analogy in learning to spell. *British Journal of Developmental Psychology, 6,* 21–33.

Graham, S., & Freeman, S. (1986). Strategy training and teacher vs. student-controlled study conditions: Effects on LD students' performance. *Learning Disability Quarterly, 9,* 15–22.

Graham, S., & Voth, V. (1990). Spelling instruction: Making modifications for students with learning disabilities. *Academic Therapy, 25,* 447–457.

Gravani, E., & Meyer, J. (2001). *Phonological awareness: Definitions and application to preliteracy skills.* Paper presented at the meeting of the New York State Speech Language & Hearing Association, Saratoga Springs, NY.

Greenhalgh, K., & Strong, C. (2001). Literate language features in spoken narratives of children with typical language and children with language impairments. *Language, Speech, and Hearing Services in Schools 32,* 114–125.

Gregg, N. (1991). Disorders of written expression. In A. Bain, L. Bailet, & L. Moats (Eds.), *Written language disorders: Theory into practice* (pp. 65–97). Austin, TX: PRO-ED.

Harste, J., Woodward, V., & Burke, D. (1984). *Language stories and literacy lessons.* Portsmouth, NH: Heinemann.

Hart, B., & Risley, T. R. (2003). The early catastrophe: The 30 million word gap by age 3. *American Educator, 27*(1), 4–9.

Hayes, J., & Flower, L. (1987). On the structure of the writing process. *Topics in Language Disorders, 7*(4), 19–30.

Henderson, E. (1990). *Teaching spelling.* Boston: Houghton Mifflin.

Hennings, D. G. (2000). Contextually relevant word study: Adolescent vocabulary development across the curriculum. *Journal of Adolescent & Adult Literacy, 44*(3), 268–279.

Hirsh, E. D. Jr. (2001). Overcoming the language gap. *American Educator, 25*(2), 4–7.

Hodson, B. (1986). *Assessment of phonological process–Revised.* Danville, IL: Interstate Printers & Publishers.

Hoggan, K. C., & Strong, C. J. (1994). The magic of "Once upon a time": Narrative teaching strategies. *Language, Speech, and Hearing Services in Schools, 25,* 76–89.

Horn, E. (1954). *Teaching spelling.* Washington, DC: American Educational Research Association.

Hyerle, D. (2004). *Student success with thinking maps: School based research, results and models for achievement using visual tools.* Thousand Oaks, CA: Corwin Press.

Individuals with Disabilities Education Improvement Act. (2004). Public Law 108-446.

Irwin, J., & Baka, I. (1989). *Promoting active reading strategies.* Newark, NJ: Prentice Hall.

Johnston, R. S., Anderson, M., & Holligan, C. (1996). Knowledge of the alphabet and explicit awareness of phonemes in pre-readers: The nature of the relationship. *Reading and Writing: An Interdisciplinary Journal, 8,* 217–234.

Juel, C. (1983). The development and use of mediated word identification. *Reading Research Quarterly, 18,* 309–327.

Juel, C. (1991). Beginning reading. In R. Barr, M. Kamil, P. Mosenthal, & P. Pearson (Eds.), *Handbook of reading research* (Vol. 11, pp. 306–317). New York: Longman.

Justice, L., Invernizzi, M. A., & Meier, J. D. (2002). Designing and implementing an early literacy screening protocol: Suggestions for the speech–language pathologist. *Language, Speech, and Hearing Services in Schools, 33*(2), 84–101.

Kahneman, D., Slovic, P., & Tversky, A. (1982). *Judgement under uncertainty: Heuristics and biases.* Cambridge, England: Cambridge University Press.

Kamhi, A. G. (2003). The role of the SLP in improving reading fluency. *ASHA Leader, 8*(7), 6–8.

Kher, U. (2001, March 26). Blame it on the written word. *Time, 157*(12), 56.

Klecan-Aker, J. (1985). Syntactic abilities in normal and language deficient middle school children. *Topics in Language Disorders, 5*, 46–54.

Knight, J. (Ed.). (2002). Adults with dyslexia: Legislation, remediation, therapy and work. *Perspectives of the International Dyslexia Association, 28*(4), 1–25.

Kroll, B. (1985). Rewriting a complex story for a young reader: The development of audience-adapted writing skills. *Research in the Teaching of English, 19*, 120–139.

Langer, J. (1986). *Children reading and writing: Structures and strategies.* Norwood, NJ: Ablex.

Larrivee, L., & Catts, H. (1999). Early reading achievement in children with expressive phonological disorders. *American Journal of Speech–Language Pathology, 8*, 118–128.

Lavine, L. (1977). Differentiation of letter-like forms in pre-reading children. *Developmental Psychology, 18*, 89–94.

Leslie, L., & Caldwell, J. (2000). *Qualitative reading inventory* (3rd ed.). Upper Saddle River, NJ: Pearson Allyn & Bacon.

Liles, B. (1985). Cohesion in the narratives of normal and language-disordered children. *Journal of Speech and Hearing Research, 28*, 123–133.

Loban, W. (1976). *Language development: Kindergarten through grade twelve.* (Research Report No. 18). Urbana, IL: National Council of Teachers of English.

Lombardino, L., & Ahmed, S. (2000). What is the role of the speech–language pathologist in assessing and facilitating spelling skills? *Topics in Language Disorders, 20*, 83–84.

Lonigan, C., Burgess, S., & Anthony, J. (2000). Development of emergent literacy and early literacy skills in preschool children: Evidence from a latent-variable longitudinal study. *Developmental Psychology, 36*, 596–613.

Lonigan, C., Burgess, S., Anthony, J., & Barker, T. (1998). Development of phonological sensitivity in 2- to 5-year-old children. *Journal of Educational Psychology, 90*, 294–311.

Luckner, J. L., & Isaacson, S. L. (1990). Teaching expressive writing to hearing impaired students. *Journal of Childhood Communication Disorders, 131*, 135–152.

Lyon, G. R., & Chhabra, V. (1996). The current state of science and the future of specific reading disability. *Mental Retardation and Developmental Disabilities Research Review, 2*, 2–9.

MacArthur, C., Graham, S., Haynes, J., & De La Paz, S. (1996). Spelling checkers and students with learning disabilities: Performance comparisons and impact of spelling. *Journal of Special Education, 30*, 35–57.

MacDonald, G., & Cornwall, A. (1995). The relationship between phonological awareness and reading and spelling achievement eleven years later. *Journal of Learning Disabilities, 28*, 523–527.

MacLean, M., Bryant, P., & Bradley, L. (1987). Rhymes, nursery rhymes, and reading in early childhood. *Merrill-Palmer Quarterly, 33*, 255–281.

Marsh, G., Friedman, M., Welch, V., & Desberg, P. (1980). The development of strategies in spelling. In U. Frith (Ed.), *Cognitive processes in spelling* (pp. 121–147). London: Academic Press.

Mason, J., & Allen, J. (1986). A review of emergent literacy with implications for research and practice in reading. In E. Z. Rothkopf (Ed.), *Review of research in education* (pp. 3–47). Washington, DC: American Educational Research Association.

Masonheimer, P., Drum, P., & Ehri, L. (1984). Does environmental print identification lead children into word reading? *Journal of Reading Behavior, 16*, 257–272.

Massey, D. D., & Heafner, T. L. (2004). Promoting reading comprehension in social studies. *Journal of Adolescent & Adult Literacy, 48*(1), 26–40.

Masterson, J. J., & Apel, K. (2000). Spelling assessment: Charting a path to optimal intervention. *Topics in Language Disorders, 20*(3), 50–65.

Mattes, L. J. (1997). *Developing language for literacy.* Oceanside, CA: Academic Communication Associates.

McCleary, J., & Tindal, G. (1999). Teaching the scientific method to at-risk students and students with learning disabilities through concept anchoring and explicit instruction. *Remedial and Special Education, 20,* 7–18.

McFadden, T. U. (1997). Sounds and stories: Teaching phonemic awareness in interactions around text. *American Journal of Speech Language Pathology, 7*(2), 5–13.

McKeown, M., Beck, I., Omanson, R., & Perfetti, C. (1983). The effects of long-term instruction on reading comprehension: A replication. *Journal of Reading Behavior, 15,* 3–18.

McLaughlin, M., & DeVoogd, G. (2004). Critical literacy as comprehension: Expanding reader response. *Journal of Adolescent & Adult Literacy, 48*(1), 52–62.

Meyer, B., & Freedle, R. (1984). Effects of discourse type on recall. *American Education Journal, 21,* 121–144.

Mezynski, K. (1983). Issues concerning the acquisition of knowledge: Effects of vocabulary training on reading comprehension. *Review of Educational Research, 53,* 253–279.

Moats, L. (1995). *Spelling: Development, disability and instruction.* Baltimore: Brookes.

Moats, L. (2000). *Speech to print: Language essentials for teachers.* Baltimore: Brookes.

Montgomery, R. (2003). Idea swap: Spellish. *Word of Mouth, 14*(5), 14.

Muter, V., & Snowling, M. (1998). Concurrent and longitudinal predictors of reading: The role of metalinguistic and short-term memory skills. *Reading Research Quarterly, 33*(3), 320–335.

National Reading Panel. (2000). *Teaching children to read: An evidence-based assessment of the scientific research literature on reading and its implication for reading instruction: Reports of the subgroups.* Washington, DC: National Institute of Child Health and Human Development.

Nation, K., & Hulme, C. (1997). Phonemic segmentation, not onset-rime segmentation, predicts early reading and spelling skills. *Reading Research Quarterly, 32,* 154–167.

Nippold, M. (1998). *Later language development: The school-age and adolescent years.* Austin, TX: PRO-ED.

Nisbitt, R., & Ross, L. (1980). *Human inference: Strategies and shortcomings of social judgement.* Englewood Cliffs, NY: Prentice Hall.

Nottingham Writing Team. (2001). High school generic rubric-6 point. *The writing process for good academic writing—Nottingham High School 2001—2002.* Syracuse NY: Nottingham High School.

Parton, T. (2002). Building language and reading for the high school student. *Perspectives on School Based Issues, 3*(1), 32–34.

Perera, K. (1984). *Children's writing and reading: Analyzing classroom language.* Oxford, England: Blackwell.

Rand Reading Study Group. (2001). *Reading for understanding: Toward an R & D Program in reading comprehension.* Arlington, VA: Rand.

Rasiniski, T. (1994). Developing syntactic sensitivity in reading through phrase-cued texts. *Intervention in School and Clinic, 29*(3), 165–168.

Reitsma, P. (1983). Printed word learning in beginning readers. *Journal of Experimental Child Psychology, 75,* 321–339.

Romero, L. (2002). At-risk students: Learning to break through comprehension barriers. In C. Block, L. Gambrell, & M. Pressley (Eds.), *Improving comprehension instruction: Rethinking research, theory, and classroom practice* (pp. 354–369). San Francisco: Jossey-Bass.

Rorabacher, L. (1956). *A concise guide to composition.* New York: Harper.

Rosenshine, B., & Meister, C. (1992). The use of scaffolds for teaching higher-level cognitive strategies. *Educational Leadership, 48*(7), 26–33.

Rubin, H., Patterson, P., & Kantor, M. (1991). Morphological development and writing ability in children and adults. *Language, Speech, and Hearing Services in Schools, 24,* 228–235.

Sanders, M. (2001). Impediments to reading comprehension. *Perspectives, 27*(2), 1–4.

Scarborough, H. (1990). Very early language deficits in dyslexic children. *Child Development, 61*(1), 1728–1743.

Scarborough, H. (1998). Early identification of children at risk for reading disabilities: Phonological awareness and some other promising predictors. In B. K. Shapiro, P. I. Accardo, & A. J. Capute (Eds.), *Specific reading disabilities: A view of the spectrum* (pp. 75–91). Timonium, MD: York Press.

Scarborough, H. (2001, November). *Linking language to literacy: Recent research.* Paper presented at the meeting of the American Speech-Language-Hearing Association, New Orleans, LA.

Scott, C. (1999). Learning to write. In H. Catts & A. Kamhi (Eds.), *Language and reading disabilities* (pp. 224–258). Boston: Allyn & Bacon.

Scott, C. (2000). Principles and methods of spelling instruction: Application for poor spellers. *Topics in Language Disorders, 20,* 66–82.

Scott, C., & Erwin, D. (1992). Descriptive assessment of writing: Process and products. In W. Secord (Ed.), *Best practices in school speech language pathology* (Vol. 2, pp. 60–75). San Antonio, TX: Psychological Corp. and Harcourt Brace Jovanovich.

Seidenberg, P. (1988). Cognitive and academic instructional intervention for learning-disabled students. *Topics in Language Disorders, 8*(3), 56–71.

Senechal, M., LeFevre, J., Thomas, E., & Daley, K. (1998). Differential effects of home literacy experiences on the development of oral and written language. *Reading Research Quarterly, 33,* 96–116.

Shaywitz, B. A, Fletcher, J. M., & Shaywitz, S. E. (1994). Issues on the definition and classification of attention deficit disorder. *Topics in Language Disorders, 14,* 1–25.

Silliman, E. R., Bahr, R., Beasman, J., & Wilkinson, L. C. (2000). Scaffolds for learning to read in an inclusion classroom. *Language, Speech, and Hearing Services in Schools, 31*(3), 265–279.

Singer, B. (1995). Written language development and disorders: Selected principles, patterns, and intervention possibilities. *Topics in Language Disorders, 16*(1), 83–98.

Singer, B., & Bashir, A. (1999). What are executive functions and self-regulation and what do they have to do with language learning disorders? *Language, Speech, and Hearing Services in Schools, 30,* 265–273.

Smith, J., & Elkins, J. (1985). The use of cohesion by underachieving readers. *Reading Psychology, 6,* 13–25.

Snow, C. E., Scarborough, H. S., & Burns, M. S. (1999). What speech language pathologists need to know about early reading. *Topics in Language Disorders, 20*(1), 48–58.

Snowling, M., Hulme, C., Smith, A., & Thomas, J. (1994). The effects of phoneme similarity and list length on children's sound categorization performance. *Journal of Experimental Child Psychology, 58,* 160–180.

Snyder, L. S., & Downey, D. M. (1997). Developmental differences in the relationship between oral language deficits and reading. *Topics in Language Disorders, 17*(1), 27–40.

SPELL–Links to Literacy. (2004). *Spelling assessment software, grade 2—adult.* Evanston, IL: Learning by Design.

Stahl, S. (1983). Differential word knowledge and reading comprehension. *Journal of Reading Behavior, 15,* 33–50.

Stahl, S., & Murray, B. (1994). Environmental print, phonemic awareness, letter recognition, mathematics and reading. *National Conference Yearbook, 42,* 227–233.

Stahl, S., Osborn, J., & Lehr, F. (1990). *Beginning to read: Thinking and learning about print by Marilyn Jager Adams: A summary.* Urbana, IL: Center for the Study of Reading.

Stanovich, K. (1986). Matthew effects in reading: Some consequences of individual differences in the acquisition of literacy. *Reading Research Quarterly, 21,* 360–406.

Stanovich, K. (2000). *Progress in understanding reading.* New York: Guilford Press.

Stanovich, K., Cunningham, A., & Freeman, D. (1984). Intelligence, cognitive skills, and early reading progress. *Reading Research Quarterly, 19,* 270–303.

Stevens, D., & Englert, C. (1993). Making writing strategies work. *Teaching Exceptional Children, 20*(1), 34–39.

Stevenson, H., & Newman, R. (1986). Long-term prediction of achievement and attitudes in mathematics and reading. *Child Development, 57,* 646–659.

Strattman, K. (2001). Phonological awareness. *Word of Mouth, 13*(1), 3–4.

Swank, L. (1997). Linguistic influences on the emergence of written word decoding in first grade. *American Journal of Speech–Language Pathology, 6,* 62–66.

Tabors, P., Patton, O., Snow, C., & Dickinson, D. (2001). Homes and schools together: Supporting language and literacy development. In D. Dickinson, P. Tabors, & O. Patton (Eds.), *Beginning literacy with language* (pp. 313–334). Baltimore: Brookes.

Templeton, S. (2002). Spelling: Logical, learnable—And critical. *ASHA Leader, 7*(3), 4–5, 12.

Tirolo-Zaleski, B. (2002). Promoting adolescent literacy: A model for implementation. *Perspectives on School Based Issues, 3*(1), 29–34.

Tolchinsky-Landsmann, L., & Levin, I. (1977). Writing in four- to six-year-olds: Representation of semantic and phonetic similarities and differences. *Journal of Child Language, 14,* 127–144.

Treiman, R. (1997). Spelling in normal children and dyslexics. In B. Blachman (Ed.), *Foundations of reading acquisition and dyslexia* (pp. 191–218). Mahwah, NJ: Erlbaum.

Treiman, R., & Bourassa, D. (2000). The development of spelling skill. *Topics in Language Disorders, 20,* 1–18.

Treiman, R., & Cassar, M. (1997). Spelling acquisition in English. In C. Perfetti, L. Rieben, & M. Fayol (Eds.), *Learning to spell: Research theory and practices across languages* (pp. 61–80). Mahwah, NJ: Erlbaum.

Treiman, R., Cassar, M., & Zukowski, A. (1994). What types of linguistic information do children use in spelling? The case of flaps. *Child Development, 65,* 1310–1329.

Treiman, R., Goswami, U., & Bruck, M. (1990). Not all non words are alike: Implications for reading development and theory. *Memory and Cognition, 18,* 559–567.

Trueba, H., & Wright, P. (1992). On ethnographic studies and multicultural education. In M. Saravia-Shore & S. Arvizu (Eds.), *Cross-cultural literacy: Ethnographies of communication in multiethnic classrooms* (pp. 299–338). New York: Garland.

van Kleeck, A. (1990). Emergent literacy: Learning about print before learning to read. *Topics in Language Disorders, 10,* 25–45.

van Kleeck, A. (1994, November). *A connectionist model of preliteracy: Reconciling the pedagogy debate.* Paper presented at a meeting of the American Speech-Language-Hearing Association, New Orleans, LA.

Vellutino, F., & Scanlon, D. (1987). Phonological coding, phonological awareness, and reading ability: Evidence from a longitudinal and experimental study. *Merrill-Palmer Quarterly, 33,* 321–363.

Venezky, R. (1976). *Theoretical and experimental base for teaching reading.* The Hague: Mouton.

Wagner, R., Torgesen, J., & Rashotte, C. (1999). *Comprehensive Test of Phonolgical Processing.* Austin, TX: PRO-ED.

Ward-Lonergan, J. M. (2002, November). *Helping older children and adolescents master the language of the curriculum.* Paper presented at the American Speech-Language-Hearing Association Convention, Atlanta, GA.

Westby, C. (1999). Assessing and facilitating text comprehension problems. In H. W. Catts & A. G. Kamhi (Eds.), *Language and reading disabilities* (pp. 154–223). Needham Heights, MA: Allyn & Bacon.

Westby, C. (2004). Evidence-based practice: A new requirement for service provision. *Word of Mouth, 16*(1), 1–3.

Whitehurst, G., & Lonigan, C. (1998). Child development and emergent literacy. *Child Development, 69,* 848–872.

Wylie, R., & Durrell, D. (1970). Teaching vowels through phonograms. *Elementary English, 47,* 787–791.

Yopp, H. (1992). Developing phonological awareness in young children. *The Reading Teacher, 45,* 696–703.

Chapter 8

Augmentative and Alternative Communication in School Settings

Ralf W. Schlosser, Donna McGhie-Richmond,
and Helen Arvidson

Augmentative and alternative communication (AAC) "is, foremost, a set of procedures and processes by which an individual's communication skills (i.e., production as well as comprehension) can be maximized for functional and effective communication. It involves supplementing or replacing natural speech and/or writing with aided (e.g., picture communication symbols, line drawings, Blissymbols, and tangible objects) and/or unaided symbols (e.g., manual signs, gestures, and finger spelling). Whereas aided symbols require some type of transmission device, unaided symbols require only the body to produce. Many individuals with severe communication and cognitive impairments can benefit from nonsymbolic forms of AAC such as gestures (reaching for a desired object) and vocalizations that convey different emotions. AAC also refers to the field or area of clinical, educational, and research practice to improve, temporarily or permanently, the communication skills of individuals with little or no functional speech and/or writing. Regardless of the mode(s) selected, AAC involves the utilization of symbols (e.g., single meaning pictures, alphabet based methods, and semantic compaction) to represent individuals' communication intents" (American Speech-Language-Hearing Association [ASHA], 2002, p. 98).

Demographic studies in North America indicate that 2.5% to 6% of all students receiving special education services have such severe communication impairments that they cannot be understood by their teachers or peers (Burd, Hammes, Bornhoeft, & Fisher, 1988; Lindsay, Cambria, McNaughton, & Warrick, 1986; Matas, Mathy-Laikko, Beukelman, & Legresley, 1985; National Institute on Disability and Rehabilitation Research, 1992). In addition to having difficulties with face-to-face communication, many of these students have multiple disabilities (e.g., perceptual, cognitive, manipulative) that may contribute to their problems using traditional writing tools, such as paper and pencils. Increasingly, such children can be helped in face-to-face communication and written communication through AAC systems (Beukelman & Mirenda, 1998; Lloyd, Fuller, & Arvidson, 1997). AAC systems may be unaided, such as manual signs and gestures, or they may be aided, involving external aids beyond the user's own body, such as communication boards, speech generating devices (SGDs), and computers. It is the aided AAC part that overlaps with the services and devices of assistive technology (Lloyd et al., 1997).

The intent of this chapter is to assist current and future speech–language pathologists in their support of students who have little or no functional speech or writing ability. The information in this chapter can help enhance children's communication, participation, and membership in school settings. We will present illustrative cases, discuss applicable research findings, and introduce, as an example of one means of assessing a student's participation patterns and levels of independence, the Participation Assessment Framework, used to devise strategies for removing identified barriers (Beukelman & Mirenda, 1998).

THE SCHOOL SETTING: COMMUNICATION, PARTICIPATION, AND MEMBERSHIP

In addition to their home surroundings, children spend their time predominantly in some sort of educational environment. Schools may focus on academic learning, but they are also about socialization, developing friendships, and establishing a sense of community. It is a given, of course, that schools have to follow academic curricula, and in order for students to succeed in school academically or socially, each student must have access to those curricula. Without access, no formal learning is likely to take place.

In the past, SLPs have understood that their primary role as professionals was to support a student's communication—and that is where it stopped. Communication, however, cannot be viewed in a vacuum; changes in communication without concomitant changes elsewhere amount to nothing more than a meaningless demonstration of the application of an AAC system in a narrow and perhaps nonfunctional set of circumstances. Ferguson (1994) asked the provocative question, "Is communication really the point?" (p. 7). She concluded that the primary purpose of our professional intervention should not be enhanced communication as much as it should be enhanced membership in society, "specifically participatory, socially valued, image enhancing membership" (p. 10). Although they are related terms, *participation* and *membership* are different concepts. As only one ingredient involved in "conferring" membership, participation must be active and socially valid for membership to occur. Membership should also be characterized by status in the group. Thus, in the world of schools, unless changes in communication skill result in better access to the curriculum, improved participation in the classroom, and a better sense of membership, we have not accomplished all that we should. We agree with this conclusion. We posit that for us to ensure the ultimate goal of participation and membership, every step we take in planning assessment and intervention within the realm of AAC will be different from those taken by the person who assumes that the goal is communication alone. Because the regular education classroom is rapidly becoming the least restrictive environment for most students with severe communication impairments (Mirenda & Calculator, 1993), we will approach this chapter within the context of students who are to be fully included in school life.

FROM PARTICIPATION IN ASSESSMENT TO ASSESSMENT OF PARTICIPATION

In common with other special services, the first step in the intervention process is assessment. In the following section, alternate assessment procedures are described, illustrated by a case study. A specific assessment approach, the participation assessment framework (PAF), is discussed in detail.

Using Alternate Assessment

There is considerable variability in the extent to which students who use AAC participate in educational activities. The Individuals with Disabilities Education Act (IDEA) Amendments of 1997 and 2004 (P.L. 105-17; P.L. 108-446) provide legislative support for districts to develop and use assistive technologies that promote the inclusion of students with disabilities in the areas of educational instruction, assessment, and accountability systems. Opportunities for participation in instruction improve with the availability and implementation of appropriate instructional and technological supports. Opportunities for participation in assessment and accountability systems, however, improve with the development and implementation of appropriate accommodations and alternate assessments specifically designed for students who cannot fully demonstrate their abilities on the standardized tests used during wide-scale assessments. The National Center on Educational Outcomes (NCEO), a collaborative organization including professionals from the University of Minnesota, the National Association of State Directors of Special Education, and St. Cloud University, was established in 1990 to work with national organizations, state departments of education, and other groups and individuals to facilitate and enhance the development and implementation of indicators of educational outcomes for students with disabilities (McGrew, Thurlow, Shriner, & Spiegel, 1992; Ysseldyke & Thurlow, 1997). Early investigations by the NCEO revealed variability in how states included students with disabilities in assessment and accountability systems. Several generalizations, however, did emerge:

- Most existing national and state data collection programs excluded large portions of students with disabilities.
- Exclusion occurred at many different points along a continuum ranging from the development of assessment instruments to the reporting of results.
- Differential guidelines for exclusion made it difficult to compare assessment results.
- A sizable portion of the students who had been excluded could have participated, some of them with accommodations and some without.

Ysseldyke, Thurlow, McGrew, and Shriner (1994) described three types of students with disabilities:

- students who can take wide-scale tests without accommodations,
- students who can take wide-scale tests with accommodations, and
- students who need a different assessment because their curriculum is different from the one being tested.

Elliott (1998) defined test accommodations as changes in ways tests are administered or variations in ways students respond to test items. He described employing test accommodations as being analogous to using corrective lenses, maintaining that one can obtain a clearer image of student performance when students are allowed to use accommodations to compensate for disabilities. Thurlow, Elliott, & Ysseldyke (1998) discussed accommodations as changes in testing materials or procedures that allow students with disabilities to demonstrate abilities rather than disabilities. They organized accommodations into six categories:

- setting
- timing
- scheduling
- presentation
- response
- other

In order that a student's performance on tests taken with accommodations can be compared with her performance on tests taken without accommodations, however, the accommodations must be valid; that is, they must make a difference only for students with disabilities, not for students without disabilities (Tindal, Heath, Hollenbeck, Almond, & Harniss, 1998).

The IDEA Amendments of 1997 mandated that all states had an alternate assessment in place by July 1, 2000, to serve the small percentage of students for whom wide-scale assessments are ineffective in determining skills or measuring achievement (e.g., students with severe physical disabilities or intellectual disabilities). Students who do not have the physical abilities to respond to test questions in the manner required by a specific standardized instrument may be able to participate in wide-scale assessments if the procedures include appropriate accommodations. Students who have not been enrolled in curricula that teach the content material that is being tested, however, are potential candidates for alternate assessment. They would be included in the small percentage (between 1% and 3%) of students identified as participating in alternate assessment according to the No Child Left Behind Act of 2001. According to IDEA (2004), an explanation of why the alternative assessment is needed must be included in the IEP.

Since this requirement has been put in place, states have been addressing a number of issues related to alternate assessment, including why students should be assessed, which students should be assessed, what knowledge or skills should be assessed, and when assessment should take place. Additional issues include how to assess, how to score, and how to report the results (Olsen et al., 1998). The IDEA Amendments of 1997 also require that student performance on alternate assessments be reported with the same degree of frequency and detail as student performance on typical standardized measures. Policies on the participation of students in wide-scale assessments vary across states as they continue to grapple with how to use assessment information and how to implement development and training (Thurlow, House, Scott, & Ysseldyke, 2000; Ysseldyke, 2001).

Alternate assessment systems typically include a variety of assessment forms (Erickson, Ysseldyke, Thurlow, & Elliott, 1998). They may include traditional forms of assessment, such as tests that require students to respond to questions using pencil and paper, but they are more likely to be based on less traditional forms of assessment, such as portfolio collections of student work and teacher ratings of essential skills. Information used in alternate assessments should be gathered from a variety of sources and settings. Sources may include but are not be limited to parents, physicians, teachers (general and learning specialists), speech pathologists, and occupational or physical therapists. Information gathered outside of the school setting may also assist the school-based team in determining the most comprehensive individual assessment—for example, home, outside clinical providers, other community resources.

Some states have been particularly active in developing and implementing alternate assessment procedures. The Indiana Assessment System of Educational Proficiencies (IASEP), a computer-based rating and documentation system developed by Purdue University and the Indiana Department of Education Division of Special Education, was designed to meet the assessment needs of students with the most significant disabilities (Bennett, Davis, Cunningham, & Arvidson, 1999). IASEP is based on an extension of Indiana's academic content standards in language arts, mathematics, science, and social studies but also includes skills in the domains of personal adjustment, social adjustment, recreation and leisure, and vocational experience. Teachers enter ratings of student performance on subdomains and skills into a computer using a rating rubric that takes into account frequency or amount, degree of support, generalizability, and quality of performance (Arvidson, Cunningham, Davis, & Bennett, 1999). Ratings are supported by electronic documentation in the form of audio recordings, scanned images, video clips, and text entries. The documentation can be used to create an electronic portfolio within the system. Alternate assessments provide a means to assess the skills of students with significant disabilities at any given point in time. IASEP, however, is designed to provide more than snapshots in time. It is based on the ongoing data input. Teachers are encouraged to rate performance on skills and enter supporting documentation any time a student makes notable progress. IASEP shows which skills students have achieved not only at the time wide-scale tests are given, but at any given point in time. It displays the skills that have been achieved up to the last entry of data. Since skills that still need to be accomplished are already listed in the system, the teacher can easily determine what needs to be worked on next. In this way, assessment and instruction are intertwined. Here, as in any area of speech–language pathology, assessment plays a role in driving instruction.

Accountability systems for students in general education and special education vary from state to state. Some states (e.g., Indiana) emphasize student accountability, whereas others (e.g., Rhode Island) put emphasis on program accountability. Still others (e.g., Illinois) stress both. In student accountability, the focus is on a student's ability to demonstrate a variety of skills in multiple environments. In program accountability, the focus is on a school's provision of educational opportunities and access. A school may provide student access to a variety of instructional approaches in a variety of environmental settings, encourage the development of social relationships and self-determination in terms of making choices and self evaluating, or concentrate on the availability and use of supports in terms of modifications and accommodations. The Assessment and Instructional Management System (AIMS), an adaptation of IASEP, is being used by a number of states that emphasize program accountability.

There are compelling reasons for including students with disabilities in wide-scale assessment programs (Salvia & Ysseldyke, 1998; Thurlow et al., 1998). Assessment programs provide a picture of how well an educational system is working. If students with disabilities are excluded, the picture is incomplete and inaccurate, and changes are likely to have little relevance. Students with disabilities are more apt to benefit from educational initiatives and reforms if their performance is included in analyses of achievement. Change can best meet the needs of all students when the needs of all students are considered.

Another reason for including students with disabilities in assessment programs and accountability systems relates to expectations (Thurlow et al., 1998). Expectations of achievement may be lower when no system for accountability is in place. Individuals and institutions can become apathetic about improvement if there is neither accountability nor accompanying consequences for lack of achievement. Since many students with disabilities are included in general education curricula, providing access to assessment emphasizes the importance of their participation and learning. Including all students in assessment programs can help promote high expectations for all students, not just those deemed "typical."

Laura: Participating in Alternate Assessment

Laura is a 12-year-old student in special education who is included in a sixth-grade elementary school classroom. When she was 5, Laura was evaluated by the school-based assessment team to determine eligibility for special education services. The team included the school psychological examiner, general and special education teachers, a speech pathologist, an occupational therapist (OT), a physical therapist (PT), an adapted physical educator, and a school nurse. The team determined that Laura was eligible for services under the diagnostic category of multiple disabilities with a secondary eligibility of communication disorders. She has a medical diagnosis of cerebral palsy and uses a wheelchair for mobility within the school environment; she employs a variety of AAC devices for communication.

Although Laura has been included in general education classrooms, her teachers and school-based OT and PT determined that she did not have the motor skills necessary to answer paper-and-pencil test questions on grade-level, wide-scale standardized tests. There was also a concern regarding her ability to read. Prior to the sixth grade, the IEP team had exempted Laura from participation in standardized assessments. With recent changes in the laws of the state in which she resides, she was no longer allowed to be exempted after she entered the sixth grade. She was required to participate in her state's alternate assessment.

Laura's teacher was responsible for rating her level of independence on skills related to state academic standards. As an initial step, her teacher used a rating rubric to indicate whether Laura's level of performance on individual skills was independent, functional, supported, or emergent. If there was no indication that a skill was emerging, Laura's performance was given a rating of "Participation" to indicate that she had participated in the presentation of a skill. Skills in the areas of personal adjustment, social adjustment, recreation and leisure, and vocational experience were similarly assessed. Ratings in these areas provided information on skills that had not been previously assessed and therefore served as a baseline for developing appropriate educational programming. Electronic documentation supported the ratings.

Laura demonstrated skills related to the state standard of reading and understanding of grade-level material. Her teacher assigned her a rating of "Supported Independence," for example, for her ability to read and understand words. The rating was supported by video documentation that showed Laura using her SGD to answer questions related to select words.

Laura was able to demonstrate many skills that she had been unable to exhibit before by participating in the alternate assessment. For the first time, her responses generated assessment data that would be reported with data from typical students participating in the wide-scale assessment. This represented a significant move toward expanding her participation in the educational process. Since Laura receives most of her instruction within the general curriculum, it is the responsibility of the IEP team to determine the appropriate accommodations and modifications that will allow her to participate. The modifications should be designed by the IEP team to specifically meet her individual educational needs.

The Participation Assessment Framework

Assistive technology, including high-tech devices and low-tech AAC systems, undoubtedly has the potential to open the door to literacy and other curricular areas for many students like Laura (Lewis, 1993; Male, 1994). This potential, however, can be realized only if SLPs, teachers, and other related service providers are trained in instructional methodologies that enable the technology to be integrated into these curricular areas in a meaningful manner (Bowser & Reed, 1995; Edyburn, 1996; Toddis & Walker, 1993). The U.S. Department of Education (1998) defined what it called a "technology based approach" as an innovative combination of technology and additional curriculum material and instructional methodologies that enable a student with disabilities to achieve educational goals. Similarly, the use of unaided forms of communication such as manual signs will be successful only if they are integrated into the everyday curriculum (Loeding, Zangari, & Lloyd, 1990).

Teachers also have indicated that they must possess both the knowledge of various technologies and training in how to integrate them into the curriculum (McGhie-Richmond & McGinnis, 1996; McGregor & Pachuski, 1996). The Participation Assessment Framework (PAF) "provides a systematic process for conducting AAC assessment and designing interventions based on functional requirements of non disabled peers of the same chronological ages as the potential AAC user" (Beukelman & Mirenda, 1998, p. 147). As such, it can be used as a framework for integrating students who use AAC into educational programs.

The framework provides variables that can be manipulated to achieve a participation pattern that is appropriate to the needs and capabilities of the student who uses AAC. The variables include three levels of overall integration (fully, selective, and none) that becomes a specific pattern related to levels of academic and social participation (competitive, active, involved, and none) and the student's level of independence. Each of these levels of participation can be charted along a continuum. The Participation Matrix is a tool for supporting a team in coming to consensus concerning a student's level of integration and participation. It also provides a baseline from which the team can discuss goals and expectations.

In the following section, we will present illustrative examples from a recent research study that examined the effects of training a school team in how to use the PAF and barrier-specific intervention as they related to the participation of a student during literacy and math activities (Schlosser et al., 2000). These examples will be supplemented with others from our collective clinical and educational experiences.

Assessing and Removing Barriers to Participation

The Activity Standards Inventory (ASI) is used to document and analyze the student's actual participation in classroom activities and to identify the barriers responsible for any discrepancies between the target student and her nondisabled peers. Once an activity is selected, the observer breaks down the activity into observable steps, similar to a task analysis. Next, the SLP chooses a peer who is judged capable of performing the activity at the expected standard. After observing the activity, the rater indicates the peer's level of participation with a "P" on a continuum from *independent* to *independent with setup,* to *verbal assistance,* to *physical assistance,* to *unable to participate.* Next, the observer rates the participation level of the target student and marks each step with a "T" at the appropriate level. Subsequently, the rater indicates whether there is a discrepancy in participation levels between the peer and the target student, and if so, what barriers might be responsible for this discrepancy. Barriers include those related to opportunity or access (Beukelman & Mirenda, 1998). Opportunity barriers may be associated with policy, practice, attitude, knowledge, or skills.

Policy barriers may include segregation policies that either prevent inclusion, or limiting policies that prevent learners from taking home AAC devices purchased with school district funds. Such barriers are difficult to overcome with technology-based interventions.

Practice barriers refer to procedures or conventions that have become commonly accepted in a setting without being "official" policies. Thus, the above examples of policy barriers may appear in a lesser form as practice barriers in some school settings.

Attitude barriers may manifest themselves when an individual's beliefs present a barrier to participation. Often, these attitudes result in limited expectations toward students with disabilities. A teacher may not want a child with disabilities as a student in his classroom despite institutional policies that say otherwise.

Knowledge barriers refer to a lack of information about AAC intervention options, instructional strategies, and AAC devices on the part of someone other than the target learner. This lack of information may result in delimited opportunities for participation.

Skill barriers occur when, despite their knowledge level, persons other than the learner have difficulty with actual implementation. It is in part due to this important difference between knowledge and skills that the American Speech-Language-Hearing Association termed recent competency documents as "Knowledge and Skills" documents (ASHA, 2002).

Access barriers "pertain to the capabilities, attitudes, and resource limitations of potential AAC users themselves, rather than to limitations of their societies or support systems" (p. 157). For example, a child with cerebral palsy may have limited use of his hand. This makes it impossible for him to raise his hand as a signal that he has something to contribute.

The team can use the ASI to develop new goals or to determine whether the student's actual participation reflects the agreed upon goals. Interventions are planned for those steps in the activity for which a discrepancy between the target student and his peers has been identified.

While these interventions readily accommodate technology-based approaches, not all interventions necessarily need to involve technology. Table 8.1 presents a summary of illustrative examples of identified barriers faced by Nick, a student with cerebral palsy and no functional speech, in the cited research project and the recommended solutions as they apply to a specific instructional format (Schlosser et al., 2000). As can be seen, some barriers are classifiable as two different types. For example, Nick's inability to manage manipulatives independently in order to solve the mathematical equations could be viewed as an access barrier because he is physically not capable of moving the manipulatives. This identification, however, might lead the team members to contemplate removing the barrier itself. Should we somehow, then, teach Nick the motoric skills necessary? Probably not. Rather, team members should classify this barrier as a team-based knowledge barrier. In reality, Nick was presented with an access barrier because the team adopted manipulatives that were inappropriate for him. The actual solution, therefore, needs to address knowledge gaps in the team. Keep in mind also that a lack of skills cannot account for barriers unless the team has demonstrated knowledge relevant to that skill.

Developing Barrier-Specific Goals

Calculator (2000) noted that instructional goals need to be written with the following in mind: "AAC can be conceptualized as a means of enhancing the number and quality of interactions students can have with a broadening array of partners in an expanding range of settings and contexts" (p. 350).

For example, when Nick's teacher directed a question to a large group, Nick was unable to raise his hand quickly enough to be called on to answer. The IEP team met to discuss possible solutions. The school-based occupational and physical therapists on the team noted that because of his motor deficits it was unlikely that he would be able to raise his hand more quickly. They suggested that an alternate method of response such as a buzzer be employed. Following a trial with several buzzers and other signaling systems, they determined that he could use an appropriate buzzer in the majority of his classes to indicate his desire to respond to questions. Therefore, the IEP team developed a goal as follows: "Nick will activate his buzzer in time to respond to questions a minimum of three times per class."

The results of the ASI and the proposed solutions represent but one of the many sources of information to assist the team in the goal-setting process. Other sources include the perspectives of the student herself and her family members regarding priorities. Calculator and Jorgenson (1991) describe several methods of "getting to know students in different ways," including the MacGill Action Planning System (Vandercook, York, & Forest, 1989), Personal Futures Planning (Mount, 1987), and Choosing Outcomes and Accommodations for Children (Giangreco, Cloninger, & Iverson, 1998). These methods are excellent means of incorporating the perspectives of the student and her family in the goal-setting process.

In addition to choosing goals that represent personal and family priorities, it has been our experience that goals will not be addressed with adequate effort and resources unless they are linked to the IEP document. Therefore, every attempt should be made to integrate the proposed solutions for the removal of barriers with the IEP goals, including the process developed to evaluate their accomplishment.

Implementing Solutions Based on Communication as a Transactional Process

Given that many of the problems we encounter represent opportunity barriers, it is essential that our solutions be based on the philosophy that communication is a transactional process.

As such, communication involves not only our target student but also communication partners such as teachers, educational assistants, peers, family members, friends, and laypeople (Light, Dattilo, English, Gutierrez, & Hartz, 1992). Many of the goals targeted for our learners using AAC are best accomplished by changing partner behavior (Schlosser & Rothschild, 1999). This approach is consistent with the systemic paradigm of service delivery whereby the learner's entire treatment system is considered (Andrews, 1994). This

Table 8.1 Illustrative Examples of Identified Barriers and Recommended Solutions by Instructional Format

Instructional Format	Context	Goal	Barrier (and Type)	Solution
Group	Teacher asks a question and expects students to raise their hands to indicate that they have an answer.	To monitor student understanding of the concepts being taught and to facilitate student learning through active participation.	The teacher did not expect Nick to be able to participate in group discussions (attitude barrier).	To expect Nick to participate at least once during classroom discussion. To assess his ability to raise his hand on his own. To give Nick time to prepare an answer when necessary.
			Nick often did not have the vocabulary he needed to answer the questions (knowledge barrier).	The teacher and educational assistant will determine appropriate vocabulary to enable Nick to participate. A theme display containing appropriate vocabulary will be developed and given to Nick.
	Teacher asks a question to the whole class that requires a communal response (e.g., yes–no question).	To monitor student understanding of concepts being taught and to facilitate student learning through active participation.	Nick had no way of verbally participating in a communal, vocal response (knowledge barrier).	To provide a small voice output communication aid programmed with yes–no and other phrases to communicate across space.
Individual	Students are working on their own to complete 3-digit addition and subtraction equations from their math textbooks. Nick is working on 1-digit addition equations using manipulatives.	To practice addition and subtraction operations.	Nick is unable to independently manage the manipulatives in order to solve the equations (access and knowledge barriers).	To provide Nick with an abacus on which he will be able to independently move the beads.
			Nick is unable to write the answers to the equations in a timely manner (access and knowledge barriers).	Nick will point to answers on a number line. The educational assistant will write the answers and have Nick confirm their accuracy.

Setting	Activity	Goal	Barrier	Solution
	Students are writing their daily entries in their journals.	To have experience writing based on their personal ideas.	Nick's communication book is not up to date in organization and vocabulary, based on recent experiences to support his writing (knowledge and practice barriers).	To redevelop Nick's communication book. To expect Nick to use his communication book during the first stage of the writing process (i.e., to generate ideas) before going to the computer to write.
			Nick's computer workstation limited his effective and efficient writing. The writing software was not appropriate. The hardware was not optimally placed (knowledge barrier).	To provide a word processor with speech feedback at the letter, word, and sentence levels. To provide a word prediction program to support his spelling. To provide Nick with a smaller keyboard that would sit on his laptray and a trackball. To attach a paper holder to the monitor at Nick's eye level.
Small group	The students are expected to work in groups of four to collect data (e.g., to record measurements of items in the class) and report their findings to the whole class.	To gain experience with the measurement of objects and with communicating measurements to the class.	The team struggled with determining an active role for Nick, which led to the educational assistant participating for Nick (practice and knowledge barriers).	Discuss with the team the role that Nick could actively take. For example, he could decide what should be measured, as well as determining whether it was longer or shorter than a meter. The other students would do the physical measuring and recording. Nick could also report back with the use of a theme display and eye gaze to indicate objects in the room. The educational assistant would be there only until the peers could take over.

Note. From "Training a School Team To Integrate Technology Meaningfully into the Curriculum: Effects on Student Participation," by R. W. Schlosser, D. McGhie-Richmond, S. Blackstien-Adler, P. Mirenda, K. Antonius, & P. Janzen, 2000, *Journal of Special Education Technology, 15*, pp. 31–44. Copyright 2000 by the Technology and Media Division of the Council for Exceptional Children. Reprinted with permission.

approach is also consistent with incorporating the perspectives of parents and other family members, who, as noted previously, are important communication partners for the target student. To date, the majority of partner instruction studies seem to have focused on adult partners rather than peers. Clearly, research on peer instruction is a timely issue that warrants immediate attention. On a practical level, peer instruction may focus on a number of strategies that help students who use AAC meet classroom demands, such as assistance with note taking, participation in "support circles," and buddy systems (Sturm, 1998). The SLP as well as other IEP team members can play a crucial role in setting up peer instruction in collaboration with the classroom teacher and educational assistant.

Considering Instructional Formats

Students may be exposed to a variety of instructional configurations, including group, small group, and individual. Although research on the role of instructional formats for including learners who use AAC is scant, it seems that some formats may lend themselves more to participation of target learners than others do. In the aforementioned study, we replicated the effect of training a school team in the PAF and technology applications across the three instructional formats listed above. The effect of eliminating barriers and increasing participation proved to be more salient as we worked with individuals or small groups (Schlosser et al., 2000). We argued that perhaps these formats were more conducive to participation because of their different instructional requirements. SLPs involved in curriculum modification together with other school personnel may therefore want to explore the use of small groups that operate using cooperative learning principles as they plan implementation (Thousand, Villa, & Nevin, 1994).

Selecting Vocabulary That Supports the Proposed Solutions

Some of the barriers identified on the ASI may be due to a lack of appropriate vocabulary, as was the case with Nick (see Table 8.1). Calculator (2000) noted, "Always ask yourself, does the student have the means and content to be an active participant in activities throughout the day" (p. 347). Involving peers, the teacher, the teacher aide, the SLP, and, if possible, the target student in planning lessons will facilitate the selection of activity relevant vocabulary. Given that we strive to reach the same participation levels as nondisabled peers in the same classroom, peers make invaluable informants for vocabulary selection. The vocabulary selected may then be arranged in topic-specific displays to facilitate easy access and support the learner's participation. In addition, peer involvement in vocabulary selection may prepare the way for increased peer interaction with the target student in a natural environment. In terms of vocabulary selection, it is important to realize that the vocabulary has to meet a student's academic participation needs *and* her social participation needs.

ILLUSTRATIVE CASE EXAMPLES OF STUDENTS

The following examples of Sam, Janelle, and Nick illustrate many of the important AAC issues in school settings, including the importance of vocabulary selection, alternate assessments, collaboration with other disciplines, family and learner involvement, advanced planning, peer interaction, and, most of all, participation as a focus of assessment and intervention.

 ## Sam

Sam is a lively 10-year-old with a medical diagnoses of mild cerebral palsy (CP) and Pervasive Developmental Disorder (PDD). Because his gross and fine motor skills are only mildly affected, he is able to walk and perform many daily living activities such as eating, dressing, and toileting independently. He is able to print using traditional writing instruments like pencils, pens, and crayons. However, he exhibits significant problems in expressive language. His speech is quite dysarthric, and he experiences particular difficulty expressing complete thoughts. These speech difficulties, compounded by a lack of understanding of how to interact socially, significantly and negatively influence his interaction with his peers.

Sam attends his neighborhood school. Although he is selectively integrated into a regular fourth-grade classroom, his frequent behavioral outbursts and noncompliance prevent him from undertaking and completing many activities within the classroom. Consequently, he receives considerable one-to-one instruction in subjects in a resource room outside of his classroom. While he is involved in the usual Grade 4 core subjects such as math, language arts, social studies, and science, his educational program is modified to meet his learning needs. Socially, he is not involved with regular peers. Since two educational assistants share responsibility for him, he is supported by one adult at all times, and he has become quite dependent on adults at school. His educational assistants, Grade 4 teacher, and program support teacher are responsible for his educational program.

The school's on-site or consulting SLPs and occupational and physical therapists provide regularly scheduled consultation support for Sam's educational program. His IEP team also receives consultive services from the AAC providers. His parents are actively involved in sharing information about Sam that assists the team in developing and supporting appropriate goals. Sam's educational program is documented in his IEP. His team has identified two goals: (a) increased participation within the regular classroom, and (b) increased independence, particularly in interaction with his peers both at home and at school.

Sam's team recognizes that much of his noncompliant behavior and outbursts appears to arise from the difficulty he experiences in attending to and processing verbal information. These problems in attending also present a barrier to his effective communication. The team has been relying on verbal communications, the very modality that is a weakness for Sam. Recognizing the barrier this represents, they have begun to incorporate AAC to augment their verbal explanations and instructions (a.k.a. aided language stimulation). As such, they are incorporating visual strategies. His team has developed a visual schedule to support Sam's understanding of the sequence of school day activities. Two visual schedules are used: One represents morning activities, and another, afternoon ones. Each subject or activity is represented by a 3/4-inch Picture Communication Symbols (PCS) symbol paired with a word. For example, Sam's morning schedule includes the following: homeroom, prayer, math, computer, recess, social studies, and lunch. The team is careful to choose symbols that are most representative of the activity or subject. The symbols are individually mounted on a piece of cardstock and laminated, and a piece of Velcro is affixed to the back of each. They are arranged sequentially to represent Sam's schedule on a Velcro strip that is attached to a length of cardstock. His educational assistant reviews the schedule with him first thing each morning for the morning activities and again first thing in the afternoon. If there is a change in his schedule, the aide takes care to show the schedule to Sam frequently as she explains the alteration in routine. In this way, he is prepared ahead of the actual change. During the period of time that the visual schedule has been consistently and repeatedly used during transitions, the team reports that Sam's disruptive behavior has decreased considerably, thereby allowing him to spend more time in his regular classroom.

Often Sam will begin an activity and then quickly want to move on to a different one. The team is therefore using another visual strategy to diminish his antsy behavior. Two symbols, representing the activity in which he is engaged (e.g., math) and the next activity (e.g., computer), are attached to a piece of cardstock and displayed on Sam's desk. For example, when he is engaged in a math activity and wants to move on to the computer, his educational assistant points to the math symbol and says, "First, math." Then the assistant points to the computer symbol, saying "Then computer." In this way, Sam is reminded visually of the sequence of activities and what is expected. PCSs representing the steps required in routine activities, such as getting ready for recess, are also used to prompt and support Sam in undertaking and completing those routines. Through consistent modeling, the team has noticed that Sam is beginning to cue himself to follow the steps. He is becoming more independent in completing some routine activities, and his noncompliant behaviors are decreasing.

Sam's team is also using visual strategies to increase his independence in social interactions with his peers during recess and gym activities. By using visuals to represent and teach appropriate social interactions (e.g., greetings, saying no) and play skills such as taking a turn, the educational assistants are able to gradually pull back from the interaction and stand on the sidelines while Sam interacts independently with his peers.

Sam is learning to expand his conversational and written communication beyond one-word utterances. People who interact with him prompt him verbally and with pictures. For writing activities, he is provided with frame sentences (e.g., "Yesterday, I _____; it was _____. On the weekend I will _____). These frames provide a scaffold for Sam, a model of correct sentence structure.

Sam's SLP and his program support teacher have collaborated in assessing his language and literacy skills. They are finding that his word recognition skills far exceed his expressive language skills. On the basis of their assessments, they are wondering whether or not he really requires the picture cues on his communication displays, as he is able to read the words the pictures represent. They have decided to develop the next communication display without the pictures to test their hypothesis. By working together to determine Sam's particular learning characteristics and needs, his classroom team has gained a more holistic understanding of him. In turn, their understanding of his overall strengths and weaknesses has influenced the interventions they have established.

Janelle

Janelle is a friendly, enthusiastic, 6-year-old girl. She experiences a sensory integration disorder, a mood disorder, and significant expressive communication difficulties. Her oral language skills do not reflect correct sentence structure. In addition, she speaks very quickly, changes topics freely, and has difficulty articulating individual sounds clearly. As a result, her intelligibility is very poor.

Janelle participates fully in a regular kindergarten classroom in her neighborhood school. Her kindergarten program is composed of a mix of teacher-directed and free-play activities. Janelle is at a competitive level of participation for most of the classroom activities. She is at an active level of participation for many structured activities such as arts and crafts and paper-and-pencil tasks, where she has difficulty following a sequence of steps. Socially, she is at an involved level with her peers. She is just beginning to show an interest in their activities. Her social interaction is passive, and she does not influence her peers through her communication.

Janelle's classroom team works together to support her learning. She receives one-to-one assistance from an educational assistant. The school's program support teacher works alongside the educational assistant and classroom teacher in the classroom on a weekly basis to support Janelle's participation in the various classroom activities. An occupational therapist and an SLP from the school board (district) provide consultation support to the school team concerning her sensory integration and speech and language needs, respectively.

In addition to providing some direct speech–language therapy, the SLP has recommended cueing Janelle to slow her speech by continual natural modeling of a slow rate of speech and correct speech sounds. Visual, auditory, and tactile cues increase her awareness of all of the sounds that she produces. She uses a topic setter book, which supports and clarifies the subject of her conversational exchange. It also provides her with a means of staying focused on a particular topic in conversation. The small, diary-sized book is organized according to themes, which reflect her home, school, and community experiences. The vocabulary is represented by 3/4-inch colored PCS with accompanying words.

Janelle's team wants to specifically target goals of successful interaction with her peers during free-play activities. They are using AAC techniques to support her in initiating and maintaining a conversation with a peer within a play situation. For example, when playing with the classroom doll house, a motivating activity for Janelle, she uses a portable communication display with vocabulary such as "Want to play?" "I need," "I want," and "I am." The words of the sentences are represented by PCS. The display provides a visual cue to full-sentence production and serves to clarify Janelle's speech. To teach Janelle how to use the display, her educational assistant engaged her in playing with the dollhouse and modeled how to use the display. This teaching and modeling occurred over several play sessions. Next, Janelle was expected to use the display independently as she and the educational assistant played with the dollhouse. Finally, a peer was engaged in the play, with the educational assistant continuing to provide modeling of how to use the display for Janelle and introducing it to the peer. The educational assistant, classroom teacher, and program support teacher are now providing support and prompts only as required, since Janelle and her peers have learned to use the display independently during some structured play activities. The team is extending the use of communication displays within other free-play activities, such as dress-up, and sand and water play.

An unexpected benefit of using the communication displays has been their role in supporting the development of Janelle's literacy skills. The pictures and accompanying words and the manner in which they are used to support her speech have also increased her developing understanding of letter knowledge and phonemic awareness, as well as skill in decoding, word recognition, spelling, and writing. In turn, her developing literacy skills have supported her oral language and communication skills.

Like many parents, Janelle's parents expressed concern over using pictures with her, believing that she would rely on pictures rather than

speech to communicate. However, as is often the case, quite the opposite has occurred. Since using the pictures, Janelle's team has noticed
an improvement in her speech in terms of overall rate, sentence structure, and clarity. There has been a further increase in Janelle initiating
interaction with her peers during play.

 ## Nick

Nick is a mischievous 12-year-old boy who has cerebral palsy. He is
independently mobile in a power wheelchair. He is dependent for most
other activities of daily living, such as eating, drinking, dressing, and
toileting. He is nonspeaking and relies on AAC to express his wants,
needs, and ideas. He uses a variety of tools for communication. He has
a communication book in which vocabulary representing his experiences
is organized. The vocabulary is represented by ³/₄-inch PCS and words.
It is arranged on each page to reflect the structure of oral language
(i.e., agent, action, and object; e.g., "John [agent] eats [action] cookies
[object]"). The communication book supports Nick's quick access to
frequently used vocabulary. Nick is independent in turning the pages
of his communication book and pointing to the symbols with the little
finger of his left hand. A small SGD provides him with a voice in the
classroom and for quick messaging and sharing of news at school and
at home.

Nick's SLP has worked closely with the program support teacher
in assessing his receptive and expressive language abilities and his literacy skills. They have taken a lead in designing his communication book
to ensure that it reflects his current vocabulary level and is supporting
the ongoing development of his language and literacy abilities.

For writing, the SLP works closely with the school's OT and PT.
The PT provides information regarding proper positioning for Nick in
his motorized wheelchair so that he can access a computer keyboard
easily. The OT provides information and specialized instruction regarding his hand and finger dexterity. Nick is able to use the middle finger
of his left hand to activate the keys on the keyboard. The PT and OT
determined that a smaller keyboard would allow him to access all of the
keys, although he is limited by his upper body mobility. A specialized
trackball is employed as an effective pointing device. Nick has access
to word-processing software with speech (sound, word, sentence)
feedback features. He also has access to word prediction software that
assists with typing speed and allows him to focus on sentence development and completion. The software is updated as necessary, and data
are collected on Nick's progress in using the software to meet his educational goals.

Nick is selectively integrated into a Grade 6 classroom at his neighborhood school. He is involved in all subjects in the class except French. During the twice-weekly French lessons, he goes to the school resource room to work with a group of students who need help in developing their English literacy skills. His educational program reflects an active level of participation. That is, the educational goals within each subject are modified to reflect his particular learning needs. He receives the support of an educational assistant for most classroom activities. The IEP team members, including Nick's mother, work together to determine and implement his educational program. Nick's progress toward meeting his specific educational goals are documented on a regular basis. The specialized materials, strategies, and methodologies employed to assist him are shared among the IEP team members to ensure consistent use across disciplines and subjects.

In addition to further developing Nick's language and literacy goals, his team wants to increase his level of independence in academic activities within his regular classroom. They are aware of the dependent relationship that often develops between students who have multiple disabilities and their educational assistants. They are determined that this will not happen with Nick and have begun to expect him to work on his own once they have ensured that he is set up with the materials he needs. For example, when his teacher is teaching a lesson, the educational assistant no longer sits with Nick during the lesson. Once he has his communication book or communication display materials that are relevant to the topic, he is able to listen to the teacher and participate in answering and asking questions. Similarly, once he is set up at the computer, he is able to work on an activity such as his weekly spelling assignment or copy typing his journal entry.

The classroom team is also pairing Nick with other students. Sometimes the other student is a higher-achieving student, and sometimes the other student requires support similar to Nick's. For example, for a language arts assignment, the class was required to complete a report on a preferred trade book. Nick's independent reading is at a Grade 2.5 level, which limits his choice of books based on his interests. For this assignment, he worked with a peer who also has reading difficulties. They chose an age-appropriate book on tape that they listened to while following along with the text. The other boy's teacher provided the assignment, including the vocabulary they needed to know from the book. Nick's family supported him in completing the reading at home. His teacher and his educational assistant worked together to provide the two boys with the appropriate supports.

Nick's teacher outlined her evaluation criteria for the project, explaining to the boys the personal goals they were to keep in mind as they completed the activity. The educational assistant created an outline of the book report on the computer to ensure that the book-related vocabulary was entered into the word prediction program. The two boys completed the assignment by taking turns answering the questions and typing the answers on the computer. The classroom teacher and educational assistant provided instruction and supports as necessary to assist the boys in meeting the goals of the activity and completing the assignment.

CONCLUSION

The purpose of this chapter was to assist current and future SLPs in their support of students who have little or no functional speech or writing in inclusive classrooms. Inclusive classrooms are rapidly becoming the least restrictive environments for most students with severe communication impairments. AAC in inclusive school settings is most productively employed when viewing communication within its broader context of participation and membership of students with disabilities in inclusive classrooms. Strategies such as alternate assessments and the Participation Assessment Framework were provided and illustrated with case examples to ensure that every step we take in planning assessment and intervention is in line with the overarching goal of participation and membership. This focus requires SLPs to avoid becoming "broom closet therapists" (Simon, 1987) and to develop into classroom-based communication specialists.

 STUDY QUESTIONS

1. Define augmentative and alternative communication in terms that a teacher, parent, or other members of the school community could understand.
2. At one time in educational history, children with severe handicapping conditions were placed exclusively in separate schools. Why has this changed?
3. What could be included in an "alternate assessment system"?
4. Discuss the different categories of barriers to participation faced by students with severe communication problems.
5. List three activities for a regular classroom and describe how you would plan for the student described in each of the cases to take part.
6. Define *inclusion* and explain how this concept may affect your role as a speech–language pathologist in the public school setting.
7. Why is the team approach essential in augmentative and alternative communication?

REFERENCES

American Speech-Language-Hearing Association. (2002, April 16). Augmentative and alternative communication: Knowledge and skills for service delivery. *ASHA Leader,* 7(Suppl. 22), 97–106.

Andrews, J. R. (1994). Human communication disorders in context and environment. In F. D. Minifie (Ed.), *Introduction to communication sciences and disorders* (pp. 279–311). San Diego, CA: Singular.

Arvidson, H. H., Cunningham, J. N., Davis, M. A., & Bennett, D. (1999). *Indiana Assessment System of Educational Proficiencies Program Manual.* West Lafayette, IN: Purdue University, Purdue Research Foundation; Indiana Department of Education Division of Special Education.

Bennett, D. E., Davis, M. A., Cunningham, J. N., & Arvidson, H. (1999). *Indiana Assessment System of Educational Proficiencies: Computer Based Rating and Documentation System.* West Lafayette, IN: Purdue University, Purdue Research Foundation.

Beukelman, D. R., & Mirenda, P. (1998). *Augmentative and alternative communication: Management of severe communication disorders in children and adults* (2nd ed.). Baltimore: Brookes.

Bowser, G., & Reed, P. (1995). Educational TECH Points for assistive technology planning. *Journal of Special Education Technology, 12,* 325–338.

Burd, L., Hammes, K., Bornhoeft, D., & Fisher, W. (1988). A North Dakota prevalence study of nonverbal school-age children. *Language, Speech, and Hearing Services in Schools, 19,* 371–383.

Calculator, S. N. (2000). Augmentative and alternative communication. In E. Pritchard Dodge (Ed.), *The survival guide for school based speech–language pathologists* (pp. 345–366). San Diego, CA: Singular.

Calculator, S. N., & Jorgenson, C. M. (1991). Integrating AAC instruction into regular education settings: Expounding on best practices. *Augmentative and Alternative Communication, 7,* 204–212.

Edyburn, D. (1996). The technology and media division. *CEC Today, 3,* 15.

Elliott, S. N. (1998). *Testing accommodations for students with disabilities: Selection, documentation, & evaluation.* Unpublished manuscript, University of Wisconsin at Madison, Wisconsin Center for Education Research, and Department of Educational Psychology.

Erickson, R., Ysseldyke, J., Thurlow, M., & Elliott, J. (1998). Inclusive assessments and accountability systems: Tools of the trade in educational reform. *Teaching Exceptional Children, 31,* 4–9.

Ferguson, D. (1994). Is communication really the point? Some thoughts on interventions and membership. *Mental Retardation, 32,* 7–18.

Giangreco, M. F., Cloninger, C. J., & Iverson, V. S. (1998). *Choosing outcomes and accommodations for children* (2nd ed.). Baltimore: Brookes.

Individuals with Disabilities Education Act Amendments of 1997. (1997). Public Law 105-17.

Individuals with Disabilities Education Improvement Act of 2004. (2004). Public Law No. 108-446.

Lewis, R. B. (1993). *Special education technology: Classroom applications.* Pacific Grove, CA: Brooks/Cole.

Light, J., Dattilo, J., English, J., Gutierrez, L., & Hartz, J. (1992). Instructing facilitators to support communication of people who use augmentative communication systems. *Journal of Speech and Hearing Research, 35,* 865–875.

Lindsay, P., Cambria, R., McNaughton, S., & Warrick, A. (1986, September). *The educational needs of non speaking students and their teachers.* Paper presented at the Fourth Biennial Conference of the International Society for Augmentative and Alternative Communication, Cardiff, Wales.

Lloyd, L. L., Fuller, D. R., & Arvidson, A. (1997). *Augmentative and alternative communication: A handbook of principles and practices.* Needham Heights, MA: Allyn & Bacon.

Loeding, B. L., Zangari, C., & Lloyd, L. L. (1990). A "working party" approach to planning in-service training in manual signs for an entire public school staff. *Augmentative and Alternative Communication, 6,* 38–49.

Male, M. (1994). *Technology for inclusion: Meeting the special needs of all students.* Boston: Allyn & Bacon.

Matas, J., Mathy-Laikko, P., Beukelman, D. R., & Legresley, K. (1985). Identifying the non-speaking population: A demographic study. *Augmentative and Alternative Communication, 1,* 17–31.

McGhie-Richmond, D., & McGinnis, J. (1996). *A survey of current practices and perceived needs in teaching literacy to students who use augmentative and alternative communication systems.* Unpublished manuscript.

McGregor, G., & Pachuski, P. (1996). Assistive technology in schools: Are teachers ready, able, and supported? *Journal of Special Education Technology, 13,* 4–15.

McGrew, K., Thurlow, M. L., Shriner, J. G., & Spiegel, A. N. (1992). *Inclusion of students with disabilities in national and state data collection programs (Technical Report 2).* Minneapolis: University of Minnesota, National Center on Educational Outcomes.

Mirenda, P., & Calculator, S. N. (1993). Enhancing curricula design. *Clinics in Communication Disorders, 3,* 43–58.

Mount, B. (1987). *Personal futures planning: Finding directions for change.* Ann Arbor: University of Michigan Dissertation Information Service.

National Institute on Disability and Rehabilitation Research. (1992, March). *Augmentative and alternative communication intervention consensus validation conference program and abstracts.* Washington, DC: Author.

No Child Left Behind Act of 2001. (2001). Public Law No. 107-110. Retrieved July 19, 2005 from the U.S. Department of Education Web site: http://www.ed.gov/nclb/landing.jhtml

Olsen, K., Bechard, S., Kennedy, S., Haigh, J., Parshall, L., & Friedebach, M. (1998). *Alternate assessment issues and practices.* Lexington, KY: Mid-South Regional Resource Center. (ERIC Document Reproduction Service No. ED 431 263)

Salvia, J., & Ysseldyke, J. E. (1998). *Assessment* (7th ed.). Boston: Houghton Mifflin.

Schlosser, R. W., McGhie-Richmond, D., Blackstien-Adler, S., Mirenda, P., Antonius, K., & Janzen, P. (2000). Training a school team to integrate technology meaningfully into the curriculum: Effects on student participation. *Journal of Special Education Technology, 15,* 31–44.

Schlosser, R. W., & Rothschild, N. (1999). Augmentative and alternative communication for persons with developmental disabilities. In I. Brown & M. Percy (Eds.), *Developmental disabilities in Ontario* (pp. 475–489). Toronto: Front Porch.

Simon, C. (1987). Out of the broom closet and into the classroom: The emerging speech–language specialist. *Journal of Childhood Communication Disorders, 11,* 41–66.

Sturm, J. (1998). Educational inclusion of AAC users. In D. R. Beukelman & P. Mirenda (Eds.), *Augmentative and alternative communication: Management of severe communication disorders in children and adults* (pp. 391–426). Baltimore: Brookes.

Thousand, J. S., Villa, R. A., & Nevin, A. I. (1994). *Creativity and collaborative learning: A practical guide to empowering students and teachers.* Baltimore: Brookes.

Thurlow, M. L., Elliott, J. L., & Ysseldyke, J. E. (1998). *Testing students with disabilities: Practical strategies for complying with district and state requirements.* Thousand Oaks, CA: Corwin Press.

Thurlow, M. L., House, A. L., Scott, D. L., & Ysseldyke, J. E. (2000). Students with disabilities in large-scale assessments: State participation and accommodation policies. *The Journal of Special Education, 34,* 154–163.

Tindal, G., Heath, B., Hollenbeck, K., Almond, P., & Harniss, M. (1998). Accommodating students with disabilities on large-scale tests: An experimental study. *Exceptional Children, 64,* 439–450.

Toddis, B., & Walker, H. (1993). User perspectives on assistive technology in educational settings. *Focus on Exceptional Children, 26,* 3.

U.S. Department of Education. (1998). *Federal Register, 63,* Number 156.

Vandercook, T., York, J., & Forest, M. (1989). The McGill action planning system: A strategy for building a vision. *Journal of the Association for Persons with Severe Handicaps, 14,* 205–215.

Ysseldyke, J. (2001). Reflections on a research career: Generalizations from 25 years of research on assessment and instructional decision making. *Exceptional Children, 67,* 295–309.

Ysseldyke, J., & Thurlow, M. (1997). The National Center on Educational Outcomes. *Diagnostique, 22,* 213–224.

Ysseldyke, J. E., Thurlow, M. L., McGrew, K. S., & Shriner, J. G. (1994). *Recommendations for making decisions about the participation of students with disabilities in statewide assessment programs (Synthesis Report 15).* Minneapolis: University of Minnesota, National Center on Educational Outcomes.

Chapter 9

Culturally and Linguistically Diverse Students

Regina B. Grantham,
Luis F. Riquelme,
and Li-Rong Lilly Cheng

The cultural composition of the United States is diverse and constantly changing. At one time the United States was considered a "melting pot," where many cultures blended into one population, each influencing the other. Because *culture* refers to the customs, beliefs, values, social conventions, and linguistic aspects of a specific group of people (Paul, 2001; Terrell, Battle, & Grantham, 1998), it helps groups to be cohesive, preserving values and beliefs over time (Paul, 2001). Most recently, the analogy used to characterize America has been a salad or soup. In a salad or stew all the ingredients (cultures) blend to form a whole but also retain their individuality. Each group has its own features, language, and traditions to contribute to enrich the salad or the stew (Goldstein, 2000; Haynes, Moran, & Pindzola, 1999; Paul, 2001).

For many culturally and linguistically diverse (CLD) populations, there is a struggle between wanting to fit into the mainstream society and enjoy its benefits, and wanting to maintain or preserve their cultural heritage, which may be in conflict with the mainstream. Speech–language pathologists and teachers can help balance this conflict for CLD populations by providing a culturally sensitive learning environment and by helping them establish effective communication to access mainstream society while retaining their cultural pride, communication style, and strategies. This approach is called bicultural education, allowing a person to successfully participate in two or more cultural styles, switching back and forth when appropriate. Bicultural education is built on the understanding and respect shown by teachers and SLPs for cultures that contrast with the mainstream culture (Paul, 2001).

Changes in demographics indicate why bicultural education is critical. In 2000, 23 of the 25 largest public school systems in the United States were composed mostly of minority students, who brought their various heritages and cultures with them. It is projected that in the 21st century, about 25% to 38% of school-age populations will be culturally and linguistically diverse (Lue, 2001). By the year 2050, people of color will constitute 47.5% of the U.S. census (Banks, 1999). Certainly, this enrichment and infusion of culture will be observed in classrooms across the country and in the caseload of the speech–language pathologist.

AFRICAN AMERICAN STUDENTS: REGINA B. GRANTHAM

African Americans share a unique history and culture that is reflected in African American English. This section of Chapter 9 will discuss that topic, as well as characteristics of African American English across the five aspects of language and its developmental trends in young children. Diagnostic considerations and intervention strategies will be addressed, in addition to cultural sensitivity or competency, a vital characteristic of successful speech–language pathologists.

African American Culture

African Americans are one of the largest culturally and linguistically diverse groups in the United States. This cultural group is well represented in the schools. Like most other groups, African Americans are not all alike. A large segment of the African American population is poor, some are wealthy, and some are middle class. The class that is noted most in research and journal articles is the lower class. However, there is a very visible African American upper class that involves debutante balls, arranged marriages, summers on Martha's Vineyard, exclusive all-black boarding schools, million-dollar homes, and membership in exclusive organizations, both black and white. This elite group dates back to the 1880s (Graham, 1999; Washington & Craig, 1999).

One cultural experience that all African Americans have in common is their history of forced abduction, the history of slavery (Paul, 2001). According to Terrell, Battle, and Grantham (1998), this was the "largest involuntary migration movement in modern times" (p. 31). People from Africa were forced to leave their homes and were sold into slavery. About 20 million people were brought from Africa to the Americas and the Caribbean (Terrell & Jackson, 2002). To add to this history, racism and discrimination, based on skin color and linguistic differences, have also left scars. Through the years, such experiences have had a profound effect on African Americans, specifically in music, religion, attitudes, and communication styles. Given their history, it is not surprising that there is often mistrust of others by African Americans (Terrell et al., 1998; Terrell & Jackson, 2002; Terrell & Terrell, 1996).

Linguistically, African Americans use a number of dialects. These include Gullah, spoken by people who live on the islands off the coast of South Carolina and Georgia; Creole such as Jamaican Creole English; and those spoken by people who have origins in African countries or the Caribbean. African American English is the most common dialect associated with African Americans (Terrell et al., 1998; Terrell & Jackson, 2002).

What Is African American English?

African American English has had various names, such as nonstandard Negro English, Black speech, Black English, Black English vernacular, Black dialect, slang, "lazy English," "broken English," Ebonics (combination of "ebony" and "phonics"), and African American language. The nomenclature indicates a search for more respect, because many of these names were derogatory and demonstrated disrespect for the people and the dialect (Seymour, Abdulkarim, & Johnson, 1999; Terrell et al., 1998; Terrell & Jackson, 2002). According to Seymour, Abdulkarim, and Johnson (1999), the preferred terminology has been Black English, African American English, or African American vernacular English. For this chapter, the terminology used will be African American English (AAE).

Although African American English is spoken by millions of African Americans, not all African Americans use it (ASHA, 2003). The use of AAE varies according to socioeconomic level (more AAE is used at lower-income levels), gender (more boys use AAE), age (its use decreases with age), geographic location, occupation, education, and condition or communicative intent (e.g., more AAE is used in describing pictures than in unstructured play) (Goldstein, 2000; Washington & Craig, 1998; Washington, Craig, & Kushmaul, 1998). Terrell and Jackson (2002) propose that intensity of commitment to or identification with the African American community and culture are factors that might influence AAE use.

Often, AAE speakers do not use all of the features of AAE in all contexts. For instance, a child may not use the copula in one context but may use it in another. School-age children seem to use more AAE features when they are excitedly talking with their peers (Wyatt, 1995). AAE usage is like a continuum that ranges from those who do not use it at all to those who use it in all communication actions (Hulit & Howard, 2001; Seymour, Abdulkarim, & Johnson, 1999; Terrell & Jackson, 2002).

According to Washington and Craig (1992), working-class African Americans use AAE, predominately. Roseberry-McKibbin and Hegde (2000) stated that middle-class African Americans use AAE less frequently than working-class African Americans, particularly when they are in formal settings. There are also Caucasians, Hispanics, Asians, and other ethnic or cultural groups that use AAE. If an individual interacts frequently with people who use AAE or lives in a community where AAE is spoken, that person may adopt or acclimatize to AAE and use the dialect to assimilate into that environment. Also, children will speak the dialect to which they are exposed. These facts indicate that learning a language or a dialect is not a biological occurrence but a product of the environment in which one lives and interacts (Goldstein, 2000; Hulit & Howard, 2001; Terrell & Jackson, 2002).

The characteristics of AAE are not the same across the country. Various types are used, depending on the geographical region. One example of an AAE variation is Southern African American English (SAAE), which combines characteristics of AAE and southern dialect (Oetting & McDonald, 2001).

Within the African American community, both AAE and Standard American English (SAE) coexist. SAE is defined as "the linguistic variety used by the government, the mass media, business, education, science and the arts in the United States" (ASHA, 2003, p. 46).

Numerous African Americans speak both AAE and SAE and are called bidialectal speakers, using two dialects. Bidialectal speakers can code switch, which is the ability to change in response to the communicative context. Everyone uses code switching to some extent, depending on the situation. For instance, you would talk differently to your roommate than you would to the president of a university. You would talk differently to a neighbor in a bar than you would at a formal occasion. Thus, an AAE speaker who is bidialectal might use AAE when talking with friends at home but switch to SAE in an academic or employment setting. AAE might also be spoken at family get-togethers, church events, and street corner discussions. Not every African American speaks the same way whether using AAE or SAE. Communication is influenced by such factors as region, community, economic level, and educational level (Goldstein, 2000; Haynes et al., 1999; Paul, 2001; Terrell et al., 1998; Van Keulen, Weddington, & DeBose, 1998; Washington & Craig, 1992).

AAE reflects the customs, sounds, life, and language of a community. It is the voice of such literary greats as Langston Hughes, Alice Walker, Toni Morrison, and August Wilson. In other words, it represents a culture—its past, present, and future (Goldstein, 2000; LeMoine, 2001; Terrell et al., 1998; Terrell & Jackson, 2002).

It should be noted that AAE "is a systematic, rule-governed, phonologic, grammatical, syntactic, semantic and pragmatic system of language" (Terrell & Jackson, 2002, p. 40). It is different from SAE but has sufficient similarities to SAE that it can be called a dialect of Standard American English. It contains patterns common to the languages of West Africa, as well as features shared by other dialects, such as southern English (Van Keulen et al., 1998). It includes not only verbal aspects, but also nonverbal factors such as body language, use of personal space, narrative sequence, eye movement and contact, facial expression, and use of silence.

As indicated before, dialects have their own set of rules that are both similar to and different from the standard form of language (Paul, 2001; Terrell et al., 1998). Originally, dialects were considered by many as a deviant, impoverished form of SAE. Since language is the mode used to express our thoughts and our abilities, speakers of dialects were also thought to have inferior intellectual abilities (Haynes et al., 1999).

However, in 1983 the American Speech-Language-Hearing Association (ASHA) created a position statement indicating that dialects were legitimate and were language differences (rule-governed language style that deviates from the standard) not language disorders (severe discrepancies in skills for a client's age or developmental level). This position statement also affirmed that a person who demonstrates a language difference could elect a bidialectical program. Through this program, the speaker would be given access to SAE, but the dialect would remain intact, valued, and respected (ASHA, 1983). The concept, in such a situation, is to add SAE to the person's linguistic repertoire rather than eliminating AAE. People would then learn to code-switch (move back and forth between AAE and SAE when appropriate). Many African American families encourage their children to learn SAE because it is the language needed to succeed in school, to succeed in a profession. The parents feel that learning the mainstream dialect will help their children avoid bias in the school and in mainstream society (ASHA, 1983; Paul, 2001). In 2003, ASHA reaffirmed its 1983 position in a technical report on American English dialects. This report indicated that a dialect was not a language disorder or a pathology. Further, the report indicated that dialects are a variety of American English and serve as communicative tools for specific speech communities (ASHA, 2003).

Supporting a similar view in 1997, the Linguistic Society of America (LSA) passed a resolution that acknowledged and recognized Ebonics as a regular, systematic, rule-governed speech variety. The society also affirmed that dialects should be maintained, that they basically support linguistic diversity (LSA, 1997).

In 1998, ASHA disseminated another position paper reinforcing the fact that a dialect is a legitimate linguistic variety. The paper was entitled "Students and Professionals Who Speak English with Accents and Nonstandard Dialects: Issues and Recommendations." This position statement indicated that speech–language pathologists and audiologists who used dialects could provide clinical services to people with communication disorders as long as they had the necessary knowledge of normal and disordered communication, diagnostic and clinical management skills, and the ability to provide the appropriate model for a target phoneme, a grammatical feature, or other linguistic characteristic. The presence of a dialect should not keep a person from enrolling in higher education, nor should it be a deterrent in employment (American Speech-Language-Hearing Joint Subcommittee of the Executive Board on English Language Proficiency, 1998).

In addition to position statements, ASHA maintains and is committed to the Office of Multicultural Affairs (OMA). OMA addresses cultural and linguistic diversity issues related to the professions of speech–language pathology and audiology. There is also the Multicultural Issues Board (MIB) composed of ASHA members from various multicultural groups, who assist the OMA in its goals and objectives. A few of the division's many charges include focusing on the unique speech and language assessment and therapeutic needs of communities of color and addressing professional development issues relating to African American speech and language service providers. One of the division's focused initiatives for 2003 was to develop an instructional CD-ROM on African American English and its implications. This CD-ROM is available for sale through ASHA's Product Sales (Adger, Schilling-Estes, & Wolfram, 2003).

In summary, it is important to remember that all dialects have the same capacity for communication, and one dialect is not better than the other. It is the attitudes and biases of people that separate one dialect from another and place negative and positive value on them (Seymour et al., 1999).

History

There are many theories or hypotheses concerning the history of AAE. One theory is called the *deficit perspective* and dates back to the early 1900s. At that time, it was felt that African slaves exhibited substandard speech and were unable to master SAE because of poor cognitive functioning. Thus, they used "broken English." It is this perception that has been responsible for bias and discriminating experiences for AAE speakers and has led to misdiagnosis of AAE speakers as disordered and overinclusion of African American children in special education programs (LeMoine, 2001).

The most common theory about AAE history is the Creolist view developed around the 17th century. This theory states that AAE has its roots in the western coast of Africa. As mentioned earlier, Africans were brought to the United States as slaves from various parts of West Africa. It is very likely that they did not speak each other's native languages, so they had no way of communicating with each other in their new environment. Actually, slaves were deliberately separated from their tribespeople so they would be isolated and alone and have limited communication with each other. This isolation was meant to keep slave rebellions at a minimum. As the speakers began to interact, they created a common language called *pidgin,* a restricted social code that facilitated communication between speakers of two or more languages. It combined elements of all the native languages involved into a simpler language with less morphology and restricted phonological and syntactic range; it began as an informal communication tool consisting mostly of nouns and gestures. As pidgin was used by members of the slave community and their children, it grew more formal and became the primary language or native language of its users. It was then called a Creole language. A Creole language is one that develops from a pidgin with expanded grammar and vocabulary and functions as a native language. As years passed, the Creole language became more and more like the language of the dominant culture, although it did keep some grammatical markers and vocabulary that had African origins, such as the habitual tense that means the activity is recurring (the *habitual be*) and *john,* which when translated from the African word means "someone who can be easily exploited" (Terrell & Jackson, 2002, p. 41). AAE also retained some of the English that was used in the 17th century, such as the multiple negation, which was acceptable at that time. The Creole languages became known as AAE, Gullah, and other Caribbean dialects (Hulit & Howard, 2001; LeMoine, 2001; Terrell et al., 1998; Terrell & Jackson, 2002).

Another hypothesis concerning the development of AAE is that European languages also had an influence on its development. The Portuguese, the Dutch, the French, and the English were all strong traders in Africa. Most of these European traders did not learn the African languages, so the African people had to develop various pidgins to communicate with this group of slave traders. These pidgins were brought to the United States and eventually evolved into a Creole. Through the years, African American English has changed as a result of social and educational pressures. African Americans who spoke AAE moved from the Southeast to the Northeast and other parts of the United States in the early 1900s and brought AAE to the urban areas of the North (Hulit & Howard, 2001).

The Oakland School Board controversy is part of AAE's more recent history. This issue is not about the origin of AAE, but is rather about the struggle to recognize AAE as a regular, systematic, rule-governed, linguistic entity. On December 18, 1996, the Oakland Unified School District Board of Education passed a policy that supported development of Standard American English proficiency for all students. The school system noticed that Oakland's African American students were not succeeding in the school system, and they felt one of the common denominators that connected these students was the fact that they used African American English. Certainly, this was not the only common characteristic, but it was a major one and needed to be addressed. The school system wished to make AAE a language and mandate a Standard English Proficiency (SEP) program. It should be noted that for at least 15 years, California had a voluntary SEP program, which educated teachers about the history and culture of African American English. The teachers were also taught techniques to facilitate code switching. This program was reported to be successful, even though African American children were lagging behind their peers in SAE proficiency. However, the key word here is *voluntary*. Teachers were not mandated to participate in this early program; rather, it was left up to their sense of commitment. The new resolution added more encouragement for teachers to embrace this program. The SEP program was a linguistically and pedagogically sound program that recognized the discontinuity between the child's linguistic code at home and the code of the schools, and proposed to make them equal. However, because of media hype, the purpose, goals, and objectives of this program were misconstrued, and opposition to the program arose. Part of the opposition came from African Americans. In many cases, they were embarrassed and concerned because AAE (Ebonics) was a reminder of old customs and highly stigmatized times. Some of the public's misconceptions about the resolution included (a) that the district had decided to teach Ebonics in place of English; (b) that the district was trying to classify Ebonics as part of the bilingual program to obtain additional monies; (c) that the district was rewarding failure and lower standards; and (d) that the district was condoning the use of slang in the schools. None of these issues of concern were valid. The Oakland Board revised its resolution. It was weaker, but the emphasis was still on SAE proficiency, using the home language as a foundation.

No matter what the opposition is to the various programs that increase English proficiency, the issue remains that there are many African American children who come to school using AAE. This dialect conflicts with the language of the schools and mainstream society. This conflict places the children at an academic disadvantage (it negatively affects reading and writing, and children who speak AAE are placed in slower education tracks or special education) and thus makes programs like Oakland's essential (Seymour et al., 1999; Wolfram, 1997).

Related to this topic, in 1997 the Board of Directors of Teachers of English to Speakers of Other Languages (TESOL) supported using the home language as a bridge for teaching Standard English. They felt that teachers should show respect for the home language. This respect is a strong foundation for a partnership between home and school. The TESOL board also stated that if children's cultures are valued, children will have more self-respect and self-confidence, which will certainly facilitate learning, and thus increase test scores. The TESOL board also issued a policy statement on African American vernacular English. It affirmed the fact that AAE, through research, has been shown to be a rule-governed linguistic system that deserves recognition (Center for Applied Linguistics, 1997).

Characteristics

As mentioned earlier, SAE and AAE have many aspects in common. They share some grammatical and phonological rules, but they also have differences.

The vocabularies share both similarities and differences, as well. These will be discussed later in this chapter.

Some AAE vocabulary terms have become widespread in American discourse, like the words *jive, cool, rap,* and *whassup.* Much of this incorporation is due to rap, hip-hop, and other crossover music that is prevalent in the media and popular with mainstream youth (Terrell & Jackson, 2002). In fact, one of the co-hosts of the television program *The Today Show* used the phrase "You da man" (meaning "You're special") in one of his interviews. A newscaster on the CNN television station commented that a particular sports figure "has his groove on" (meaning that he's successful in his profession). A newscaster on a different television station stated that astronaut John Glenn was "good to go" (meaning ready to go, prepared) in his second trip to the moon. These are all phrases used in AAE but comfortably assimilated into the mainstream discourse.

The SLP must effectively determine whether a speaker has a communication disorder or a language or dialectal difference, and therefore must know the similarities and contrasting features of AAE and SAE (Paul, 2001). A complete analysis of all aspects of AAE would require volumes, so selected characteristics from each of the five aspects of language will be addressed.

Phonology. Phonology refers to the sound system of a language or dialect, the study of speech sounds in a spoken language. The rules are the same in AAE and SAE for combining phonemes into words (Stockman, 1996; Terrell & Jackson, 2002); the differences occur in the positional distribution of particular consonants. There are more consonant differences than vowel differences (Stockman, 1996). There are three differences in cluster production for AAE versus SAE: *thr* (voiceless) becomes /r/; *shr* becomes /sr/, and *str* becomes /skr/ (Terrell & Jackson, 2002).

According to Terrell et al. (1998), there are three major AAE phonological rules. The first rule is the elimination or substitution of the medial or final consonant in a word. Usually, voiced and voiceless fricatives are affected by this rule, as are voiced stops in the final positions. For instance, AAE speakers would say "nofin" for *nothing,* "teef" for *teeth,* and "wif" for *with.* The second major phonological rule is the silencing of unstressed initial phonemes and unstressed initial syllables. An AAE speaker might say "bout" for *about,* "cause" for *because,* and "this un" for *this one.* The last rule is the silencing of the final consonant so that, for example, *bad* becomes "ba," and *good* becomes "goo" (Haynes & Moran, 1989; Terrell et al., 1998). Another rule in AAE is consonant cluster reduction at the end of a word. Examples of this rule would be "pes" for *pest* and "was" for *wasp* (Terrell & Jackson, 2002). Other phonological differences include the following: "n" for *ng* substitution (*walking* becomes "walkin" and *thinking* becomes "thinkin"); *b/v* substitution (*vase* becomes "base"); metathesis (switching the order of phonemes, as "axe" for *ask*); and dipthong simplification, as "pond" for *pound* (Goldstein, 2000; Roseberry-McKibbin, 1995; Terrell & Jackson, 2002).

Morphology. Morphology is concerned with the structure of words and how it represents meaning, including use of suffixes, prefixes, plurality, and various other grammatical tenses. There are many differences in this component of language between AAE and SAE. In AAE, the past tense of regular verbs is not used. An AAE speaker would say "move" for *moved* or "jump" for *jumped*. Another grammatical feature of AAE is the use of "seen" for *saw* and "done" for *did* (Terrell & Jackson, 2002, p. 43). In SAE, use of past tense is obligatory. In SAE, plurality and possession are obligatory as markers; in AAE, the possessive *s* may be omitted when the possessor is included, such as "It John house." Similarly, AAE speakers omit the plural *s* marker when the quantity is included, such as, "He gave me two candy bar." In addition, in SAE, the copula and auxiliary forms of *to be* are required, but in AAE, they are often omitted. So utterances such as "He a happy man" or "The two girl runnin fast" are produced in AAE. Those sentences would be "He is a happy man" and "The two girls are running fast" in SAE (Hulit & Howard, 2001; Terrell & Jackson, 2002). AAE speakers also use the "habitual" or "aspect" tense, which indicates a continuous or permanent quality or condition, so the sentence "She be married" in AAE indicates "She has been married for a while." AAE speakers have rules for comparatives and superlatives that differ from SAE irregular forms, such as "worstest" or "worser," "baddest," and "mostest" (Goldstein, 2000; Terrell & Jackson, 2002).

Pragmatics. Pragmatics involves the way language is used in context. There are specific AAE pragmatic characteristics, such as code switching. This is when AAE speakers increase the use of SAE or AAE depending on the person with whom they are speaking, the communicative intent, or the environment. AAE speakers also might style-shift (change the use of AAE features between literate and oral styles).

African Americans also use a high-context communication style. That means that they depend greatly on group identity and shared meaning among speakers. Wit and sarcasm are pragmatic aspects used in AAE and present in many forms. One of the most popular forms is "playing the dozens." This is a game that is usually played with friends, males. The first friend insults the second friend's mother, and the second friend tries to think of a better insult about the first friend's mother. Upon first glance, this game of disrespecting mothers seems like the beginning of a disagreement. However, Terrell and Jackson (2002) indicate that the players have great love for their parent and withstanding the insults is a way to teach the players how to handle future negativism. They also note that it is a wonderful exercise to develop outstanding social and verbal skills.

Use of eye contact also differs. SAE speakers use direct eye contact when they are either the speaker or listener. AAE speakers use direct eye contact when they are speakers but indirect contact when they are listeners. This behavior is a sign of respect.

Originally, research found that AAE speakers used a topic-associated narrative style (ideas generated from statements that precede them). However, further research indicated that AAE speakers vary their narrative style depending on the task demand. Turn-taking rules differ in SAE and AAE. In SAE, one waits her turn before talking in a conversation. AAE speakers do not have to wait until the other person has finished—interruptions are perfectly acceptable and expected. The stronger, more aggressive speaker obtains the conversational floor. Other pragmatic differences are that although approval and positive energy are conveyed by an AAE speaker through touching a person's hand or arm, touching other parts such as someone's hair might not be as positively received—in fact, that action might be misconstrued as an insulting gesture (Quails & Harris, 1999; Terrell et al., 1998; Terrell & Jackson, 2002).

Syntax. Syntax refers to the rules for sentence construction and usage. AAE shares the same fundamental sentence structure as other English varieties, such as word order, but there are some differences. One difference is the zero copula or auxiliary in AAE; the copula or auxiliary is omitted as in "This his toy." In SAE, the structure is always used ("This is his toy"). In AAE, subject-verb agreement is not always required (so the subject and verb can differ in either number or person), for example, "The boy need some pants." In SAE, there is always subject-verb agreement in a sentence ("The boy needs some pants") (Jackson & Roberts, 2001; Washington & Craig, 1994). In AAE, forms are shortened or abbreviated, for example, *want to* becomes "wanna," *supposed to* becomes "sposeta," *fixing to* becomes "fitna," and *about to* becomes "bouta." The complete forms are used in SAE. Another syntactic difference is AAE's use of multiple negatives, with more than one negative marker allowed in a sentence, such as "He don't wanna do nothing." In SAE, only one negative maker is included per utterance—the use of more than one negative sometimes makes an utterance positive. In AAE, the use of multiple negatives strengthens the negative sentiment. In AAE, *ain't* is used as a negative auxiliary ("They ain't playing no cards"); the word *ain't* does not exist in SAE.

The use of the reflexive pronouns *himself* and *themselves* change to "hisself" and "theyself" in AAE—"He went all by hisself." In AAE, the indefinite article *a* is used regardless of the vowel context—"This is a umbrella," whereas in SAE, one would use *a* when a consonant followed ("a horse") and *an* when the article is followed by a vowel ("an umbrella"). The use of future tense is different in AAE, as the contraction for *will* is silent. Examples of this difference are "He work with you" for "He will work with you." Unlike SAE speakers, AAE speakers also use appositive pronouns (a pronoun and a noun referring together to the same person or object)—"The boy he's gonna eat." In SAE, either a pronoun or a noun is used but not both—"The boy is going to eat." For AAE speakers, nominative, objective, and demonstrative pronouns are used interchangeably, so "Him singin" is appropriate (Goldstein, 2000; Jackson & Roberts, 2001; Terrell & Jackson, 2002; Washington & Craig, 1994).

Semantics. *Semantics* refers to the study of word meaning. Word meaning and vocabulary are culturally influenced. The vocabulary of AAE speakers is influenced by many factors, such as geographic region, economic level, and the passing of time. The word *tonic* is used to indicate a carbonated soft drink in areas around Boston. The same carbonated drink is called "pop" in Pittsburgh,

"Coke" in Dallas, and "soda water" in Gainesville, Florida (Terrell & Jackson, 2002, p. 46). As time passes, each generation creates a new set of words and meanings. Often these creations are called slang. Terrell and Jackson (2002) indicate that slang is very prominent among African American youth. They suggest that it may be a way for African American youth to feel special and unique, since they are not always accepted into the social activities of Caucasian youth. Some examples of the generation-changing terms for *good* or *great* are "crazy" (1950s), "boss" (1970s), "phat" and "stompin" (1990s), and "representin" (2001) (Terrell & Jackson, 2002, p. 47). Other examples of differences in vocabulary and meaning between AAE and SAE include: "bad" (good), "cat" (friend), "cool" (calm), "dig" (comprehend), "bogus" (false or fake), "true dat" (agree), "change up" (change), "chillin" (relaxing), "dissin" (disrespecting), and "crib" (home or parent) (Terrell et al., 1998; Terrell & Jackson, 2002).

African Americans also use figurative language to maintain their cultural and social identity. Some examples of figurative language in AAE to mean *good* or *great* are "kick it to the curb," "put your foot in it," "off the hook," and "you be trippin." Other examples are "get my groove on" (feel romantic, have a good time), and "flip the script" (change) (Quails & Harris, 1999; Terrell & Jackson, 2002). The vocabulary and meanings change quickly, so the examples provided here may already be passé.

Acquisition and Development

Like all language acquisition, the development of AAE is a complex process that involves social, environmental, biological, and cognitive factors (Wyatt, 1998). It is important for the SLP to recognize these factors and know a few facts about the acquisition of AAE. There are still broad gaps in research on AAE development; however, Stockman's (1986, 1996) research has given us some guidelines. She noted that the acquisition of AAE is developmental, just like SAE and other linguistic systems. AAE speakers acquire the same semantic (action existence, location, attribution, notice, negation, recurrence, possession, time) and pragmatic categories at similar stages of development and in the same sequence as speakers of SAE (Battle, 2002a; Stockman & Vaughn-Cooke, 1982). Terrell and Jackson (2002) noted that between the ages of 18 months and 2 years, AAE-speaking children develop some functions such as informative, requestive, regulative, imaginative, affective, participative, and attentive the same as children learning other languages. Mean length of response and semantic and pragmatic categories increase with age. Again, this developmental trend is similar to that of SAE. Stockman (1986, 1996) also stated that there is tremendous variation in the acquisition of AAE features among children. It is often difficult to detect differences in the language development of AAE speakers and SAE speakers before the age of 3 years, particularly in morphosyntactic development (Stockman, 1986). This difficulty arises because the forms that are associated with AAE, such as omission of the copula and past tense markers, occur in SAE speakers in the early stages of language development. Between the ages of 3 and 5 years, AAE speakers increase their use of AAE characteristic features, while SAE speakers of those ages tend to decrease use of those forms (Battle, 1996; Wyatt, 1995, 1998).

Goldstein (2000) created an acquisition table for AAE morphosyntactic features. By age 3, the AAE speaker is using the present tense copula, regular past tense, remote past, and third-person singular. The indefinite article regularization, multiple negation, and mean length of C-units (words 3.14, morphemes 3.48) are used at 4 years. By 5, the AAE speaker is using the demonstrative pronoun, a mean length of utterance of 3.36 words (or 3.76 morphemes in C-units), and reflexive and pronominal regularization ("He asked can he ride with us"), plurals, present and past tense copula, and increased mean length of utterance.

The phonemic inventory of AAE is similar to that of SAE except for the voiced interdental fricative. Children speaking AAE progress through the same phonological process stages as SAE speakers, except that final consonant deletion persists longer in AAE (Goldstein, 2000; Haynes & Moran, 1989). AAE speakers produce most initial consonants the same as SAE speakers. Specifically, by the age of 3, speakers of both dialects produce the following phonemes: /m/, /n/, /p/, /k/, /g/, /h/, /j/, /t/, /d/, /b/, and /s/ (Battle, 2002b; Stockman & Settle, 1991). Just like SAE speakers, speakers of AAE correctly produce consonants and vowels by 8 years of age.

Pragmatically, by 5 years of age, many African American children who are exposed to both SAE and AAE are already code switching between the two dialects depending upon the topic, listener, and communicative intent. By this age, children are already aware of the social significance of the use of AAE in social and educational situations (Battle, 1996; Goldstein, 2000; Wyatt, 1998).

Also in the area of development, Craig and Washington (2002) have provided some useful information about the "typically developing African American child." In their study of 100 African American preschool and kindergarten students, they found that typically the African American student will be an AAE speaker. The AAE will be characterized by copula or auxiliary deletions and inconsistent use of number agreement markers for verbs. These young AAE speakers will use conjunctions and simple infinitives to combine clauses. Using C-units as a measurement, the AAE-speaking student will use phrase lengths ranging from 2.5 words to 4 words. Craig and Washington also found that these students will be able to understand requests for information and active statements but not passive ones. Yet given this information, the SLP must always remember that there are no stereotypes. Not all traits, including use of AAE, can be applied to every African American. Each person is a unique individual and should be treated as one.

Assessment

The challenge to the SLP is to appreciate our multicultural society and to help our clients and students participate in it. Specifically, the primary job of the

SLP, when serving children from culturally and linguistically different backgrounds, is to determine a child's natural language or dialect and accurately and sensitively diagnose and treat language disorders. The SLP must distinguish language disorders (severe discrepancies in skill per culture and developmental level) from language differences (rule-governed communication that deviates from the mainstream) by providing a nonbiased assessment (Battle, 2000; Paul, 2001; Seymour et al., 1999).

Frequently, SLPs use standardized tests as part of their assessment battery. For the culturally and linguistically diverse population, they must use tests that are designed specifically for the language or dialect of the speaker they are testing. People who use the dialect or language of the client must have been included in the test norms. The SLP must know both the communication patterns of the client's culture and the communication problems experienced by the client.

Until recently there were no complete standardized tests specifically for speakers of AAE. Dr. Harry Seymour of the University of Massachusetts was awarded a 6-year multimillion-dollar grant by the National Institutes of Health to develop and validate a speech and language test for children who speak nonstandard English. In conjunction with the Psychological Corporation and a team of specialists, Dr. Seymour developed a series of assessments that have been tested across the United States. Two of these tests were published in 2003—the *Diagnostic Evaluation of Language Variation* (DELV)–*Screening Test* and the *Diagnostic Evaluation of Language Variation–Criterion-Referenced Test*. The third test, *Diagnostic Evaluation of Language Variation–Norm-Referenced*, was published in 2005. The DELV screening tool takes 15 to 20 minutes to administer and has two parts. Part I, Language Variation Status, distinguishes those children who speak SAE (Seymour refers to it as mainstream American English, MAE) from those who use another dialect; it is appropriate for children ages 4 to 12. Part II, Diagnostic Risk Status, distinguishes students who are developing normal language from those who might be at risk for a language disorder; this section is appropriate for ages 4 through 9. The DELV Criterion-Referenced Test is administered to children who fail the screening test. It is a comprehensive evaluation designed to separate those children who are developing normally in communication from those who are not. The test takes approximately 45 to 50 minutes and is appropriate for ages 4 through 9. The test includes semantics (verb contrasts, preposition contrasts, quantifiers, fast mapping–real verbs, fast mapping–novel verbs), pragmatics (communication role taking, short narratives, question asking), syntax (wh-questions, passive, articles), and phonology (25 target phonemic clusters, age-appropriate cut-off scores, initial and medial positions of words only, cluster targets—two and three elements). The DELV Norm-Referenced version is currently the only test normed on African American children (ASHA, 2002; Seymour, Roeper, deVilliers, & deVilliers, 2003). This test is for children ages 4 through 9 years. The standardization sample was based upon the 2000 U.S. Census. It assesses syntax, pragmatics, semantics, and phonology (Seymour, Roeper, deVilliers, & deVilliers, 2005).

There are other strategies to use when assessing AAE speakers. One strategy considered in addressing the issue of nonbiased assessment is the modification of existing standardized tests. Generally, credit is given for test items that are potentially affected by AAE use or other cultural influences. SLPs should check the tests they are using to see if this modification process is available (Washington & Craig, 1999). Another form of this process is to first give the test according to the standardized procedure in SAE, then check the responses, comparing to the general AAE dialect and to the AAE characteristics used in the child's community, and giving credit for the correct AAE responses (Battle & Grantham, 1997).

Yet another strategy for the SLP to use is to make certain the test is nonbiased. While reviewing the test, the SLP should look at the conceptual basis for the test, the standardization sample (does it include your client's culture or language or dialect?), the responses of the groups that are within the sample (any groups similar to your client?), and finally review each item in the test for potential bias against the client or his culture (Battle, 2002a). Vaughn-Cooke (1983) also suggests that the SLP ask the following questions when deciding on a nonbiased test:

- Can the test tell the difference between actual errors and responses attributed to dialectal or cultural differences?
- Does the test include dialect variation?
- Is there an adequate description of the dialect?
- Do the results of the test include dialectal differences?
- Can the test tell the difference between a child with a language difference and a child with true language pathology?

Washington and Craig's (1999) study found an established standardized test that was culturally fair to use with African Americans who are AAE speakers—the *Peabody Picture Vocabulary Test–Third Edition* (PPVT–3). The subjects used in their study spoke AAE, and they were considered at risk because of their low income level, family density, or teenage parents. It was felt that all culturally biased pictures and responses had been removed from this standardized norm-referenced test (Washington & Craig, 1999).

Seymour et al. (1999) suggest creating simple diagnostic tests. For instance, a prominent feature of AAE is the absence of the *to be* verb. In AAE, a person might say "She bad" or "They silly." AAE speakers delete *is* and *are* but rarely delete *were, was,* or *am*. The AAE speaker usually says, "He was good" or "They were good" or "I am fine." Thus, if an AAE speaker deleted *was* or *were* in her speech, an SLP might become suspicious that a disorder was present. Seymour et al. (1999) also noted that *is* is more likely to be omitted when proceeded by the pronoun *he* than when it is preceded by a word ending in *t*. Therefore, a diagnostic procedure might be to present a picture of an orange and say, "This is a plum." Children love to correct their teachers, so they will more than likely reply, "That is not a plum, that [it] is an orange." If the child says "is," it is obvious that he has the *is* form, even though he may omit it in the sentence "He bad." If the child omits *is* after both the *t* and *he,* it may be a sign that he has language problems. Of course, other similar tasks must be performed to verify that (Seymour et al., 1999).

Criterion-referenced measures have also been suggested as helpful in a culturally and linguistically sensitive assessment. Terrell, Arensberg, and Rosa (1992) offer the SLP a systematic, criterion-referenced method for assessing a person's dialect, termed Parent–Child Comparative Analysis (PCCA). This method uses the client's parent or caregiver as a language referent. Speech and language tests are administered to both the parent and the child. The child's speech and language patterns are compared to the parent's responses. Those responses that are not similar to the parent's responses are compared to normal expectations for the child's chronological age (via charts, scales, tables). If divergent language patterns remain after this process, there is a high probability of speech or language problems (Terrell et al., 1992).

Seymour, Bland-Stewart, and Green (1998) and Battle (1996, 2002a) suggest that in order to determine a disorder from a difference, the SLP should assess the language features that are not contrastive. In other words, assess the language areas that AAE and SAE have in common (noncontrastive). Language features of AAE and SAE that are noncontrastive include early semantic functions (existence, state, locative state, action, locative action, specification, possession, time, negation), articles, conjunctions, prepositions, demonstratives, subjective marking of pronouns, and complex sentences (Battle, 2002a; Seymour et al., 1998). Jackson and Roberts (2001) also found complex syntax to be non-contrastive. They found that MLU for words was related to complex syntax, so it also might be a useful measurement tool. Phonological noncontrastive features between AAE and SAE include "the use of more than one or two stop errors, initial word position errors, glide errors in children over age 4, more than a few cluster errors and fricative errors other than" the voiceless *th* (Battle, 1996, p. 25).

Using an interpreter, translator, family friend, or other culturally sensitive individual is another method that has been suggested as a way to facilitate a culturally and linguistically fair assessment. The SLP must use these assistants with caution. Sometimes they do not accurately reflect the intent of the test item and thus compromise standardized protocol (Battle & Grantham, 1997).

Use of a language sample and observational techniques has also been suggested as a nonbiased assessment method. For this to be an effective process, developmental data and cultural communication behavior along with the expectations for AAE speakers must be available (Battle & Grantham, 1997).

Craig and Washington (2000) recommend a nonbiased assessment battery for African American school-age children who use AAE. They found this test battery distinguished a disorder from a difference. The battery consisted of spontaneous language sampling in which the mean length of C-units in either words or morphemes was calculated, along with the number of different words used in the language sample (measured expressive vocabulary), the frequency of complex syntax use (measured morphologic and syntactic growth), responses to *wh*-questions or requests for information and to active and passive sentence constructions (measured comprehension). In addition, the results of the PPVT–3 (which measured receptive vocabulary) and the *Arizona Test of Articulation Proficiency–Second Edition* (which distinguished articulation and phonological disorders from normally developing errors) should be reviewed. The average length of C-units, the complex syntax task, the number of different words used, and the responses to reversible sentences consistently distinguished the language-impaired student from the chronologically (typically) developing student. Craig and Washington note that future research should pursue normative data to assist with the interpretation of student performances.

Gutierrez-Clellen and Peña (2001) found that the test–teach–retest aspect of dynamic assessment was a good tool to use to differentiate language differences from disorders in various language areas, such as vocabulary, narrative, synonyms, and antonyms. Using this method, the SLP first identified deficient or emerging skills that may be due to lack of experiences. The assumption was that poor performance may be due to limited experience with the test situation and items or culturally based language differences. After testing, the SLP provided activities so that the student could learn the deficient skills. The activities were not the actual test items or materials. A retest was given. Gutierrez-Clellen and Peña found that typical language learners made significant changes in their test scores. Qualitative responses were better, as well. Those learners who had actual disorders scored low at the beginning and made only minimal gains on the posttest after the teaching intervention. These results have been obtained with several different cultural groups and show promise for a bias-free assessment.

SLPs who are culturally sensitive also use the ethnographic method of gathering data. They observe as much as possible without making early judgments, carefully reviewing the detained descriptions, making interpretations (looking for themes and patterns), and then drawing conclusions (making sense from themes and patterns) (Stone-Goldman & Olswang, 2003).

Another assessment strategy noted by Peña and Quinn (1997) is to use familiarity as a tool in assessment. They found that test performance is influenced by a person's experience, general knowledge, and familiarity with the task. They tested African American children who were in a Head Start program, using unfamiliar and familiar test tasks. The familiar test tasks were from a subtest of the *Stanford-Binet Intelligence Scale* and involved describing use of objects, naming body parts, and answering "why" questions. The unfamiliar task was labeling from the *Expressive One-Word Picture Vocabulary Test*. In this study, the African American children performed better on the familiar test tasks. The familiar test task was also more sensitive in differentiating typically developing children from low-language-ability children. Based on these results, it would appear that use of familiar test tasks might obtain more valid assessment information (Peña & Quinn, 1997).

It is obvious that there is no one way to assess AAE speakers. To provide an accurate, culturally sensitive, and nonbiased assessment of AAE speakers, many methods and tools must be used. This will help the SLP achieve the goal of differentiating a language disorder from a language difference. This differentiation can only be achieved by careful comparison of language structures and analysis of features. SAE cannot be used as a comparison for a child who speaks AAE and hears it in her home and community (Battle, 2002b).

Intervention

Once a nonbiased assessment has been accomplished, the service delivery options are (a) no communication disorder and thus no intervention, or (b) a communication disorder, which would necessitate treatment. If intervention is needed, several questions arise:

- What is the best treatment?
- Who will provide the therapy? A monodialectal SLP? Will an interpreter, translator, or family friend be used?
- What is the best language or dialect for intervention? (Battle, 2002a)

Although the "rule of thumb" is to provide intervention in the language or dialect of the home, the responses to these questions must be answered on a case-by-case basis, depending on the family's or caretaker's wishes, the cognitive level of the child, the motivation of the child, and the learning skills of the child. Some intervention strategies might include previewing lessons, going over previously learned material, using a multisensory approach, highlighting salient words, decreasing speaking rate, paraphrasing and restating information, concentrating on the communication of meaning, using scaffolding, making sure that questions and comments are understood, and using cooperative or group learning (Battle, 2002a; Battle & Grantham, 1997).

The SLP should be certain that the objectives and outcomes of therapy are consistent with the expectations of families, teachers, and clients and involve the parents and the teachers in the intervention process. Use of vocabulary and real-life situations based on the client's culture would be culturally sensitive and appropriate. Adapting a cultural style similar to the client's—such as a more animated instructional style for African Americans who use AAE— would also be culturally sensitive. Understanding the differences in eye contact and other nonverbal cues is also critical in intervention (Battle & Grantham, 1997). In addition, the SLP should be aware of the client's learning and cognitive styles. In general, African Americans are thought to have a field-dependent learning style. This would then be true for African Americans who use AAE. Field-dependent learners are cooperative and strongly influenced by their peers and authority figures. They view group achievement as important and thus like to work with others. This means that the SLP should adapt a field-dependent teaching style (encourage cooperation, encourage group achievement, show confidence in the student's ability to complete the task, instruct by modeling, personalize concepts) (Battle & Grantham, 1997; Terrell & Jackson, 2002).

The SLP must also use therapy materials and activities that are culturally relevant and that present the African American culture in a positive light. When possible, the SLP should use the dialect or language of the client or obtain the assistance of an interpreter or translator. Appropriate use of the dialect or language demonstrates the SLP's caring and willingness to learn (ASHA, 2001; Battle & Grantham, 1997). Another helpful hint is to play music in the waiting room of the office or clinic that is more appropriate to African American culture, such as jazz (perhaps the most appropriate because it is accepted by many cultures). This consideration might make the client feel more comfortable (Terrell & Jackson, 2002).

The Culturally Competent Speech–Language Pathologist

To accomplish culturally and linguistically sensitive assessment and intervention, the SLP must be culturally and linguistically competent. Before addressing the specific characteristics of a culturally competent speech–language pathologist (CCSLP), it is appropriate to look at the major attributes of "good teachers" of African American students. Two recent articles by Tatum (2000) and Hefflin and Barksdale-Ladd (2001) discuss the characteristics of good teachers working with young African American elementary and middle school students. These teachers were concerned about the students' social, affective, and emotional development, as well as their cognitive development. They used a culturally relevant approach to teaching. African American community norms were included in the classroom instruction. Cooperation was emphasized more than competition, and learning was formulated as a social activity. With such an approach, students experienced academic success; maintained their cultural competence; and had a foundation that allowed them to critique cultural norms, values, mores, and institutions that support and maintain inequities. Another key to this successful approach was using culturally relevant literature in the teaching process. Students need to see positive images of their culture in books and materials. It allows them to connect with the material and authenticates their world (Hefflin & Barksdale-Ladd, 2001; Tatum, 2000).

Battle (2000) defines cultural competence as "a process through which one develops an understanding of self, while developing the ability to develop responsive, reciprocal, and respectful relationships with others" (p. 20). Therefore, CCSLPs should have all of the attributes of the good teachers mentioned above and more to successfully serve AAE speakers. They must understand, accept, and support the dialect of their students. They must be introspective and look at their own beliefs and ideas. They must eliminate negativism, biases, and other misperceived concepts about culture, language, and dialects, because these characteristics might negatively influence the client–clinician interaction. CCSLPs should not immediately assume that because a person is an African American that he must use AAE as his primary language. They should be knowledgeable about dialect features, different cultures, and use of code switching. Increasing their knowledge and understanding of the clients' culture and language or dialect might involve spending time in the client's community or having discussions with experts on the culture and linguistic expectations of the client's community. Becoming familiar with the cultural customs, values, and beliefs of the clients and demonstrating appreciation for the differences provides a comfort level for both the SLP and the client. Once children know you care and are accepting of them for who they are, it is easier to obtain a more culturally sensitive assessment and provide culturally sensitive intervention (ASHA, 2001; Battle, 2000; Battle & Grantham, 1997; Owens, 1999; Seymour et al., 1999).

Battle (2002a) suggests that the CCSLP is a good listener who attends to what the client says and does, who attends to them as people. She also states that the CCSLP notes important events and behaviors; describes salient, language features; appropriately requests information; and investigates and seeks answers using all available methods (i.e., asks the right questions). Battle also presents the antithesis. She describes the characteristics of a non–culturally competent SLP: a poor listener, self-centered, poor observer of client communication, poor communicator with the client or family caregivers, poor evaluator of communication ability; does not ask for clarification of what is seen and heard; relies totally on norm-referenced tests; and does not include life history in the evaluation process.

CCSLPs should learn the appropriate greetings and forms of address and contrastive and noncontrastive features of AAE and other languages or dialects. They should also avoid the use of professional jargon (Owens, 1999). "They should consider each client as an individual with unique experiences and beliefs that affect clinical service" (Uffen, 2001, p. 1). Most important, the CCSLP should demonstrate sensitivity and respect by not scheduling assessments and therapy sessions on religious holidays or when students are scheduled to participate in religious activities. They should be aware of and respect the appropriate dress, food, and other cultural variables of religious practices (Battle & Grantham, 1997).

In addition, ASHA has several required competencies for the SLP, which are included in the technical report on American English Dialects (ASHA, 2003). The competencies include (a) "recognizing all American English dialects as rule-governed linguistic systems"; (b) "understanding the rules and linguistic features of American English dialect(s) represented by their clientele"; and (c) "being familiar with nondiscriminatory testing and dynamic assessment procedures such as the following: identifying potential sources of test bias, administering and scoring standardized tests in alternative manners, using observation and nontraditional interview and language sampling techniques, and analyzing test results in light of existing information regarding dialect use" (p. 46). The report also states that the SLP has a "social and ethical responsibility" (p. 46) to discuss the use the dialect and the social and educational implications with the client or caregiver.

Conclusion: African American Students

AAE is a dialect of SAE with both similarities and differences to SAE. It has a unique history and foundation that include a way of life and a specific culture.

It has its own linguistic rules, which encompass pragmatics, semantics, syntax, morphology, and phonology. Mostly, African Americans speak it, but other people who are exposed to or immersed in a community that uses AAE, regardless of their race or ethnicity, use it as well. SLPs must be culturally competent and provide nonbiased assessment and intervention for AAE speakers. The culturally competent SLP must treat AAE-speaking clients with respect and be nonjudgmental, knowing that there might be cultural as well as linguistic differences between them. CCSLPs must know how to determine a dialectal or language difference from a language disorder and treat only a disorder. This chapter has provided some guidelines for the evaluation of AAE speakers. More research is needed to further knowledge about nonbiased assessment and intervention procedures, as well as to increase cultural competence for the SLP and other professionals who will work with AAE speakers.

HISPANIC AND LATINO STUDENTS: LUIS F. RIQUELME

Currently, the Hispanic–Latino population is the largest minority group in the United States (U.S. Bureau of the Census, 2000a). Hispanics are the fastest-growing ethnic minority in this country. In 2004, Latino children are already a majority among racial and ethnic minority children in the schools nationwide. Also of note among language minority groups is the fact that Latinos tend to retain their "mother tongue" (Spanish) more than other non–English-speaking groups in this country.

Hispanics–Latinos are people of primarily Spanish descent representing Spain, Portugal, Mexico, Central America, South America, and parts of the Caribbean (Cuba, Dominican Republic, Puerto Rico). They are a heterogeneous group of people, as they come from over 20 different countries. This serves to highlight differences in culture, as well as differences in immigration patterns and attitudes toward living in the United States.

This section of the chapter will focus on providing the reader with a brief synopsis of Hispanic cultures and relevant clinical assessment and intervention issues, as they relate to communication sciences and disorders.

Heterogeneity

According to the last U.S. Census, in 2000, Mexicans remain the largest Latino group (58.5%), followed by Puerto Ricans (9.6%), Cubans (3.5%), Dominicans (2.2%), Central Americans (4.8%), South Americans (3.8%), and other Hispanics (17.3%) in this country. The majority of Central Americans in the United States are from El Salvador, Guatemala, and Honduras. The majority of South Americans in the United States are from Colombia, Ecuador, and Peru. The term "other Hispanic" was used in the 2000 Census for those persons not identifying their country of origin, and for those of mixed Hispanic backgrounds (e.g., a person of Puerto Rican and Colombian descent). Hispanics and Latinos are, of course, culturally and ethnically diverse, as well as racially heterogeneous. For example, Latinos from the Caribbean islands of Puerto Rico, Cuba, and the Dominican Republic represent a mixture of White (European descent), Indian (native to the islands), and Black (African slaves brought to the islands). Other parts of Latin America with a similar mixture include the eastern coast of Mexico and the northern coasts of Colombia and Venezuela. Mixtures of Indian and White can be seen in the remaining countries of Latin America. Furthermore, different Indian tribes inhabited different parts of Central and South America, and so different physical features exist, making the mixture of White and Indian in a person from Mexico different from the same mixture in a person from Chile.

Within the United States, as of the year 2000, 43.5% of Hispanics lived in the West, 32.8% lived in the South, 14.9% in the Northeast, and 8.9% in the Midwestern United States. Approximately 87% of the Hispanic population in the United States is concentrated in 10 states: California, Texas, New York, Florida, Illinois, New Jersey, Arizona, New Mexico, Colorado, and Massachusetts (U.S. Bureau of the Census, 2000b). Hispanics are the majority of the population in East Los Angeles (96.8%), El Paso (76.6%), and San Antonio (58.7%). Over the last 5 years, however, a greater spread of Latinos across the United States has been noted, with Hispanic communities present in a wide variety of states, including Georgia, North Carolina, Arkansas, Minnesota, and Nebraska.

Heterogeneity regarding language dominance and use is also evident in the Hispanic–Latino community. While most Hispanics may speak Spanish as their primary language, not all do. Some Hispanics speak primarily Portuguese. Moreover, some are second- or third-generation Hispanics, with little, if any, knowledge of the Spanish language. The speech–language pathologist in the schools will encounter children across a continuum, from the child who is a monolingual Spanish speaker, to the child who is bilingual and English or Spanish dominant, to the child who is a monolingual English speaker.

Hispanic or *Latino:* **What's in a Name?**

This primarily political argument dates back to the early 1980s. Some people feel strongly about which term is used. Of note is the population on the West Coast, where the majority prefers the term *Latino*. For example, the *Los Angeles Times* exclusively uses the term *Latino,* not *Hispanic.* That does not hold true on the East Coast of the United States. To understand this, one must first understand the use of the term *ethnic. Ethnic* is defined as pertaining to a particular race, culture, or nationality, or any combination of these. The term was originally used in the United States for a diverse group of second- and third-generation European immigrants living in inner-city neighborhoods. It was later used for recent immigrants from Latin America and Puerto Rico (even though the latter were, and are, American citizens). Because of difficulties in identifying persons from Latin America, the U.S. Office of Management and Budget created the term *Hispanic* in 1970. It was operationalized as "a person of Mexican, Puerto Rican, Cuban, Central or South American or other Spanish culture or origin, regardless of race." Subsequently, other definitions arose, and so did confusion regarding nomenclature to be used for Brazilians, Spaniards, and Filipinos. The term *Hispanic* is used by the U.S. Census Bureau.

Today, it is most commonly acknowledged that the term *Hispanic* includes people from Latin America, as well as Spain and Portugal. The term *Latino* is accepted as that used only for people of Latin American descent.

Arguments for the use of both exist. Treviño (1987), of the University of Texas, states that the advantages of continuing to use the term *Hispanic* include the following:

- *Hispanic* provides more universal coverage of the population than is possible with *Latino,* as it includes Spanish and Portuguese.
- The term has worked well in studies conducted in New Mexico for identification of Hispanics.
- Most of the professional literature uses the term *Hispanic*. Treviño argues that continuing to use the term would allow for better follow-up studies and continued research.
- The term *Hispanic* presents with the most "user friendliness" among people in the group. Treviño states that the term *Latino* still presents with uncertain stereotypes, as some believe the term arose in "trendy" California.

On the other hand, Hayes-Bautista and Chapa (1987) offer the following arguments in support of the term *Latino:*

- Immigrants from Latin America to the United States have very different experiences upon arrival, compared to Europeans (Spanish, Portuguese). Europeans do not experience the level of discrimination that Latinos do. Spanish and Portuguese come to this country without Indian blood. Their countries are not desperately poor or viewed as inferior by many U.S. citizens.
- *Latino,* according to Hayes-Bautista and Chapa, states a national origin better than *Hispanic* does.

It should be noted that other authors, for example, Yankauer (1987), state that the two terms connote socioeconomic differences, with Latino being the "ordinary, middle or low status" individual. For some, there is humor in the distinction: "A Hispanic is like a Latino Yuppie."

One may ask, "Why the need for a collective term?" Some argue that most Hispanics choose their country of origin when asked to classify themselves. Other Hispanics, however, see the collective designation as a way of establishing their commonality with Hispanics who have more clout. This is similar to the notion of "situational ethnic identity" in which individuals shift their claims to ethnic membership as the advantages or disadvantages dictate. This is reportedly mostly seen in complex urban environments.

In summary, it appears that the terms *Hispanic* and *Latino* carry different meanings for different people, but these terms certainly allow for greater political power within the U.S. society, as there is more power in numbers. The common term, whichever is used, also allows for clearer accountability of the "other" categories that result from intermarriage among Hispanics and Latinos. For purposes of this chapter, the terms *Latino* and *Hispanic* will be used interchangeably.

Assimilation and Acculturation

Culture is always an interesting term to define. It is a set of values, beliefs, and behaviors shared by a group of people. Most think of culture as attributed only to a person's ethnic background, yet culture entails other groups of people as well. Religious beliefs, lifestyles, and work all influence the places people can come together by their commonality.

When attempting to understand the Latino culture, the speech–language pathologist needs to be aware of a variety of factors. Of note to any clinician working with diverse populations are the concepts of assimilation and acculturation. *Assimilation* is the process of someone in a new environment totally embracing the host culture. *Acculturation* is the integration of the host culture with the native culture to varying degrees. In reality, we all experience and practice acculturation within the variety of environments in which we exist (e.g., work, social, educational) (Riquelme, in press).

General Religious Beliefs

Historically, groups that immigrated to the United States from Europe brought their clergy, who often served as the "brokers" between immigrants and the host society. Priests acted as political and economic community leaders, as well as educators. In contrast, most Latino groups come to the United States without accompanying clergy. Although Hispanics may also be Catholic, the Catholic church in the United States is institutionally quite different from that of the native country. It is often assumed that all Latinos are Catholic. This has not been substantiated. According to Doyle (1982), in the 1950s approximately 50% of Puerto Rican marriages in New York City were performed in Protestant churches. It is noted, however, that Mexicans remain the least affected group by Protestant sects. Some studies show that Catholicism, rather than Protestantism, is associated with upward mobility for Mexican Americans.

It is important to note that while Hispanics are not exceptionally devout in an institutional sense (not frequent mass attenders), they nonetheless value the church greatly and are comfortable in seeking it out for assistance. Euro-American Catholics, in contrast, have focused on Mass attendance as a measure of devotion. Other aspects of spirituality will be discussed under the following section on health care.

General Health-Care Practices

The speech–language pathologist may encounter families who believe in the following health-care practices to varying degrees. This has an effect on the professional's role in providing appropriate remediation. The perception of illness among some Hispanic groups may be related to psychological states, environmental or natural causes, or supernatural causes. Psychological states may include embarrassment, envy, anger, fear, excessive worry, turmoil in the family, improper behavior, or violations of moral or ethical codes. For example, a headache or an upset stomach may be related to a mother's excess worry over a son's impending divorce. Another perceived causal factor for illness may be environmental or natural conditions, which includes bad air, germs, dust, excess cold or heat, bad food, or even poverty. An example of a natural cause may include becoming ill after opening the refrigerator door without a shirt on (cold). Illness may also be believed to be related to supernatural causes, such as malevolent spirits, bad luck, witchcraft, or living enemies (believed to cause harm out of vengeance or envy). Often seen on Hispanic children are *manos de azavache* (small charms of a hand or amulet) believed to protect them from the "evil eye" (envy of others).

For some Latino families, the health subculture includes belief in folk diseases and in special healers. Folk diseases may include *mal de ojo* (evil eye), *susto* (fright), *empacho* (upset stomach), or hot or cold diseases (remedies are selected to keep the body "in balance," so as not to have too much cold or too much heat). Healers include the *curandero,* who is usually an herbalist or "general practitioner." This person prepares home remedies using herbs for internal or external injuries. There is also the *espiritista,* who is like a high-ranking curandero, one who can handle folk diseases and physical ailments and is also believed to have the power to communicate with the spirits.

Again, belief in these practices varies by individual, especially among the younger generations of Latinos in this country. It should be noted that other traditional health practices may include herbs, teas, and home remedies (e.g., using mentholated alcohol on the forehead to relieve a headache).

Hispanic Family Life

The importance of family is a Hispanic cultural value; individuals have a strong identification with and attachment to their nuclear and extended families. With this comes values of solidarity, loyalty, and reciprocity among family members (Marin & Marin, 1991). The Hispanic family structure provides a strong source of social and emotional support (Dikeman & Riquelme, 2002). Family members are seen to be dependable and reliable; there's a sense of duty toward each other and a sense of willingness to give (often with the idea that one may someday be in a position of needing family help).

Family members include parents and children, as well as aunts and uncles, cousins, and *compadres* (godparents). In more traditional families, the father remains the authority figure. It is also important to acknowledge that experience associated with age is highly regarded, and so children are expected to show respect toward elders, regardless of status or formal education. Also of note is the fact that in some families, children are raised to value cooperation within the family unit more than individual achievement (Langdon & Cheng, 1992). Furthermore, many Hispanic children are taught to listen, obey, and not challenge authority. Rodriguez and Olswang (2003) note that, in their study, although Mexican American mothers differed from Anglo mothers concerning some beliefs and values on child rearing and education, beliefs and values varied based on the level of acculturation to the U.S. culture.

Other Cultural Values

In his recent book, Brice (2002) notes the following cultural values and implications for health-care and educational professionals (p. 7):

- Elders, experts, and those with curing powers (e.g., curanderos) are respected.
- The concepts of circularness, wholeness are important—this means to work with the student and his family in a team effort.
- Silence is valued.
- Privacy for personal matters is respected.
- Congeniality and graciousness are cherished.
- Health problems are the result of past behaviors; one must accept what is.
- Illness is supernatural.
- Negative thoughts or actions may cause them to occur.
- Time is viewed differently. Family events take precedence over appointments with speech–language pathologists.
- Healers give tangible objects. Leave something for the family at the end of the meeting—for example, a pamphlet or a small toy.

Gathering Information

In order for the speech–language pathologist to provide culturally sensitive services to individuals from Hispanic backgrounds, appropriate information regarding cultural practices, beliefs, and communication patterns needs to be gathered. Wallace (1997) provides an excellent framework for the clinician working with culturally and linguistically diverse populations to organize this information. The following areas are part of her framework for organizing information:

- overall impression of culture and history
- generational status

- communication patterns
- social organization
- time concept
- spiritual orientation
- health practices
- food preferences
- risk factor for communication impairments or dysphagia

Wallace identifies these areas as a primary focus for the clinician attempting to gather information regarding a culture he is not familiar with. She states that this greater understanding of the culture will allow for improved service delivery.

The manner in which to gather the information is also of importance. *Ethnographic interviewing* is a technique that has gained much attention over the past 2 decades or so. One can think of the ethnographic approach as a personalized method of exploration that provides the clinician with an opportunity to obtain a deep, true, and naturalistic understanding of the behavior or culture under study. This interview approach is appropriate for people from backgrounds other than that of the clinician who may not be as responsive to the direct questioning format used by clinicians in traditional interviews. The goal in this technique is to obtain information about a culture from the perspective of a member of that culture and not from that of the interviewer. It conveys empathy and acceptance of the world as defined by the informant; allows information necessary for generating appropriate support and clinical practice to be collected; helps equalize the power differential; provides a means for the professional to discover the culture of the family and their strengths and needs; provides a means for focusing on the perspective of the informant; helps reduce potential bias in assessment and intervention; and allows the data to be collected in a more ecologically valid framework (Westby, 1990). During ethnographic interviewing, the clinician has a general set of questions at the outset, but the flow of questioning is molded by the scope and depth of information obtained as the interview unfolds. The clinician is also advised to pay attention to the wording of questions; use open-ended rather than closed-ended questions; use presupposition questions effectively; ask one question at a time; make use of preliminary statements; and maintain control of the interview. Other essential elements of effective ethnographic interviewing include the following (Wallace, 1997; Westby, 1990):

- establishment of rapport;
- good listening skills;
- a clear set of goals for information to be obtained;
- skill in selecting the appropriate types of questions (e.g., grand tour, mini tour, example, experience, or native-language questions);
- skill in framing questions, so that they are open ended yet targeted to probe into key areas of interest;

- skill in looking for patterns and common theme expressions as an essential key to detecting critical concerns of interest to the client or patient and family.

It is important for the speech–language pathologist conducting the interview to realize that his background will affect the kinds of questions to be presented, the way the questions are posed, and the way answers are interpreted.

Dialectal Variations of Spanish

Spanish dialects can differ markedly from each other in terms of lexicon, phonology, morphology, syntax, semantics, and pragmatics. It is important to note, however, that most speakers of Spanish are able to communicate with each other because of the use of a core Spanish language. This is unlike dialects in other languages, where communication between users of different dialects is close to impossible. For the speech–language clinician, the existence of differences between Spanish dialects further complicates the process of characterizing phonological patterns in Spanish-speaking children. Unlike English, where dialectal variations are generally defined by variations in vowels, Spanish dialectal differences primarily affect consonant sound classes (Goldstein, 1995).

Because speech–language pathologists may not be aware of important phonological or phonetic differences among the predominant dialects of Spanish spoken in the United States, additional information should be obtained from sources listed in the bibliography (see Goldstein, 1995, 2000; Iglesias & Goldstein, 1998). Goldstein and Iglesias (1996) provide several characteristics of Spanish-speaking children with phonological disorders. In addition, Goldstein and Iglesias (2001) discuss the possibility of misdiagnosis if a child's productions are compared to an incorrect or inappropriate dialect.

It is also important to note that the production of Spanish-accented English does not signify a communication disorder. In such an event, the aspect of intelligibility needs to be addressed. If the child is intelligible, then no remediation is necessary, unless accent modification is sought.

Other Spanish-Language Influences

It is important for professionals working with Latino children to understand language differences that are commonly observed when acquiring English. According to Roseberry-McKibbin (1995, p. 67), these include the following:

- Adjective comes after noun (e.g., "The house green …").
- S is often omitted in plurals and possessives (e.g., "The girl book is …").
- Past tense *ed* is often omitted (e.g., "We walk yesterday").

- Double negatives are required (e.g., "I don't have no more").
- Superiority is demonstrated by using *mas*, "more" (e.g., "The cake is more big").
- The adverb often follows the verb (e.g., "He drives very fast his motorcycle").

Restrepo (1997) reported that the most common errors produced by Spanish-speaking children with language impairment included omission of preposition and articles, person agreement in verbs, and gender agreement in articles. She also noted that Spanish-speaking children with language impairment are more likely to exhibit errors in noun phrases than in verb phrases.

Peña, Bedore, and Rappazzo (2003) discuss the area of semantics. They note the need to look at a variety of tasks when assessing semantics (e.g., characteristics, similarities and differences, functions) rather than simply examining receptive vocabulary with a pointing task or expressive vocabulary with labeling.

Second-Language Acquisition: An Overview

Understanding how a person acquires a second language is of great importance to the speech–language pathologist working with children from bilingual backgrounds. Many Latino children first learn Spanish at home and subsequently begin the acquisition of English, their second language. It is important to note that assessment of the child may be conducted at any point along the continuum of acquiring the second language. It is therefore possible to see children whose scores may be depressed in their native language, L1, because they have stopped developing in that area so as to commence acquiring the second language, L2. At the time of testing, such a child may present with depressed scores for both L1 and L2. Does this indicate a communication disorder? No, it does not. The clinician needs to be aware that this is part of the typical process of acquiring a second language.

Some clinicians will look at *communicative competence,* which lies in the student's ability to communicate messages effectively. When looking at communicative competence, the speech–language pathologist should differentiate among the following: (a) *grammatical competence:* phonological, syntactic, and lexical skills; (b) *sociolinguistic and sociocultural competence:* the use of language and communication rules appropriate in one's language; (c) *discourse competence:* the skills involved in the connection of a series of utterances to form a conversation or narrative; and (d) *strategic competence:* the strategies used by the bilingual person to compensate for breakdowns in communication that may result from imperfect knowledge of the rules or fatigue, memory lapses, distraction, or anxiety. Evaluating the child in a variety of communicative contexts may allow the clinician to observe competence in different areas.

When addressing the critical period for second-language acquisition, consensus has been reached on the following three points:

- Adults proceed more quickly through the very early stages of phonological, syntactical, and morphological development.
- When time and exposure are controlled, older children move through the stages of syntactical and morphological development faster than do younger children.
- Those who begin to acquire L2 as young children usually achieve higher levels of oral proficiency in accent and syntax than those who begin as adults. The prepubescent and postpubescent periods have been identified as major markers in this area.

Code switching and code mixing are also part of the language proficiency continuum of the bilingual student or child. *Code switching* is understood to mean the alternation of English and Spanish (in the case of the Latino child) at the intersentential level (e.g., "Give me something to eat. *Tengo hambre.*"—that is, "Give me something to eat. I am hungry."); or at the intrasentential level (e.g., "Give me *un papelito.*"—"Give me a little piece of paper."). The switches are not random; they are governed by constraints such as the free morpheme constraint and the equivalency constraint (C. Crowley, personal communication, 2003). *Code mixing* refers to the use of mixed-language utterances, usually at the lexical level, within a sentence. Many argue over the difference between code mixing and code switching. In any event, these forms of language alternation are considered part of the typical process of acquiring a second language, as well as part of the typical language usage of a bilingual speaker, as they allow for a combination of the pragmatic, syntactic, and morphological dimension of both languages. Indicators of possible deficiencies in code switching (Brice, Roseberry-McKibbin, & Kayser, 1997) may consist of long pauses indicating word searching and retrieval difficulties; inability to switch and mix between the two languages with ease; and an overpreponderance of one language.

It is also important for the speech–language pathologist working with the Hispanic/Latino child to understand that there are similarities as well as differences in the first- and second-language acquisition process. Brice (2002), outlines both. He states that developmental similarities when a person is acquiring English or Spanish include the following (a) easier sound forms and words are acquired before more complex forms; (b) labels are acquired first; and (c) it is common for errors to occur in learning L1 and L2. However, he also notes some differences in L1 and L2 acquisition. The following characteristics are not prevalent in first-language acquisition: (a) Children learning a second language may avoid certain topics, tenses, words, situations. Children learning a first language do not avoid certain syntactic tenses, morphological constructions, or word choices; (b) Spanish–English-speaking children may also use social and cognitive strategies not typically used by monolingual children. For example, repeating to oneself and starting and stopping a sentence several times is seen with bilingual children; (c) Children learning a second language can often experience certain psychological barriers, such as fatigue; and (d) If Spanish is not maintained while English is being acquired, it may atrophy and be lost.

Collaborating with Interpreters and Translators

Regulations on the use of interpreters and translators for speech–language assessment and intervention vary by state. In some states, every bilingual child referred for a speech–language evaluation is required to undergo the assessment performed only by a clinician who is bilingual in the child's native language. Needless to say, this is sometimes quite difficult to achieve, as a match between the child's native language and the clinician's bilingual proficiency is not always possible. According to recent demographics, fewer than 2% of ASHA members identify themselves as bilingual or multilingual (ASHA, 2002).

In other states, interpreters and translators are often used by the speech–language pathologist for assessment and intervention. Often the interpreter or translator is hired as support personnel if the need is great (Kayser, 1995). This underscores the need for all clinicians to become culturally competent, as even a monolingual English speech–language pathologist will have bilingual children in his caseload. Recall that the bilingual child may be dominant in English. The clinician treating this child may be a monolingual English professional, who will need to be sensitive to the cultural and linguistic differences of the child. It would be inappropriate to measure this bilingual child's communication skills and style against that of a monolingual English language speaker.

An *interpreter* is a person specially trained to transpose oral or signed text from one language to another. A *translator* is a person trained to transpose written text from one language to another. Speech–language pathologists most often require the services of an interpreter. It should be understood that not every bilingual person has the ability to be an interpreter. In addition to proficiency in two languages, skills needed by an interpreter include the ability to say the same things in different ways; the ability to shift styles; the ability to retain chunks of information while interpreting; and familiarity with medical, educational, and professional terminology (Langdon, 2002). The interpreter should not be a friend or family member, as information may be misunderstood, relayed inaccurately, or purposely omitted (Kayser, 1995b).

Even if a professional interpreter is used, training by the speech–language pathologist will be required. The clinician needs to introduce the interpreter to the goals of assessment and intervention and the importance of accurate and direct interpretation, because of the complexity of speech–language diagnostics. It serves to highlight how the clinician reaches an impression based on what may be interpreted. If a professional interpreter is not available, another professional may be trained to assist the speech–language pathologist. Again, the use of a family member or friend should be avoided.

During the session it is important that the clinician maintain eye contact, or a direct connection, with the student or client and not with the interpreter.

Other modifications to testing procedures include the following:

- Reword instructions, as needed.
- Allow for additional response time.
- Record all responses, for later analysis.
- Accept culturally appropriate responses.
- Repeat stimuli as needed.
- Use culturally appropriate pictures and themes.

Langdon (2002) has developed a handbook with procedures and training exercises for the interpreter collaborating with the speech–language pathologist. Additional guidelines and suggestions are offered in Wallace (1997) and Kayser (1995b).

Implications for Assessment

In general, the bilingual speech–language evaluation entails gathering additional information on development of L1, acquisition of L2, parents' knowledge of L1 and L2, and the child's preferred language. This is in addition to information usually obtained regarding the child's health status, educational placement and progress, and so forth. The examiner or diagnostician then conducts the testing in both languages. Results are subsequently reviewed to determine whether the child presents with a communication disorder, delay, or difference. In the case of a communicative difference, the clinician determines if it is part of the process of acquiring a second language or not. The examiner is cautioned that, depending on when in the second-language acquisition period the child is tested, she may display depressed scores in both L1 and L2. It is normal for the child's L1 to stop developing while the acquisition of L2 is in progress.

It is also of note that conducting a bilingual speech–language assessment is quite a challenge. Not only, as mentioned above, is the evaluation conducted in two languages, but the examiner also needs to obtain additional background information, qualitatively analyze the data (formal and informal), and make diagnostic decisions regarding the child's performance. Just as with monolingual evaluations, a bilingual speech–language evaluation is only as good as the evaluator conducting it.

Formal Testing

The use of formal tests for bilingual children is an interesting challenge for any speech–language pathologist. First, the examiner needs to find the most appropriate test for the child, depending on the goals of the assessment. Then, the examiner needs to become familiar with the normative sample used, in addition to the chronological age ranges of the test battery. Subsequently, the examiner needs to review the stimuli used in the test battery to assess the cultural relevance of the pictures and tasks presented. While so far these appear to be tasks every speech–language pathologist employs when selecting a formal test battery, they are a bit more complex when assessing a child from a bilingual or multicultural background. Looking at cultural relevance and the normative sample of a test battery appears to be a common procedure for any examiner. In this case, however, speech–language pathologists must understand that any formal test battery employed presents with inherent linguistic and cultural biases (Anderson, 2002). Anderson then describes *linguistic bias* as the language used during testing or the language expected in the child's responses. This is often quite subjective, as is the examiner's acceptance of responses from the child being tested. She further describes *cultural bias* as referring to the use of activities and items that do not correspond to the child's experiential base.

Since the testing will be conducted in English and Spanish, the examiner needs to determine how the Spanish version of the test was developed. Was it translated or adapted? What norms were developed for use with the Spanish version? Was the sample used for the normative data a monolingual Spanish population, or a bilingual English–Spanish population? To date, few formal test batteries have even attempted to specify the development of norms and the population (monolingual vs. bilingual) included in the sample.

Another aspect to consider is that most children being tested are bilingual to differing degrees. Norm-referenced tests look at each language as a separate entity and do not assess the relationship between the two languages.

Research has shown that formal tests tend to overidentify Hispanic children as language-learning disabled (Kayser, 1995a; Peña, Quinn, & Iglesias, 1992). Unfortunately, in spite of these findings, many examiners and school districts continue to rely on the results of norm-referenced tests for the identification of children with communication disorders (Kayser, 1995a).

Psychometrics

Understanding the psychometrics of a formal test battery becomes increasingly relevant when conducting a bilingual speech–language evaluation. While it would be ideal to avoid using norm-referenced or formal test batteries with bilingual children, the reality is that many clinicians have no experience in other forms of assessment and are also often required by school districts and administrators to provide "numbers." Until these issues are addressed at all levels of administration and practice, speech–language pathologists will continue to be required to present some formal test validation for their impressions.

The examiner is therefore cautioned that the literature does not support the use of norm-referenced or formal tests for the assessment of Hispanic children, because great knowledge of psychometrics is required. Speech–language pathologists should report results carefully, use only relevant data, and therefore avoid the overidentification of children into speech–language programs.

Some examiners include a disclaimer statement in their reports, noting the reduced validity of the formal tests employed. However, many then go on to report derived scores, such as age equivalents, percentile ranks, and standard scores. These data place the validity and reliability of other measures (e.g., criterion-referenced or informal testing) in question. Depending on who is reading the report, and for what purpose, the impressions reached by the examiner may be at risk of being invalidated or weakened.

Validity (whether the test measures what it is designed to measure) and *reliability* (whether the test measures a given attribute or behavior consistently) are test construction criteria that each examiner reviews on a regular basis. Validity is known to be a subjective measure, regardless of the often ample data offered by the developers. In the case of its use with bilingual populations, validity remains relative, because the particular construct may be valid for one population but not for another. To further highlight psychometric criteria required in norm-referenced tests, the reader is referred to McCauley and Swisher (1984a, 1984b). To further understand aspects of cultural and linguistic bias in norm-referenced tests, the reader is referred to Anderson (2002, pp. 157–163). She provides ample examples of biases and cautionary notes to the examiner.

Normative Sample

In looking at the psychometric construction of the test, the normative sample, or who was used to norm the test, needs to be reviewed carefully. As mentioned earlier in this section, the examiner must attempt to match the normative sample with the child being tested. If every examiner were to follow this rule, formal tests would not be used at all with bilingual children. That is, there is no one test that offers norms that are directly relevant to the child about to be tested. There are many reasons for this. In addition to the realities of every child's differences in communicative development, the examiner needs to address the fact that each bilingual child is at a different point along the language acquisition continuum. For example, two 6-year-old children who arrived in the United States at age 4 and live in Spanish-speaking households may present varying levels of proficiency in Spanish and in English, according to their exposure to L2 and where they may be along the second-language acquisition continuum. This is one of the reasons the goal of developing a formal test with "bilingual norms" may never be achieved. Other statistical approximations are currently being offered. Clinical practice will decide whether these approximations are a help or a hindrance to the examiner and, most important, to the bilingual child being tested.

Derived Scores

Understanding and reporting derived scores is a difficult issue for many speech–language pathologists assessing bilingual children. In addition to understanding the statistical construct behind each score, the examiner must clearly understand the impact these numerical scores have on the child being tested.

The most commonly used derived scores are age equivalents or developmental scores, percentile ranks, and standard scores. *Age equivalents* or *developmental scores* provide the examiner with information about the test taker's performance in relation to the performance of other children of the same chronological age. These scores present several difficulties, including not taking into account individual differences. In light of what we have discussed thus far regarding the bilingual second-language acquisition continuum, this can potentially be a dangerous score to rely on when testing a bilingual child. *Percentile ranks* indicate the percentage of individuals in the normative group whose test scores fell below a given value. Percentiles indicate the position of a test taker's score relative to the scores of the normative sample. *Standard scores*, often thought of as the most satisfactory kind of derived score, can be used to estimate the position of a test taker's score relative to the scores obtained by the normative sample, so as to compare one person's score on two different tests and to compare one person's score to someone else's in a meaningful way.

When testing Hispanic children, or any other children from bilingual backgrounds, the following formal test modifications should be considered (adapted from Erickson & Iglesias, 1986; Kayser, 1989; Kayser, 1995a):

- Reword instructions.
- Provide additional time to respond.
- Continue testing beyond the ceiling.
- Record all responses, particularly when the child changes an answer, explains, comments, or demonstrates.
- Compare the child's answers to dialect or to first- or second-language learning features.
- Develop several more practice items, so as to establish the process of "taking a test."
- On picture vocabulary tests, have the child name the picture in addition to pointing, so as to ascertain the appropriateness of the label presented.
- Have the child explain why the "incorrect" answer was chosen.
- Have the child identify the actual object, body part, action, etc., particularly if she has had limited experience with books, line drawings, or whatever materials are being used.
- Complete the testing in several sessions.
- Omit items you expect the child to miss because of age, language, or culture.
- Change, as needed, the pronunciation of vocabulary.
- Use different pictures, as needed.
- Accept culturally appropriate responses as correct.
- As appropriate, consider having a parent or another trusted adult administer the test items.
- Repeat the stimuli more than specified in the test manual.

Informal Testing

Many examiners consider informal testing an important part of the assessment process; however, when reporting results, it appears they lack objectivity. Of greater validity are *criterion-referenced procedures*. These procedures provide the examiner with information that cannot be obtained from formal tests. They assess an individual's performance of a particular skill, structure, or concept. The fundamental purpose of criterion-referenced procedures is to distinguish between levels of performance (McCauley, 1996). Examples within our field include obtaining a percent of syllables stuttered during a speech, maximum phonation time, percent of consonants correct and mean length of utterances (McCauley, 1996). Criterion-referenced measures are relatively narrow in focus, as they are used to differentiate among levels of performance. Anderson (2002) offers the following example.

An example of a criterion-referenced measure would be a child's ability to use episodic structure in a story-telling task. As such, it is developed so that the particular relevant aspects of the episodic structure during a retelling task can be scrutinized. The clinician may establish how many stories the child will retell, how many episodes each story contains, and the expected performance level, such as number of complete episodes produced.

An obvious advantage of these measures is that they can be tailored to each individual child. Procedures and materials can be used that are familiar to the child, and thus responses are not affected by the child's lack of experience with the materials or by cultural differences in interaction (Anderson, 2002).

Another alternative or adjunct to testing Hispanic children is the use of *ethnographic observations*. This allows the examiner to observe the child in a variety of communicative contexts and determine his competence. The examiner is cautioned, however, to observe in a variety of settings (e.g., one or more classrooms, the playground). Another cautionary note is to understand that this type of observation is colored by the examiner's view of the world. If the examiner interprets the child's behavior incorrectly, that may result in misdiagnosis of the child. In order to prevent as much examiner bias as possible, it is suggested that clear objectives or goals for the observation be established (Anderson, 2002; Kayser, 1995a) and that a cultural informant is used to review results.

Language sampling is another available technique for the assessment of bilingual children. This is a well-known technique in our field. For specific suggestions on conducting language sampling with Latino children, the reader is referred to Anderson (2002) and Kayser and Restrepo (1995).

One further option for informal testing is *dynamic assessment*. This procedure assesses not only the child's current performance level, but also how the child can learn. Because dynamic assessment provides information on the child's ability to learn, it provides the examiner with great insight for both identifying a language disorder and planning intervention. Peña, Quinn, and Iglesias (1992), Ukrainetz, Harpell, Walsh, and Coyle (2000), and Peña, Iglesias, and Lidz (2001) have documented the benefits of using this procedure. They tested children on a particular task, then taught it to the children, and subsequently retested the children on the task without using cues or other supports. The studies documented that children who were language impaired failed to evidence learning in the same manner as children who demonstrated typical language skills. This certainly appears as a viable procedure to be used by speech–language pathologists assessing the communicative skills of Hispanic children.

In general, speech–language pathologists are cautioned not to label Latino children as disordered if the deficits are apparent in only one language. As has been noted, the examiner is expected to consider language differences, issues of language loss, and second-language acquisition.

Treatment Considerations

Deciding on the language of treatment with Hispanic children has been a highly debated issue in the bilingual education literature, as well as in that of speech–language pathology. Many questions arise when deciding how to approach remediation of the Hispanic bilingual child with a language disorder: Will intervention in L1 retard the progression of L2? Should treatment be provided only in L2? Will treatment in both L1 and L2 be too "taxing" to the child? Gutierrez-Clellen (1999) provides an excellent review of these and other issues and their clinical implications. To date, no study has been able to support an "English only" (L2) approach. Most studies have focused on bilingual or monolingual L1 intervention. In reviewing the literature, it appears to be understood that children's language learning can be maximized when the language of instruction or treatment matches the child's languages and L1 is used as an organizational language framework to facilitate second-language learning (Gutierrez-Clellen, 1999). Children with a language impairment who are learning a second language compose a heterogeneous group. This is evidenced by the different types of deficits presented (e.g., phonological, pragmatic, morphosyntactic), the severity of the disorder, the modality of the disorder (e.g., receptive, expressive, both), the language experiences of the child in L1 and L2, and where along the second-language acquisition continuum the child may be. These factors will affect the rate of learning each language, as well as the progress in an intervention program.

Of great importance to the treating clinician working with Hispanic children is the joint work with ESL teachers, classroom teachers, and parents. The speech–language pathologist's success in treatment with a Latino child who is language impaired hinges on this collaboration and on developing culturally relevant strategies, tasks, and materials.

Another factor that influences the success of the Latino child with a language impairment is the type of service delivery models available. This is largely determined by the resources of the particular school district, as well as the underlying philosophy on bilingual and special education of that school district.

Providing optimal treatment to the Hispanic child is a multifaceted endeavor that requires commitment to working with families, students as individuals, and school team members to foster success for the child (Roseberry-McKibbin, 2002).

Conclusion: Hispanic and Latino Students

As speech–language pathologists continue to practice in a multicultural world and continue to provide services to Latino children, the increasing need to become culturally competent becomes paramount. Cultural competence will allow the speech–language pathologist to provide services to children from all cultural and linguistic backgrounds with as little bias as humanly and clinically possible.

This chapter has presented only a brief overview of the complexities of providing culturally competent services, specifically in working with Hispanic/Latino children. It is hoped that the reader will use the references provided to continue developing the skills and knowledge base needed to make appropriate clinical decisions.

The challenges that lie ahead are many, mostly caused by a culture that originally intended to be homogeneous (e.g., the old notion of America as a melting pot). Providing culturally competent services to children of all backgrounds should be a challenge all clinicians engage in with enthusiasm and passion. Until misdiagnosis because of cultural differences is a thing of the past, speech–language pathologists cannot stop learning and challenging their clinical practices.

ASIAN PACIFIC ISLANDER AMERICAN STUDENTS: LI-RONG LILLY CHENG

Asian Pacific Islander Americans (APA) people have been immigrating to the United States for more than two centuries. Most early immigrants were laborers from China, Japan, Korea, and the Philippines. They first went to Hawaii and the U.S. West Coast. The earliest immigrants were few in number. A recent book by Iris Chang, *The Chinese in America: A Narrative History* (2003), discusses the Chinese immigration and treatment in the United States.

After World War II, many Filipinos and Koreans began to immigrate in large numbers to the U.S. mainland. In 1975, following the Vietnam War, the first wave of Southeast Asian refugees came, and since then more than a million refugees from Vietnam, Laos, and Cambodia have settled in the United States. In recent years, the shortage of professionals in high technology prompted the United States Immigration and Naturalization Service to admit thousands and thousands of professionals from India to fill the shortage of high-technology jobs. Not only have the profiles of APA changed significantly, but the numbers have increased as well. By 2010, the National Center for Education Statistics (1997) estimates there will be significant increases in the number of Hispanic, APA, American Indian, and Alaska Native students in the public schools, whereas the monolingual (English) white student population will decrease by more than 10%.

The APA population in the United States increased from less than 1% in 1970 to 4% in the year 2000, a growth of 400% in 30 years. The population is a diverse group from Southeast Asia, Hong Kong, China, India, Pakistan, Malaysia, Indonesia, and other Pacific Rim and Pacific Basin areas. In addition, the APA school-age population has increased more than sixfold, from 212,900 in 1960 to almost 1.3 million by 1990. In 1990, 40% of Asian Pacific American children were first generation, 44% were second generation, and 15% were third generation. By the year 2020, Asian American children in U.S. schools will total about 4.4 million (Jiobu, 1996).

Where Is Pacific Asia?

Pacific Asia is divided into the following regions: East Asia (China, Taiwan, Japan, and Korea); Southeast Asia (Philippines, Vietnam, Cambodia, Laos, Malaysia, Singapore, Indonesia, Thailand); Indian Subcontinent or South Asia (India, Pakistan, Bangladesh, Sri Lanka); and Pacific Islands (Polynesia, Micronesia, Melanesia, New Zealand, and Australia). These countries and regions are connected to the Pacific Ocean; thus, the term *Pacific Asia* is used to describe this large region. The countries of Asia are listed in Figure 9.1 and the countries of the Pacific Islands are listed in Figure 9.2.

In addition to population growth through live births, refugees in large numbers have come to the United States. Table 9.1 shows the largest refugee source countries. Refugees tend to go through a process called secondary migration and congregate where there is a large population from their own place of origin. Table 9.2 shows the top ten states of refugee resettlement.

Afghanistan	Israel	Pakistan
Armenia	Japan	Qatar
Azerbaijan	Jordan	Saudi Arabia
Bahrain	Kazakhstan	Singapore
Bangladesh	Korea, North	Sri Lanka (Ceylon)
Bhutan	Korea, South	Syria
Brunei	Kuwait	Taiwan
Burma	Kyrgyzstan	Tajikistan
Cambodia (Kampuchea)	Laos	Thailand
China	Lebanon	Turkey
Cyprus	Macao	Turkmenistan
Hong Kong	Malaysia	United Arab Emirates
India	Maldives	Uzbekistan
Indonesia	Mongolia	Vietnam
Iran	Nepal	Yemen
Iraq	Oman	

Figure 9.1. Asian countries.

American Samoa	Marshall Islands	Papua New Guinea
Cook Islands	Micronesia	Solomon Islands
Easter Island	Nauru	Tonga
Fiji	New Caledonia	Tuvalu
French Polynesia	Northern Mariana	Vanuatu
Guam	Islands	Wallis and Futuna
Kiribati	Palau	Western Samoa

Figure 9.2. Pacific Islands.

Who Are Asian Pacific Islander Americans?

APA are extremely diverse in all aspects of their ways of life, including language, culture, religion, attitudes toward education, childrearing practices, and roles within the family. At the same time, they share many similarities. Those who have lived in the United States for more than two generations share a common history of being Asian Pacific Americans. Others who are recent immigrants or refugees share the newcomer status. There are clear generational differences, which will be delineated in the following section.

Generational Differences

Among the APA populations, there are many who have lived in the United States for generations. They do not speak the language of their ancestors and do not practice the "old ways." They are mainstreamed into the U.S. culture and are not familiar with the home culture of their grandparents or great grandparents. The term *ABC* is used, for example, to describe Americans born Chinese, and the term *FOB* is used to describe those fresh off the boat. The ABCs do not identify with the FOBs. Refugees and immigrants from the Asian

Table 9.1 Ten Largest Refugee Source Countries, 2003

Former U.S.S.R.	8,728
Liberia	2,915
Former Yugoslavia	2,500
Iran	2,428
Sudan	2,090
Somalia	1,708
Ethiopia	1,669
Vietnam	1,461
Afghanistan	1,446
Sierra Leone	1,350

Note. From *Report to the Congress: Proposed Refugee Admissions for FY 2005.* 2004, Washington, DC: Department of State, U.S. Department of Homeland Security, U.S. Department of Health and Human Services.

Table 9.2 Refugee Resettlement: Top Ten States with Percent of Total Refugees to U.S. (2003)

California	15%
Washington	10%
New York	8%
Minnesota	6%
Texas	5%
Pennsylvania	4%
Georgia	4%
Florida	3%
Illinois	3%
Arizona	3%

Note. From *Report to the Congress: Proposed Refugee Admissions for FY 2005.* 2004, Washington, DC: Department of State, U.S. Department of Homeland Security, U.S. Department of Health and Human Services.

Pacific Island regions come from a variety of historical, social, educational, and political backgrounds. Voluntary *immigrants* are usually prepared for their move, are psychologically motivated, and are prepared linguistically and culturally to succeed in their new country. But *refugees* are forced to leave their country because of adverse domestic, social, or political conditions. Most refugees enter their adopted country without knowledge of the language or the culture. They generally go through a long and arduous process of adjustment. Many refugees may not achieve high levels of acculturation into their host country and continue to live in isolation, mainly staying in their cultural or ethnic enclaves (Cheng, 1990, 1995).

It is extremely difficult to make generalizations about APA populations when there are clear generational differences. Takaki's book *Strangers From a Different Shore* (1989) and Liu's *Accidental Asian* (1998) are two good examples of the differences in APA identities. The word *nisei* refers to "second-generation Japanese American" and the word *san sei* refers to "third-generation Japanese American." The terms connote multiple identities and hyphenated identities (Young, 1998). Cheng (2004) discusses the concept of multiple or hyphenated identities and the cultural and linguistic considerations of these hyphenated identities.

Multiple Identities

Many immigrants identify with their home culture and their new host culture. Those born in the United States find it difficult to accept their hyphenated existence. They often say things like "Why do you think I speak Japanese? I am an American." Hyphenated identities may be a source of identity confusion and crisis. One of the critical elements of one's identity is one's language. Since the second- and third-generation APAs generally do not speak the mother tongue of their parents, they are sometimes embarrassed by the lack of linguistic and sociocultural knowledge of their parents.

The notion of multiple consciousnesses works best with individuals who grow up with diverse experiences. An example is a fifth-generation Chinese American veteran who grew up in San Diego, fought in the Second World War, and won three purple hearts. He speaks no Chinese but goes to a Chinese Community Church, volunteers at the Chinese Center, and views himself as a San Diegan. Another example is a Chinese Mexican woman who grew up in Mexicali speaking fluent Spanish and English but cannot speak much Mandarin. On the one hand, such people are trying to cope with their given hyphenated identity; on the other hand, their parents and grandparents may stress the importance of maintaining their home culture.

Maintenance of the Home Culture

Many second-, third-, and fourth-generation immigrants experience "push and pull" conflicts. The "push" to be mainstreamed conflicts with a "pull" to retain cultural roots and traditions. Recent literature provides rich examples of this. *The Joy Luck Club* by Amy Tan (1989) and *The Woman Warrior* by Maxine Hong Kingston (1976) described the struggles of American-born Chinese. *The First Suburban Chinatown,* by Timothy Fong (1994), tells the story of recent Chinese immigrants in Monterey Park, California, and *The Gangster We Are All Looking For,* by Le Thi Diem Thuy (2003), describes a young Vietnamese girl and her parents settling in the United States. Many feel marginalized, and yet some have gained not only political clout but also political position. Norm Menita and Elaine Chow were named as the secretaries of transportation and labor, respectively, by President George W. Bush and are two examples of mainstreamed APAs in politics.

Some of the newcomers find their new homes comfortable and welcoming; others have very different experiences. Research on adjustment problems has recurrently addressed the question of why some refugees and immigrant groups adapt readily to the American way and others have tremendous difficulty making the adjustment. Trueba, Jacobs, and Kirton (1990) studied the Hmong community in California and found that the adjustment was extremely difficult and painful. Many immigrant parents are faced with the need to make decisions about what parts of their home culture must be preserved and what must be "let go" (Cheng, 2004). Since culture is what sustains a group of people, a discussion of the key cultural APA themes may be helpful to the readers.

APA Culture

APA culture is not one but many. What they share is ancestry from either the continent of Asia or islands in the Pacific Ocean. Some have a very long cultural tradition, such as those from India and China; others have been isolated because they are from islands in the middle of the Pacific. Their cultural views are pertinent to our understanding of the way of life in Pacific Asia. Clearly, intra- and intergroup differences exist among the Asian and Pacific Islander immigrant and refugee groups. These people represent diverse social, cultural, and linguistic backgrounds. They offer opportunities to understand cultures, languages, and peoples. For example, due to Singapore's history of repeated colonization, its culture is a mosaic, with input from the British, American, Chinese, Malay, Indian, and other cultures. The multicultural influences on Singapore make the country unique and fascinating. The Polynesian, Melanesian, and Micronesian cultures have some similarities. They believe in collectivism rather than individualism. Families are usually large and extended.

Folk Beliefs, Religions, and Philosophical Views

The APA new immigrant populations hold a variety of religious and philosophical beliefs. They include Buddhism, Confucianism, Taoism, Shintoism, animism, and Islam. Christianity is also practiced. There are many Catholic churches in the Philippines and across the Pacific Islands. Many Pacific Islanders consider the Bible a major source of inspiration.

People from urban and rural areas and those with different levels of education, exposure to Western cultures, and personal experiences vary in their reactions to folk beliefs. Attitudes toward disabilities are a reflection of current and historical beliefs about the nature of handicapping conditions. Illness is usually treated with all available methods, including consulting with the priest, clansmen, and elders before a licensed physician is consulted. For example, the Hmong people view surgical intervention as invasive and harmful. They believe that spirits may leave the body once the body is cut open, causing death (Fadiman, 1997).

Treatments vary a great deal, ranging from surgery, medication, and therapy to acupuncture, massage, cao (coin rubbing), bat gio (pinching), giac (placing a very hot cup on the exposed area), steam inhalation, balm application, herbs, inhaling smoke or ashes from burnt incense, and the ingestion of hot or cold foods (Cheng, 1995; Fadiman, 1997).

Key APA Cultural Perceptions of Disabilities

A definition of what constitutes an impairment is critically dependent upon the values of a particular cultural group. The treatment of birth defects and other disabilities is influenced by cultural beliefs and by the socioeconomic status of the individual and the family within society (Cheng, 1990; Chinn, 1990; Gollnick & Chinn, 1990; Ortiz-Monasterio & Serrano, 1971; Strauss, 1985). There are broad similarities and differences between Western and non-Western belief systems and practices. In all Asian Pacific Islands cultures, attitudes toward disabilities can be traced, in part, to folk beliefs and superstitions. Folk belief may conflict with the way medication is used, and often Eastern and Western medicines are combined. For example, acupuncture may be used for pain or injuries in addition to antibiotics.

Invisible disability, such as a speech, language, or learning disability, is generally not regarded as the same as physical disability (e.g., blindness, multiple handicaps, cerebral palsy, cleft palate). Many APA immigrants view a disabling condition as the result of wrongdoing of the individual's ancestors, resulting in guilt and shame. The cause of disabilities can be explained through a variety of spiritual or cultural beliefs, such as an imbalance of inner forces, bad wind, spoiled foods, gods, demons or spirits, or hot or cold forces.

Languages and Dialects

There are approximately 6,500 languages in the world, and hundreds of distinct languages are spoken in Pacific Asia. They can be classified into five major families: Malayo-Polynesian (includes Tagalog, Ilocano), Sino-Tibetan (includes Thai, Yao, Mandarin, Cantonese), Austro-Asiatic (includes Vietnamese, Khmer), Altaic (includes Japanese, Korean), and Dravidian (includes Tamil, Telugu). There are also 15 major languages in India from four language families (Shekar & Hegde, 1996), namely, Indo-Aryan, Dravidian, Austro-Asiatic, and Tibeto-Burman. Furthermore, over 1,200 indigenous languages belonging to the Austronesian language family are spoken among the 5 million inhabitants of the Pacific Islands. The five lingua francas, also called hybrid languages or language mixtures, used by the Pacific Islanders are French, English, pidgin, Spanish, and Bahasa. Table 9.3 shows the nine language families of Pacific Asia.

These languages differ a great deal—from being tonal, monosyllabic, and logographic (a property of a writing system) to being intonational, polysyllabic, alphabetic, and agglutinational. Tonal languages such as Mandarin, Lao, and Vietnamese rely on tonal differences for meaning. The highlights of selected languages follow.

Hindi and Kannada

There are four major language families represented on the Indian subcontinent: Indo-Aryan (Indic), Dravidian, Austro-Asiatic, and Tibeto-Burman. The Indian branch of the Indo-European family contains Hindi, Marathi, Punjabi, Gujarati, Sindhi, Oriya, and Assamese. These languages are spoken in northern India, Pakistan, and Bangladesh. The Dravidian language family has four major languages: Kannada, Malayalam, Tamil, and Telugu. Approximately 95% of the people in southern India speak these languages. Most of the immigrants from South Asia to the United States speak a language of the Indic or the Dravidian family, and many also speak English very well. Hindi and Kannada have similar vowel systems. Each has five short vowels /a/, /e/, /i/, /o/, and /u/ and their long counterparts. Vowel length is phonemic in Hindi and Kannada. Hindi also has nasalized vowels (Shekar & Hegde, 1995).

Aspiration on a phoneme is often a phonemic difference. So, for example /b/, a voiced bilabial stop is a separate phoneme from an aspirated voiced bila-

Table 9.3 Asian Pacific Languages by Family

Language Family	Languages and Regions
Austroasiatic	• Mon-Khmer branch: Vietnamese, Khmer (Cambodian), and various minority and tribal languages of Southeast Asia • Munda branch: tribal languages of eastern India
Austronesian (also known as Malayo-Polynesian)	• Malay, Indonesian, other languages of Indonesia (Javanese, etc.) • Philippine languages: Tagalog, Ilocano, Bontoc, etc. • Aboriginal languages of Taiwan (Tsou, etc.) • Polynesian languages: Hawaiian, Maori, Samoan, Tahitian, etc. • Micronesian languages: Chamorro (spoken in Guam), Yap, Truk, etc. • Malagasy (spoken in Madagascar)
Altaic	Japanese, Korean
Dravidian	Languages of southern India, including Tamil, Telugu
Mongol	Mongolian, Buryat, Kalmuck, etc.
Sino-Tibetan	• Sinitic branch: Han—several dialects: Mandarin, Wu (Shanghai), Min (Hokkien [Fujian], Taiwanese), Yue (Cantonese), Hakka, Gan, Xiang • Tibeto-Burman branch: Tibetan, Burmese, Hmong, various languages of Burma, China, India, Nepal, and Hindi
Tai-Kadai	Thai, Laos, and other languages of southern China and northern Burma
Turkic	Turkish, Azerbaijani, Kazakh, and other languages of Central Asia
Papuan	Tok Pisin, Motu (in Papua New Guinea)

bial stop [bʰ]. Other phonemes that this may occur for are *t, th, ch, sh, j, d,* and *g*. Additional Indic and Dravidian consonants (not differentiated by aspiration) are also not present in English.

Japanese

Japanese, like Korean, is part of the Altaic language family. It uses five vowels: /a/, /i/, /u/, /e/, /o/, varying in duration; /i/ and /u/ vowels are silent when located between voiceless consonants such as /f/, /h/, /k/. There are 18 consonants, some doubled, as in /kk /and /pp/, and a single final consonant: /n/. The consonants include /k/, /s/, /t/, /n/, /h/, /m/, /ʒ/, /dʒ/, /r/, /w/, /g/, /d/, /b/, /z/, /p/, /ʧ/, /j/, and /ʃ/). Varying combinations of consonants and vowels are used in the formation of syllables. Japanese is polysyllabic and has an elaborate inflectional system. It is not tonal. Every syllable is given equal stress. There are no consonant clusters in initial or final positions of words, or labiodental, interdental, or palatal fricatives. Japanese uses three kinds of stops and fricatives: voiced, tense voiceless, and lax voiceless. The sounds /r/ and /l/ belong to the same phonemic category in allophonic variation. This presents difficulties in English, which uses /l/ and /r/ as two distinct phonemes. Other difficulties encountered by Japanese people learning English are substitutions (s/θ, z/th, j/ʃ, and b/v); addition of vowels to words ending in consonants (desker/desk, milku/milk); and approximations of phonemes (/f/ phoneme is pronounced between /f/ and /h/ such that food sounds similar to hood).

Japanese has numerous grammatical differences with English. The Japanese writing system, which was adopted from the Chinese system, uses characters in writing called Kanji. The Japanese modified the Chinese symbols for phonetic purposes, organizing a syllabary called Kana (Cheng, 1991).

Khmer
This language includes 85 initial consonant clusters, largely different from those of English; aspirated and nonaspirated stops; and two fricatives. Vowels are divided into short and long. Khmer uses sentential intonation patterns, with a steep fall in intonation on final syllables to denote simple affirmative, negative, and interrogative statements. Words are monosyllablic or disyllabic with stress on the second syllable. Syllable types include variable combinations of consonants and vowels. Fifty different vowels and diphthong sounds occur in Khmer, as compared to 17 in English. Even though the vowels are divided into short and long, as in English, the sounds differ in the two languages. Thus, Khmer speakers will have to learn the differences between similar sounds and learn to hear and produce those that are new to them. Khmer speakers learning English will have difficulty with substitution of k/g, v/w, f/b, tʃ/ʃ, s/θ, and t/θ. The /r/ will be approximated as a trill /r/. Many final consonants, such as /r/, /d/, /g/, /s/, /b/, and /z/, will be omitted. The /b/ and /d/ will be implosive, and there will be possible vowel distortion of /ʊ/, /i/, /u/, and /æ/.

Korean
The Korean language belongs to the Altaic family. Koreans in North and South Korea speak the same language with some variations among the various regional dialects. The dialects, however, are mutually intelligible. The Korean written language has 19 consonants and 8 vowels. The sound of a letter is pronounced differently depending upon its location in a word. The phonetic systems of English and Korean are quite different and cause difficulty for Koreans learning to speak English. There are no consonant clusters in the initial and final positions of words in Korean, fricatives and affricates do not occur in the final position of words, and final stops are often nasalized when they occur before a nasal sound (e.g., banman/batman). Korean does not have contrasting vowel length, so the following vowels are problematic: /i/, /I/, /u/, /ʌ/, and /ɔ/. Because there are no labiodental, interdental, or palatal fricatives in Korean, speakers may make the following substitutions: b/v, p/v, s/ʃ, s/z, t/tʃ, and dʒ/ʒ. Because /r/ and /l/ belong to the same phonemic category, they may be used interchangeably (e.g., r/l and l/r).

Laotian or Lao

The Laotian language belongs to the Tai-kadai group. It is unstressed, with six tones (five denoting syllables), including high, rising, rising-falling, falling-rising, falling, and short. There are three syllable types (cvc, cvvc, cvv). Laotian has numerous morphological and syntactical differences with English.

Mandarin

This is the national language of China and is a tonal language. It belongs to the Sino-Tibetan group. Mandarin has 35 initial sounds and 32 final sounds; two sonorants /n/ and /ŋ/, which are final sounds; and no consonant blends.

More than 80 languages and hundreds of dialects are spoken in China. In Mandarin Chinese, there are four tones (and a neutral tone). The first tone has a high level; the second tone is rising; the third tone is falling-rising; and the fourth is falling. The same spoken syllable will have different meanings, depending on the tone and the various characters that the syllable represents. Each Mandarin dialect has its own tonal system with differing numbers of tones. A syllable in Mandarin and Cantonese consists of both segmental and suprasegmental features. Segmental features include an initial consonant (optional) and a final sound. Suprasegmental features include the distinct tones that are an intrinsic part of the phonological makeup of a Chinese syllable. Each character is phonetically represented by a single syllable, and each syllable has a tone mark.

Tagalog and Filipino

Authorities disagree on the exact number of Philippine languages. The Philippine census of 1970 listed 75 mother tongues. All of the languages are from the Malayo-Polynesian group. The major languages are Tagalog, Ilocano, and Visayan. Tagalog is spoken by 25% of the population; Ilocano by 16%; and Visayan by 44% of the total population. There are 27 phonemes in Tagalog: 16 consonant sounds, including the glottal stop ('), 5 vowel sounds, and 6 diphthongs. There is also large-scale borrowing from Spanish and English. A complex system of affixation is used. Words consist of roots, either substantive, verbal, or adjectival, and affixes, which show respect, focus, and mode. The root and affix together are determinants of word meaning. An example of this is plurality, which is marked by the word *mga* placed before the pluralized nominal (e.g., *mga bata* / children) or by another word carrying the concept of plurality (e.g., *dalawang bata* / two child). The Filipino speaker learning English will have difficulty with the marking of plurality, particularly when it is redundant to the context (e.g., "many friends").

Tagalog is a polysyllabic language with its own dialectal variations. The phonetic and syntactical differences between English and Tagalog cause many frustrations for the native Filipino learning English. While many of the Tagalog phonemes are similar to those used in English, nine English phonemes do not occur in Filipino: /v/, /z/, /dʒ/, /θ/, /j/, /f/, /ʃ/, /tʃ/, and /ʒ/. The Philippine speaker substitutes /p/, /b/, /s/, and /t/ for /f/, /v/, /z/, and /ʒ/, respectively, because these sounds closely resemble sounds produced in the Filipino language. Differences in vowel boundaries lead Philippine speakers to have difficulty distinguishing between words like *lift* and *left*.

Vietnamese

Vietnamese is a tonal language that is essentially monosyllabic. It is in the Austro-Asiatic group. There are three dialects: Northern, Southern, and Central. Proficient and educated speakers speak in two forms of Vietnamese, the high (formal) form and the vernacular (informal) form (Chuong, 1990). By comparing English and Vietnamese phonetic systems, the following differences are found: (a) consonant blends occur in all word positions in English, whereas there are no consonant blends in Vietnamese; (b) syllabic stress is used for contrastive purposes in English but is not phonemic in Vietnamese, as lexemes in Vietnamese are typically monosyllabic; (c) English uses many final consonants, whereas Vietnamese uses only a limited number of final consonants, including /p/, /t/, /k/, /m/, /n/, and /ʃ/ (Te, 1987). In the early part of the 20th century, the Vietnamese adopted a modified Romanized alphabet system to replace the old writing system that was based on Chinese characters. Diacritical marks are used to signify the tone of each word. A more indepth review of Vietnamese phonology can be found in an article by Hwa-Froelich, Hodson, and Edwards (2002).

Implications for Education and Assessment

The prevailing views toward education in most Asian Pacific cultures present challenges for American educators and speech–language pathologists. The so-called chopstick cultures (China, Korea, Japan, Vietnam) tend to view education as the most important thing one can achieve in life. This is due largely to the influence of the teachings and principles of Confucius (Cheng, 1993). Others, such as the Lao and Pacific Islanders, do not generally view education as supremely important. The Asian groups often have different approaches to learning, and these approaches have implications for the strategies Asian students use to learn.

Standardized formal assessment procedures are designed to measure discrete areas of language. These procedures are not effective in accounting for cultural and linguistic diversities. The translation of standardized tests into other languages to accommodate the needs of culturally and linguistically diverse students is also inappropriate because many words cannot be translated into another language without losing meaning. Certain key concepts that may be considered common in English may not be common at all in another language. Thus, formal assessment instruments, translated tests, and their interpretive scores are inappropriate for the APA. The following section offers brief principles and guidelines for assessing the APA population. The main purpose of assessment is to identify strengths and weaknesses of the individual, so that appropriate clinical intervention can be provided.

Recommended Procedures

The following are general guidelines for diagnosis, often referred to as the RIOT procedure (Cheng, 1995), adapted here for APA populations:

1. *Review* all pertinent documents and background information:
   - school records (Many Asian countries do not have cumulative school records, and, when available, they would not be in English.)
   - reports (Oral reports are sometimes unreliable, yet they may be the only way to find information, for example, from refugee parents.)
   - medical records (Records may be difficult to obtain; pregnancy and delivery records might not have been kept, especially if the birth was a home birth or in a refugee camp.)
   - teacher's comments
   - social and family background (An interpreter may be needed for this procedure due to the lack of English proficiency of the parents or guardians.)
   - previous therapy or testing results
2. *Interview* teachers, peers, family members, and other informants. Interview questions are available from multiple sources (Cheng, 1990, 1991; Langdon, 1992; Langdon & Saenz, 1996; Westby, 1990).
3. *Observe* student in multiple contexts with a variety of people:
   - Observe interactions at school, both in the classroom and outside.
   - Observe interactions at home. (Some APA families may find it embarrassing to show their home to the visitors and may not be clear on why such a visit is crucial.)
   - Observe interactions in the community.
   - Observe verbal input and comprehension. (Does the parent demonstrate limited proficiency in L1 or in English?)
   - Observe verbal output and language expression. (Does the student mix languages or code-switch?)
   - Observe language preference and dominance. (Do the student's two languages perform different functions—e.g., one performing social functions?)
   - Observe overall level of cognitive function.
   - Observe peer interaction.
   - Observe family dynamics.
4. *Test* both school language and home language:
   - Use informal assessment.
   - Obtain language samples in both languages.
   - Select instruments for assessment battery.

- Adapt formal testing procedure.
- Use alternative scoring.
- Use dynamic assessment.
- Use the portfolio approach by keeping records of the client's performance over time.

The assessment must also consider the child's educational style and history with American teaching style as important factors in adjustment to school and performance on standardized tests. In addition to the general guidelines, the clinician must attempt to collect data that are truly representative of the student's background and experience. In the assessment of a child's communicative competence, educators should view communication as an interactive and dynamic process by addressing the following areas (Langdon & Saenz, 1996):

- curriculum
- language development opportunities
- language competence in both the primary language and the school language
- family communication
- school communication
- health-related problems
- general program options

Within various communicative contexts, the following questions should be answered:

1. How does the client use his language?
2. What purposes do the client's communications serve?
3. Is the client successful in expressing his needs?
4. Are the client's needs met?
5. What is the quality of communication between the client and his communication partners within the family?
6. What kind of communications are present?
7. What is the client capable of communicating?
8. Are there other factors that should be taken into consideration?

Intervention Strategies

What clinicians learn from the assessment should be integrated into their intervention strategies. Intervention should be constructed based on what is most productive for promoting communication and should incorporate the client's personal and cultural experiences. Salient and relevant features of the client's culture should be highlighted to enhance and empower the client. Cheng (1989b) provided culturally relevant strategies for intervention. The following questions provide some insight for clinicians to evaluate the appropriateness of their own strategies:

- Are topics that have social and cultural relevance being used?
- Is the strategy based on the culture and experience of the client?
- How does the strategy help the client develop her communication skills?
- Is the strategy interactive and stimulating?
- Are rules explained explicitly?
- Does the strategy promote a positive attitude toward linguistically and culturally diverse clients?
- Is the family involved in the intervention?

The above questions provide a framework for judging the appropriateness of intervention. Clinicians need to be cognizant of the multiple sociological and psychological difficulties that arise in the conflict of culture, language, and ideology between APA students, their parents, and the American educational system. Cheng (1994, 1999) has provided some helpful strategies for intervention:

- Intervention activities and materials may be selected based on the child's family and cultural background, using activities that are culturally and socially relevant. In addition to traditional intervention techniques of modeling and expansion, the speech–language pathologist may use the following strategies, as discussed by Cheng (1989b) and Heath (1985).
- Alternative strategies may need to be offered when parents are reluctant to sign the IEP forms for services. Inviting them to special classes or speech and languages sessions may be a useful way to provide the needed information.
- Assistance from community leaders and social service providers may also be necessary to convince the parents of the importance of therapy or recommended programs.
- Parents from diverse backgrounds may also be asked to work with parents who are reluctant to accept the school's recommendations. Other parents may be more effective in sharing their personal stories about their children.
- The SLP must have patience with the parents, as they think through the problem, and wait for them to make the decision.

The following sections provide guidelines for therapy sessions.

Personal Life History

SLPs can arouse the interest and attention of their students by sharing a piece of their personal life history. A photograph from childhood, an item from home, or a letter from a friend could spark great interest and curiosity of the students. Students should be encouraged to share their personal life stories using maps, photographs, drawings, and items from home such as food, photographs, and letters.

Narratives

A narrative is a type of expanded discourse, classified as a recounting, an account, an event cast, or a story (Heath, 1983). Narratives can occur in oral or written form. The construction and discussion of narratives is a current popular methodology in language intervention. Students can work together on a collective narrative for group presentation. A shared experience, such a field trip or a school game, can be used to provide a topic of discussion and writing. Computers can be used to help store and retrieve the stories, as well as to make changes. The speaker may also provide information that is new to the listener. Activities such as "Show and Tell" are a type of narratives called accounting. Objects from home can be useful intervention materials. Clients could bring special items of clothing and explain how the items are worn and what they may symbolize. The class could take turns trying on and modeling the different clothes. Other items for sharing include recipes, games, jewelry, and artwork or crafts.

During or before a play activity, the speaker can be encouraged to provide a narrative of an event currently shared with the listener. For example, children may talk about what is happening as they play with toys.

Children's literature is currently serving a major function in language intervention. The child is asked to talk about, retell, fill in blanks, or answer questions about a story. For example, folk tales, fairytales, stories about historical figures and events, biographical and current events stories are all materials for teaching children about human experiences (Cheng, 1999; Van Dongen & Westby, 1986). Stories relevant to the client's experiences should be used so that the client is not expected to retell a story that uses concepts and terms with which he is not familiar.

Cultural and Linguistic Capsules and Clusters

Capsules are unique elements of a culture, and clusters are activities and events that are practiced in a culture, such as Easter. Capsules and clusters are inherent within each culture. Although they may appear to be obvious examples of familiar elements and events, children with language disorders can benefit from additional structuring and organization (Cheng, 1989a). The concepts of capsules and clusters can be applied to language structure. For example, a cluster could be organized around a core verb such as *run* ("run for office," "runner," "running," etc.). A capsule could be represented by the word *shower* ("baby shower," "sudden shower," "cold shower," etc.).

Role Playing

The following roles are suggested, each of which might be tailored to reflect important aspects of the child's new environment: teacher–student, salesperson–customer, parent–child, older sibling–younger sibling, and child–child. Role playing will allow the child to learn routine exchanges, practice language skills, and change roles so that she can experience an exchange from different perspectives.

Script Writing for Pragmatic Activities

The following are suggestions for event scripts that can be used for therapy: attending a birthday party, sharing a story, asking for direction, greeting a friend, accepting compliments, making telephone calls, and joint activities such as games (e.g., Monopoly, Scrabble). In sum, the following are specific guiding principles to enrich language learning in real-life contexts (Cheng, 1994, 1999):

- Language learning is continuous, and students should be encouraged to participate in high-interest activities with low risk and low anxiety context.
- Language activities should be experiential and relevant.
- Natural support systems should be sought out, and students should be allowed to have self-selecting cooperative groups.

Conclusion: Asian Pacific Islander American Students

As the nation becomes more diverse, better understanding of the challenges facing speech–language pathologists is of paramount importance. This chapter attempted to answer the following questions:

- Who are the APA?
- What are APA cultures?
- Where is Asia Pacific?
- What are the main languages spoken in Asia Pacific?
- What are the guiding principles for assessment?
- What are the implications for intervention?

It is hoped that the information presented will help readers to lay a solid foundation for further exploring the client's strengths and weaknesses. When assessment procedures are guided by the general principles given here, and when assessors take into consideration the cultural and pragmatic variables of an individual's background and culture, the results should be less biased. When culturally relevant and appropriate approaches are employed, the outcome of enhancing appropriate language and communication behaviors, home language, and literacy can be achieved.

The following Web sites are resources for APA populations:

- http://www.krysstal.com
- http://www.dictionaries.travlang.com

- http://www.sil.org/ethnologue/com
- http://www.zompist.com/langfaq.html

Web site information was verified July 26, 2005.

CHAPTER CONCLUSION

This chapter has presented information concerning the linguistic character-istics, culture, and family values of African Americans, Hispanic/Latinos, and Asian Pacific Americans. Across the three sections, there is valuable informa-tion regarding the diagnostic process and intervention. The information pro-vided is not all inclusive. Not all languages were included (for example, only selected Asian Pacific Island languages were covered), nor were all dialects con-sidered. Information will continually be added as more studies are completed. As noted in the introduction, the demographics of the United States are chang-ing, and this is clearly reflected within our public schools. In its document "Knowledge and Skills Needed by Speech–Language Pathologists and Audi-ologists To Provide Culturally and Linguistically Appropriate Services," ASHA defines key terms and outlines the knowledge base necessary for diagnosis and treatment of culturally and linguistically diverse clients (ASHA, 2004). Ad-ditional information can be found on the ASHA Web site or by using a search engine like Google or Yahoo.

STUDY QUESTIONS

African American Students
1. Name an existing standardized test for receptive vocabulary that is consid-ered by some researchers to be culturally fair for AAE speakers.
2. Discuss one way in which the language development of an AAE speaker is different from that of an SAE speaker. Discuss one way they are similar.
3. Name some characteristics of a CCSLP.
4. What are some strategies for providing a culturally competent assessment? Culturally sensitive intervention?
5. What are some questions that a CCSLP must ask when selecting a standardized test for administration to an AAE speaker?

Hispanic and Latino Students
1. List the arguments supporting the use of each term, *Latino* and *Hispanic*.
2. List five cultural values described by Brice and indicate their implications for you as a professional.
3. Describe ethnographic interviewing.
4. What are three differences in Spanish and English that may present diffi-culty to children learning English as a second language?

5. What are some testing modifications that can be used?
6. What are issues to consider when using a Spanish version of a standardized test?
7. Describe two informal testing procedures.

Asian Pacific Islander American Students

1. Describe the "push–pull" dilemma often experienced by APA individuals.
2. Explain why it would be important to have knowledge of religion, folk beliefs, and views on medicine when interacting with APA families. Give a specific example.
3. Describe the RIOT strategy for evaluation and how you would implement it.
4. Describe four intervention strategies for APA and how they would be used.
5. List three specific ways that a child's culture can be incorporated into therapy.

REFERENCES

African American Students

Adger, C. T., Schilling-Estes, N., & Wolfram, W. (2003). *African American English: Structure and clinical implications.* Retrieved on September 2, 2005 from http://www.asha.org/about/continuing-ed/ASHA-courses/CDR7120.htm

American Speech-Language-Hearing Association. (1983). Position paper: Social dialects and implications of position on social dialects. *Asha, 25,* 23–27.

American Speech-Language-Hearing Association. (2001). *Serving a multicultural population.* Retrieved October 18, 2005, from http://www.asha.org

American Speech-Language-Hearing Association. (2002). Assessment tool offers culturally fair evaluation. *ASHA Leader, 7*(23), 17.

American Speech-Language-Hearing Association. (2003). Technical report: American English dialects. *ASHA Supplement, 23,* 45–46.

American Speech-Language-Hearing Joint Subcommittee of the Executive Board on English Language Proficiency. (1998). Students and professionals who speak English with accents and nonstandard dialects: Issues and recommendations. Position statement and technical report. *Asha, 40*(Suppl. 18), 28–31.

Banks, J. (1999). Multicultural education in the new century. *School Administrator, 56,* 4–7.

Battle, D. (1996). Language learning and use by African American children. *Topics in Language Disorders, 16*(4), 22–37.

Battle, D. (2000). Becoming a culturally competent clinician. *Language Learning and Education, 7*(3), 20–23.

Battle, D. (2002a, March). *Developing culturally competent clinicians.* Paper presented at the Annual Spring Conference, State University College of New York at Cortland, Cortland, NY.

Battle, D. (2002b). Language development and disorders in culturally and linguistically diverse children. In D. Bernstein & E. Tiegerman-Faber (Eds.), *Language and communication disorders in children* (5th ed.; pp. 354–386). Boston: Allyn & Bacon.

Battle, D., & Grantham, R. (1997). Serving culturally and linguistically diverse students. In P. O'Connell (Ed.), *Speech language and hearing programs in schools: A guide for students and practitioners* (pp. 345–371). Gaithersburg, MD: Aspen.

Center for Applied Linguistics. (1997). *Policy statement of the TESOL board on African American vernacular English.* Retrieved July 25, 2005, from http://www.cal.org/ebonics/tesolebo.html

Craig, H., & Washington, J. (2000). An assessment battery for identifying language impairments in African American children. *Journal of Speech, Language and Hearing Research, 43,* 366–379.

Craig, H., & Washington, J. (2002). Oral language expectations for African American preschoolers and kindergartners. *American Journal of Speech–Language Pathology, 11,* 59–70.

Gardner, M. F. (1990). *Expressive One-Word Picture Vocabulary Test.* Novato, CA: Academic Therapy.

Goldstein, B. (2000). *Cultural and linguistic diversity resource guide for speech–language pathologists.* San Diego, CA: Singular.

Graham, L. (1999). *Our kind of people: Inside America's black upper class.* New York: Harper Collins.

Gutierrez-Clellen, V., & Peña, E. (2001). Dynamic assessment of diverse children: A tutorial. *Language, Speech, and Hearing Services in Schools, 32,* 212–224.

Haynes, W., & Moran, M. (1989). A cross-sectional developmental study of final consonant production in southern Black children from preschool through third grade. *Language, Speech, and Hearing Services in Schools, 20,* 400–406.

Haynes, W., Moran, M., & Pindzola, R. (1999). *Communication disorders in the classroom: An introduction for professionals in school settings.* Dubuque, IA: Kendal/Hunt.

Hefflin, B., & Barksdale-Ladd, M. (2001). African American children's literature that helps students find themselves: Selection guidelines for grades K–3. *The Reading Teacher, 54,* 810–819.

Hulit, L., & Howard, M. (2001). *Born to talk: An introduction to speech and language development.* Needham Heights, MA: Allyn & Bacon.

Jackson, S., & Roberts, J. (2001). Complex syntax production of African American preschoolers. *Journal of Speech, Language and Hearing Research, 44,* 1083–1096.

LeMoine, N. (2001). Language variation and literacy acquisition in African American students. In J. Jarris, A. Kamhi, & K. Pollock (Eds.), *Literacy in African American communities* (pp. 169–194). Mahwah, NJ: Erlbaum.

Linguistic Society of America. (1997). *LSA resolution on the Oakland "Ebonics" issue.* Retrieved July 25, 2005, from http://www.lsadc.org/resolutions/ebonics.htm.

Lue, M. (2001). *A survey of communication disorders for the classroom teacher.* Needham Heights, MA: Allyn & Bacon.

Oetting, J., & McDonald, J. (2001). Nonmainstream dialect use and specific language impairment. *Journal of Speech, Language and Hearing Research, 44,* 207–228.

Owens, R. (1999). *Language disorders: A functional approach to assessment and intervention* (3rd ed.). Needham Heights, MA: Allyn & Bacon.

Paul, R. (2001). *Language disorders from infancy through adolescence, assessment and intervention* (2nd ed.). St. Louis, MO: Mosby.

Peña, E., & Quinn, R. (1997). Task familiarity: Effects on the test performance of Puerto Rican and African American children. *Language, Speech, and Hearing Services in Schools, 28,* 323–332.

Quails, C., & Harris, J. (1999). Effects of familiarity on idiom comprehension in African American and European American fifth graders. *Language, Speech, and Hearing Services in Schools, 30,* 141–151.

Roseberry-McKibbin, C. (1995). *Multicultural students with special language needs.* Oceanside, CA: Academic Communication Associates.

Roseberry-McKibbin, C., & Hegde, M. N. (2000). *An advanced review of speech–language pathology: Preparation for NESPA and comprehensive examination.* Austin, TX: PRO-ED.

Seymour, H., Abdulkarim, M., & Johnson, V. (1999). The Ebonics controversy: An educational and clinical dilemma. *Topics in Language Disorders, 4*, 66–77.

Seymour, H., Bland-Stewart, L., & Green, L. (1998). Difference versus deficit in child African American English. *Language, Speech, and Hearing Services in Schools, 29*, 96–108.

Seymour, H. N., Roeper, T., deVilliers, J., & deVilliers, P. (2003). *Diagnostic evaluation of language variation–Criterion referenced.* San Antonio, TX: Harcourt Assessment.

Seymour, H. N., Roeper, T. W., deVilliers, J., & deVilliers, P. (2005). *Diagnostic Evaluation of Language Variance (DELV)–Norm Referenced.* San Antonio, TX: Harcourt Assessment.

Stockman, I. (1986). Language acquisition in culturally diverse populations: The Black child as case study. In O. Taylor (Ed.), *Nature of communication disorders in culturally and linguistically diverse populations* (pp. 117–155). San Diego, CA: College-Hill Press.

Stockman, I. (1996). Phonological development and disorders in African American children. In A. Kamhi, K. Pollock, & J. Harris (Eds.), *Communication development and disorders in African American children* (pp. 117–153). Baltimore: Brookes.

Stockman, I., & Settle, S. (1991, November). *Initial consonants in young Black children's conversational speech.* Poster presented at the meeting of the American Speech-Language-Hearing Association, Atlanta, GA.

Stockman, I., & Vaughn-Cooke, F. (1982). Semantic categories in the language of working-class Black children. *Proceedings of the Second International Child Language Conference, 1*, 312–327.

Stone-Goldman, J., & Olswang, L. (2003). Learning to look, learning to see: Using ethnography to develop cultural sensitivity. *ASHA Leader, 8*(5), 6–7, 14–15.

Tatum, A. (2000). Breaking down barriers that disenfranchise African American adolescent readers in low-level tracks. *Journal of Adolescent and Adult Literacy, 44*, 52–56.

Terrell, S., Arensberg, K., & Rosa, M. (1992). Parent–child comparative analysis: A criterion-referenced method for the nondiscriminatory assessment of a child who spoke a relatively uncommon dialect of English. *Language, Speech, and Hearing Services in Schools, 23*, 34–42.

Terrell, S., Battle, D., & Grantham, R. (1998). African American cultures. In D. Battle (Ed.), *Communication disorders in multicultural populations* (2nd ed.; pp. 31–71). Newton, MA: Butterworth-Heinemann.

Terrell, S., & Jackson, R. (2002). African Americans in the Americas. In D. Battle (Ed.), *Communication disorders in multicultural populations* (3rd ed.; pp. 33–70). Woburn, MA: Butterworth-Heinemann.

Terrell, S., & Terrell, F. (1996). The importance of psychological and sociocultural factors for providing clinical services to African American children. In A. Kahmi, K. Pollock, & J. Harris (Eds.), *Communication development and disorders in African American children* (pp. 55–72). Baltimore: Brookes.

Thorndike, R. L., Hagen, E. P., & Sattler, J. M. (1986). *Stanford-Binet Intelligence Scale.* Chicago: Riverside.

Uffen, E. (2001). Becoming a culturally competent clinician. *Asha Leader, 6*(6), 1, 8.

Van Keulen, J., Weddington, G., & DeBose, E. (1998). *Speech, language, learning and the African American child.* Needham Heights, MA: Allyn & Bacon.

Vaughn-Cooke, F. B. (1983). Improving language assessment in minority children. *Asha, 25*, 29–34.

Washington, J., & Craig, H. (1992). Articulation test performances of low-income African-American preschoolers with communication impairments. *Language, Speech, and Hearing Services in Schools, 23*, 203–207.

Washington, J., & Craig, H. (1994). Dialectal forms during discourse of urban, African American preschoolers living in poverty. *Journal of Speech and Hearing Research, 37*, 816–823.

Washington, J., & Craig, H. (1998). Socioeconomic status and gender influences on children's dialectal variations. *Journal of Speech and Hearing Research, 38,* 618–626.

Washington, J., & Craig, H. (1999). Performances of at-risk, African American preschoolers on the Peabody Picture Vocabulary Test–III. *Language, Speech, and Hearing Services in Schools, 30,* 75–82.

Washington, J., Craig, H., & Kushmaul, A. (1998). Variable use of African American English across two language sampling contexts. *Journal of Speech and Hearing Research, 38,* 1115–1124.

Wolfram, W. (1997). *Ebonics and linguistic science: Clarifying the issues.* Retrieved July 25, 2005, from the Center for Applied Linguistics Web site: http://www.cal.org/ebonics/wolfram.html

Wyatt, T. (1995). Language development in African-American English child speech. *Linguistics and Education, 7,* 13–15.

Wyatt, T. (1998). Children's language development. In C. Seymour & E. H. Nober (Eds.), *Introduction to communication disorders: A multicultural approach* (pp. 58–69). Newton, MA: Butterworth-Heinemann.

Hispanic and Latino Students

American Speech-Language-Hearing Association. (2002). *Communication development and disorders in multicultural populations: Readings and related materials.* Retrieved October 18, 2005, from http://www.professional.asha.org

Anderson, R. T. (2002). Practical assessment strategies with Hispanic students. In A. Brice (Ed.), *The Hispanic child* (pp. 143–184). Boston: Allyn & Bacon.

Brice, A. (2002). *The Hispanic child.* Boston: Allyn & Bacon.

Brice, A., Roseberry-McKibbin, C., & Kayser, H. (1997, November). *Special language needs of linguistically and culturally diverse students.* Paper presented at the annual meeting of the American Speech-Language-Hearing Association, Boston, MA.

Dikeman, K., & Riquelme, L. F. (October, 2002). Ethnocultural concerns in dysphagia management. *Perspectives on Swallowing and Swallowing Disorders, 11*(3), 31–35.

Doyle, R. (1982). *Hispanics in New York: Religious, cultural and social experiences* (Vol. 1). New York: Office of Pastoral Research, Archdiocese of New York.

Erickson, J. G., & Iglesias, A. (1986). Assessment of communication disorders in non–English proficient children. In O. Taylor (Ed.), *Nature of communication disorders in culturally and linguistically diverse populations* (pp. 181–218). San Diego, CA: College-Hill Press.

Goldstein, B. (1995). Spanish phonological development. In H. Kayser (Ed.), *Bilingual speech–language pathology: An Hispanic focus.* San Diego, CA: Singular.

Goldstein, B. (2000). *Cultural and linguistic diversity resource guide for speech–language pathologists.* San Diego, CA: Singular.

Goldstein, B., & Iglesias, A. (1996). Phonological patterns in Puerto Rican Spanish–speaking children with phonological disorders. *Journal of Communication Disorders, 29,* 367–387.

Goldstein, B., & Iglesias, A. (2001). The effects of dialect on phonological analysis: Evidence from Spanish-speaking children. *American Journal of Speech–Language Pathology, 10,* 394–406.

Gutierrez-Clellen, V. F. (1999). Language choice in intervention with bilingual children. *American Journal of Speech–Language Pathology, 8,* 291–302.

Hayes-Bautista, D. E., & Chapa, J. (1987). Latino terminology: Conceptual bases for standardized terminology. *American Journal of Public Health, 77,* 61–68.

Iglesias, A., & Goldstein, B. (1998). Dialectal variations. In J. Bernthal & N. Bankson (Eds.), *Articulation and phonological disorders* (4th ed.). Needham Heights, MA: Allyn & Bacon.

Kayser, H. (1989). Speech and language assessment of Spanish–English-speaking children. *Language, Speech, and Hearing Services in Schools, 20,* 226–244.

Kayser, H. (1995a). *Bilingual speech–language pathology: An Hispanic focus*. San Diego, CA: Singular.

Kayser, H. (1995b). Interpreters. In H. Kayser (Ed.), *Bilingual speech–language pathology: An Hispanic focus*. San Diego, CA: Singular.

Kayser, H., & Restrepo, M. A. (1995). Language samples: Elicitation and analysis. In H. Kayser (Ed.), *Bilingual speech–language pathology: An Hispanic focus*. San Diego, CA: Singular.

Langdon, H. W. (2002). *Interpreters and translators in communication disorders: A practitioner's handbook*. Eau Claire, WI: Thinking Publications.

Langdon, H. W., & Cheng, L. L. (1992). *Hispanic children and adults with communication disorders: Assessment and intervention*. Gaithersburg, MD: Aspen.

Marin, G., & Marin, B. (1991). Hispanics: Who are they? In G. Marin and B. Marin (Eds.), *Research with Hispanic populations* (pp. 1–17). Beverly Hills, CA: Sage.

McCauley, R. J. (1996). Familiar strangers: Criterion-referenced measures in communications disorders. *Language, Speech, and Hearing Services in Schools, 29*, 3–10.

McCauley, R. J., & Swisher, L. (1984a). Psychometric review of language and articulation tests for preschool children. *Journal of Speech and Hearing Disorders, 49*, 34–42.

McCauley, R. J., & Swisher, L. (1984b). Use and misuse of norm-referenced tests in clinical assessment: A hypothetical case. *Journal of Speech and Hearing Disorders, 49*, 338–348.

Peña, E., Bedore, L., & Rappazzo, C. (2003). Comparison of Spanish, English, and bilingual children's performance across semantic tasks. *Language, Speech, and Hearing Services in Schools, 34*, 5–16.

Peña, E., Iglesias, A., & Lidz, C. S. (2001). Reducing test bias through dynamic assessment of children's word learning ability. *American Journal of Speech–Language Pathology 10*, 138–154.

Peña, E., Quinn, R., & Iglesias, A. (1992). The application of dynamic methods to language assessment: A non-biased procedure. *Journal of Special Education, 26*, 269–280.

Restrepo, M. A. (1997). Guidelines for identifying primarily Spanish-speaking preschool children with language impairment. *ASHA Special Interest Division 14 Newsletter, 3*, 11–12.

Riquelme, L. F. (in press). Multicultural issues and aging. *Perspectives on Geriatrics*.

Rodriguez, B. L., & Olswang, L. B. (2003). Mexican-American and Anglo-American mothers' beliefs and values about child rearing, education and language impairment. *American Journal of Speech–Language Pathology, 12*, 452–465.

Roseberry-McKibbin, C. (1995). *Multicultural students with special language needs—Practical strategies for assessment and intervention*. Oceanside, CA: Academic Communication Associates.

Roseberry-McKibbin, C. (2002). Principles and strategies in intervention. In A. Brice (Ed.), *The Hispanic child*. Boston: Allyn & Bacon.

Treviño, F. M. (1987). Standardized terminology for Hispanic populations. *American Journal of Public Health, 77*, 69–72.

Ukrainetz, T. A., Harpell, S., Walsh, C., & Coyle, C. (2000). A preliminary investigation of dynamic assessment with Native American kindergarteners. *Language, Speech, and Hearing Services in Schools, 31*, 142–154.

U.S. Bureau of the Census. (2000a). *Population estimates*. Retrieved on August 31, 2005, from http://www.census.gov/prod/cen2000/dpl/2k00.pdf

U.S. Bureau of the Census. (2000b). *Statistical abstract of the United States* (119th ed.). Washington, DC: U.S. Department of Commerce.

Wallace, G. L. (1997). *Multicultural neurogenics: A resource for speech–language pathologists*. San Antonio, TX: Communication Skill Builders.

Westby, C. E. (1990). Ethnographic interviewing: Asking the right questions to the right people in the right ways. *Journal of Childhood Communication Disorders, 13*(1), 101–111.

Yankauer, A. (1987). Hispanic/Latino: What's in a name? *American Journal of Public Health, 77*, 15–17.

Asian Pacific Islander American

American Speech-Language-Hearing Association. (2004). Knowledge and skills needed by speech–language pathologists and audiologists to provide culturally and linguistically appropriate services, *ASHA* (Suppl. 24). Retrieved September 1, 2005, from http://www.asha.org/NR/rdonlyres/BA28BD9C-26BA-46E7-9A47-5A7BDA2A4713/0/v4scultlinguistic2004.pdf

Chang, I. (2003). *The Chinese in America: A narrative history*. New York: Viking Press.

Cheng, L. L. (1989a). Intervention strategies: A multicultural approach. *Topics in Language Disorders, 9*(3), 84–91.

Cheng, L. L. (1989b). Service delivery to Asian/Pacific LEP children: A cross-cultural framework. *Topics in Language Disorders, 9*(3), 1–14.

Cheng, L. L. (1990). The identification of communicative disorders in Asian-Pacific students. *Journal of Child Communicative Disorders, 13*, 113–119.

Cheng, L. L. (1991). *Assessing Asian language performance: Guidelines for evaluating LEP students* (2nd ed.). Oceanside, CA: Academic Communication Associates.

Cheng, L. L. (1993). Deafness: An Asian/Pacific Island perspective. In K. M. Christensen & G. L. Delgado (Eds.), *Multicultural issues in deafness* (pp. 113–126). White Plains, NY: Longman.

Cheng, L. (1994). Difficult discourse: An untold Asian story. In D. N. Ripich & N. A. Creaghead (Eds.), *School discourse problems* (2nd ed., pp. 155–170). San Diego, CA: Singular.

Cheng, L. L. (Ed.). (1995). *Integrating language and learning for inclusion: An Asian-Pacific focus*. San Diego, CA: Singular.

Cheng, L. L. (1999). Sociocultural adjustment of Chinese-American students. In C. Par & M. M. Chi (Eds.), *Asian-American education*. Westport, CT: Bergin & Garvey.

Cheng, L. L. (2004). The challenge of hyphenated identity. *Topics in Language Disorders, 24*, 216–224.

Chinn, P. (1990, June). *Multiculturalism in California*. Paper presented at the Conference on Multicultural Deafness, San Diego, CA.

Chuong, C. (1990, September). *The speech island: A Vietnamese perspective*. Paper presented at the Asian Language Conference, Hacienda Heights, CA.

Fadiman, A. (1997). *When the spirit catches you and you fall down*. New York: Noonday Press.

Fong, T. (1994). *The first suburban Chinatown*. Philadelphia: Temple University Press.

Goldstein, B., & Iglesias, A. (2001). The effects of dialect on phonological analysis: Evidence from Spanish-speaking children. *American Journal of Speech-Language Pathology, 10*, 394–406.

Gollnick, D. M., & Chinn, P. C. (1990). *Multicultural education in a pluralistic society*. New York: Merrill/Macmillan.

Heath, S. B. (1983). *Ways with words*. New York: Cambridge University Press.

Heath, S. B. (1985, November). *Second language acquisition*. Paper presented at the American Speech-Language-Hearing Association Convention, San Francisco, CA.

Hwa-Froelich, D., Hodson, B. W., & Edwards, H. T. (2002). Characteristics of Vietnamese phonology. *American Journal of Speech–Language Pathology, 11*, 264–273.

Jiobu, R. M. (1996). Recent Asian Pacific immigrants: The Asian Pacific background. In B. O. Hing & R. Lee (Eds.), *The state of Asian Pacific America: Reframing the immigration debate* (pp. 59–126). Los Angeles: Leadership Education for Asian Pacifics.

Kingston, M. H. (1976). *The woman warrior: Memoirs of a girlhood among ghosts*. New York: Random House.

Langdon, H. (1992). Language communication and sociocultural patterns in Hispanic families. In H. Langdon, & L. L. Cheng (Eds.), *Hispanic children and adults with communication disorders: Assessment and intervention* (pp. 99–131). Gaithersburg, MD: Aspen.

Langdon, H. W., & Saenz, T. I. (1996). *Language assessment and intervention with multicultural students: A guide for speech-language-hearing professionals.* Oceanside, CA: Academic Communication Associates.

Liu, E. (1998). *Accidental Asian.* New York: Random House.

National Center for Education Statistics. (1997). *The condition of education, 1997.* Washington, DC: U.S. Department of Education.

Ortiz-Monasterio, F., & Serrano, R. A. (1971). Cultural aspects of cleft lip and palate treatment. In W. C. Grabb, S. W. Rosenstein, & K. R. Bzoch (Eds.), *Cleft lip and palate: Surgical, dental, and speech aspects* (pp. 130–141). Boston: Little, Brown.

Report to the Congress: Proposed Refugee Admissions for FY 2005. (2005). Washington DC: U.S. Department of State, U.S. Department of Homeland Security, U.S. Department of Health and Human Services, 2004.

Shekar, C., & Hegde, M. N. (1995). India: Its people, culture, and languages. In L. L. Cheng (Ed.), *Integrating language and learning for inclusion* (pp. 125–148). San Diego, CA: Singular.

Shekar, C., & Hegde, M. N. (1996). Cultural and linguistic diversity among Asian Indians: A case of Indian English. *Topics in Language Disorders, 16*(4), 54–64.

Strauss, R. P. (1985). Culture, rehabilitation and facial birth defects: International case studies. *Cleft Palate Journal, 22,* 56–62.

Takaki, R. (1989). *Strangers from a different shore.* Boston: Little, Brown.

Tan, A. (1989). *The joy luck club.* New York: Putnam.

Te, H. D. (1987). *Introduction to Vietnamese culture.* San Diego, CA: Multifunctional Resource Center, San Diego State University.

Thuy, L. T. D. (2003). *The gangster we are all looking for.* New York: Knopf.

Trueba, H. T., Jacobs, L., & Kirton, E. S. (1990). *Cultural conflict and adaptation: The case of Hmong children in American society.* New York: Falmer.

Van Dongen, R., & Westby, C. (1986). Building the narrative mode of thought through children's literature. *Topics in Language Disorders, 7*(1), 70–83.

Westby, C. (1990). Ethnographic interviewing: Asking the right questions to the right people in the right ways. *Journal of Childhood Communication Disorders, 13*(1), 101–111.

Young, R. (1998). Becoming American: Coping strategies of Asian Pacific American children. In V. O. Pang & L. L. Cheng (Eds.), *Struggling to be heard.* Albany: State University of New York Press.

Chapter 10

◆ ◆

Third-Party Payments, Supervision, and Support Personnel

Mary Ann O' Brien

The purpose of this chapter is to acquaint the reader with several key areas of current concern. The three topics of third-party payments, supervision, and support personnel share a core of administrative involvement. They are also important for the school practitioner. Each one provides evidence of the increasing complexity of the school environment as a service delivery site, as well as the concomitant demands on the school speech–language pathologist to be a broadly educated and well-informed professional.

THIRD-PARTY REIMBURSEMENT

Although the intent of the laws that enable government-supported education for children with disabilities is noble, the reality is that Congress has never adequately provided the needed level of funding to support services and programs. This has created financial difficulty for local school districts. Out of need, schools have had to seek alternative methods of funding programs to help defray expenses for providing education and services to students with disabilities. Billing third-party payers for speech–language pathology and audiology services has long been an accepted practice in health-care agencies and in private practice. In 1976, the federal government legislated access to third-party money for these services in schools. Although the possibility of bringing in additional funding for overburdened educational systems was enticing, it took several years for schools to understand the law and to undertake the complicated processes involved in collection and billing.

History

In 1975, Public Law No. 94-142, the Education for All Handicapped Children Act, was passed. It ensured the provision of a free and appropriate public education for all children at no cost to parents. The key phrase is "at no cost to parents." In 1977, the regulations interpreting the act were published. They indicated that states could use whatever state, local, federal, and private monies were available to meet the requirement of providing a free and appropriate public education. In spite of this clearly articulated intent, many third-party payers interpreted the law and regulations to mean that provision and funding of services were the responsibility of the schools and responded by discontinuing payment for services for children. Medicaid specifically denied payment for any services required in a child's Individualized Education Program (IEP), even if the child was eligible for Medicaid services (Wolf, 1991). This refusal to reimburse extended to the hospital and private practice settings, where it was Medicaid's position that speech–language pathology and audiology services for school-aged children were automatically educational and thus should be funded by education rather than health-care funds.

In 1980, the Office of Special Education and the Office of Civil Rights, both in the U.S. Department of Education, jointly published a *Notice of Interpretation* saying that private insurance could be used by an educational agency only if parents incurred no financial loss and if their participation was voluntary. The inference was that private insurance could be used with parents' consent if they suffered no financial loss. Using this interpretation, a private agency in Illinois, the Trans-Allied Medical Educational Services, Inc. (TAMES), was established and worked very successfully with school districts in the state to obtain reimbursement for speech–language and audiology services provided in an education setting. The use of private insurance, however, can be hazardous. We will discuss this later in this section.

In 1986, Congress passed Public Law No. 99-457, the Education of the Handicapped Act Amendments (title changed in 1991 to Individuals with Disabilities Act—IDEA). It addressed the Medicaid funding issue and expanded special education and related services to children ages 3 to 5 years. It also added a new part, the Handicapped Infants and Toddlers Early Intervention Program (Part H), which encouraged states to provide early intervention services for handicapped infants and toddlers at no cost. Congress indicated that with the passage of Public Law No. 99-457, it was the policy of the United States to provide financial assistance to states to facilitate the coordination of payment for early intervention services from federal, state, local, and private sources, including public and private insurance coverage (American Speech-Language-Hearing Association [ASHA], 1991). Part H also indicated that Part H funds were to be used as the "payer of last resort." No one was volunteering to be the payer of first resort.

In 1988, Public Law No. 100-360, the Medicare Catastrophic Coverage Act, was passed. Its purpose was to establish catastrophic coverage to pay for extended hospital stays and prescription drugs for older people. Unfortunately, the cost was prohibitive, and the act was eventually repealed. However, that act contained a Medicaid technical provision that was not overturned when the act was repealed. It notes that state education agencies are financially responsible for educational services. In the case of a Medicaid-eligible handicapped child, state Medicaid agencies remain responsible for the "related services" identified in the child's IEP if those services are covered under the state's Medicaid plan. Clearly, Congress is saying that Medicaid has to pay.

The last barrier to payment of Medicaid money for provision of certain related services in schools was eliminated in 1990, when the Health Care Financing Administration (HCFA) reversed its 1984 stance and proposed regulations that would cover services that are medical and remedial in nature. It still held that educational services are not reimbursable but defined educational services as pertaining to traditional academic subjects, such as science, history, literature, foreign language, and mathematics, and also talked about vocational services. This change in position was triggered by both the passage of Public Law No. 99-457 and a lost lawsuit in Massachusetts, in which the court ruled that determination of whether a service is educational should rest on the nature of the service and not on the state's method of administering the service (ASHA, 1992b).

Informed Consent

In its 1990 report to its Legislative Council, ASHA's Governmental Affairs Committee recommended that speech–language pathologists and audiologists know about informed-consent procedures and promote the use of the following guidelines by school administrators for informing parents:

- The IEP must be developed and signed before the family is requested to authorize third-party payments.
- The parent must grant informed written consent to allow the school to bill medical insurance.
- The family should be informed in writing of the following facts:
    1. There is a risk to their lifetime health insurance cap if their insurance is used to pay for services in the schools.
    2. Consent to bill third-party payers is purely voluntary.
    3. Consent or lack of consent to bill third-party payers will not alter the quality, type, duration, or manner of speech–language pathology or audiology services that the child needs and receives.
    4. The child will receive all necessary speech–language pathology or audiology services even if the parents deny consent to bill third-party payers.
- Speech–language pathologists and audiologists should recommend that as part of the informed-consent process, schools provide families with a written projection of the amount expected to be billed to the family insurance. In addition, the amount actually billed to the insurance company must be disclosed to the family.

Private Third-Party Payers

Initially, there was confusion about whether and when schools could access private insurance money, but in 1980, through a *Notice of Interpretation*, the U.S. Department of Education notified states that Part B of IDEA and Section 504 of the Rehabilitation Act of 1973, and their implementing regulations, allow use of private insurance when parents incur no financial loss and when the use of that insurance is voluntary.

Wolf (1991) wrote that private health insurance carriers will not allow their potential liabilities to increase and that the billing of private third-party payers for "related services" in the schools has had negative repercussions. He noted that health insurance plans that do provide coverage designate limits on the amount of treatment. Insurance plans also have a lifetime cap specifying the total dollar amount that the plan will cover over an individual's lifetime. If payments for "related services" in the schools reach the lifetime cap, a child may be left without health care coverage for the rest of his life. Wolf and others argued that risking the lifetime cap in this manner violates the child's right to free public education. Accessing private health insurance remains voluntary for the parents and a risk to future insurance benefits.

Inasmuch as federal law allows the billing of private insurance companies, and inasmuch as Medicaid is the payer of last resort, many schools are investigating the use of private insurance before accessing Medicaid monies. However, it should be noted that many insurance companies (third-party payers) have policies that state that services provided by schools under IDEA are not covered, and therefore reimbursement requests are denied (ASHA, 2003). When dealing with insurance, speech–language pathologists and audiologists must be aware of coinsurance and deductible insurance requirements. School districts must absorb these costs for children ages 3 through 21 years, on the basis of the "free and appropriate public education" language in Public Law No. 94-142 (ASHA, 1991). Speech–language pathologists and audiologists must also know individual state requirements for students from birth to 2 years 11 months (early intervention). If insurance problems occur for an individual family, that family may have to bring suit against the school district to attempt to recoup damages. Employees of that district should be as aware of the requirements of the law in these cases as is the administration. Ignorance is never an excuse.

Issues

No radical change of national proportions flows smoothly at its onset. Third-party billing for certain related services in schools is no exception. Speech–language pathologists and audiologists have become competitors for third-party funds. Members of the professions "took sides," depending on their work site. Those in favor of schools' billing said that the possible benefits included

- additional money for an overburdened educational system
- money for schools and programs in need
- more favorable budgetary consideration for speech–language pathologists and audiologists because of the funds resulting from their work
- increased number of qualified providers, triggered by the incentive to raise the requirements for school speech–language pathologists in states that do not require a master's degree
- more service for rural and other underserved populations
- a new market for practitioners who can bill directly and serve as consultants—a new career track for school speech–language pathologists and audiologists
- increased attention to the parameters of informed consent
- better accountability practices

Those opposed to schools' billing said the most negative issues were

- increased insurance claims and private insurance companies dropping coverage of speech–language and audiology services
- haphazard policies and procedures established by states and resulting ethical problems
- paucity of supervisors and monitors

- professional liability involving physician referral, credentials, and service
- increased documentation, decreased child contact time
- the possible bankruptcy of two underfunded and overextended systems (education and Medicaid)
- caseload management: needs versus available time
- parents not fully informed
- the money generated flowing into the general fund and not into the speech–language pathology and audiology program
- different standards for determining service needs in private practice and public school settings

School districts or individuals in schools may be certified as Medicaid providers. It seems appropriate in most cases that the school district be certified, because you as an individual are not keeping the reimbursed funds. In order to be certified, federal and state provider qualifications need to be met (ASHA, 2003). For individuals, federal Medicaid regulations stipulate that a speech–language pathologist or audiologist is an individual who has:

- obtained an ASHA certificate of clinical competence (CCC);
- completed the equivalent requirements for CCC in terms of education and work experience; or
- completed the academic program and is being supervised in work experience in order to qualify for CCC.

If the school district is the enrolled provider, it must ensure that services are provided by staff who meet state licensure and other payer credential requirements. If these requirements are not met, the school district will not be reimbursed. This fact has both positive and negative aspects. The positive is that states may look to a master's entry requirement for speech–language pathologists who choose to work in the schools. The negative aspect is that licensed or ASHA-certified speech–language pathologists will be asked to direct or supervise practitioners who do not meet minimum requirements.

Concerns about adequate supervision of unlicensed or non-ASHA-certified providers of speech–language or audiology services are long standing. Federal Medicaid regulations state that services for individuals with speech, hearing, and language disorders means diagnostics, screening, and preventative or corrective services provided by or under the direction of a speech–language pathologist or audiologist, for which a patient is referred by a physician (*Code of Federal Regulations,* Title 42, section 440.110(c)). Accordingly, Medicaid programs may pay for services provided "under the direction of" qualified personnel.

There is no clear federal guidance for determining the extent of supervision that meets the definition or interpretation of "under the direction of." The Centers for Medicare and Medicaid Services (CMS) provided some guidance on a case in 1992. It interpreted the "direction" requirement to mean that a qualified (ASHA-certified or equivalent) speech–language pathologist "must see the patient at least once, prescribe the type of care provided, and periodically review the need for continuing services.... the speech–language pathologist accepts ultimate responsibility for the care provided and should maintain close oversight of any services for which he or she agrees to assume direction" (ASHA, 2003, p. 8).

In the absence of federal direction, states are left to determine what "equivalent" (to ASHA CCC) means and how much is "as much time as necessary" related to the review of services. States solemnly proclaim that "under the direction" is not the same as "supervision." As long as the word games continue, *it is essential that speech–language pathologists and audiologists working in the school setting make themselves very familiar with the regulations of the state in which they work and the district that employs them.* ASHA has provided a Position Statement and Technical Report (2004a, b) in the absence of guidelines from Medicaid.

In its 1990 report to the Legislative Council, the ASHA Governmental Affairs Committee outlined 16 issues and guidelines that covered the pros and cons of the highest-qualified provider and responded effectively to the many questions raised by the committee and by members. These were broken into two topic areas: (a) child and family issues and (b) professional issues.

Child and Family Issues and Guidelines

- Issue 1: *Eligibility criteria used by education agencies may cause services in noneducational settings to be disallowed by third-party payers.* The guidelines state that although a student may not be eligible to receive special education or related services in the school, that student may be eligible to receive services outside the school from a private provider or in-an agency or hospital clinic. When writing the evaluation report, the speech–language pathologist or audiologist should indicate the nature of the student's disability and the reason that student was ineligible for service in the school. Furthermore, the parents must be informed of their rights to pursue services elsewhere, services possibly covered by third-party payers.

- Issue 2: *Parents' rights to informed consent is unclear to many service providers and parents.* According to the guidelines, speech–language pathologists and audiologists must know about informed-consent procedures and promote the use of the guidelines outlined previously in this chapter.

- Issue 3: *Parents may have insufficient information about third-party reimbursement processes.* According to the guidelines, the responsibility for acquiring the necessary information to provide parent education rests squarely on the speech–language pathologist or audiologist. ASHA suggests use of its summary of relevant federal regulations and details the necessity of obtaining state-specific information on third-party billing for speech–language pathology and audiology in the schools.

- Issue 4: *Children should receive uniform speech–language pathology and audiology services from qualified personnel, regardless of funding source.* The guidelines stress the necessity for providers to maintain at least minimum qualifications for practice as defined by federal and state regulations. They state that no child should be denied services or have services reduced in any form or manner because of the funding source and state that speech–language pathologists should use available resources to ensure consistency of care within all settings.

• Issue 5: *Confidentiality of school records may be compromised by allowing third-parties to see all information in the educational record when they make coverage judgments.* According to the guidelines, providers must know the confidentiality requirements of the state in which they practice, and parents should be informed of those requirements.

Professional Issues and Guidelines

• Issue 1: *There is confusion about the documentation procedures required for special-education–related services and health insurance.* According to the guidelines, the documentation must meet the requirements of the payer. Administrators and providers should collaborate to avoid duplication of effort and paperwork.

• Issue 2: *Speech–language pathologists and audiologists may be unaware of billing collection results, especially denials and appeals.* The guidelines state that providers should have a right to obtain feedback on denials and unpaid claims. (Note: That "right" can probably be accessed by collaborating with administrators and suggesting that good feedback will result in fewer rejected claims.)

• Issue 3: *Schools, as providers of health-insurance–reimbursable services, must meet certain requirements.* The guidelines state that schools must secure and meet personnel and organization requirements before submitting any claims.

• Issue 4: *Third-party reimbursement may influence the need for qualified personnel in the schools.* The guidelines state that providers must meet the requirements of the payer. (Note: If the private insurer or the state Medicaid authority requires the provider of services to have a state license or ASHA certification, the school must meet that requirement.)

• Issue 5: *Federal regulations require providers to access other third-party payers prior to billing medicaid.* According to the guidelines, the Medicaid statute requires that Medicaid be the payer of last resort. (Note: Providers should investigate the requirements of the state in which they are practicing. Some states require districts to pursue private monies; others discourage it.)

• Issue 6: *Health insurance policies generally include limitations on the number of hours, units of service, or maximum benefits paid (i.e., yearly or lifetime).* According to the guidelines, speech–language pathologists and audiologists should have knowledge of Public Law No. 94-142 regulations and the requirement that schools ensure that there will be no reduction in a child's or family's health insurance coverage, whether measured in hours, units of service, or lifetime caps.

• Issue 7: *The establishment of fees and billing procedures may be unfamiliar to speech–language pathologists and audiologists in the schools.* The guidelines state that speech–language pathologists and audiologists should know about proper methods for determining fees. Interested members should contact Publication Sales at the ASHA national office. Professionals also should know that Medicaid is not mandated by law to cover the usual and customary charges of providers. (Note: In the schools, the business officer and immediate supervisor usually oversee the specific processes and procedures involved with data collection. Fees are most often regulated by the state Medicaid authority.)

- Issue 8: *An additional source of funds may influence the level of service in the schools.* According to the guidelines, the level of service is determined by the child's IEP or Individual Family Service Plan (IFSP) for children from birth to 2 years 11 months, regardless of funding source.

- Issue 9: *Services will be subject to deductibles and coinsurance.* The guidelines state that speech–language pathologists and audiologists should be aware of coinsurance and deductible insurance requirements. The school districts must absorb these costs for children ages 3 through 21 years on the basis of the "free and appropriate public education" language in Public Law No. 94-142. Speech–language pathologists and audiologists should also be knowledgeable about individual state differences for children from birth to 2 years 11 months regarding practices or coinsurance and deductibles.

- Issue 10: *Schools may appear to be double-billing or even multiple-billing—that is, using education and health funds for the same service.* The guidelines state that although schools may receive funding from multiple sources to pay for services, this is legal financing and is not considered "double-billing." Federal statutes allow schools to seek funding from all public and private sources to provide a free appropriate public education. Some schools may use private billing services to obtain third-party funds. Such billing practices should be used only when they are cost effective and reflect actual services provided.

- Issue 11: *Some school districts will be required to bill health maintenance organizations (HMOs), preferred provider organizations (PPOs), and self-insured plans.* The guidelines state that speech–language pathologists and audiologists should be familiar with all forms of health insurance and managed care. Cornett (1988), the ASHA Web site, and *Governmental Affairs Review* are excellent resources for information on these systems for financing services. (Note: In most schools, speech–language pathologists and audiologists are charged with quality service provision and accurate data collection. Business officials work with payers.)

- Issue 12: *When there is a third-party billing for speech–language pathology and audiology services in the schools, supervision requirements exist for supportive personnel.* According to the guidelines, speech–language pathologists and audiologists should read and be familiar with the articles "Guidelines for the Employment and Utilization of Supportive Personnel" (ASHA, 1981) and "Position Statement on Training, Credentialing, Use, and Supervision of Support Personnel in Speech–Language Pathology" (ASHA, 1995, 2004b).

• Issue 13: *The sale of products may become an issue for school-based speech–language pathologists and audiologists.* The guidelines state that the federal regulations for special education and related services do not include the sale of products. Assistive technology used in the schools is not for sale to children through third-party payers. (Note: School districts often exercise the option of purchasing assistive technology equipment for students. Speech–language pathologists and audiologists should become familiar with procedures in their assignment.)

• Issue 14: *Third-party reimbursement may bring additional professional liability to speech–language pathologists and audiologists.* The guidelines state that speech–language pathologists and audiologists providing service should obtain adequate and appropriate professional liability insurance in addition to the general liability insurance coverage carried by their employer.

• Issue 15: *The provider, for reimbursement purposes, can be the speech–language pathologist or audiologist or the educational agency itself.* According to the guidelines, speech–language pathologists and audiologists should know about the ramifications of being the enrolled provider. The enrolled provider should be the school district, because it is the school district that receives the reimbursement.

• Issue 16: *There may be an impact on other service providers as a result of health insurance coverage of services provided in schools.* According to the guidelines, eligibility of schools to receive third-party reimbursement does not change the mission of school-based services—that is, to provide appropriate special education and related services. Availability of funding should not be interpreted as an incentive to expand services to children who are not eligible for special education and related services and whose services are not otherwise covered by other education funds.

ASHA Policy

In November 1990, the ASHA Legislative Council approved the following five points as ASHA's official policy on third-party reimbursement:

1. That necessary services shall be provided regardless of funding source, location, or parental authorization.
2. That services shall be provided at no cost to individuals or families.
3. That providers must be clinically competent.
4. That treatment standards must be equal and treatment may be appropriately delivered in both educational and health-care settings.
5. That a family's refusal to authorize use of private insurance does not relieve public agencies of their responsibility to provide appropriate services. (ASHA, 1990, p. 54)

If assigned to a school district that bills Medicaid or other third-party payers, a speech–language pathologist or audiologist should do some groundwork to ensure professional and personal integrity:

- Immediately look into personal liability insurance above that carried by the agency.
- Know the interpretations of federal, state, and local laws and regulations that govern the practice of speech–language pathology and audiology in the schools.
- Know the scope of practice of the state license and the definition of the state certification.
- Understand the ASHA Code of Ethics and its application to the performance of responsibilities.
- Research third-party reimbursement options in your state and in your area.
- Research the differences in documentation needed for related services provided under special education regulations and those provided under Medicaid regulations.
- Be certain that the school district, not the individual, registers as the service provider when third-party money is claimed.
- Be familiar with various forms of health insurance and managed care.
- Know your administrator or supervisor and collaborate on implementation processes and on streamlining paperwork.

School districts that decide to bill Medicaid for speech–language pathology and audiology must adapt their documentation to include Medicaid requirements. The basic requirements, at least for the federal Medicaid reimbursement process (ASHA, 1992b), are as follows:

1. The IEP must require the service.
2. Parental consent must be obtained.
3. There must be some form of physician authorization (required by Medicaid, but not always by other third-party payers).
4. Services provided must be documented in some way.
5. There must be some form of progress summary completed at set intervals—monthly or quarterly, for example.
6. There must be some form of daily documentation. School attendance records for providers and students can be used, but personal documentation gives the provider an excellent grasp of time and progress. A daily note or some form of documentation about what was done with the child not only enhances professional performance but serves the purposes of accountability and protection from liability. The information accumulated serves the basis for district billing and must be totally accurate.

Third-party billing in schools has created an acute awareness of the importance of accurate, meaningful documentation. Long, beautifully written reports may make the provider appear erudite but may not document change and growth in a measurable fashion. Evaluation reports may be comprehensive but may not sufficiently document the medical need for service. The focus is now on accuracy and outcomes, not length and excessive narrative. This focus must change the way record keeping is taught in colleges and universities. It must change the way school providers think about therapy and record keeping.

As of 2003, ASHA reported that 47 states permit schools to bill Medicaid for speech–language pathology services and audiology services provided in schools. In 2000, the U.S. General Accounting Office noted that school districts billing Medicaid report receiving an average of $2,000 per student (ASHA, 2003). Even if Medicaid accepts school billing for reimbursement of speech–language and audiology services, there is no guarantee that the reimbursement will be returned by the school district to the speech–language pathology and audiology program. In some states, the union or other bargaining unit can lead to an agreement with the district that the funds be spent to benefit the speech–language and audiology program.

Estomin (2004) relates her experience in the Pittsburgh Public School System with the Medicaid program. She indicated that her three most significant challenges were:

- to understand the Medicaid program;
- to gain assurances that funds generated would be returned to the speech–language pathology budget; and
- to develop a proposal for the union, balancing the increased paperwork with benefits for the speech–language pathologists.

She reported favorable results with increased funds for professional development, larger inventory of current diagnostic and therapy materials, more assistive devices, and updated laptop computers (Estomin, 2004).

Not all districts return funds to directly benefit speech–language services. The majority of Portland, Oregon's public schools' Medicaid funds go to the school district's general fund, but special education receives some of the money. That has been used to purchase tests and technology. Also, a few positions are primarily funded from the Medicaid payments (Annett, 2002).

However, school districts may not receive some of the Medicaid money. A General Accounting Office report on Medicaid in the schools indicated that 18 states kept a total of $324 million (34%) of Medicaid funds intended to reimburse school districts. Private firms hired by school districts for assistance with Medicaid billing received from 3% to 25% of the claim (U.S. General Accounting Office, 1999).

A U.S. General Accounting Office (GAO) report in 2000 indicated problems with Medicaid school billing. This report specified that the Centers for Medicare and Medicaid Services (CMS) had not provided adequate monitoring. Excessive claims and undocumented claims also were noted. The GAO has been conducting audits in a variety of states and cities. More than 20 federal audits indicated that the federal government was overbilled for millions of dollars (U.S. General Accounting Office, 1999).

The importance of detailed documentation, appropriate referrals, and use of qualified providers is highlighted by audits of the Office of Inspector General (OIG) for the Department of Health and Human Services. Over the past

5 years, approximately 20 audits of school-based Medicaid programs have been conducted. OIG found in at least five of these audits that "speech–language services were not compliant with federal provider qualification requirements" (Boswell, 2005).

One example is an audit of the New York City Department of Education (Department of Health and Human Services, 2005). The New York City audit focused on the early to mid 1990s. Following the review, OIG reported the following deficiencies. Of the 100 claims for speech services in the sample, 86 did not comply with federal and state requirements. Additionally, 68 of the sampled claims had two or more deficiencies. The report states, "Specifically: (1) For 42 claims, we were unable to verify that the services billed were rendered. (2) For 47 claims, we were unable to verify that a minimum of 2 speech services were rendered during the month billed … (7) For 76 claims, the services were not provided by or under the direction of an individual certified by the American Speech-Language-Hearing association or a similarly qualified person. As a result, we estimate that the State improperly claimed $435,903,456 in Federal Medicaid funding during our audit" (Department of Health and Human Services, 2005, p. 1).

Boswell (2005) noted that many school administrators and agents responsible for billing are not well-informed about the requirements for provider qualification, supervision, and documentation that are necessary for Medicaid reimbursement. Medicaid does not stipulate the amount of direction to be provided nor the qualifications of the individual who is providing services under the direction of a qualified provider. ASHA has developed a Position Statement and Technical Report titled "Medicaid Guidance for Speech-Language Pathology Services: Addressing the 'Under the Direction of' Rule" (2004c). It outlines the minimum qualifications of both the qualified speech–language pathologist and the lesser qualified individual. Also the amount and type of supervision or review deemed necessary are specified (ASHA, 2004a, 2004b).

An additional difficulty is that "Medicaid requirements follow a medical model, which is unfamiliar to many education personnel" (Power-deFur in Boswell, 2005). This is illustrated by a lawsuit (*United States of America ex rel. Toni R. Barron and Vicky J. Scheel v. Deloitte and Touche, LLP, et al.*) originally filed in 1998, which alleges fraudulent billing to Medicaid. In 2003, it was under appeal in the Fifth Circuit Court of the U.S. (Moore, 2003). Barron notes that she was supervising assistants who were "asked to bill for services that weren't medically necessary" (Moore, 2003, p. 13).

Some of the alleged Medicaid violations include the following:

- Inadequate documentation: Federal law requires service dates, listing services at each contact, and noting the child's progress relative to the medical services. Some school districts had been advised that attendance records were sufficient.
- Unqualified providers and unsupervised assistants.
- Billing for individual services when group services were provided.
- Transportation billing.

Both Barron and Scheel had experience in medical settings and were familiar with the specific requirements for Medicaid (Moore, 2003).

ASHA's 2005 Focused Initiative on Health Care Reimbursement is working to develop tools to access information and navigate Medicaid program requirements. Information on Medicaid regulations and billing is available for ASHA members at www.asha.org/members/issues/reimbursement/medicaid/. Information is also available for members of Division 16, the Special Interest Division concerned with school-based issues.

SUPERVISION

Supervision can be broadly defined as any activity or process intended to improve an individual's skills, attitudes, comprehension, and performance as related to employment roles and responsibilities. It is part of professional preparation and practice. It is an important factor in facilitating a growth process that should continue throughout an individual's education and professional career (ASHA, 1993). ASHA requires it for acquisition of the Certificate of Clinical Competence (CCC). State licensure boards require it for practicum and initial work experience. Most national regulatory bodies require a mechanism for ongoing supervision throughout professional careers. And education agencies usually base continued employment and often pay increases on supervision reports. A good supervision process validates and supports the changing, expanding roles and responsibilities necessarily assumed by speech–language pathologists and audiologists who choose to work in the school setting. These professionals are no longer just making decisions about the mouth and the ear. They are involved in making decisions about a student's total educational program. They are essential members of an educational team.

One of the most widely used supervisory models in speech–language pathology and audiology today is the Anderson model (Papir-Bernstein, 1995). It identifies a continuum of three stages of supervision based on the professional development of the supervisee:

1. The evaluation–feedback stage gives the supervisor a more dominant role. It is effective with individuals who are just starting their careers or with those who have more experience but may be undergoing burnout and need some direct clinical input.
2. The transitional stage is used effectively with experienced, competent individuals who are becoming more personally involved in their own professional growth. The supervisor must be careful not to move too quickly to this stage and cause frustration and discouragement.
3. The self-supervision stage is used with individuals who are searching for personal mastery and who have the ability to self-analyze and truly alter their clinical attitudes and behaviors. (Not everyone reaches this stage.)

None of the stages is time bound or evolves through natural progression. Individuals can be at any stage and can move between stages at any time in their careers. Their position depends on a variety of situational and personal variables.

There are almost as many supervisory styles as there are supervisors. Anderson identified three that include most of them. They can all facilitate growth if matched effectively with the development of the supervisee:

1. The *direct-active style* is often called the traditional supervision style and is the one most frequently used. It works well with the individual who is new to the field and requires ample guidance and input. The supervisor carries the more dominant role and exercises more control. The supervisee takes a more passive and subordinate role. This model takes less time and is easier for the supervisor. There is no collaboration. It is effective when it is used appropriately to facilitate the growth of the supervisee.

2. In the *collaborative style,* the supervisor and the supervisee work together and make mutually agreeable decisions. The supervisee has more involvement in and ownership of the process.

3. In the *consultative style,* the supervisee sets goals, continues to search for appropriate professional growth activities, and identifies personal strengths and weaknesses. The supervisor is an active listener, helps in problem solving, and gives direct clinical assistance as asked or as deemed necessary.

Throughout the supervision process, the relationship changes between the supervisor and the supervisee. As the individual moves from dependence to independence, the supervisor should move from direct to indirect supervision. Research indicates that this does not always happen. Unfortunately, some supervisors have one style of supervision, and that style does not necessarily facilitate the growth and professional development of the supervisee.

ASHA Statements

In 1978, the ASHA Committee on Supervision in Speech–Language Pathology and Audiology defined supervisors as individuals who engage in clinical teaching through observation, conferences, review of records, and other procedures related to the interaction between a clinician and a client and to the evaluation or management of communication skills. The implication of clinical teaching as an integral part of supervision is critical.

In 1985, the ASHA Committee on Supervision outlined 13 tasks basic to effective clinical teaching in the distinct area of practice that comprises communication disorders (ASHA, 1985). When students, speech–language pathologists, and audiologists investigate the tenets of the supervision process under which they must function, they can measure it against these 13 tasks:

1. establishing and maintaining an effective working relationship with the supervisee;
2. assisting the supervisee in developing clinical goals and objectives;
3. assisting the supervisee in developing and refining assessment skills;
4. assisting the supervisee in developing and refining clinical management skills;
5. demonstrating for and participating with the supervisee in the clinical process;
6. assisting the supervisee in observing and analyzing assessment and treatment sessions;
7. assisting the supervisee in the development and maintenance of clinical and supervisory records;
8. interacting with the supervisee in planning, executing, and analyzing supervisory conferences;
9. assisting the supervisee in evaluation of clinical performance;
10. assisting the supervisee in developing skills of verbal reporting, writing, and editing;
11. sharing information regarding ethical, legal, regulatory, and reimbursement aspects of professional practice;
12. modeling and facilitating professional conduct; and
13. demonstrating research skills in the clinical or supervisory processes.

The committee enumerated from 4 to 10 competencies under each task. Knowledge and skill in supervision, as well as in the professions and in the area of practice, are essential for an effective supervisor.

Performance appraisal, sometimes a synonym for the supervisory process, was defined by the ASHA Committee on Professional Appraisal in 1992 as "the practice of evaluating job-related behaviors" (ASHA, 1993, p. 11). The position developed by this committee and adopted by the 1992 Legislative Council reads,

> It is the position of the American Speech-Language-Hearing Association that professional performance appraisals of speech–language pathologists and audiologists who are engaged in the delivery of clinical services should include an assessment of the clinical skills that are unique to the employee's profession. This component of the performance appraisal should be conducted by people who hold ASHA certification (and licensure where appropriate) in the employee's professional area. In cases in which organizational structure precludes adoption of this position, participatory approaches (peer evaluations and/or self-evaluations) should be instituted as components of the performance appraisal process.

The committee's technical report noted that a good performance appraisal (a) improved the quality of client care, (b) maintained or improved performance,

(c) facilitated professional growth and development, and (d) provided feedback about the potential for increased job responsibilities.

Supervision and performance appraisal focus on two kinds of employee behaviors, those relating to general responsibilities and those relating to professional skills. The general responsibilities may include attendance, dependability, meeting participation, adherence to employer policies and procedures, punctuality, and appropriate use of resources. These aspects of professional performance can be effectively evaluated by any competent administrator.

Professional skills, however, involve competencies defined by specific education, knowledge, and experience. A supervisor outside the profession can judge interpersonal skills, ability to control a group, planning skills, and timely submission of reports but would experience difficulty evaluating the ability to select, administer, and interpret diagnostic tasks that lead to differential diagnoses of speech, language, or hearing disorders; the ability to implement specialized treatment strategies; and the ability to document the relationship of the student's educational needs to the need for therapy. These job functions are unique to the professions of speech–language pathology and audiology and must, when possible, be evaluated by persons with the same professional background as the employee.

It is a common occurrence, however, that speech–language pathologists and audiologists who work in an educational agency are supervised by an administrator or supervisor outside the professions. They may be evaluated by special education directors, school principals, occupational or physical therapists, or psychologists. It may therefore fall to the employee to develop or assist in the development of a supervision process that in some manner reflects professional as well as generalized and administrative responsibilities. ASHA's Committee on Performance Appraisal (1993) suggested two add-ons that can help speech–language pathologists and audiologists design discipline-specific programs or units to meld into their supervision process: peer appraisal and self-appraisal.

Peer Appraisal

Peer appraisal (peer coaching, peer partnering, etc.), the process whereby colleagues rate or enhance each other's job performance, is a well-accepted supervisory tool. It was developed to enhance instruction, not to supersede the evaluation process. It facilitates the autonomy of participants by enabling them to improve their ability to self-monitor, self-analyze, and self-evaluate. It fosters independence and decision making. To be effective and efficient, peer partners must be trained in the process, which, of course, has been approved by the administration of the employing agency. Peer partners, with input from the supervisor, must first decide whether they will analyze or coach one another. Although peer analysis and peer coaching are closely related, there are differences.

- Peer analysis involves clarification of therapy or evaluation activities and practices. Peer partners share implementation of strategies and interpretation of results and engage in self-analysis and problem-solving techniques.

- Peer coaching strives for the improvement of therapy or evaluation activities and practices. This partnering is usually entered with the express goal of improving a specific skill or process by working with a peer who has mastered that skill or process.

Roles must be clarified to avoid possible conflict. Peer partnering can solidify the skills and expand the repertoires of the partners, and it promotes cooperative problem solving. A preobservation form can set the scene and facilitate achievement of the session's goal.

Self-Appraisal

Self-appraisal is a process of taking responsibility for developing a program of professional growth, for developing and following professional improvement goals, and for using a wide variety of resources to achieve those goals. One form of self-appraisal is self-directed study or self-managed professional development. It is encouraged by advocates of coaching and mentoring; and it is indicated by the changing standards and criteria of educational evaluation; by the increased and more complex roles and responsibilities in which providers in the schools are involved; and by research in the fields of education, psychology, business management, religion, and self-help. It must become an integral part of the professional development of speech–language pathologists and audiologists, whatever their practice site. It allows an employee to enter into a contract with herself to study new facts, acquire a specific skill in a particular domain of practice, keep abreast of current research and literature, and, when applicable, meet state certification and licensure continuing education requirements. In addition to measuring one's own growth, the process and the results can and should become part of the supervision process. The self-directed process is defined in four steps (Papir-Bernstein, 1995):

1. formulation of an open-ended list of potential professional growth objectives;
2. completion of a professional growth plan that includes both a self-evaluation and targeted areas for growth;
3. completion of an action plan that breaks down areas into performance objectives, methods, resources, and time lines needed to achieve the objectives; and
4. completion of a summative conference or self-evaluation.

There are many sources of information on and resources for self-directed study. They include undertaking independent studies under the sponsorship of ASHA or many state professional associations, participating in workshops and conferences, taking or auditing a course, forming or joining a journal study club, engaging in computer searches on relevant topics, joining a Special Interest Division (SID) through ASHA, and taking self-study "courses" through journals such as *Topics in Language Disorders*. Most of these activities are or can be designed to be eligible for ASHA continuing education units (CEUs). Acquisition of seven CEUs earns an Award for Continuing Education (ACE) from ASHA. Following issuance of the award, the ASHA national office sends a letter to the recipient's supervisor or employer lauding the accomplishment.

Continuous learning is not optional. The proliferation of journals and research in the professions of speech–language and audiology, the increasing client base, the multiple service delivery models, and the expanding role of the speech–language pathologist and audiologist in the schools require continuous learning to remain current. Self-managed study is an excellent method of accomplishing this goal. And if speech–language pathologists and audiologists in schools are supervised by individuals outside the professions, self-directed study, incorporated into the supervision process with the approval of that supervisor, is an excellent way of educating the supervisor and keeping discipline-specific activities in the supervisory process.

A Model Process

In 1992, in response to concerns about the existing supervision process expressed by staff and administrators at the Monroe No. 1 Board of Cooperative Education Services (BOCES) in upstate New York, a volunteer committee was organized to look at the role of supervision in the teaching–learning process. The committee was made up of an assistant superintendent, a school principal, a program director, a teacher of the deaf, a speech–language pathologist, a vision teacher, and a classroom teacher. Members met monthly through one school year. The process was piloted in several departments, including the Department of Speech–Language Pathology and Audiology, and in one school building. It was included in union bargaining sessions the following year and was approved as part of the teacher contract.

The stated purpose of the adopted supervision–evaluation structure is the promotion of the ongoing development of each staff member. Such development is possible only when mutual trust and respect exist between those being supervised and evaluated and those who supervise and evaluate. It was the goal of the committee to create a structure that makes possible productive, constructive interactions between professionals, both peers and supervisors. The process is based on eight components of professional behavior (Chirico et al., 1992). (Components 7 and 8 are considered part of a staff member's daily routine and are not the focus of the formalized observation.)

> 1. *Communication*. Professionals understand that communication is a two-way process that involves both verbal and nonverbal components. They question and answer openly, and they accurately impart specific knowledge, information, and emotion.

2. *Understanding and knowledge of the field.* Professionals are proficient in their particular discipline and in learning theory. They avail themselves of resources, internal and external, to increase knowledge and to improve the practice of their professions. They know the purpose of the organization that employs them and the range of services offered within that organization.

3. *Management of the professional environment.* Professionals are well organized and consistent, as is their environment. They make good use of time, act independently, and use available resources.

4. *Planning.* Professionals understand that planning is a process that precedes instruction and therapy and involves long-term goals as well as short-range objectives. Planning includes a determination of strategies and resources and requires knowledge of assessment methods and various learning styles.

5. *Instructional strategies.* Professionals understand the most productive ways to interact with students–clients. They implement appropriate objectives, provide opportunities for active involvement, continually evaluate progress, incorporate practice, use creative and varied methods, and provide ongoing feedback.

6. *Interpersonal skills.* Professionals within the schools and the community demonstrate respect and empathy for others and behave in ways that foster collaboration.

7. *Professional responsibilities.* Professionals execute routine matters such as attending meetings, keeping records, contributing to the organization's positive public relations, and maintaining confidentiality whenever appropriate. Within this component, it is understood that a professional is punctual, is reliable, and acts in an ethical manner.

8. *Willingness to grow.* Professionals stay current with their field and take the initiative to become continually more proficient at their work. Such professionals evaluate their needs, establish clear development goals, seek feedback and support, and are receptive to ideas and suggestions.

The second component, "Understanding and knowledge of the field," was included after it was introduced and rationalized by the speech–language pathologist member of the committee. For that component, individual departments, including classroom teachers, are required to develop knowledge-of-field documents for new and for experienced staff. The speech–language pathology and audiology documents were developed by department committees and form the basis for that part of their supervision process (Babiarz et al., 1991; Greer, Newman, & Towsley, 1991). At Monroe No. 1 BOCES, the processes of supervision and evaluation are kept totally separate.

The *purpose of supervision* is to enhance professional growth through an interactive, ongoing process that focuses on the components of professional behavior listed previously. In the related services departments, such as speech–language pathology and audiology, the supervision is provided by a certified or licensed professional in the same field. Multiple observations occur annually, as agreed upon by the supervisor and supervisee. A preconference prior to an observation is optional, but it is useful to clarify what, specifically, will be observed and discussed. A postconference follows each observation, in which observer and person observed discuss the session with the goal of improving professional competence. The written summary of each observation is not part of the supervisee's permanent record. Peer coaching is an option for nonevaluation years.

The *purpose of evaluation* is to provide a periodic summative statement of the performance of a staff member based on the same components of professional behavior. It reflects input from both evaluator and evaluatee. Evaluation occurs annually for nontenured staff, and every 3 years for tenured staff. An evaluation conference precedes the writing of an evaluation, and the written evaluation reflects this conference. The written evaluation is in a personal letter format and becomes part of the evaluatee's permanent record.

Mentoring

Mentoring is an informal process of support among co-workers, between professionals, and between a supervisor and a supervisee. It is not a supervisory process. It is an alliance that facilitates growth. Mentors must be willing to make a commitment of time to work with an individual new to the department, new to an assignment area, or just wanting additional support. Mentors should have basic conferencing skills, be nonjudgmental and supportive, be able to share information, have experience or expertise in a given assignment area, and maintain confidentiality. Again, mentoring is not supervising.

Matching mentors and mentees is critical to the success of the venture. Allowing professional staff to choose a volunteer mentor for a designated period of time is one way to do it. Sharing a mentor's role before the time period begins is advisable. The mentor should not address issues of performance unless responding to a specific question. The mentor can be involved in assisting the mentee in problem solving by sharing strategies, ideas, and new research; discussing diagnostic batteries; helping administer evaluation tools; developing intervention strategies; scheduling, organizing, and planning; helping the mentee understand agency or department policies and procedures; and sharing information about resources and materials (Huffman & Russell, 1992).

Mentoring can be on a volunteer or paid basis. Some states define and encourage mentoring. Their districts employ full- or part-time paid mentors. The time that mentoring requires will vary depending upon the amount of support a mentee requests or the amount of time a district requires.

Students

Students at both the undergraduate and graduate levels should be keenly aware of the supervision requirements necessary for state licensure and ASHA Certificates of Clinical Competence. Specific standards for supervision of students can and do differ depending on work or practicum site. Students should know at the onset of their work or practicum experience that supervised clinical experiences will satisfy ASHA (CCC) requirements only if the supervision is provided by ASHA-certified personnel (ASHA, 1994b).

It is incumbent upon each individual to ask for specific information on the supervision process used in the agency or school where practicum experience or employment will occur. As it is understood, that process can be used for professional growth and self-improvement. In whatever setting the speech–language pathologist or audiologist works, strategies can be employed to enhance professional knowledge; improve skills; and make supervisors, evaluators, and administrators aware of the professional activities that make up the practice of speech–language pathology or audiology in that setting. These strategies require professional energy, time, and occasionally ingenuity, but they result in a work environment that promotes job satisfaction and allows for professional growth and development.

SUPPORT PERSONNEL

The role of support personnel in speech–language pathology and audiology (presently referred to as speech–language pathology assistants, or SPLAs) and the guidelines governing their use in schools, agencies, and hospitals have long been controversial issues. In 1967, John P. Moncur, chair of the first Committee on Support Personnel appointed by ASHA, noted that the question of support personnel was not a future issue but one that needed immediate attention. The ASHA Ethical Practices Board published an *Issues in Ethics* statement, which became effective in June 1979 (ASHA, 1992a). It highlighted the professional and ethical responsibilities of the supervising professional and emphasized the dependent role of the "communication aide." Werven (1993) noted that the support personnel issue has sparked strong discussion between advocates, who cite increased caseloads, underserved populations, and a diminishing professional work force, and opponents, who express concerns about job security, quality of care, and ethics. The debate continues, and the problems proliferate.

Use of support personnel in schools has been declared successful in several states. Many titles are used. They include assistant, aide, communication assistant, speech–language pathology aide, speech–language assistant, audiometrist, audiometric technician, communication helper, speech aide, and many more (ASHA Task Force on Support Personnel, 1992a; Paul-Brown & Goldberg, 2001). Support personnel's responsibilities may range from clerical work through data collection to maintenance of corrected articulation and implementation of a feeding plan. Freilinger (1992) supported use of support personnel in the Iowa schools. He stated that the Iowa schools' motive was to employ someone to do the routine activities that did not require a person with a master's degree. He believed that the support personnel program was efficient, effective, and economical and could complement a school's speech and language program—if it was thought through and planned, if goals and responsibilities were clearly articulated, and if the support personnel were carefully supervised.

A 1993 study by Nancy Striffler of the National Early Childhood Technical Assistance System (NECTAS) in Chapel Hill, North Carolina, looked at the use of support personnel in early childhood and preschool services in 31 states. Several of these states had developed new occupational categories to ensure services to children and parents at this level. Many of these categories were for support personnel. In Illinois, teacher aides, child development associates, developmental education associates, and family support associates work in early intervention programs. In Utah, early intervention aides and three levels of early interventionists are active. Striffler noted that some of the factors that influence the establishment of a new occupational category include (a) a commitment to include parents as service providers and a desire to employ individuals who are responsive to the culture they serve; (b) the need to extend the services of professionals, especially allied health professionals; and (c) a commitment to provide services in varied environments and service settings, including the home and child care centers.

Striffler (1993) reported that the most severe professional shortages are in the areas of the allied health services of occupational and physical therapy and speech–language pathology. But using support personnel to provide services in the areas of motor and language development requires careful consideration. When, for instance, does one cross the line from appropriate developmental activities to therapeutic intervention? What specific activities, and at what level, violate state licensure laws? Why is it appropriate to give developmental recommendations to parents for implementation but not to support personnel? With no professional service providers in many remote areas throughout the country, how do we meet the needs of individuals and groups within those areas who need speech–language and audiology services?

Both opponents and proponents of the use of support personnel have many concerns. They worry about the qualifications and availability of supervisors, the amount of supervision, and the supervisor–support personnel ratio. They express concern about educational and training standards, scope of practice, ethical considerations, reimbursement issues, and the question of who will monitor the credentialing process.

ASHA Statements

ASHA attempted to clarify the use of support personnel in 1969, when the Legislative Council adopted the first guidelines. ASHA's *Rule of Ethics II.D* states in part that support services may be provided by uncertified persons only when a certificate holder provides appropriate supervision. That paper was not specific in setting ratios or in delineating activities. In 1981, ASHA's second Committee on Supportive Personnel published "Guidelines for the Employment and Utilization of Supportive Personnel." The issues underlying those guidelines were as follows:

1. The legal, ethical, and moral responsibility to the client for all services provided cannot be delegated; that is, they remain the responsibility of the professional personnel.
2. Support personnel may be permitted to implement a variety of clinical tasks, given that sufficient training, direction, and supervision are provided by the audiologist or speech–language pathologist responsible for those tasks.
3. Support personnel should receive training that is competency-based in character and specific to the job performance expectations held by the employer.
4. The supervising audiologist or speech–language pathologist should also be trained in the supervision of support personnel.
5. The supervision of support personnel must be periodic, comprehensive, and documented to ensure that the client receives the high-quality services needed.

These guidelines allow trained speech–language pathology and audiology support personnel to assist in the delivery of services and to augment program and treatment activities under the direct supervision of ASHA-certified speech–language pathologists and audiologists.

Since 1981, the use of support personnel in speech–language pathology and audiology has increased throughout the professions. Several factors have influenced that increase:

- The passage of Public Law No. 94-142 in 1975 increased the mandated responsibilities of the speech–language pathologists in the schools. Children with severe disabilities, formerly evaluated and treated elsewhere, are now mandated to be evaluated and serviced by the speech–language pathologists in the schools.
- The passage of Public Law No. 99-457 in 1986 mandated service to the preschool population. Children's disabilities are now identified and treated earlier.
- Technological advances made possible the mainstreaming and inclusion of students who are severely disabled—that is, students who did not participate in public education at an earlier time. The increase of these students has necessitated the increase of service providers to serve them. The technology necessary to allow these students access to public education demands increased and specific expertise of the service provider.
- Personnel shortages and underserved populations across the country have caused administrators and supervisors to look at alternatives to traditional service delivery.

Use of support personnel with underserved populations may include the expansion of services in rural areas. In addition, a bilingual speech–language pathology assistant may be able to assist with bilingual clients (ASHA, 1988; Paul-Brown & Goldberg, 2001).

In 1994, ASHA's Task Force on Support Personnel prepared a position statement and guidelines for one category of support personnel. These guidelines included a recognized credentialing process and an outcome-based evaluation system. The 1994 Legislative Council adopted the position statement (ASHA, 1995). It was reviewed and updated in 2003. The position statement reads,

> It is the position of the American Speech-Language-Hearing Association (ASHA) that support personnel may be used to perform activities adjunct to the primary clinical efforts of speech–language pathologists. ASHA supports the establishment of categories of support personnel for the profession of speech–language pathology. Appropriate training and supervision must be provided by speech–language pathologists who hold ASHA's Certificate of Clinical Competence in Speech–Language Pathology. Activities may be assigned only at the discretion of the supervising speech–language pathologist and should be constrained by the job responsibilities for support personnel. The communication needs and protection of the consumer must be held paramount at all times. (ASHA, 2004d)

In 1995, the Legislative Council approved new guidelines for the training, credentialing, use, and supervision of speech–language pathology and audiology assistants. In 1996, the Legislative Council approved a strategic plan for implementing that credentialing process. Later, the Legislative Council charged the Council of Professional Standards in Speech–Language Pathology and Audiology to develop a credentialing process for assistants in speech–language pathology and to then administer it (ASHA, 2000a). The document, concerned with criteria for approval of the associate degree in technical training, was developed in October 2000 and revised in April 2001. The criteria for registration of speech–language assistants were approved in September 2000 (Moore & Pearson, 2003). However, ASHA's Legislative Council voted to discontinue the registration process due to financial concerns. There is no formal registry of SPLAs or recognition of training programs by ASHA. Information on SPLAs can be obtained at the ASHA Web site under Frequently Asked Questions (ASHA, 2004a).

It is critical to remember that speech–language pathologists and audiologists are legally bound to follow the licensure laws that regulate them and their practice in the state where they work. Use of support personnel is not permitted in some states. The ASHA Web site lists information about states that officially regulate use of support personnel.

Licensure

In 2001, Paul-Brown and Goldberg reported that six states used licensure to regulate support personnel. In addition, 23 states use registration to regulate support personnel. Seven other states acknowledge support personnel but do not officially regulate them.

The common thread through the various rules and regulations is that of training these individuals according to the 1981 guidelines. There is wide variability throughout the state requirements. One example is the state requirements for education and experience. Requirements range from a bachelor's degree with graduate credit hours to a bachelor's degree with practicum, to an associate's degree, to a high school diploma and additional training (Paul-Brown & Goldberg, 2001).

Regulated or licensed support personnel perform a variety of roles within a broad range of employment settings. The typical scope of responsibilities includes screening, reinforcing, and maintaining improved or corrected articulation; conducting oral exercises; implementing computer simulation programs and programmed instruction; recording and displaying data that reflect a student's performance; filing clinical records and making progress notes; reporting changes in student behavior to the speech–language pathologist; working with parents on carryover activities; demonstrating select assistive listening devices; creating therapy materials; and maintaining the equipment and materials inventory. Some "out-of-the-box" thoughts include employing support personnel to work in such areas as inclusion, research, grant writing, reading, and multicultural domains (Mullins, 2000). Prohibited activities are typically those that require the formal education and credentialing of a speech–language pathologist or audiologist, including, but not limited to, diagnostic evaluations, caseload selection, interpretation and dissemination of clinical information, writing reports, determining related services, and determining dismissal from therapy. ASHA provides guidelines for the use of support personnel within the schools (ASHA, 1996, 2000b).

Supervision requirements vary across states according to demographics. Rural areas usually require fewer on-site hours and more readily accept audio and videotapes for review. Most states require support personnel to practice only under the supervision of a licensed, certified speech–language pathologist or audiologist who maintains legal accountability and responsibility for all activities and services provided. Also, in most states where there is regulation of support personnel, a formal plan of supervision is required, and the number of support personnel who can be supervised by one speech–language pathologist or audiologist is specified.

Some who object to the development of support personnel in the professions cite proposals that replace professional personnel with trained "aides." The most radical proposals involve something called institutional licensure. Under such a system, an institution would be regulated by a state agency, such as a state education department, which could essentially decide who is competent to discharge what duties. Proponents of licensing support personnel say this could not happen if licensure defined their scope of practice. In some states, licensure is not required in schools, or schools are exempt from state licensure. In those states, licensure would provide no protection against the misuse of support personnel.

Proponents of the use and regulation of speech–language pathology assistants as support personnel say that the practice is operational and that it is up to "us" to regulate it so as to avoid abuse. They say that as speech–language and audiology professionals, we must regulate our own support personnel or risk the possibility that diverse agencies such as state education departments will regulate them for us. Use of SPLAs

- frees the speech–language pathologist to perform higher-level activities that require the education and expertise of the professional;
- relieves the professional from routine, clerical, and time-consuming tasks that do not require discipline-specific expertise;
- has proved cost effective in places where large and diverse populations require service;
- provides a career ladder both for the support personnel who continue into the professions of speech–language pathology and audiology and for the speech–language pathologist or audiologist wishing to move into an administrative or supervisory role; and
- has proved effective in areas where readily available support personnel are used to reinforce or maintain recommended activities.

Opponents to the use and regulation of support personnel are very vocal. They ask the following questions:

- Will the use of support personnel downgrade the professional status of speech–language pathology and audiology?
- Will support personnel take over the role of speech–language pathologists—especially in the schools?
- Will jobs be lost? Will support personnel replace instead of assist?
- Will consumers be confused over differences in provider qualifications?
- Will schools provide adequate release time for training and supervision?
- Will it be possible to implement supervision by a speech–language pathologist or audiologist in a system that clearly allocates supervision to school administrators?
- Will appropriate supervisor–supervisee ratios be enforced?
- Will quality of service be maintained?
- Will there be adequate training of both the support personnel and the supervisor?
- Will abuses occur, especially in schools where cost containment is critical?
- Will third-party payers accept two different levels of reimbursement?
- Does this profession really need another layer of service provider?

ASHA's Special Interest Division 11 is concerned with these matters, as well as others related to supervision. If you are interested, you may want to look at the information available on the ASHA Web site and possibly join this division.

The practice of audiology in the schools is an area that lends itself easily to the use of support personnel. In the educational milieu, many students with hearing loss are mainstreamed. The troubleshooting and management of frequency-modulated (FM) systems and other assistive listening devices are responsibilities that could be performed by individuals other than licensed or certified audiologists. Under the supervision of an audiologist, support personnel could be trained to troubleshoot and manage that equipment. Viable activities include conducting listening checks on FM systems and hearing aids; communicating with vendors; providing in-service training on troubleshooting techniques; arranging annual service maintenance; making minor repairs; managing records and maintaining files; monitoring service contracts and purchase orders; ordering equipment and parts; and updating information on product lines, parts, and prices. Credentials could be minimal. Money could be saved. The SLP and audiologist could be relieved from the performance of tasks that can be done easily and well by less credentialed individuals.

CONCLUSION

The use of speech–language pathology assistants as support personnel in speech–language pathology and audiology is here. It is not a future possibility about which we have the luxury of pondering. It is something we need to acknowledge, accept, and integrate as necessary into the practice of our professions. Given the expanding role of speech–language pathologists in schools, use of support personnel is one way to facilitate improved services to students. Assistants can be used to increase the intensity, efficiency, and availability of services, particularly in remote areas and with underserved populations. As more support personnel become recognized members of service provision teams, more professionals will be called upon to train and supervise them. The role of supervision and the supervisory skills needed to carry out this function are critical. The quality of training, support, and supervision provided to support personnel will influence their success in providing quality services to the children in our schools and to their parents.

Individuals who enter the professions of speech–language pathology and audiology see themselves as future professionals. They take on the ethics and responsibilities that go with their chosen professions. They do the right thing whether anyone is watching or not. They think first of the client, of the student. They possess a sense of public responsibility, a code of ethics, a sense of duty beyond self. This could be lost if we were to place our responsibilities in the hands of assorted support personnel with no unifying philosophy. However, we know that our professions are dynamic. We know they change and grow. We know that over time they acquire new and more complex responsibilities at the upper end of their scopes of practice, while activities at the lower end tend to drop out of the scope. If we are flexible about recognizing selected responsibilities for which support personnel can be responsible, we are more likely to be taken seriously by policy makers when we object to the delegation of professional duties that expose our consumers to serious risk.

STUDY QUESTIONS

1. List some of the advantages of third-party payments for school services, and be prepared to discuss some of the serious obstacles to their use.
2. What has ASHA said about third-party payments?
3. If you work for a school system that bills Medicaid or other third-party payers, what are some of the things that you should know?
4. Why do some school districts have difficulty with audits for Medicaid billing? How could you protect against such difficulty?
5. What is performance appraisal, and how is it related to supervision?
6. Differentiate between supervision, evaluation, and mentoring.
7. What forces have led to the inclusion of speech–language pathology assistants in school services for children with handicapping conditions?
8. What services do you think would be appropriate for speech–language pathology assistants to perform in speech and language?

REFERENCES

American Speech-Language-Hearing Association. (1981). Guidelines for the employment and utilization of supportive personnel. *Asha, 23*, 165–169.

American Speech-Language-Hearing Association. (1985). Clinical supervision in speech–language pathology and audiology. *Asha, 27*, 57–60.

American Speech-Language-Hearing Association. (1988). Utilization and employment of speech–language pathology supportive personnel with underserved populations. *Asha, 30*, 55–56.

American Speech-Language-Hearing Association. (1990). *Utilization of Medicaid and other third-party funds for "covered services" in the schools: Report to the 1990 American Speech-Language-Hearing Association Legislative Council as required by LC 42-89*. Rockville, MD: Author.

American Speech-Language-Hearing Association. (1991). Utilization of Medicaid and other third-party funds for "covered services" in the schools. *Asha, 33*(Suppl. 5), 51–58.

American Speech-Language-Hearing Association. (1992a). ASHA policy regarding support personnel. *Asha, 34*(Suppl. 9), 18.

American Speech-Language-Hearing Association. (1992b). *Third-party reimbursement in the schools: Teleconference report*. ASHA Transcript Series: Focus on School Issues.

American Speech-Language-Hearing Association. (1993). Professional performance appraisal by individuals outside of the professions of speech–language pathology and audiology. *Asha, 35*(Suppl. 10), 11–13.

American Speech-Language-Hearing Association. (1994a). National Medicaid issues for public school practioners. *Asha, 36,* 31–32.

American Speech-Language-Hearing Association. (1994b). Supervision of student clinicians. *Asha, 36*(Suppl. 13), 13.

American Speech-Language-Hearing Association. (1995). Position statement on training, credentialing, use, and supervision of support personnel in speech–language pathology. *Asha, 37*(Suppl. 14), 21.

American Speech-Language-Hearing Association. (1996). Guidelines for the training, credentialing, use, and supervision of speech–language pathology assistants. *Asha, 38,* 21–34.

American Speech-Language-Hearing Association. (2000a). *Council on academic accreditation in audiology and speech–language pathology: Criteria for approval of associate degree technical training programs for speech–language pathology assistants.* Rockville, MD: Author.

American Speech-Language-Hearing Association. (2000b). *Use and supervision of speech–language pathology assistants in schools.* Rockville, MD: Author.

American Speech-Language-Hearing Association. (2003). *Medicaid and third-party payments in the schools.* http://www.asha.org/members/issues/reimbursement/medicaid/thirdparty-payment.htm

American Speech-Language-Hearing Association. (2004a). *Frequently asked questions speech–language pathology assistants.* www.asha.org/about/membership-certification/faq-slpasst.htm

American Speech-Language-Hearing Association. (2004b). Medicaid guidance for Speech-Language Pathology Services: Addressing the "under the direction of" rule [*Position Statement*]. Retrieved January 9, 2006, from http://www.asha.org/members/deskref-journals/deskref/default

American Speech-Language-Hearing Association. (2004c). Medicaid guidance for Speech-Language Pathology Services: Addressing the "under the direction of" rule [*Technical Report*]. Retrieved January 9, 2006, from http://www.asha.org/members/deskref-journals/deskref/default

American Speech-Language-Hearing Association. (2004d). *Training, use and supervision of support personnel in speech–language pathology.* [Position statement]. http://www.asha.org/members/deskref-journals/deskref/default

American Speech-Language-Hearing Association Task Force on Support Personnel. (1992). *Support personnel: Issues and impact on the professions of speech–language pathology and audiology. A technical report.* Rockville, MD: Author.

Annett, M. M. (2002). *Billing Medicaid for school-based services.* Retrieved August 20, 2005, from http://www.asha.org/about/publications/leader-online/archives/2002/q2/020416.htm

Babiarz, B., Bergin, M., Corea, M. A., Corwley, E., Hooey, K., Oglia, D., et al. (1991). *Knowledge and skills in speech–language pathology.* New York: Board of Cooperative Educational Services, First Supervisory District, Monroe County.

Barron & Scheel v. Deloitte & Touche, L.L.P.; Deloitte & Touche Consulting Group, L.L.C.; Deloitte & Touche Consulting Group Holding, L.L.C.; Medicaid Claim Solutions of Texas, Inc.; National Heritage Insurance Co. Available at: http://caselaw.findlaw.com/data2/circs/5th/0350507p.pdf

Boswell, S. (2005). New York City Medicaid program faulted by the Inspector General. *ASHA Leader, 10*(10), 1 & 28.

Chirico, P., Byrne, P., Cullings, J., Diesenberg, V., Keller, S., Lynch-Nadich, K., et al. (1992). *Amended supervision and evaluation process.* New York: Board of Cooperative Educational Services, First Supervisory District, Monroe County.

Cornett, B. S. (1988). Speech–language pathologists, audiologists, and HMOs: Status and outlook. *Asha, 30,* 64–67.

Department of Health and Human Services. (2005). Review of Medicaid speech claim made by New York City Department of Education. Retrieved January 9, 2006, from http://oig.hhs.gov/oas/oas/cms.html

Estomin, E. (2004). *Success story: Returning SLP-generated Medicaid funds to the SLP budget.* Retrieved August 20, 2005, from http://www.asha.org/members/slp/schools/salaries/success-estomin.htm

Freilinger, J. J. (1992). Support personnel. *Asha, 34,* 51–53.

Greer, C., Newman, S., & Towsley, M. (1991). *Knowledge and skills in audiology.* New York: Board of Cooperative Educational Services, First Supervisory District, Monroe County.

Huffman, N., & Russell, L. (1992). *Mentoring: Staff directory for speech–language pathology and audiology.* New York: Board of Cooperative Educational Services, First Supervisory District, Monroe County.

Moore, M. (2000). Putting Medicaid to work in schools. *ASHA Leader, 5,* 21.

Moore, M. (2003). Medicaid school billing under fire. *ASHA Leader, 8,* 1, 12–15.

Moore, S. M., & Pearson, L. D. (2003). *Speech–language pathology assistants.* Clifton Park, NY: Delmar Learning.

Mullins, J. M. (2000, Sept. 18). *Out-of-the-box tasks for speech-language-pathology assistants.* Retrieved August 20, 2005, from http://speech-language-pathology-audiology.advance web.com/common/EditorialSearch/AViewer.aspx?AN=SP_p.5html&AD=09-18-2000

Papir-Bernstein, W. (1995, March). *Supervision for the twenty-first century: Facilitating self-directed professional growth.* Miniseminar presented at the annual meeting of the New York State Speech-Language-Hearing Association, New York.

Paul-Brown, D., & Goldberg, D. (2001). Current policies and new directions for speech–language pathology assistants. *Language, Speech, and Hearing Services in Schools, 32,* 4–17.

Striffler, N. (1993). *Current trends in the use of paraprofessionals in early intervention and preschool services.* Chapel Hill, NC: National Early Childhood Technical Assistance System.

U.S. General Accounting Office. (1999). *Medicaid and special education—Coordination of services for children with disabilities is evolving.* (No. GAO/HEHS-0020). Retrieved August 20, 2005, from http://www.gao.gov.new.items/he00020.pdf

Werven, G. (1993). Support personnel: An issue for our times. *American Journal of Speech–Language Pathology, 2,* 9–12.

Wolf, K. E. (1991). Third-party billing for school services: The healthcare provider's perspective. *Asha, 33,* 45–48.

SECTION IV

The Roles of Related Professionals in School-Based Practice

Section IV is based on the recognition that speech–language pathologists are not alone in assisting students with differences and disabilities within the school environment. These final two chapters of the text describe other professionals in the school setting with whom school-based speech–language pathologists can expect to interact. Both chapters stress the need for honest communication and true collaboration as we seek to provide the best services possible to the children who rely on all of us.

Chapter 11 describes the role of the audiologist in the schools and addresses for the first time the student who has received a cochlear implant. As in the case of speech–language pathology, the accelerating rate of change has affected our sister profession in both assessment and provision of services. Improvement in audiological technology has added a dimension that directly affects our services as SLPs.

Chapter 12 allows other professionals—classroom and special education teachers, the school psychologist, the school-based librarian, and occupational and physical therapists—to answer in their own words the question often asked of SLPs, "What is it that you people do?" Issues include training, educational background, duties, and specific ways in which SLPs and these colleagues can effectively collaborate.

Chapter 11

Audiology Services in the Educational Setting

Nancy P. Huffman,
with Arlene Balestra-Marko

P rior to 1975 and the passage of the Education of the Handicapped Act, children with disabilities were not routinely visible in public school classrooms. In many instances, the identified disability determined the educational program, placement, technique, and personnel. Minimal attention was given to the least restrictive environment (LRE) or a continuum of services as we know it today. Local school districts had little if any involvement with or ownership of the identification and placement of students with disabilities. Children went to special schools for the blind, deaf, physically handicapped, or mentally retarded. They were instructed solely by special teachers—teachers of the deaf, blind, or mentally retarded. They had no involvement with non-disabled peers, for the most part. Large school districts may have had buildings dedicated to exceptional children or special programs for the "trainable" or "educable" retarded. Preschool programs for children with disabilities, if they existed at all, were privately funded, perhaps associated with residential schools, but certainly not accessible through publicly supported systems.

Children regarded as deaf may have attended a school for the deaf. For many children with hearing loss, a school for the deaf was the only option, so it is probable that the definition of *deaf* was broad in terms of the range of hearing loss acceptable for entrance. Many students who today might not be regarded as deaf received their education in schools for the deaf. Children with milder hearing problems went to public schools, but they may not even have been identified as having a hearing problem. The hearing problem often was invisible. They may have been treated as they were perceived by the current teacher, possibly as strange, unable to speak clearly, retarded, or having a behavior problem.

During this period the still young audiology profession was growing and changing. For many years, audiologists could only prescribe hearing aids. They could not dispense them. They tested hearing, determined hearing aid candidacy, and made recommendations for the type of hearing aid, which was then fit and managed by the individual selling the hearing aid (not the audiologist). The idea of an audiologist's dispensing hearing aids was unthinkable in terms of professional ethics. With regard to children, hearing aid use and technology was in its infancy compared with the amplification and sensory options available today for virtually every kind of hearing loss. Body-type hearing aids were the norm, over-the-ear hearing aids were improving, and in-the-ear hearing aids were being developed. Completely-in-the-canal (CIC) aids, programmable aids, digital technology, and cochlear implantation were unheard of. It was not uncommon for experts to suggest waiting before fitting amplification to see if the child was ready. What a contrast to today's thrust for early diagnosis and early amplification.

ENABLING LEGISLATION AND REGULATION

The Education for All Handicapped Children Act of 1975 (now known through its reauthorizations as the Individuals with Disabilities Education Act—IDEA) had a significant impact on the audiology profession and the services that were and are now provided in schools. The legislation gave birth to the expansion of audiology services in schools, defined the practice of educational audiology, and placed school audiology services in the public sector.

Prior to the opportunities created by the act, children in schools with hearing loss and listening disorders had access to audiology services primarily through clinics, community agencies, university facilities, physicians, and some private practices. Unfortunately, the providers often had little familiarity with issues of the educational setting. Except for schools for the deaf and some forward-thinking school systems, audiology services in public school agencies were rare.

The Education of the Handicapped Amendments of 1986 created new opportunities for infants, toddlers (Part H), and preschoolers (Part B) with disabilities to access service and education. Under this legislation, mandated services and protections were extended downward to cover children with disabilities ages 3–21. States were given incentives to develop early intervention (birth–2) programs. The effect of the legislation was to create additional responsibilities and involvement for audiologists, speech–language pathologists, and other related service providers in all kinds of educational and early intervention programs for children ages birth through 5 and their families.

The reauthorization in 1990 responded to public sentiment, which recognized that people with disabilities were not necessarily handicapped. The law was amended as the Individuals with Disabilities Education Act (IDEA). In changing the words and the word order, it reinforced that people with disabilities are first individuals, who, second, have a disability. The new IDEA placed renewed focus on a free and appropriate education (FAPE) in the least restrictive environment and required states to defend pull-away services in the federal compliance reviews.

The most recent reauthorization of IDEA occurred in 2004, with regulations proposed. This reauthorization, like the 1997 reauthorization, focused on the next step in the concept of the least restrictive environment—the access of children with disabilities to general education, the premise being that special education is a service and not a place. Today we have in place regulations, policies, procedures, programs, accommodating facilities, and a myriad of professional services related to early intervention and special education to fulfill the goal of access to public education.

We cannot forget other legislation that today affects access to audiology services in schools. Section 504 of the Rehabilitation Act of 1973 prohibits discrimination and requires accommodation of students with disabilities in any program or activity receiving federal financial assistance. Broadly stated, it prohibits denial of participation in public education or enjoyment of the benefits offered by a public school system to a student with a disability. A student who does not qualify for services under IDEA may qualify for services under Section 504. The Americans with Disabilities Act (ADA) passed in 1990 also prohibits discrimination and requires accommodation of students with disabilities in any state or local government program or activity *whether or not* it receives federal financial assistance. Both sets of legislation deal with access. Under both ADA and Section 504, the definitions of disability and who qualifies are much broader than under IDEA. Because not all students with hearing loss may qualify under IDEA, and because hearing loss can affect access to communication and learning, audiology services in schools have an important role to play.

The regulations for IDEA put into print the definition of audiology as a related service. The Regulations for Preschool and School Age (ages 3–21) state that audiology includes the following:

- identification of children with hearing loss;
- determination of the range, nature, and degree of hearing loss, including referral for medical or other professional attention for the habilitation of hearing;
- provision of habilitative activities, such as language habilitation, auditory training, speech reading (lipreading), hearing evaluation, and speech conservation;
- creation and administration of programs for prevention of hearing loss;
- counseling and guidance of children, parents, and teachers regarding hearing loss; and
- determination of the children's needs for group and individual amplification, selecting and fitting an appropriate aid, and evaluating the effectiveness of amplification.

The IDEA regulations for the Early Intervention Program for Infants and Toddlers with disabilities include a definition of audiology similar to that for children ages 3–21 years, but there are differences. The definition currently states that audiology includes the following:

- identification of children with auditory impairment using at-risk criteria and appropriate audiologic screening techniques;
- determination of the range, nature, and degree of hearing loss and communication functions, by use of audiological evaluation procedures;
- referral for medical and other services necessary for the habilitation or rehabilitation of children with auditory impairment;
- provision of auditory training, aural rehabilitation, speech reading and listening device orientation and training, and other services;
- provision of services for prevention of hearing loss; and
- determination of the child's need for individual amplification, including selecting, fitting, and dispensing appropriate listening and vibrotactile devices, and evaluating the effectiveness of those devices.

IDEA's regulations also provide definitions for the disability categories of deaf and hearing impairment as follows: *Deafness* means a hearing impairment that is so severe that the child is impaired in processing linguistic information through hearing, with or without amplification, that adversely affects a child's educational performance. *Hearing impairment* means an impairment in hearing, whether permanent or fluctuating, that adversely affects a child's educational performance but that is not included under the definition of deaf in this section.

The significant role of the audiologist is implicit in these definitions in the need to determine the presence of hearing loss, whether it is permanent or fluctuating, the effect of hearing loss on the processing of spoken language, the effectiveness of amplification, and the need for assistive technology to access the learning environment. Further, regulations state that "each public agency shall ensure that the hearing aids worn in school by children with hearing impairments, including deafness, are functioning properly." Again the responsibility of the school district and the role of the audiologist are acknowledged and reinforced.

Turning Regulation Into Reality

Although federal regulations establish parameters, as in defining audiology services, states have the responsibility to develop their own regulations to comply with federal mandates. Many states do not have requirements for credentials to be held by audiologists who practice in schools, nor do they define roles. Only a few states have guidelines for audiology services in the schools. Many have licensure requirements for audiologists, but public schools are often exempt from those requirements. Audiology services, then, are sometimes defined and delivered by individuals who are not audiologists. DeConde Johnson (1991) in a survey conducted for the Educational Audiology Association, found that ASHA audiology certification or state licensure was required in all but 14 states for individuals who provided audiology services in schools. However, four years later, in regards to services, English (1995) reported that still "most states do not have established guidelines for providing audiology services in schools" (p. 216). Further, she stated that "many school professionals do not have basic information regarding the impact of hearing impairment on learning, nor are they aware of the contributions and expertise of the educational audiologist" (p. 216). Thirty-two states and Washington, D.C. have school requirements for audiologists. These include state licensure, teacher certification, and ASHA certification. Eighteen states have no requirements (M. Mannebach, personal communication, September 7, 2005).

Professional Qualifications and Competencies

Most states require audiologists who work in schools to hold the Certificate of Clinical Competence in Audiology (CCC-A) from ASHA or to be licensed as an audiologist in the state in which they are practicing. Licensure requirements differ from state to state, and some states have separate credentialing or certification requirements for audiologists who work in schools (DeConde Johnson, 1991). There are indeed unique competencies for educational audiology practice beyond those considered traditional for the practice of audiology. Such competencies include knowledge of the structure of the learning environment, including classroom acoustics and implications for learning; skill in the selection and management of assistive listening devices for use in the school setting; skill in consultation and collaboration with teachers (particularly in general education) regarding the relationship of hearing and hearing loss to academic achievement; knowledge of regulatory processes dealing with IDEA and the development of the Individualized Family Service Plan (IFSP) and the Individualized Education Program (IEP); strategies for determining eligibility, evaluation, placement, and performance monitoring of students under IDEA; familiarity with legal issues and procedures surrounding services to students; knowledge of general education curricular requirements for students; skill in using evaluative tools pertinent to listening skills necessary for success in school; sensitivity to family systems, diversity, and cultures, including deaf culture; knowledge of communication systems and language used by individuals who are deaf and hard of hearing; and ability to participate in team processes (Educational Audiology Association, 1994).

AUDIOLOGY RESOURCES

There are now a wide variety of professional and grassroots organizations for children who are deaf and hard of hearing, their families, and the professionals who work with them. A list of these organizations is provided in Appendix 11.A. A list of professional resources related to cochlear implants and therapy materials is provided in Appendix 11.B. ASHA has published numerous position papers, guidelines, policy statements, and reports for the professional audiologist; many of these are cited in the reference section for this chapter. The Educational Audiology Association (EAA) has also published position statements that relate directly to audiology services in schools. These are listed in Appendix 11.C.

THE HEARING NEEDS OF STUDENTS

Although IDEA focuses on students who meet eligibility requirements for one of the 13 disability classifications defined in its regulations, it is important to understand that audiology services in schools need not be focused solely on students with hearing loss or other disabilities. Audiology services touch and benefit all students, nondisabled and disabled, in a variety of ways.

Identification and Screening

Prior to entering school (formal education as defined by each state), most, if not all, children experience some kind of screening that may place them on a high-risk register for hearing loss, or rule out hearing loss, or identify them as having a hearing loss. The Newborn and Infant Screening and Intervention Act of 1999 created funds for state grants to develop infant hearing screening and intervention programs. At the time of this writing, over 40 states have enacted legislation that will provide universal hearing screening to newborns. A list of states that have passed legislation pertaining to newborn hearing screenings can be found on the ASHA Web site (http://www.asha.org). Thus, a child may be identified by a universal newborn infant screening program as having a hearing loss. Or, perhaps as part of a high-risk register, a child may be identified at birth or in infancy as being at risk for hearing loss and therefore be involved in periodic audiologic evaluation and monitoring. As a toddler or preschooler, a child may be a participant in a number of health-related screening programs that typically include hearing screening.

Screening and early identification are so important because it is now widely understood and accepted that hearing is a critical factor for the development of speech and language, communication skills, and learning. The presence of hearing loss of any kind, including minimal or fluctuating loss, is a form of sensory deprivation. It is also widely recognized that the most common etiology of hearing loss in young children is otitis media, which causes a conductive type of loss that is usually fluctuant. Otitis media most frequently occurs during the first 3 years of life (Bluestone & Klein, 1995) yet can continue through ages 8 to 10 (Davis, Shepard, Stelmachowicz, & Gorga, 1981). It is critical that any hearing loss be identified early and appropriately managed.

Many, if not all states, require schools to carry out hearing screening on a periodic basis as students begin, move through, and complete their formal education. All states do not, however, follow the same guidelines. Speech–language pathologists and audiologists working in schools should familiarize themselves with their state's requirements for hearing screening.

Typically, it is required that all children be screened for hearing loss either prior to or upon entry into formal education at age 5 (or the age at which education is mandatory in a particular state) and at regularly defined intervals thereafter. The screening usually occurs at frequent intervals in the elementary grades, followed by a screening at least once during high school. In New York State, for example, hearing screening must be administered at least annually to students in Grades K through 7 and in Grade 10 and to all new entrants into the school district (New York State Education Department, 1992). It is not commonly required by states that all children be screened for middle ear disorders, although some states, such as New York, suggest that it be done on an optional basis or if available. Immittance measures identify individuals with potentially medically significant ear disorders, which may have accompanying hearing loss.

It should be noted that screening programs may not specify who performs the hearing screening. In most cases, screening procedures are performed by nonaudiologist personnel, such as nurses, speech–language pathologists, and technicians. Best practice would warrant that any program conducting screening for hearing loss or middle ear dysfunction be supervised and managed by a licensed and certified audiologist. Regarding screening for hearing loss and middle ear function, speech–language pathologists should be aware of the Scope of Practice statements in speech–language pathology and in audiology published by the American Speech-Language-Hearing Association (ASHA, 1996, 2001). Speech–language pathologists should also be familiar with the ASHA Issues in Ethics statement "Clinical Practice by Certificate Holders in the Profession in Which They Are Not Certified" (ASHA, 2004b).

All identification and screening programs require systematic procedures for protocol, interpretation, referral, follow-up, and management. ASHA has published guidelines for audiologic screening that are a valuable reference for speech–language pathologists in school practice. ASHA guidelines require monaural presentation of pure tones at 500, 1,000, 2,000, and 4,000 Hz at 20 dB (ASHA, 1985; ASHA Panel on Audiologic Assessment, 1997).

Assessment

Audiologists in educational practice are involved in assessment and evaluation of students for a number of reasons. Hearing screening programs operate according to pass–fail and refer criteria. They simply separate individuals into two groups: those who passed (and are therefore presumed to have no hearing loss) and those who failed (and are presumed to have hearing loss) and must be referred for further testing. Children who fail a hearing screening must have an audiological assessment performed by a licensed and certified audiologist to determine the degree, nature, and extent of the suspected hearing loss. The evaluation results may document that no hearing loss exists and the screen failure was a false positive.

The evaluation will yield data that allow the audiologist to describe the degree, nature, and extent of the hearing loss. With regard to degree of hearing loss, the audiologist is looking for quantitative information. Hearing levels are expressed in decibels based on a pure tone average for the frequencies 500 to 4,000 Hz and discussed using descriptors related to severity: normal hearing (−10 to +15 dB HL), borderline hearing loss (16–25 dB HL), mild hearing loss (26–40 dB HL), moderate hearing loss (41–55 dB HL), moderate to severe hearing loss (56–70 dB HL), severe hearing loss (71–90 dB HL), and profound hearing loss (91 dB HL or greater).

With regard to the nature of hearing loss, the audiologist is looking for the type of hearing impairment and information suggesting the site of lesion. The loss may be conductive (a temporary or permanent hearing loss typically due to abnormal conditions of the outer or middle ear), sensorineural (typically a permanent hearing loss due to disease, trauma, or inherited conditions affecting the sensory or nerve cells in the cochlea or inner ear, or conditions affecting the eighth cranial nerve), mixed (a combination of conductive and sensorineural components), or due to an auditory processing disorder (a condition that typically is found in the presence of normal hearing but may occur in combination with conductive, sensorineural, and mixed hearing loss such that there is difficulty processing audible signals).

With regard to extent of hearing loss, the audiologist is looking at qualitative attributes such as bilateral versus unilateral hearing loss; symmetrical versus asymmetrical hearing loss; high-frequency versus low-frequency hearing loss; flat versus sloping versus precipitous hearing loss; progressive versus sudden hearing loss; and stable versus fluctuating hearing loss.

Assessment for the Purpose of Monitoring a Condition

Once a particular hearing loss has been identified, a treatment and management plan is put into place. The plan may include medical or surgical intervention, prescription of personal hearing aids, prescription or provision of assistive listening devices, skills development through aural (audiologic) habilitation or rehabilitation, or simply monitoring of the condition through periodic assessment. It is important, however, for a student's hearing loss to be checked periodically to determine its stability: Is it fluctuating? Has it improved as a result of medical intervention? Is it progressing? Have new conditions come into play that have affected the original condition? It is also important that a student's ability to hear using amplification (i.e., personal hearing aids and any assistive listening devices that are used in place of, or in conjunction with, personal amplification) be monitored and documented. This monitoring would include functional gain assessment, real ear measurement, electroacoustic analysis, listening check, and informal "functional" assessment in the listening environment in which the student operates (i.e., the classroom, the work–study placement, the home).

Assessment Because of Suspected Hearing Loss

Students who have successfully passed periodic school hearing screenings may experience a change in hearing as a result of an event or a particular condition that causes concern. Perhaps a concern has been raised about a student's ability to listen, or the student has had an illness or been treated with a medication that is known to cause hearing loss. There are any number of reasons to suspect hearing loss.

Assessment To Determine Eligibility for Various Programs

As students move through their school careers, they are often required to have reports of hearing testing before they can participate in certain contact sports (some state laws and regulations may require this as a part of a health examination), as part of an application for certain vocational and postsecondary programs, as part of an application to qualify for supplemental security income (SSI), or to demonstrate eligibility for 504 or ADA accommodations and IDEA programs.

Assessment as Part of a Multidisciplinary Team Evaluation

Audiologists are a frequent resource for school placement teams as part of the evaluation process for students who are suspected of having a disability. Sometimes the purpose of the audiological assessment is to confirm the presence of normal hearing. Sometimes the purpose is to conduct tests of auditory processing. A team of professionals is involved in analyzing the listening and auditory processing behaviors of a student and the impact those behaviors have on her learning. Sometimes as part of early intervention (birth to age 3) and early childhood (ages 3 to 5) assessment teams, the purpose is to determine eligibility for services and a description of services needed.

Prevention

An oft-forgotten "hearing need" of students in educational settings is the need to be educated and informed about how to prevent hearing loss. The educational setting is an ideal and natural forum to introduce values and practices relative to hearing hygiene and prevention of hearing loss. It is interesting to note that although schools typically have health education curricula and provide health education, health educators, when surveyed, were shown to have deficiencies in knowledge of hearing, hearing loss, hearing health practices, and, in particular, the effect of noise on hearing (Lass et al., 1990). There is no question that information about methods of prevention, as well as causes and effects, of hearing loss needs to be provided not only to students but also to teachers and administrators.

Hearing hygiene and hearing preservation require education not only on diseases and medical conditions that place one at risk for hearing loss but also on the effects of drugs and over-the-counter medications on hearing. Approximately 200 drugs have been identified as being ototoxic; that is, having the potential to cause toxic reactions to structures of the inner ear, including the cochlea, vestibule, semicircular canals, and otoliths (ASHA, 1994; Miller, 1985). Audiologists are prepared to develop curricula or assist in the development of curricula pertaining to hearing, hearing health, and hearing hygiene as part of school health education programs.

There is ongoing concern about the high prevalence of high-frequency sensorineural hearing loss in school-age students, particularly older students (Anderson, 1967; Woodford, 1973, 1980, 1981; Woodford & O'Farrell, 1983). Researchers have concluded that exposure to excessive noise levels in the educational setting and during recreational activities such as listening to music, riding snowmobiles and motorcycles, and using power tools appears to be the primary etiology of high-frequency hearing loss in older school-age students (Clark, 1991; Katz, Gertsman, Sanderson, & Buchanan, 1982; Woodford & O'Farrell, 1983). The educational setting as an environment for hazardous noise exposure might come as a surprise to many, yet the demonstration of noxious noise levels in vocational and industrial arts classes led the state of Iowa to adopt a law requiring that hearing protection be worn in all educational classes in which noise levels exceed Occupational Safety and Health Administration (OSHA) guidelines for excessive noise (Plakke, 1985, 1991). Audiologists in the educational setting are equipped to determine noise levels, recommend and provide ear protection for both students and staff, and carry out education programs with regard to noise.

Treatment and Management

The educational audiologist, traditionally linked with providing services to students with hearing loss, is an increasingly visible member of school district teams involved in educational programs and placement planning for all students, with and without disabilities. The use of the plural "teams" is deliberate because often there are a number of teams on which an audiologist might participate. They may have differing composition, and they may operate in sequence, at different times, or simultaneously. The audiologist's and speech–language pathologist's need to participate productively on school teams cannot be overstated.

Let us look at this complex and dynamic team process. In a school setting, when a child's needs become apparent or a concern emerges, there is usually a resource team within the building to address concerns, solve problems, and identify areas in which testing is necessary. The resource team typically includes the school psychologist, the speech–language pathologist, a teacher, a school nurse, a social worker, a reading or curriculum specialist, and a school administrator. They are responsible for a student's initial testing and for referral, perhaps to an intermediate unit or an evaluation center familiar with educational contexts, for testing to be done in specific areas such as audiology, occupational therapy, or others. In addition to a building resource team and consistent with IDEA regulation, there is also the school district's placement team. In some states, such as New York, this is called the Committee on Special Education. Its membership consists of persons mandated by federal and state regulation and others selected by the district who work with the family and the building resource team in developing a child's IEP, determining related services, and making placement decisions. Finally, regardless of whether the student has a disability or not, there is the team of educators, related services providers, and school administrators who, with the support of the parents, work together to implement the student's education program wherever it is located.

It is critical that a team work together under administrative leadership to create goals and objectives for a particular student or to implement the goals and objectives that have been created by someone else. This is a dynamic process because team members share their various perspectives (English, 2002). Team members may identify different goals and objectives. Perhaps members agree on the goals and objectives but rank them differently in priority. Team members may have differing perceptions of time frames in which goals can be achieved. They may have differing perceptions as to who is responsible for a particular goal or objective. And they may have different ideas for methods and techniques to use to achieve a goal or objective. The team members around the table are at the same time experts (in their particular field) and novices (in the fields of the other team members). Further, they may not know each other. And finally, they must work together.

In looking at the needs of students with hearing and listening problems, the audiologist's priority may not be the same as that of the teacher of the deaf, which may be different still from the priority of the speech–language pathologist, which may not satisfy the priority of the parents. Each team member, including the parent, sees herself as a key stakeholder. Goals and objectives for a particular student must be a common focus, and the roles of the audiologist, speech–language pathologist, teacher of children who are deaf and hearing, interpreter, note taker, classroom teacher, parent, and any others involved in program implementation must be clearly defined and understood by all. It must also be recognized and understood that under IDEA, special education and related services are to be designed to promote the student's success in the context of the general education curriculum.

Team members must recognize and acquire the necessary skills that allow them to work as a team to identify, work toward, and achieve the student's desired outcome. These skills include collaboration, consensus building or whole-group support, collaborative problem solving, conflict resolution, capitalizing on divergent thinking, collecting and analyzing data, nonjudgmental information sharing, and finally, understanding what is and what is not under the control of the team or an individual member of the team (Katzenbach & Smith, 1994; Kayser, 1994). It is critical that the educational audiologist be seen not only as a team member but also as a team player in this process.

The Audiologist and Students with Hearing Loss

As they participate on teams developing and carrying out treatment and management plans for students with hearing loss, audiologists and speech–language pathologists know that hearing loss negatively affects the development of receptive and expressive language skills, which in turn causes learning problems, which then jeopardizes and often lowers academic achievement. In fact, the relationship between hearing loss and poor academic performance has been documented over the years (Bess, 1985; Brackett & Maxon, 1986; Davis, 1977). Further, Bess (1985) has shown that even a mild hearing loss or a unilateral hearing loss can result in academic failure. The student's communication difficulties frequently lead to social isolation and poor self-esteem. Often the student's vocational choice and vocational success are affected.

As a first step, the audiologist may have a lead role in determining candidacy for and prescribing personal amplification (i.e., hearing aids). When possible, the audiologist prescribes hearing aids that can easily connect to assistive listening devices (ALDs), using audio input and telecoil options. The hearing aid–assistive device combination should allow for various listening options: (a) listening only through the hearing aid microphone (thus able to hear close sounds), (b) listening only to the signal coming in via audio input or through the telecoil (thus able to hear only the teacher's voice being transmitted and shutting off close sounds), and (c) listening to the signals coming from both the hearing aid microphone and the signal from the telecoil or audio input (thus able to hear the teacher as well as close sounds). As a team member, the audiologist is also prepared to design and carry out programs to assist students in developing listening skills, managing their hearing aids, managing various listening situations and environments, and managing communication environments. The audiologist, in partnership with parents, speech–language pathologists, and others working with the student, is prepared to assist those partners in recognizing when amplification may not be working, to perform listening checks, and to do basic troubleshooting. This is consistent with the federal regulation cited earlier that requires school districts to ensure that hearing aids worn in school by hard-of-hearing and deaf students are working properly.

With cochlear implantation becoming an increasingly viable alternative for children with severe to profound hearing loss, the educational audiologist would be a key member of the implant team, especially at the local school district level. A section on cochlear implants is at the end of the chapter.

For students who are deaf it is necessary for the school team to have particular sensitivity to issues pertaining to educational placement, amplification, communication methods, the cultural aspects of deafness, and the deaf community. The deaf community has been defined as "the community of people whose primary mode of communication is signed language and who share a common identity, a common culture and a common way of interacting with each other and the hearing community" (National Association of State Directors of Special Education [NASDSE], 1994, p. 78). It is again crucial that the team work together to identify needs and resources consistent with the family's expectation of outcome. Team members such as the audiologist, the teacher of the deaf and hard of hearing, and the speech–language pathologist are valuable resources for further understanding of philosophies of education of the deaf; communication modes (American Sign Language [ASL], cued speech, signed English, signing exact English, finger spelling, total communication); and, depending on the placement and communication system used, the need for educational interpreters or transliterators, note takers, and other supports required to achieve outcomes identified for the student. These specialists have unique preparation, certification, and roles.

Teachers of children who are deaf and hard of hearing have preparation in general education and additional special education preparation and expertise in the learning needs of children who are deaf. They should be able to communicate proficiently in the primary language and preferred mode of communication of their students. They are skilled in using technology that is known to enhance instruction for students who have hearing loss, they can modify curriculum and apply instructional techniques for clearer presentation and ease of comprehension of information in specific content areas, they carry out appropriate test modification, and they are frequently the coordinators of educational programs for students in mainstreamed settings. It should be noted that the title for these teachers used throughout this chapter is consistent with the terminology in a position paper developed by a joint committee of ASHA and the Council on Education of the Deaf (ASHA, 2004d).

The note taker is trained to take notes for students who have hearing loss and are unable to simultaneously participate in instruction and take notes. (If a student with hearing loss is trying to listen, follow a visual media presentation, read lips, or attend to an interpreter, taking notes becomes virtually impossible.) More recently, note takers have been providing services for students with other disabilities who for various reasons are unable to take class notes. The note taker attends classes with the student, takes notes, and provides copies of the notes to the student, the classroom teacher, and the teacher of children who are deaf and hard of hearing, who may be providing support.

Educational interpreters and transliterators facilitate communication exchanges between students and others, including teachers, service providers, and peers within the educational environment (NASDSE, 1994, p. 66). They interpret for the student the spoken communication of the teacher, using the student's preferred communication mode. For the teacher and others who are not fluent in the student's preferred communication mode, they interpret into spoken English the student's communication. Educational interpreters are trained and must meet competencies. The Registry of Interpreters for the Deaf, the Council of Education of the Deaf, and the National Cued Speech Association have standards and ethics codes that all interpreters must meet.

The speech–language pathologist provides communication services to children who are hard of hearing and deaf. These include language development, auditory perception and listening training, speech therapy, speech reading training, and communication situation management. The term *communication services* is purposefully used here because the specific areas of skills training mentioned are integrated to focus on communication in the education environment and success in the general education curriculum.

The Audiologist and Students Whose Primary Disability Is Not Hearing Loss

Audiologists are involved in developing treatment and management plans for students whose primary disability is not hearing loss. They collaborate with speech–language pathologists in the assessment and intervention of central auditory processing disorders (CAPDs) in cases where there is evidence of speech, language, or other cognitive communication disorders (ASHA, 1996). There has been disagreement over use of the word *central*. Keith (1999) notes that the original use of the word in *CAPD* was meant to indicate that the processing difficulty occurred at the brain stem or cortical levels, while auditory processing disorders would originate in the peripheral auditory system (cochlea and auditory nerve). Central auditory processes include sound localization and lateralization, auditory discrimination, auditory pattern recognition, temporal aspects of audition, auditory performance with competing acoustic signals, and auditory performance with degraded acoustic signals (ASHA Task Force on Central Auditory Processing Consensus Development, 1996). Friel-Patti (1999) noted that the Task Force did not provide specific criteria for the diagnosis of CAPD, and therefore the group of children diagnosed with CAPD is heterogeneous. Although the term *CAPD* is still used, the term *auditory processing disorder* (APD) is frequently used now. An example of this is in ASHA's *Guidelines for Audiology Service Provision in and for Schools* (2002a). These guidelines note the 1996 descriptors used by the Task Force. They note that the communication, academic, and psychosocial characteristics of children with APD are similar to those demonstrated by children who have language-learning disabilities, hearing impairment, and attention deficit disorder. A listing of these characteristics is included in the guidelines (ASHA, 2002a).

ASHA (2005d) uses the term *central auditory processing disorder* (CAPD) and defines it as an auditory deficit diagnosed by an audiologist. The Position Statement and Technical Report list the characteristics and indicate that professionals such as speech–language pathologists collaborate with the audiologist when "speech-language and/or cognitive disorders" (ASHA, 2005c, p. 1) are present.

It should be noted that neither APD nor CAPD is a category of disability recognized by IDEA. Children with APD may sometimes be classified as having a language impairment or learning disability under IDEA when receiving services for special education. They may also receive services under Section 504.

Students with auditory processing disorders have difficulty paying attention (particularly in the presence of background noise), following spoken directions, remembering heard information, and performing fine sound analyses and discrimination. In an attempt to overcome listening problems associated with background noise and poor attending, a first intervention strategy is signal enhancement (Palacio, 2000). Educational audiologists are prepared to explore assistive listening devices; improve signal-to-noise ratio, such as large-area soundfield classroom amplification systems; and individually prescribed assistive listening systems. Audiologists can also assist teachers and staff in modifying their presentation and instructional style so the student can more easily process spoken information. Audiologists can assist in making environmental modifications to improve the listening situation. They can also provide auditory training and instruction to the student in managing his listening habits and skills. Any amplification device used with children with normal hearing should be prescribed and managed by an audiologist.

Audiologists may be consultants for classroom acoustics. A variety of studies have indicated that young listeners have more difficulty in noisy situations than adults. There appears to be a trend of the ability to listen with noise in the background improving from childhood to the teen years (Gravel, Fausel, Liskow, & Chobot, 1999; Soli & Sullivan, 1997; Stelmachowicz, Hoover, Lewis, Kortekaas, & Pittman, 2000). In addition to younger listeners, other groups that may be at risk in noisy environments are children with hearing losses (even minimal), children with otitis media, children learning English as a second language, and children with learning disabilities or attention disorders (ASHA, 2005a). Nelson, Kohnert, Sabur, and Shaw (2005) noted that in their study second graders learning English as a second language had more difficulty with word recognition tasks in a +10 dB signal-to-noise ratio than did their English-only peers. ASHA (2005a) makes the following recommendations for the acoustics of educational settings: a signal-to-noise ratio greater than +15 dB (at the child's ear); background noise levels (for unoccupied rooms) no greater than 35 dB; and reverberation times (for unoccupied classrooms) greater than .6 seconds for smaller classrooms (volume less than 10,000 cubic feet) and .7 seconds for larger classrooms (10,000–20,000 cubic feet in volume). The ASHA position statement indicates that the criteria listed are virtually identical to ANSI standards (American National Standards Institute, 2002) and that the ANSI standards have guidelines for larger areas (ASHA, 2005b).

A recent article by Knecht, Nelson, Whitelaw, and Feth (2002) examined 32 empty classrooms for noise levels and reverberation times. Only one classroom complied with both the noise and reverberation levels recommended by ASHA. Classrooms with the lowest reverberation levels and noise levels tended to be in newer buildings. The ASHA (2005) "Guidelines for Addressing Acoustics in Educational Settings" addresses the importance of classroom acoustics and issues for both new construction and corrective work on existing classrooms (ASHA, 2005a).

Audiologists also have responsibilities to groups whose members may not have a diagnosed hearing impairment. Students with mental retardation and other developmental disabilities have a higher incidence of hearing loss than the general pediatric population (ASHA, 1983; Fulton & Lloyd, 1969). They have a particularly high incidence of conductive hearing loss (for example, as a result of craniofacial anomalies and other medical conditions), which requires management and monitoring. The audiologist is prepared to explore a number of strategies in addition to personal amplification and assistive listening systems to make the listening environment more accessible to students with mental retardation and developmental disabilities.

Audiologists are involved on teams that design services for students with vision impairments. Hearing loss and impairments of vision and blindness frequently have a common etiology—as, for example, in the cases of Usher syndrome and maternal rubella. It is important that a student with vision disabilities have audiologic evaluation that includes a detailed case history. Monitoring and documentation of vision and hearing status on a periodic basis are necessary. Students with dual-sensory disabilities of vision and hearing (deaf-blindness or visual impairment–hearing impairment) require joint, collaborative management between the audiologist, the vision specialist, and the speech–language pathologist, particularly in the prescription and management of assistive technology for learning and for environmental control.

In the early 1990s, students with autism became the focus of a novel listening treatment program called *auditory integration training* (AIT), and audiologists became visible members of the team of professionals providing services to those students. AIT was developed in the 1960s in France by a physician, Guy Berard. He used the program with individuals who had a number of disabling conditions, such as dyslexia, depression, learning problems, and autism (Veale, 1994a, 1994b). The use of AIT was controversial, and no scientific studies supported its use. In response to the controversy regarding AIT, the 1994 ASHA subcommittee on AIT recommended that ASHA develop a position statement and guidelines when more research was available. ASHA has since developed a position statement on AIT indicating that it is an experimental approach and has not met scientific standards as a treatment. This position paper encourages more research to address the efficacy of this treatment approach (ASHA, 2004a).

Promoting Learning Access and Success

When working with students with hearing losses in an educational setting, we must consider several variables that will have significant impacts upon their learning. One of the primary factors is the hearing loss. This encompasses not only the degree of hearing loss but also the nature and the extent of the hearing loss. The physical setting and context for learning are also important, as are the instructional dynamics and instructional tools. Each of these factors will be discussed in the following section.

Consider the Hearing Loss

Although it may be obvious (and may risk being too simplistic), the primary difficulty for students with hearing loss is that they cannot hear in their instructional settings. They are unable to access spoken and other acoustic information to benefit from instruction because they cannot hear it. Let us now look at some examples of hearing loss and the problems they pose in hearing and ability to benefit from instruction. Earlier in this chapter, hearing loss was discussed with regard to its degree, nature, and extent. The examples here are discussed in terms of those attributes.

Degree of Hearing Loss. A student whose average hearing, between 500 and 2,000 Hz on the audiogram, lies in the mild loss range (26–40 dB hearing level) will probably not hear 25% to 40% of speech signals under ideal conditions (Anderson & Matkin, 1991). Successful hearing is dependent upon the level of noise present, the distance from the speaker, and the specific configuration (across all frequencies) of the hearing loss. In instructional settings, the student may miss up to 50% of class discussions because (a) distances vary between the classmates and teachers who are speaking to the student who is trying to hear, (b) communication exchanges and contributions occur and shift rapidly, (c) speakers have different volumes and rates of speaking, and (d) background noise is usually present. Because hearing ability is inconsistent based on specific conditions of communication experience, a mild hearing loss may go undetected. Instead, the student is seen as not paying attention, having selective hearing, or daydreaming.

A student whose average hearing (between 500 and 2,000 Hz) lies between 41 and 55 dB HL may understand conversation (a) within a distance of 3 to 5 feet, (b) when it is face to face, and (c) when it occurs with carefully controlled speaking and vocabulary (Anderson & Matkin, 1991). Those around the child would most likely suspect hearing loss because inability to hear would demonstrate itself in most situations. The child would be expected to have speech–language problems involving articulation, sentence structure, use of syntax, limited vocabulary both receptively and expressively, and self-monitoring of voice loudness and quality.

A child with a severe hearing loss can hear conversational speech only with amplification or a cochlear implant. Losses are between 70 dB and 85 dB HL. Discrimination of speech even with amplification may be significantly affected. If the hearing loss occurs before language develops, oral language and speech will not develop spontaneously. Speech intelligibility will be significantly affected. A child with a severe hearing loss often has an initial educational placement in a specialized classroom setting. She may receive instruction in oral communication or manual communication and develop skills that would provide success in other educational settings.

A child with a hearing loss greater than 90 dB is classified as profoundly deaf. Children in this category may use a combination of hearing aids and frequency modulation (FM) systems. They may use oral or manual communication. Typically, even with amplification, speech intelligibility is poor. Children with severe and profound hearing losses may be considered candidates for cochlear implants. This will be discussed in the section at the end of the chapter.

Nature of Hearing Loss. Fluctuating hearing loss commonly occurs in young children secondary to otitis media with effusion, which is the accumulation of fluid in the middle ear. If hearing is typically within normal range without fluid, the presence of fluid may create a conductive hearing loss of mild or moderate degree. When the fluid dissipates, hearing returns to previously normal levels. Hearing loss that fluctuates causes the student to have inconsistent ability to "hear." On some days the student may perform consistently in terms of response to instructional expectations. Yet at other times, he will simply not hear or will respond inappropriately in comparison to previously demonstrated behaviors and responses in similar situations.

In unilateral hearing loss, hearing levels in one ear are within normal range and in the other ear there is a hearing loss of mild or greater severity. Individuals with unilateral hearing loss cannot "hear" conversation or sounds originating on the "bad" side. They have the greatest difficulty locating and localizing sound source and direction. They have difficulty in noisy situations, particularly when the noise source is on the "good" side. Because one ear is normal, this type of loss may go undetected for quite some time or, if detected, may be regarded as insignificant. The child might be viewed as having selective hearing or poor attention or as hearing only what he wants to hear.

Extent of Hearing Loss. High-frequency hearing loss refers to a situation in which hearing levels in the low to middle frequencies (250–1,000 Hz) lie within normal limits but hearing drops off to mild and greater loss levels in the higher frequencies (1,500–8,000 Hz). There are variations, but the essence is that lower pitches (frequencies) are easily heard, and high pitches are not heard. This causes distortion in hearing because the student may hear the vowel and some voiced consonant portions of what is said but not the unvoiced consonants. The unvoiced consonants are markers of verb tense, possession, gender, plurality, and so on; if they are not heard, the intended message may be confused or misconstrued. For example, "What time is it?" might be heard as "What kind is it?" or "I passed the test" might be heard as "I packed the rest." Words like *paint, painting,* and *painted* might all sound like "ain't." The result is miscommunication and a response that to the listener is not appropriate or related to the topic. Depending on the degree and configuration of the high-frequency loss, the student will demonstrate articulation errors, poor receptive and expressive language development and skills, and inappropriate responses in instructional and social contexts.

These are but a few examples of the various kinds and types of hearing loss that are managed in educational settings. As stated earlier, there are variations. Of course, the attributes of degree, nature, and extent or configuration of hearing loss, though separated here, become inextricably intertwined as we study a particular student's situation. In addition to these attributes, other important features of the hearing loss, such as age of onset, age of discovery, etiology, and age at which intervention was introduced, influence decisions about instruction and access to instruction. Mark Ross, an audiologist who himself has a severe to profound hearing loss, suggested that the problem with having a hearing loss is that (a) you hear what you think you hear, (b) you don't know what you didn't hear, and (c) you don't know what you misheard because you didn't hear it correctly in the first place (Ross, Brackett, & Maxon, 1991). Any student with hearing loss requires a carefully designed and monitored management program based on the attributes of the hearing loss that are unique to that individual student and on the demands of the instructional program.

Consider the Setting and Context of Instruction

The setting influences access to spoken and other acoustic information that enhances instruction. Instruction today occurs in a multitude of places. For most, the traditional school classroom immediately comes to mind, the kind that houses 20 to 25 desks in rows, chairs, a few small tables, and a teacher's desk. Today, that layout may not be the norm. Our classrooms are divided into instructional centers, technology centers, and pull-aside therapeutic centers. What remains the norm is that classrooms exist in buildings that could be as old as 70 years or brand new, or may be stand-alone portable rooms. The buildings exist in urban, suburban, and rural areas. They are subject to air, ground, and underground traffic noise and other external acoustic factors that are completely out of our control. Unfortunately, even the most recently constructed buildings have been designed without consideration of the acoustics necessary for learning. Classrooms vary in function and therefore may be large, with specialized equipment and workstations, as in a shop, a kitchen, or a gymnasium. Or they may be rather small, as in a room in which small-group instruction or therapy occurs. It can be stated with confidence, however, that most classrooms are subject to external noise (street traffic, construction, air traffic), internal building noise (ventilation and heating systems, toilets, adjacent classrooms, entryways, workshops), and room activity noise (computers, talking, shuffling feet, desk movement, paper noise).

Instruction today also occurs in naturalistic and functional settings. These include the student's home, day care centers, nursery schools, work–study placements, and field placements. Some unique, alternative general and special education programs provide full-time instruction in settings such as farms, greenhouses, and carpentry shops, where the setting is the "classroom" and academics are integrated into the functional instructional activity. Instruction occurs in hospitals, jails, and other specialized settings. For some, the classroom might be at home, where a student engaged in distance learning receives instruction via computer and telephones, and in the case of children who are home schooled. The list is endless, as are the acoustic challenges posed by the settings. The point is that the physical setting and context of instruction today extend far beyond our traditional paradigm and perception of the classroom with walls as boundaries. For a student with hearing loss, the setting and context of instruction pose access challenges that must be recognized and addressed in educational planning.

Consider the Instructional Dynamics

Our discussion of instructional dynamics focuses on (a) instructional staff (teachers, related service providers, support staff) and their interaction as an instructional team, (b) instructional models and strategies or the techniques of instruction, and (c) the tools used as part of instruction. The dynamics of instruction vary widely and change constantly as a function of the contexts and settings described above. Hence, the emphasis on dynamics.

Instructional Staff. Instructional staff may operate in instructional contexts in a variety of ways, a few of which are described here:

- Single teacher with a class of 25 students in a "traditional" classroom.
- Co-teacher, in a situation in which two teachers together provide instruction.
- Teacher with classroom aides or paraeducators. (Some regulated special education classroom ratios provide for an aide or even an aide for every 4 students in a classroom that has a maximum capacity of 12. It is therefore possible for a teacher and up to four paraeducators to be providing an instructional program. This does not include related services providers delivering service within the classroom.)
- Teacher with one or more students in a class who have an assigned one-to-one aide.
- Teacher and related service providers participating in integrated instruction in which therapies and related services such as occupational

therapy, physical therapy, and speech–language pathology occur within the context of the classroom for extended periods of time.

- Related or special instructional services delivered by providers outside of the classroom context (as when the student leaves the classroom for resource room service, instruction from a teacher of children who are deaf or hard of hearing, speech–language services, occupational therapy, physical therapy, tutoring, or audiology services). (The classroom instruction continues while the student is out of the class receiving related or special instructional services. The related service providers and the classroom instructional staff are expected to keep in touch with each other to coordinate services that are relevant to the student's educational program.)
- Single teacher who instructs students who cannot be seen (as in a distance-learning instructional context, in which the class may include many students from a wide geographical area).

Models and Strategies of Instruction. Staff who provide instruction use a number of models and strategies. Again, the traditional model comes to mind of a teacher instructing from the front of the room, a class of 25 students sitting at desks in rows. Instruction today is highly interactive and may include the following:

- cooperative learning strategies, in which small groups of students work with each other under the guidance of a teacher who may be cruising, monitoring, and prompting;
- blended classrooms, in which teachers and aides are instructing simultaneously and moving among students to monitor, target, and assist;
- instruction that combines lecture with periodic small-group interaction and reporting; and
- instruction that is highly interactive, such as large-group discussion, debate, questioning, and clarifying.

In any model or strategy that involves more than one adult, an additional dynamic of adult interaction or adult talk becomes a factor. Adult talk means the communication between and among instructional staff to manage and coordinate the instruction as it is occurring. Adult talk may come from a teacher who advises an aide to change technique, a one-to-one aide who is providing feedback to the teacher, or an interpreter who is working with a student who is deaf. Unfortunately, all too often the adult talk may be irrelevant social talk that distracts from instruction and has a negative effect on students.

Instructional Tools. Finally, the tools and technology used in instruction are extensive, expanding in scope, and constantly changing. Instructional tools include computers (with and without speakers), televisions and VCRs, film projectors, overhead projectors, tape recorders, compact disc players, and telephones. We use these tools to enhance an instructor's presentation as it is happening, to substitute for the in-person instructor, and to offer optional enrichment programs for self-study.

Contexts, settings, and instructional dynamics present significant access issues for students who have hearing loss or listening disorders (hearing problems occurring in the absence of hearing loss, such as auditory processing disorders). According to Berg (1987), students spend at least 45% of the school day engaged in listening activities. That is confirmed by teachers, who, when asked to name a crucial skill necessary for classroom success, usually resoundingly reply, "Listening." Yet we as an educational team of speech–language pathologists, audiologists, teachers of children who are deaf or hard of hearing, and classroom teachers often fail to recognize the importance of structuring and enhancing the listening environment within the instructional setting. Often, in the midst of instruction, we ask the student with limited hearing, "Can you hear me?" And what does the student automatically reply? "Yes." As Flexer, Wray, and Ireland (1989) pointed out, one would not expect the student to state the real answer: "I hear your voice, but I can't hear the unstressed linguistic markers of plurality and tense; nor can I hear articles, voiceless consonants or new vocabulary words clearly enough to distinguish them from other known words" (p. 17). Because instruction today is so dynamic, it is essential that access considerations be included in planning for a student with hearing loss.

Facilitating Listening in Instructional Settings

Typically, the effort to facilitate listening focuses first on assistive listening devices. Assistive listening devices maintain optimal signal-to-noise ratio for the student. They minimize the effects of distance, surrounding noise, and reverberation on the student's ability to receive the desired signals (e.g., the instructor's voice).

The availability of assistive listening systems as an easy and accessible tool to overcome poor listening and instructional environments has increased the value of educational audiologists. Many well-intended school districts, in seeking to provide listening accessibility for their students with hearing loss, made purchases of equipment without the advice of an audiologist. Many invested in equipment that they came to perceive as nonfunctional, with no one on site who understood its fitting or operation. Although the number of educational audiologists and audiologists practicing in educational settings is growing, it is still the exception rather than the rule for a school district to have its own audiologist. The audiologist who is familiar with instructional settings, instructional models, and instructional tools is increasingly seen as a valuable and cost-effective resource to a school district in the prescribing, procuring, fitting, troubleshooting, and managing of assistive listening system programs in educational settings.

The educational audiologist is the architect and overall manager of a school assistive listening device program. All assistive listening systems attempt to eliminate the listening problems created by poor acoustics: noise, distance, and reverberation. Although there are several kinds of assistive listening systems, frequency modulation (FM) systems are most commonly used. The FM system operates like a miniature radio station. A transmitter or microphone is placed at the sound source (the teacher wears a small microphone 3–5 inches from her mouth). The signal is transmitted to a receiver worn by the student; then it is changed back to an audio signal and routed to the ear through the student's hearing aid or through a receiver (a speaker or earphone).

Some still believe that a hearing aid performs the same function as an assistive listening system, but it does not. Students who use only hearing aids are still subject to listening problems created by distance, noise, and reverberation. The following list gives the requirements for assistive listening systems and indicates how FM systems and hearing aids (HAs) compare (ASHA, 2002b; Fettinger & Huffman, 1994; Huffman, 1982, 1985):

- The system must allow the student to receive the teacher's voice at a constant intensity level, regardless of the distance between the student and the teacher. (FM—Yes; HA—No)
- The system must allow the teacher's voice to be heard more prominently than background noise (such as papers rustling, chairs scraping, whispering, footsteps, outside noises), even when the background noise is closer to the student than the teacher's voice. (FM—Yes; HA—No)
- The system must allow the student to hear his own voice and the voices of other students who are close by in small-group discussion. (FM—Yes; HA—Yes)
- The system must be easily wearable and must allow the student and teacher to move about freely. (FM—Yes; HA—Yes)
- The system must be adjustable in frequency response and maximum power output to suit the individual student's hearing loss. (FM—Yes; HA—Yes)
- The system must be sturdy and convenient to use. (FM—Yes; HA—Yes)

The application and use of assistive listening systems in the instructional setting is both art and science.

Communication Management

Whereas the educational audiologist is the architect and manager of an assistive listening device program, the speech–language pathologist is the architect of the communication management program. More often than not, there is a strong joint partnership between the educational audiologist and the speech–language pathologist because one management program cannot happen without the other. In designing programs for students with hearing loss, it is important pragmatically to think in terms of "listening" and "communication" instead of "hearing" and "speaking." By adopting this frame of reference, we broaden our thinking to tie listening into the receiving of information, and speaking into the sending of information. This creates roles and responsibilities for all members of the team who may be involved in instruction—the teacher, aide, related services providers, speech–language pathologists, teachers of children who are deaf or hard of hearing, interpreters—to craft a learning environment in which the student can successfully receive and send information as part of instruction regardless of the mode she uses.

Questions of Management

Answers to these questions will help plan an appropriate management program for a student.

- What is the student's primary communication mode? How does the student receive information? through hearing? a manual language system? a total communication system? a vibrotactile system? Is communication mediated through an interpreter or a transliterator?
- How will multitalker instruction be handled so the student can "hear" or receive the information from each talker when that talker speaks? How will the student know to whom she should attend?
- How will adult talk (noninstructional talk among adults in the classroom) be managed?
- How will assistive listening devices be used in each of the instructional models in which the student participates? How will interpreters, note takers, and so forth be used within instructional models?
- Can the tools used in instruction be accessed by the student with hearing loss? What will the plan be for each of the tools typically used in the student's particular instructional context?

In working to design a communication management program, the speech–language pathologist's goal is for the student to engage successfully in academic conversation and social conversation. If speaking is an element of that "conversation," intervention must include helping the student to receive speech. This involves working with the audiologist to make sure the student has appropriate hearing aids and assistive listening devices. It also involves learning how to determine whether hearing aids and listening devices are working. Speech–language pathologists have indicated that they have little or no experience in inspecting hearing aids (Lass et al., 1989). This is not necessarily surprising because students with hearing losses are a low-incidence population. But this documented information is a signal to both speech–language pathologists and audiologists that together they must ensure that the speech–language pathologist, and ideally others on site, will have the demonstrated capability to complete listening checks and basic troubleshooting of the student's amplification devices. In addition to carrying out listening checks, the Five-Sound Test, attributed to Ling and described by Berg (1987), is a highly functional tool that can be easily employed by the speech–language pathologist in a variety of listening settings. Speech sounds representing energy in low, middle, and high frequencies are used. They are /u/, /a/, /i/, /ʃ/, and /s/. If the student can hear these 5 sounds, it can be assumed that he can hear all 40 speech sounds in the English language. The test can first be administered in a quiet setting. The speaker should be within 3 feet and behind the student or seated so that the student cannot see the speaker's face. The student is instructed to raise his hand when he hears the sound. The speaker proceeds to present the sounds in the order presented above. Raising the hand upon hearing the sound is a "detection" response. If the student can repeat the sound, the student is demonstrating "recognition." The task can be altered to provide additional information. For example, speaker distances can be varied, the order of sounds can be changed, and the test can be administered in different types of listening environments. Information provided by this test helps the teacher determine optimum speaking distances in different listening settings. It can also be a way to help the student begin to learn how to position himself in different settings. If the student knows that he cannot hear when the speaker is beyond 5 feet, then he can begin self-advocacy by requesting optimal seating.

In addition to working to have the student receive speech optimally, the speech–language pathologist designs programs to ensure that the student understands the speech that she receives (i.e., the focus is on receptive language development, vocabulary skills, and processing of conversation that occurs in the context of instruction). Representative examples of activities that address the understanding of speech might include training the student to recognize her name when called upon during play; word and phrase recognition and understanding; training the student in listening for and identifying tense markers (/t/ and /d/) in sentences; preteaching of vocabulary words; vocabulary expansion; use of context clues to anticipate the outcome of a story; awareness of conversational rules (recognizing that someone is talking, waiting one's turn to speak); training the student to recognize and understand routine; "unique to the teacher" phrases and directions that the teacher uses as part of instruction; recognizing and applying contextual clues; and helping the student to understand her hearing loss and what she is unable to hear because of it. The speech–language pathologist also designs programs to help the student generate messages that express the intended idea (i.e., with a focus on expressive language): use of correct vocabulary, form, and sentence structure within the pragmatic context. Representative examples of activities that focus on generating messages might include paraphrasing sentences, requesting clarification, providing more than one meaning for common words, generating sentences, object identification, action–agent activities, maintaining noun–verb agreement and topic, and successfully negotiating problem solving with peers. The speech–language pathologist designs programs to ensure that the student can produce speech that is intelligible to others—hence the focus on articulation, phonological development, rate, prosody, and temporal aspects of speaking. Representative activities might include teaching sound production, drill and practice activities, transfer of skills into context, identifying feedback mechanisms, developing an oral report, and application of pronunciation rules for letter combinations. Finally, the speech–language pathologist provides training in communication and conversation management (Tye-Murray, 1998), assisting the student to assertively manage the environment, to use expressive repair strategies in the role of speaker, to use receptive repair strategies in the role of listener, to capitalize on contextual clues in the communication situation, and to use anticipatory strategies in preparation for the communication situation.

Lasting Partnerships

As educational audiology services continue to grow and become more visible in schools, the speech–language pathologist continues to be the advocate and is often the first to be involved in issues of hearing and listening in school. It is important for both the educational audiologist and the speech–language pathologist to recognize and use each other as resources in planning and implementing programs for the hearing and listening needs of all children in school. From the points made in this chapter, some guidelines for speech–language pathologists in school practice emerge:

1. Determine the requirements in your state for audiologists who work in schools.
2. Determine if your state has requirements for the kinds of audiology services to be provided by school districts.
3. Determine your state's hearing screening requirements and who is responsible for screening.
4. If there is any question whatsoever about a student's hearing (even if the student has passed a school screening), advocate for an evaluation to be done by an audiologist.
5. Determine your audiology resources and develop a strong working partnership with an audiologist.
6. Make sure that any assistive listening system provided to a student is prescribed, fitted, and managed by a licensed audiologist.
7. Make it your priority to be able to perform a listening check on the hearing aids and assistive listening devices that your students use.
8. Work with your audiologist to develop student education programs on hearing, hearing loss, hearing hygiene, the protection of hearing, and the prevention of hearing loss.
9. Develop your teamwork skills so that all on the instructional team will be working toward common outcomes related to the student's success in the general education curriculum.
10. Broaden your thinking to include the concepts of listening and communication.
11. Familiarize yourself with curricular requirements for listening at every grade level.

12. Familiarize yourself with district-wide and statewide assessment tools and the listening requirements for students to be successful.

13. Be aware of technology used in the general education classroom and the ability of the student who is hard of hearing to access that technology using a hearing aid or assistive listening device.

14. Use listening inventories and teacher checklists as methods of gathering information on a student's ability to hear and listen in instructional settings.

15. Familiarize yourself with Scopes of Practice in speech–language pathology and audiology in order to effectively collaborate with audiologists in designing services for students with hearing loss.

16. Check for additional information on the ASHA Web site, which includes a list of questions for the evaluation of products or programs (ASHA, 2004c).

AN OVERVIEW OF COCHLEAR IMPLANTS: ARLENE BALESTRA-MARKO

The history of electrical stimulation of the hearing mechanism dates back to as early as the 19th century; however, it was not until the 1960s that research groups had an active interest in and a design of electrical stimulation of the cochlea. By the 1970s, William House, Blair Simmons, and Robin Michelson had cochlear implant research programs in place with subsequent studies of their efficacy. Fast forward 20 years, with vast amounts of research supporting implant efficacy, implant design enhancements, and FDA approval for use in adults and children, and the multichannel cochlear implant has now become an accessible and successful tool providing access to spoken language for children and adults who are deaf. More than 8,000 infants and children have received cochlear implants nationwide, and with newborn hearing screening and early intervention, the numbers are expected to grow significantly. Children with implants are beginning to appear on the caseloads of speech–language pathologists in local school districts.

Cochlear Implant Components

The multichannel cochlear implant system is composed of both external and internal components. The internal components consist of an electrode array that is inserted into the cochlea and a receiver that is placed just under the skin and housed upon the temporal bone in a recess where it rests almost directly behind the ear. The external components are those that can be seen on the child and consist of a microphone, speech processor, and transmitter. Today's technology has greatly refined the form and function of the cochlear implant, allowing consumers a choice between ear-level and body-worn processors and numerous processing strategies and rates designed to enhance overall speech discrimination. For children, the addition of special stickers and color choice individualizes their implant and promotes acceptance of the device.

The cochlear implant delivers sound to the cochlea in the following manner: The sound is captured by the microphone and travels through a cable into the speech processor, where it is rapidly converted into electrical signals. Those signals are then sent to the transmitter, which is held in place by a small magnet. Via radio transmission, the transmitter relays its information through the skin and into the receiver, where it is sent to the electrode array within the cochlea. Depending on the manufacturer, the electrode array comes in various sizes, straight or curved, and varies in number of electrodes on the array.

Surgery

Cochlear implant surgery is essentially the same regardless of device chosen. The skin is prepared just behind the ear of implantation, and an incision is made to expose the mastoid bone. A mastoidectomy (drilling of the mastoid bone) is performed. A tunneling approach is used until the cochlea is reached. Once reached, the electrode array is inserted into the scala tympani of the cochlea; then the receiver is placed in a small bed drilled within the temporal bone (Nevins & Chute, 1996). Once everything is in place, the audiologist will perform an evaluation of the system to ensure that it is working properly.

The surgery often takes 2–4 hours to complete, with a hospital stay of as little as one day. Typically, the child is recovered within a day or two. Most often, within 3–5 weeks, the child returns to see the audiologist for an initial programming of the speech processor, often called a "mapping." The audiologist details how and where along the electrode array the processor will convert sound. There are several different processing strategies to choose from, to which each child responds uniquely. Generally, the audiologist will program two distinct levels within each electrode, a comfort level and a threshold level (i.e., the minimal amount of current needed for a child to respond and the maximum that can be tolerated).

Candidacy

The determination of an appropriate candidate for a cochlear implant involves many variables. This decision does not depend solely upon the child's audiogram to measure post-implant success. It takes into consideration the expectations of the family, the educational environment post-implant, and the motivation of the family to provide and support the intensive therapy required for the child to make the necessary move to spoken language. Candidacy for a pediatric cochlear implant requires a careful team approach and assessment of many aspects of the child's life. The decision to insert an implant in a child involves a multidisciplinary team of physicians, audiologists, speech–language pathologists, social workers, and educational consultants. Considerations of medical contraindications, audiologic data, speech and language abilities, the child's mode of communication, the expectations of the parent, and a child's post-implant educational environment must all be factored into the decision. The FDA has introduced broad guidelines for candidate selection for cochlear implantation in children. These include profound deafness, little or no benefit from hearing aids, and a chronological age of at least 12 months. For children with severe to profound hearing loss, implantation may take place from 2 years and above. However, the decision to implant can be greatly influenced by the etiology of deafness. Children who have contracted meningitis are at risk of cochlea ossification, thereby challenging the insertion of the electrode array. Such children are typically given implants sooner to avoid that situation. Discolo and Hirose (2002) provide a review of the evaluation before surgery and the surgical procedures. The recent ASHA technical report on cochlear implants also provides a review of the evaluation, candidacy, and surgery (ASHA, 2004e). The American Academy of Audiology also has a position statement on the benefits, candidacy, and management (American Academy of Audiology, 1995).

Success and Outcomes

Whether a child is entering a typical school setting for the first time or has been mainstreamed for years, each child with a cochlear implant (CI) brings a unique background of variables that contributes to his success. No two children have the same capacity for learning spoken language through listening. Success with an implant has considerable variability. Duration of deafness, cognitive skills, mode of communication, and integrity of the cochlea all influence the outcome for a child with a cochlear implant.

Since FDA approval, a decade of research has now shown how well these children are learning spoken language compared with their peers who are deaf and who hear normally. On average, children make 1 year of language progress per year of implant use (Bollard, Chute, Popp, & Parisier, 1999; Robbins, Svirsky, & Miyamoto, 2000; Svirsky, Robbins, Kirk, Pisoni, & Miyamoto, 2000). Not unlike normal hearing children, children with cochlear implants manifest great variability in language and communication abilities (Fryauf-Bertschy, Tyler, Kelsay, Gantz, & Woodworth, 1997; Hasenstab & Tobey, 1991; Kirk, 2000; Meyer, Svirsky, Kirk, & Miyamoto, 1998; Pyman, Blamey, Lacey, Clark, & Dowell, 2000; Tomblin, Spencer, Flock, Tyler, & Gantz, 1999). Variability can be accounted for by factors related to the implant itself, processing strategies, and etiology of the loss; however, other factors are now found to account for the individual differences in communication skills, language environment, and aural rehabilitation (Geers, 2002; Moog & Geers, 1999; Tomblin et al., 1999). Age of implantation has been found to be a prominent factor in affecting the outcome (Gordon, Daya, Harrison, & Papsin, 2000; O'Donoghue, Nikolopoulos, Archbold, & Tait, 1998). As suspected, several researchers have found that earlier implantations yield better results. Kirk et al. (2002) found that children implanted prior to 2 years of age had significantly faster rates of receptive vocabulary growth and language development than peers who received implants at a later age. Svirsky and colleagues (2000) found that prior to implantation, children with profound, prelingual deafness developed language skills at half the rate of their peers with normal hearing, but after the cochlear implant, the average learning rate was similar to that of their normal-hearing peers. The ASHA (2004e) technical report on cochlear implants delineates these outcomes, with gains noted for speech intelligibility and language.

Open-set speech recognition within the first year of receiving the device is now proven to be attainable for some young CI recipients (Miyamoto, Kirk, Svirsky, & Sehgal, 1999; Osberger, Fisher, Zimmerman-Phillips, Geier, & Barker, 1998), with skills continuing to develop after 5 years of use (Miyamoto, Kirk, Robbins, Todd, & Riley, 1996). A child's mode of communication also plays a role in speech recognition and speech intelligibility. Speech perception and production studies, illustrating that how children speak affects their speech perception abilities, have provided promising potential for conversational competence of children with cochlear implants. However, to acquire spoken language to its fullest, children must build on their perception and production skills as necessary tools for the further development of the pragmatic, semantic, syntactic, and morphological skills that are necessary for conversation (Hasenstab & Tobey, 1991; Tomblin et al., 1999).

Communication Philosophies

The ever debated question of which philosophy best suits the education of a child who is deaf has been in the forefront of deaf education for decades. Parents have choices concerning how to raise and teach their child, but finding what suits a particular family often becomes a conflict among the professionals involved, resulting in confusion for the family. Unfortunately, not all parents have all the available options, just because of location and local resources.

Among the several options of teaching children who are deaf, the choice between oral and manual communication has certainly driven current research with respect to cochlear implants. Whether to incorporate sign language into the intensive auditory rehabilitation required after implant activation depends on individual circumstances—no one philosophy is best for all children. The most recent data suggest that children who use oral communication achieve higher levels of speech perception and production (intelligibility) levels than children who use total communication (a simultaneous use of sign and voice) (Geers, Spehar, & Seday, 2002; Kirk et al., 2002; Osberger & Fisher, 2000; Tobey et al., 2000; Young, Grohne, Carrasco, & Brown, 2000). The value of sign language is supported by many respected clinicians as a component to bridge to spoken language. Koch (1999) suggests that signs may be critical to the development of a symbolic code that allows children to create linguistic networks necessary for organization, storage, and retrieval of concepts.

The Educational Team

Working with a child with a cochlear implant is typically not exclusive to one therapist. A child will likely enter school with a host of multidisciplinary professionals who have followed her from infancy through preschool. These clinicians will serve as a resource for the therapist and an asset to the new educational team. Some may continue working with the child in school and be part of the IEP team. The disciplines discussed in the following paragraphs are likely to be included in the IEP of an implanted child:

- *Speech–language pathologist.* Depending on the needs of the child, speech and language services will vary. Some children will have an auditory–verbal therapist, who specializes in the acquisition of spoken language through audition, as well as a speech–language pathologist. In such a case, the school therapist may provide less service. If the speech–language pathologist does provide the service, Schery and Peters (2003) have written a helpful article on developing auditory learning in children with cochlear implants.

- *Auditory–verbal therapist.* An auditory–verbal therapist is a certified clinician who specializes in the acquisition of spoken language through hearing alone. She does not use formal sign language. She has a wide range of experience in the cognitive, social, emotional, linguistic, and communicative needs of children who are hearing impaired. Based upon the Auditory–Verbal Philosophy, articulated in Auditory–Verbal International's Position Statement (1991), parent involvement in all sessions is one of the primary tenets of this approach.

- *Educational audiologist.* An audiologist who specializes in the diagnosis, management, and treatment of children with hearing impairments in schools will have a variety of responsibilities. These include conducting classroom acoustic analyses, selecting and maintaining assistive devices, and collaborating with the implant audiologist and in-service staff on the unique auditory needs of a child with a cochlear implant in the classroom, as well as identifying equipment needs and, in some areas, programing the speech processor (Educational Audiology Association, 1998).

- *Teacher of children who are deaf or hard of hearing.* Specializing in the education of children with hearing impairments, this teacher will serve as the "eyes and ears" in the classroom. Typical responsibilities include collaborating with the classroom teacher, providing pre- and postteaching of core vocabulary, and monitoring the child's progress educationally.

- *Educational consultant.* Many larger implant facilities employ a liaison between school and implant center. Such a person can be a valuable part of the team. His extensive knowledge of cochlear implants, education of the hearing impaired, special auditory needs of a child with a cochlear implant, and strategies for "raising the bar" for these children can be beneficial to both the implant center and the school teams.

Of course, depending on the child's current mode of communication and age level, a speech–language pathologist may also encounter the following individuals: sign language interpreter, cued speech transliterator, teaching assistant, and CART (communication access real-time translation) translator.

Besides mainstream settings, in which the child is among hearing peers with support personnel providing service on an itinerant basis, a child may be educated in a self-contained classroom within a hearing-impaired program, in a residential school for the deaf, or in a combination of self-contained and mainstreamed settings. In each case, speech services are typically provided by a speech–language pathologist employed by the program or school, who has experience with children who have a hearing impairment.

Educational Considerations

A child with a cochlear implant will require a carefully controlled acoustic environment to help overcome the listening challenges he faces. An FM system will likely be needed in all academic settings. Although an implant is a very effective device, a child does *not* hear normally with it. With children who do not use a hearing aid on the unimplanted ear, you must keep in mind that the child hears from only the one ear. Therefore, localization of sound and discrimination of speech in the presence of background noise is extremely challenging. For children who do use a hearing aid, discrimination may be better, but they continue to require that noise levels be minimized. The educational audiologist will become the key source of information on this topic. An article by Iglehart (2004) highlights the difficulties students with cochlear implants may have with speech perception in classrooms. He examined the use of wall-mounted and desktop sound field systems in a noisy, reverberant classroom and in a quiet classroom. Use of either system was related to improved scores for phoneme recognition in the quiet classroom. In the noisy, reverberant classroom, the desktop system resulted in improved phoneme recognition scores.

The speech processor is affected by ESD (electrostatic discharge), and modifications should be made accordingly. Large plastic play equipment (including slides), computers, and carpeting can adversely affect the speech processor if the child is in contact with them. A few quick modifications will ensure that it will not become a problem.

The importance of parents as the child's advocates and partners in the educational programming cannot be overstated. Parents must work with school personnel to provide the child who has an implant with the necessary home experiences to enhance what the child is learning in school. Furthermore, it is critical that parents be advocates for the child. Cochlear implants are relatively new to school districts, and many educators and administrators have minimal experience with them (Roeser, Terry, & Sweeney, 2002).

Although the cochlear implant is a very reliable and effective device, it, like all other electronics, is not infallible. Maintaining the implant during school is essential in order for the child to have consistent, quality input. Spare batteries, cords, microphones, and, in some cases, spare processors must be accessible to the educational team during school hours. Troubleshooting should be an important part of in-servicing the school team in case of breakdown.

Final Thoughts on Cochlear Implants

The needs and services of a child with a cochlear implant vary greatly, as does the experience level of the clinicians involved. It is expected that a school-based speech–language pathologist will see more children with cochlear implants entering regular, mainstream settings as they continue to make outstanding progress acquiring spoken communicative competence. Chute and Nevins (2003) provide an overview of some of the educational challenges that these children may face. The information provided in this section hopes to serve as a broad overview of some of the issues involved in working with these dynamic children. It is certainly not exhaustive, as the issues encompassing pediatric cochlear implantation are ever changing. This is truly an exciting time for professionals who work with children with cochlear implants. There is no doubt that as technology continues to improve and the benefits of these remarkable devices are further researched, children with severe to profound hearing losses will achieve higher levels of performance with hearing aids than ever imagined.

CONCLUSION

This discussion of audiology services in educational settings focused on the needs of children with hearing loss or listening disorders who spend major portions of their day in instructional experiences and settings. Some children are in these instructional programs for as long as 21 years. They enter the system as infants and "age out" at the end of their 21st year. In schools, the instructional milieu is highly linguistic, and student success is highly dependent upon a student's ability to hear and process spoken information. Audiologists are key players and a critical resource for ensuring optimum listening environments conducive to learning, ensuring optimum hearing among children who must function in those environments, and ensuring that the professionals who work in these environments understand the listening needs of their students.

 STUDY QUESTIONS

1. What are the purposes of audiological assessment and the rationale for each?
2. IDEA defines the disability categories of "deaf" and "hearing impairment." Some think the definitions lack guidelines. How would you expand upon the definitions to add greater clarity? What might be indicators that a child's disability is deafness? What might be indicators that a child's disability could be classified under "hearing impairment"?
3. What would be indicators that a child's educational performance was being adversely affected by hearing loss?

4. How, in your state, would you find out what the guidelines are for audiology services delivered in schools?
5. As a communication specialist, what strategies would you provide a teacher to use to determine whether a child is having difficulty listening?
6. How would you go about setting up a system in your school for daily checks of hearing aids and assistive listening systems?
7. What are potential issues for a student with hearing loss in each of the instruction models and staff combinations discussed in this chapter?
8. How would you go about determining whether a new treatment protocol or intervention for listening is appropriate to use?
9. How would you go about analyzing curricular requirements for listening?
10. How would you modify an instructional environment to optimize listening for a student with hearing loss?
11. What are the cochlear implant components?
12. What are some factors that may affect the success of the implant?
13. Why might localization of sound be an issue for children with cochlear implants?

REFERENCES

American Academy of Audiology. (1995). Position statement: Cochlear implants in children. *Audiology Today, 7,* 14–15.

American National Standards Institute. (2002). *S1260-2020, Acoustical performance criteria, design requirements, and guidelines for schools.* Melville, NY: Author.

American Speech-Language-Hearing Association. (1983). *The hearing impaired mentally retarded: Recommendations for action.* Washington, DC: Department of Health, Education and Welfare, Social and Rehabilitative Services.

American Speech-Language-Hearing Association. (1985). Guidelines for identification audiometry. *Asha, 27*(5), 49–52.

American Speech-Language-Hearing Association. (1994). Guidelines for the audiological management of individuals receiving cochleotoxic drug therapy. *Asha, 36*(Suppl. 12), 11–19.

American Speech-Language-Hearing Association. (1996). Scope of practice in audiology. *Asha, 38*(Suppl. 16), 12–15.

American Speech-Language-Hearing Association. (2001). *Scope of practice in speech–language pathology.* Retrieved July 28, 2005, from http://www.asha.org/NR/rdonlyres/4FDEE27B-BAF5-4D06-AC4D-8D1F311C1B06/0/19446_1.pdf

American Speech-Language-Hearing Association. (2002a). *Guidelines for audiology service provision in and for schools.* Rockville, MD: Author.

American Speech-Language-Hearing Association. (2002b). Guidelines for fitting and monitoring FM systems. *ASHA Desk Reference.*

American Speech-Language-Hearing Association. (2004a). Auditory integration training. *Asha* (Suppl. 24).

American Speech-Language-Hearing Association. (2004b). Clinical practice by certificate holders in the profession in which they are not certified. *Asha* (Suppl. 24), 39–40.

American Speech-Language-Hearing Association. (2004c). *Questions to ask when evaluating a procedure, product or program.* Retrieved on August 27, 2005 from http://www.asha.org/members/evaluate

American Speech-Language-Hearing Association. (2004d). Roles of speech–language pathologists and teachers of children who are deaf and hard of hearing in the development of communicative and linguistic competence. *Asha* (Suppl. 24).

American Speech-Language-Hearing Association. (2004e). Technical report: Cochlear implants. *Asha* (Suppl. 24).

American Speech-Language-Hearing Association. (2005a). *Acoustics in educational settings: Position statement.* Retrieved on August 27, 2005 from www.asha.org/members/desk-ref-journals/deskref/default

American Speech-Language-Hearing Association. (2005b). Guidelines for addressing acoustics in educational settings. *Asha* (Suppl. 25).

American Speech-Language-Hearing Association. (2005c). *(Central) auditory processing disorders—The role of the audiologist [Position Statement].* Retrieved on August 27, 2005 from www.asha.org/members/desk-ref-journals/deskref/default

American Speech-Language-Hearing Association. (2005d). *(Central) auditory processing disorders—The role of the audiologist [Technical Report].* Retrieved on August 27, 2005 from www.asha.org/members/desk-ref-journals/deskref/default

American Speech-Language-Hearing Association Panel on Audiologic Assessment. (1997). *Guidelines for audiologic screening.* Rockville, MD: Author.

American Speech-Language-Hearing Association Task Force on Central Auditory Processing Consensus Development. (1996). Central auditory processing: Current status of research and implications for clinical practice. *American Journal of Audiology, 5*(2), 41–54.

Anderson, K., & Matkin, N. (1991). Relationship of degree of loss to psychosocial and educational needs. *Educational Audiology Newsletter, 8*(2), 11–12.

Anderson, U. M. (1967). The incidence and significance of high-frequency deafness in children. *American Journal of Diseases in Children, 113,* 560–565.

Auditory–Verbal International. (1991). *Auditory–verbal position statement.* Retrieved on August 27, 2005 from http://www.learntolisten.org.avtherapy2.php

Berg, F. S. (1987). *Facilitating classroom listening.* Boston: College-Hill.

Bess, F. H. (1985). The minimally hearing-impaired child. *Ear and Hearing, 6,* 43–47.

Bluestone, C. D., & Klein, J. O. (1995). *Otitis media in infants and children* (2nd ed.). Philadelphia: W. B. Saunders.

Bollard, P., Chute, P., Popp, A., & Parisier, S. (1999). Specific language growth in young children using the Clarion cochlear implant. *Annals of Otology, Rhinology and Laryngology, 108*(4), 119–123.

Brackett, D., & Maxon, A. B. (1986). Service delivery alternatives for the mainstreamed hearing-impaired child. *Language, Speech, and Hearing Services in Schools, 17,* 115–125.

Chermak, G. D., & Musiek, F. E. (1997). *Central auditory processing disorders: New perspectives.* San Diego, CA: Singular.

Chute, P. M., & Nevins, M. E. (2003). Educational challenges for children with cochlear implants. *Topics in Language Disorders, 23,* 57–67.

Clark, W. (1991). Noise exposure from leisure activities: A review. *Journal of the Acoustical Society of America, 90,* 175–181.

Cochlear Implant Association. (1997). *What is a cochlear implant?* Retrieved on August 20, 2005 from http://www.cici.org.whatis.html

Davis, J. (Ed.). (1977). *Our forgotten children: Hard-of-hearing pupils in the schools.* Minneapolis, MN: Department of Health, Education and Welfare, Bureau of Education of the Handicapped, National Support Systems Project and Division of Personnel Preparation.

Davis, J., Shepard, N., Stelmachowicz, P., & Gorga, M. (1981). Characteristics of hearing impaired children in the schools: Part I. Demographic data. *Journal of Speech and Hearing Disorders, 46,* 123–129.

DeConde Johnson, C. (1991). The "state" of educational audiology: Survey results and goals for the future. *Educational Audiology Monograph, 2,* 74–84.

Discolo, C. M., & Hirose, K. (2002). Pediatric cochlear implants. *American Journal of Audiology, 11,* 114–118.

Education of All Handicapped Children Act. (1975). Public Law 94-142.

Education of the Handicapped Amendments of 1986. (1986). Public Law 99-457.

Educational Audiology Association. (1994, Fall). Minimum competencies for educational audiologists. *Educational Audiology Association Newsletter, 11,* 4, 7.

Educational Audiology Association. (1998). *EAA position statement: Educational audiologists and cochlear implants.* Retrieved July 28, 2005, from http://www.edaud.org

English, K. M. (1995). *Educational audiology across the lifespan: Serving all learners with hearing impairment.* Baltimore: Brookes.

English, K. (2002). Why AR services are required in school settings. In R. L. Schow & M. A. Nerbonne (Eds.), *Introduction to audiologic rehabilitation* (4th ed.; pp. 247–274). Boston, MA: Allyn & Bacon.

Fettinger, M., & Huffman, N. P. (1994). *A teacher's guide to FM assistive devices (Revised).* Unpublished manuscript.

Flexer, C., Wray, D., & Ireland, J. (1989). Preferential seating is not enough. *Language, Speech, and Hearing Services in Schools, 20,* 11–21.

Friel-Patti, S. (1999). Clinical decision-making in the assessment and intervention of central auditory processing disorders. *Language, Speech, and Hearing Services in Schools, 30,* 345–352.

Fryauf-Bertschy, H., Tyler, R. S., Kelsay, D. M. R., Gantz, B. J., & Woodworth, G. G. (1997). Cochlear implant use by prelingually deafened children: The influences of age at implant and length of device use. *Journal of Speech, Language and Hearing Research, 40,* 183–199.

Fulton, R. T., & Lloyd, L. L. (Eds.). (1969). *Audiometry for the retarded: With implications for the difficult-to-test.* Baltimore: Williams & Wilkins.

Geers, A. E. (2002). Factors affecting the development of speech, language and literacy in children with early cochlear implantation. *Language, Speech, and Hearing Services in Schools, 33,* 172–183.

Geers, A. E., Spehar, B., & Seday, A. (2002). Use of speech by children from total communication who wear cochlear implants. *American Journal of Speech-Language Pathology, 11,* 50–58.

Gordon, D. A., Daya, H., Harrison, R. V., & Papsin, B. C. (2000). Factors contributing to limited open set speech perception in children who use a cochlear implant. *International Journal of Pediatric Otorhinolaryngology, 56,* 101–111.

Gravel, J. S., Fausel, N., Liskow, C., & Chobot, J. (1999). Children's speech recognition in noise using omni-directional and dual-microphone hearing aid technology. *Ear and Hearing, 20,* 1–11.

Hasenstab, M. S., & Tobey, E. A. (1991). Language development in children receiving Nucleus multichannel cochlear implants. *Ear and Hearing, 12,* 55S–65S.

Huffman, N. P. (1982). *A teacher's guide to educational amplification.* Unpublished manuscript.

Huffman, N. P. (1985). *A teacher's guide to assistive devices.* Unpublished manuscript.

Iglehart, F. (2004). Speech perception by students with cochlear implants using sound–field systems in classrooms. *American Journal of Audiology, 13,* 62–72.

Individuals with Disabilities Education Act Amendments of 1997. (1997). Public Law 105-17.

Kahmi, A. C. (1995). Defining, developing, and maintaining clinical expertise. *Language, Speech, and Hearing Services in Schools, 26,* 353–356.

Katz, A., Gertsman, H., Sanderson, H., & Buchanan, R. (1982). Stereo headphones and hearing loss. *New England Journal of Medicine, 307,* 1460–1461.

Katzenbach, J. R., & Smith, D. K. (1994). *The wisdom of teams: Creating the high-performance organization.* New York: HarperCollins.

Kayser, T. A. (1994). *Building team power: How to unleash the collaborative genius of work teams.* Burr Ridge, IL: Irwin.

Keith, R. W. (1999). Clinical issues in central auditory processing disorders. *Language, Speech, and Hearing Services in Schools, 30,* 339–344.

Kirk, K. I. (2000). Cochlear implants: New developments and results. *Current Opinion in Otolaryngology and Head and Neck Surgery, 8,* 415–420.

Kirk, K. I., Miyamoto, R. T., Ying, E., Lento, C., O'Neill, T., & Fears, F. (2002a). Effects of age at implantation in young children. *Annals of Otology, Rhinology, and Laryngology, 111,* 69–73.

Kirk, K. I., Miyamoto, R. T., Ying, E., Lento, C., O'Neill, T., & Fears, F. (2002b). Effects of age at implantation in young children with cochlear implants: Contributing factors. *Current Opinion in Otolaryngology and Head and Neck Surgery, 121,* 31–34.

Knecht, H. A., Nelson, P. B., Whitelaw, G. M., & Feth, L. L. (2002). Background noise levels and reverberation times in unoccupied classrooms: Predictions and measurements. *American Journal of Audiology, 11,* 65–71.

Koch, M. (1999). *Bringing sound to life.* Baltimore: York Press.

Lass, N. J., Woodford, C. M., Pannbacker, M., Carlin, M., Saniga, R., Schmitt, J., et al. (1989). Speech–language pathologists' knowledge of, exposure to, and attitude toward hearing aids and hearing aid wearers. *Language, Speech, and Hearing Services in Schools, 20,* 115–132.

Lass, N. J., Woodford, C. M., Schmidt, J. F., Pannbacker, M., Lundeen, C., & English, P. J. (1990). Health educators' knowledge of hearing, hearing loss, and hearing health practices. *Language, Speech, and Hearing Services in Schools, 21,* 85–90.

Meyer, T. A., Svirsky, M. A., Kirk, K. I., & Miyamoto, R. T. (1998). Improvements in speech perception by children with profound prelingual hearing loss: Effects of device, communication mode, and chronological age. *Journal of Speech, Language, and Hearing Research, 41,* 846–858.

Miller, J. J. (1985). *Handbook of ototoxicity.* Boca Raton, FL: CRC.

Miyamoto, R. T., Kirk, K. I., Robbins, A. M., Todd, S. L., & Riley, A. I. (1996). Speech perception and speech production skills of children with multichannel cochlear implants. *Acta Otolaryngologica, 116,* 240–243.

Miyamoto, R. T., Kirk, K. I., Svirsky, M. A., & Sehgal, S. T. (1999). Communication skills in pediatric cochlear implant recipients. *Acta Otolaryngologica, 119,* 219–224.

Moog, J. S., & Geers, A. E. (1999). Speech and language acquisition in young children after cochlear implantation. *Early Identification and Intervention of Hearing Impaired Infants, 32,* 1127–1141.

National Association of State Directors of Special Education. (1994). *Deaf and hard of hearing students: Educational service guidelines.* Alexandria, VA: Author.

Nelson, P., Kohnert, K., Sabur, S., & Shaw, D. (2005). Classroom noise and children learning through a second language: Double jeopardy? *Language, Speech, and Hearing Services in Schools, 36,* 219–229.

Nevins, M. E., & Chute, P. (1996). *Children with cochlear implants in educational settings.* San Diego, CA: Singular.

New York State Education Department. (1992). *School hearing screening guidelines.* Albany, NY: Author.

O'Donoghue, G. M., Nikolopoulos, T. P., Archbold, S. M., & Tait, M. (1998). Speech perception in children after cochlear implantation. *American Journal of Otology, 19,* 762–767.

Osberger, M. J., & Fisher, L. (2000). Preoperative predictors of post operative implant performance in children. *Annals of Otology, Rhinology, and Laryngology, 109*(12), 44–46.

Osberger, M. J., Fisher, L., Zimmerman-Phillips, S., Geier, L., & Barker, J. J. (1998). Speech recognition performance of older children with cochlear implants. *American Journal of Otology, 19,* 152–157.

Palacio, M. (2000, September 25). Gauging efficacy of CAPD treatment. *Advance for Speech–Language Pathologists and Audiologists, 10*(38), 10, 50.

Plakke, B. L. (1985). Hearing conservation in secondary industrial arts classes: A challenge for audiologists. *Language, Speech, and Hearing Services in Schools, 16,* 75–79.

Plakke, B. L. (1991). Hearing conservation training of industrial technology teachers. *Language, Speech, and Hearing Services in Schools, 22,* 134–138.

Pyman, B. C., Blamey, P. J., Lacey, P., Clark, G. M., & Dowell, R. (2000). The development of speech perception in children using cochlear implants: Effects of etiologic factors and delayed milestones. *American Journal of Otology, 21,* 57–61.

Robbins, A. M., Svirsky, M., & Miyamoto, R. (2000). Language development in profoundly deaf children with cochlear implants. *Psychological Science, 11,* 153–158.

Roeser, R. J., Terry, D., & Sweeney, M. (2002, March–April). The impact of cochlear implants in schools: A new era for aural (re) habilitation. *Volta Voices, 9,* 12–16.

Ross, M., Brackett, D., & Maxon, A. (1991). *Assessment and management of mainstreamed hearing impaired children.* Austin, TX: PRO-ED.

Schery, T. K., & Peters, M. L. (2003). Developing auditory learning in children with cochlear implants. *Topics in Language Disorders, 23,* 4–15.

Soli, S. D., & Sullivan, J. A. (1997). Factors affecting children's speech communication in classrooms. *Journal of the Acoustical Society of America, 101,* S3070.

Stelmachowicz, P. G., Hoover, B. M., Lewis, D. E., Kortekaas, R., & Pittman, A. L. (2000). The relation between stimulus context, speech audibility, and perception for normal-hearing and hearing-impaired children. *Journal of Speech, Language, and Hearing Research, 43,* 902–914.

Svirsky, M., Robbins, A. M., Kirk, K. I., Pisoni, D., & Miyamoto, R. (2000). Language development in profoundly deaf children with cochlear implants. *Psychological Science, 11,* 153–158.

Tobey, E. A., Geers, A. E., Douek, B. M., Perrin, J., Skellet, R., Brenner, C., et al. (2000). Factors associated with speech intelligibility in children with cochlear implants. *Annals of Otology, Rhinology, and Laryngology, 109*(12), 28–30.

Tomblin, J. B., Spencer, L., Flock, S., Tyler, R., & Gantz, B. (1999). A comparison of language achievement in children with cochlear implants and children using hearing aids. *Journal of Speech, Language, and Hearing Research, 42,* 497–511.

Tye-Murray, N. (1998). *Foundations of aural rehabilitation.* San Diego, CA: Singular.

U.S. Department of Education. (1999). 34 C.F.R. Parts 300 and 303: Assistance to states for the education of children with disabilities and early intervention program for infants and toddlers with disabilities. *Federal Register.* Vol. 64, No. 48. March 12, 1999, p. 12406–12672.

Veale, T. K. (1994a). Auditory integration training: The use of a new listening treatment within our profession. *American Journal of Speech–Language Pathology, 3,* 12–15.

Veale, T. K. (1994b). Weighing the promises and the problems: AIT may be a risk worth taking. *American Journal of Speech–Language Pathology, 3,* 35–37.

Woodford, C. M. (1973). A perspective on hearing loss and hearing assessment in school children. *Journal of School Health, 43,* 572–576.

Woodford, C. M. (1980, July). Notes on audiology in the public schools. *Hearing Aid Journal,* 5–9.

Woodford, C. M. (1981). Hearing protection in the shop. *School Shop, 41,* 17–18.

Woodford, C. M., & O'Farrell, M. L. (1983). High frequency loss of hearing in secondary school students: An investigation of possible etiological factors. *Language, Speech, and Hearing Services in Schools, 14,* 22–28.

Young, N. M., Grohne, K. M., Carrasco, V. N., & Brown, C. J. (2000). Speech perception in young children using Nucleus or Clarion cochlear implants: Effects of communication mode. *Annals of Otology, Rhinology, and Laryngology, 109*(12), 77–79.

Appendix 11.A

◆◆◆◆◆◆◆◆◆◆◆◆◆◆◆◆◆◆◆◆◆

Audiology Organizations and Resources

Alexander Graham Bell Association for the
    Deaf and Hard of Hearing
3417 Volta Place NW
Washington, DC 20007-2778
www.agbell.org

American Academy of Audiology
11730 Plaza America Dr., Suite 300
Reston, VA 20190
www.audiology.org

American Society for Deaf Children
P.O. Box 3355
Gettysburg, PA 17325
www.deafchildren.org

American Speech-Language-Hearing Association
10801 Rockville Pike
Rockville, MD 20852
www.asha.org

Auditory–Verbal International, Inc.
1390 Chain Bridge Rd., #100
McLean, VA 22101
www.auditory-verbal.org

Cochlear Implant Association, Inc.
5335 Wisconsin Ave. NW, Suite 440
Washington, DC 20015-2052
www.cici.org

Council for Exceptional Children
1110 North Glebe Rd., Suite 300
Arlington, VA 22201-5704
www.cec.sped.org

Educational Audiology Association
13153 North Dale Mabry Hwy., Suite 105
Tampa, FL 33618
www.edaud.org

National Association of the Deaf
814 Thayer Ave.
Silver Spring, MD 20910-4500
www.nad.org

Self Help for Hard of Hearing People
7910 Woodmont Ave., Suite 1200
Bethesda, MD 20814
www.shhh.org

ADDITIONAL WEB SITE RESOURCES

AudiologyNet: Audiology Information
    for the Masses
www.audiologynet.com

Deaf Linx
www.deaflinx.com

Deaf Mall
www.deafmall.net

Hearing Education and Awareness
    for Rockers (H.E.A.R.)
www.hearnet.com

National Cued Speech Association
www.cuedspeech.org

Net Connections for Communication
    Disorders and Sciences
www.mnsu.edu/dept/comdis/kuster2/
    welcome.html

Oral Deaf Education
www.oraldeafed.org

Searchwave: Your Digital Hearing Aids Guide
www.searchwave.com

Appendix 11.B

◆ ◆

Cochlear Implant Resources

WEB SITES

Advanced Bionics
www.cochlearimplant.com

Alexander Graham Bell
www.agbell.org

Auditory-Verbal International, Inc.
www.auditory-verbal.org

Boys Town National Research Hospital
www.babyhearing.org

Cochlear
www.cochlear.com

Cochlear Implant Association, Inc.
www.cici.org

Information Center on Disabilities and Gifted
    Education
www.ericec.org

John Tracy Clinic
www.johntracyclinic.org

Listen-Up Web
www.listen-up.org

National Association of the Deaf
www.nad.org

Oral Deaf Education
www.oraldeafed.org

Learning to Listen Foundation
www.learningtolisten.org

BOOKS

Children with Cochlear Implants in Educational Settings
Nevins, M. E., & Chute, P. M. (1996)
Delmar Health Care–Singular Publishing Group, Inc., 800/347-7707

Cochlear Implants for Kids
Estabrooks, W. (1998)
Alexander Graham Bell Association, 202/337-5220

Facilitating Hearing and Listening in Young Children
Flexer, C. (1994)
Delmar Health Care–Singular Publishing Group, Inc., 800/347-7707

Speech and the Hearing Impaired Child
Ling, D. (1974)
Alexander Graham Bell Association, 202/337-5220

THERAPY RESOURCES

Bringing Sound to Life: Principles and Practices of Cochlear Implant Rehabilitation
Koch, M. (1998)
York Press, 410/560-1557

Cochlear Implant Auditory Training Guidebook
Sindrey, D. (1997)
Word Play Publications, 415/397-3716

Guide for Optimizing Auditory Learning Skills (GOALS)
Rirszt, J., & Reeder, R. (1996)
Alexander Graham Bell Association, 202/337-5220

Listening Games for Littles
Sindrey, D. (1997)
Word Play Publications, 415/397-3716

Play It by Ear! Auditory Training Games
Lowell, E. L., & Stoner, M. (1960)
John Tracy Clinic, 213/748-5481

Speech Perception Instructional Curriculum and Evaluation (SPICE)
Moog, J. S., Biednestein, J., & Davidson, L. (1995)
Central Institute for the Deaf, 314/977-0223

*Word Associations for Syllable Perception (W*A*S*P*)*
Koch, M. (1998)
York Press, 410/560-1557

Appendix 11.C

◆ ◆

Position Statements of the Educational Audiology Association

- Auditory Integration Therapy (1998)
- Early Detection and Intervention of Hearing Loss: Roles and Responsibilities for Educational Audiologists (2002)
- Educational Audiologists and Cochlear Implants (1998)
- Minimum Competencies for Educational Audiologists (1994)
- Recommended Professional Practices for Educational Audiology (1997)

All available online at www.edaud.org/position.asp

Chapter 12

◆ ◆

The Roles of Teachers, Psychologists, Librarians, and Occupational and Physical Therapists

Jill Modafferi, Joseph Sheedy,
Linda Robinson, Karen Browning,
and Kim M. Nevins

n the preceding chapters, authors have stressed how important it is for
students with speech, language, and hearing problems to receive services
from qualified SLPs and audiologists within the school environment. But
SLPs and audiologists do not work alone. In Chapters 3, 5, and 8, we referred
parenthetically to other professionals. It is the rare undergraduate or graduate
program that discusses the issue, particularly as it applies to possible fragmentation of student needs, "turf" issues, and the possibility of real collaboration
with individuals in other fields.

In this chapter, some of those other professionals respond to the question that members of the school community often ask us, "What is it that you
people do?" Included as authors in this chapter are a classroom teacher who
has also worked in the area of special education, physical and occupational
therapists, a librarian, and a school psychologist. We asked them to provide an
overview of their role in the schools, their educational training, and how they
see the interface between their roles and ours. All of the authors are currently
working in the schools and their responses reflect, we feel, an in-the-trenches
perspective. You may be surprised to see how often our roles overlap.

CLASSROOM AND SPECIAL EDUCATION TEACHER: JILL MODAFFERI

In any school environment it is imperative that all support personnel involved
in a student's education, as well as the classroom teacher, coordinate their
delivery of services for students. As an educator for more than 20 years, I have
been responsible for the instruction of many students with handicapping conditions. For 15 years, as a special education teacher, I worked with children
who had a wide variety of learning problems; currently, I am a fifth-grade regular
teacher in a small school setting in an urban area in central New York state.

Background and Training

The training I received over 20 years ago is probably somewhat different from
the training college students receive today. I received my BA in special education and elementary education from Wittenberg University in Springfield,
Ohio. At that time, P.L. 94-142 had just become effective, and the need for
special education teachers was great. The ideal in public schools was to have
pupils in need of special help receive services within their "home" districts,
but the schools were expected to provide a separate education for them in
a resource room setting. At the beginning of my career, my students were in
regular classrooms for part of the day but received their support services outside of that class.

As a dually certified teacher, I was trained in reading for elementary students, plus grade-appropriate content and methods courses in math, social stud-

ies, and science. The special education part of my certificate included coursework in behavior modification, theory of learning disabilities, and instruction in basic testing and assessment theory and procedures. It was not until I started to work on my master's degree at Syracuse University, however, that I made the connection between learning disabilities and language impairment. During my studies there, I took a course in the speech and language development of typically developing children and an additional course addressing abnormal speech and language issues. For the first time, I realized that the special education teacher, the remedial reading teacher, and the classroom teacher must all understand the needs of the student with disabilities, particularly in the language area, and work together to deliver a cohesive education plan. In retrospect, my years of experience and education have led me to realize one paramount point: All instructors need to work side by side in order to provide the most meaningful instruction to children.

Overlapping Goals and Services

Conceivably, an elementary student with language difficulties can receive services from three or four different adults in a school setting. The ideal situation involves having all instructors work on the child's goals simultaneously. This type of instruction will happen only if the instructors are all "on the same page"—that is, if they fully understand what skills the student needs to master, in what order those skills should be addressed, and which teacher will focus on what skills.

As a special education teacher, I became aware of overlapping services and goals quite by accident. I happened to notice the bulletin board display outside the speech–language therapist's room. The SLP had been working on sentence types with "her" children, many of whom were also "my" students. My first thought was, "How could I have expected my students to punctuate a variety of sentences correctly when the speech–language therapist was having to instruct the same youngsters on how to formulate these different sentence types?" I was well aware that my students' written expression was weak, but I suddenly realized that the mastery goals I had set for them in writing were totally unrealistic until they were capable of verbal expression. From that day on, I knew that the first order of business for any student with speech or language disorders was for me to sit down with the therapist and discuss what goals we could work on simultaneously.

In general, children receiving intervention in the area of language will have weaknesses that play out in the academic areas of written expression, reading comprehension, and mathematical conceptualization. I have to know what those weaknesses are, and the speech–language professional has to understand the educational implication of those deficits as the children attempt work in the classroom.

Suggestions for Collaboration Between SLPs and Teachers

How might that initial meeting between the special education teacher and the SLP begin? I hope it would start out with some dialogue about the child's receptive and expressive language levels. It is important, however, to make sure that every elementary or special education teacher with whom you interact has an understanding of basic language development and some familiarity with terminology. For example, when you discuss an individual student's strengths or weaknesses in "receptive language," it is important that the teacher recognize that you are talking about the child's ability to understand language, not use it. Similarly, when the discussion turns to increasing a child's "expressive skills," the teacher should understand that you are talking about a student's ability to put thoughts into words, either orally or in writing.

Suggestions of how best to meet the student's individual language needs is important information to share at this time. As an SLP, you may have very specific suggestions, such as preferred seating arrangements, the child's body position, and the length of oral directions given by the teacher. During the meeting, it will also be necessary to determine how modifications will be made for the student to become more successful in class. For example, if the special education teacher hears something similar to "John's receptive language is like that of a 6- or 7-year-old," and the student is in fifth grade, the special ed teacher realizes that she needs to plan how to modify directions and reinforce comprehension in all subject areas. Both teacher and SLP will have insights into the best ways to accomplish this.

Early in the process I have also found it beneficial to assign a case manager to every student, particularly for those who are seen by a number of different specialists. The case manager is responsible for overseeing the student's program; all questions and concerns are filtered through him.

Some basic communication questions the speech–language therapist and the special education teacher may address include the following:

- What areas of weakness does the child have in written expression?
- What are some ways that we could deliver instruction on the concept at the same time?
- Are there some skills that could be pretaught in order to enhance instruction?
- What is the student's reading comprehension level? Could some vocabulary be taught explicitly to enhance comprehension?
- Are there other children who have similar needs who could be grouped with these particular students?
- What is a convenient time for the instructors involved with the delivery of instruction to meet? (This needs to be a regular weekly time.)
- Is there a way we could instruct these students by using a similar theme or content from the classroom? (Themes could include topics that are schoolwide, such as respect, manners, or community service.

Content could include specific literature, ecology, Native Americans, pioneers, inventions, etc.)

The relationship between the regular classroom teacher and the speech–language pathologist must be open, as well. Good communication is key. The speech–language goals on the IEP must be clearly explained to the classroom teacher in terms of the student's weaknesses and strengths, and how to modify typical classroom procedures. It is imperative that both instructors make the delivery of instruction as meaningful and concise as possible. This can happen only if there are regularly scheduled meeting times. At these meetings, the teacher should provide both an overview and pertinent details about what information and skills will be taught in various content areas.

The classroom teacher has the greatest appreciation of what information and skills are necessary for a student to be successful in a particular class. The student may be receiving a variety of support services, but the bottom line for him is appearing successful in front of his peers. He may enjoy succeeding in the reading lab or the speech therapy room, but ultimately his success in his classroom is the most reinforcing. Therefore, any opportunities that can be crafted to result in classroom success are powerful incentives for him to keep working.

It is important for the SLP to understand clearly what the expectations are within the classroom; only the classroom teacher can provide that information for specialists. In New York state, for example, not only does the student with disabilities need to achieve in the classroom, but like typical students, she must pass the fourth-grade English language arts test; the fourth-grade math test, which consists of many multistep word problems and requires explanations of how the student arrived at an answer; the fifth-grade social studies test, which requires interpretation of documents, essay writing, and general social studies knowledge; and any variety of other tests that the school district may use as "benchmarks." The school's SLP must be very familiar with such requirements and with the state learning standards on which they are based, so that he can teach the underlying skills that will allow students to be successful when they face these required state assessments.

Some initial questions the speech–language professional could ask the teacher may include the following:

- What concepts will you be working on in social studies? Is there specific vocabulary you want the students to master? (At this point you could volunteer to create a learning center or to go into the classroom and conduct a vocabulary activity that would be beneficial to the entire class.)
- Is there a test or quiz you will be giving? Could we look at it together and modify it if necessary?
- What book are you reading now? Could I take a small group and illustrate a chapter, make a character sketch, or create a time line? Could I review the comprehension questions verbally?

Other considerations might include a discussion of seating preferences; asking the teacher to make sure directions are simplified or repeated; or modifying the directions on specific worksheets, tests, or quizzes.

The most important thing to keep in mind is the question "How can the student's IEP goals be met in the most effective and meaningful way?" The special education teacher must keep the order of goal instruction clearly in mind. She must also coordinate the goals under a common theme or content. The classroom teacher must know what specific content the students will be responsible for and how the SLP can be most helpful delivering that instruction, addressing underlying weaknesses, and assisting in modifying curriculum and assessment when deemed necessary.

Conclusion: Classroom and Special Ed Teacher

Clearly, the most common thread among all professionals should be a conscious effort to work together. When this is done well, not only do the students benefit, but the teaching staff does, as well. As professionals grow accustomed to talking together, it changes the way they see a specific student and deepens their potential understanding of children they may see in the future. Sometimes insights can be quite dramatic, such as when I took a look at the SLP's bulletin board. Other times the learning curve is more gradual, but understanding is always enhanced.

SCHOOL PSYCHOLOGIST: JOSEPH SHEEDY

Early school psychology was exactly as its title implied—the practice of psychology in a school setting. While it had been a professional entity since the turn of the century, the number of practitioners was small, and the field was not well defined until P.L. 94-142 was enacted in 1975. As a natural condition of the law's multidisciplinary requirement and the professional's presence in a school setting, universities throughout the country developed specific training curricula for the school-based psychologist. Assuming a prerequisite foundation in basic psychology, graduate coursework for prospective school psychologists now typically includes the study of personality theory, family systems, learning theory, tests and measurement, advanced statistics, research design, and counseling practica and internships. Although some programs focus their training on only one or two of these areas, all school psychologists are trained to view each child or student as unique, each exhibiting a dynamic array of intellectual, sensory, and emotional strengths and weaknesses in his adjustment to school environments (Thomas & Grimes, 1990).

Primary Functions of the School Psychologist

Ideally, school psychologists deliver services in each of the following seven domains, although they commonly complain that their skills are not divided equally among them:

- diagnostic testing and reporting,
- consulting,
- acting as agency liaison,
- participating as a multidisciplinary CSE (committee on special education) team member,
- acting as a facilitator,
- providing supportive counseling, and
- engaging in staff development.

Historically, the primary function of the psychologist has been to provide diagnostic testing of children suspected of having an educationally handicapping condition. Performing this task at a level of excellence still demands a significant percentage of the psychologist's time, especially during the months of the academic year when referrals to the CSE increase dramatically.

Diagnostic Testing and Reporting

Diagnostic testing is requested when a teacher, a concerned professional, or a parent suspects that a student is unable to learn effectively during typical classroom instruction in one or more academic areas. Testing requires an in-depth study of a child's strengths and weaknesses. Although the process is as diverse as the individuals being tested, there are several questions that are addressed in virtually all school psychological assessments:

- What is the intellectual potential of the student?
- In what academic, social, or behavioral areas does the student deviate from the expectations predicted by her intelligence?
- What is the student's preferred style of learning?
- What is the nature of the instructional methods to which she is being exposed?
- What is the student's proficiency in processing basic and complex stimuli via visual, auditory, tactile, and motor modalities?
- What is the family history with regard to school success?
- What medical and developmental factors exist that could contribute to learning inhibition?
- What is the nature and status of the student's overall personality development?
- What emotional factors exist that affect readiness for learning?

Other diagnostic questions and hypotheses are generated as the school psychologist attempts to address these basic areas and discover the inevitably complex nature of the individual. For example, a highly intelligent sixth-grade student, referred for testing because he fails to demonstrate his knowledge in formal classroom discussions and tests, may have significant comprehension deficits that in turn are the result of a specific language weakness in understanding inferences and verbal abstractions. Testing establishes the student's intellectual potential, highlights his learning strengths and weaknesses, calculates the nature and degree of his deficient academic performance, and begins the process of identifying instructional modifications that will increase a likelihood of success.

Let us assume that testing reveals that the student is a concrete learner. He will require demonstration rather than lecture in order to acquire new information. He will benefit from visual cueing. The task of meeting his needs, however, is complicated by his practice of avoiding complex verbal exchanges with teachers. His uninterested and defiant demeanor is a direct reflection of how he copes with his fear of appearing incompetent in the presence of peers in the classroom. A fairly clear language-based learning disability that could be therapeutically or logistically managed in a straightforward manner becomes complicated by the development of poor self-esteem and resultant defensive acting-out behaviors. In a final report, these issues are clearly outlined for teachers and parents. Recommendations generated in this report begin the ongoing consultative process of helping teachers and specialists make decisions that will coax this troubled student away from his defensiveness and fear of failure into a successful learning experience.

Consulting

The consultative process begins with promoting the student's understanding of both the testing process and the meaning of its results, taking care to consider the student's developmental and emotional readiness in the process. The psychologist's consultation with parents is aimed at educating them about their child's learning ability, as well as encouraging them to inform and collaborate with their child's teachers regarding her nature and her response to school instruction. This shared information is fundamental to the dynamic process of styling a student's instruction according to her strengths. The student's response to, or acceptance of, a particular instructional method is not always obvious; a parent's insight is extremely valuable.

At best, consultation with teachers is an ongoing process of applying diagnostic information to the search for instructional methods and interpersonal approaches that promote student success. It can take many forms, from hallway dialogue to formally scheduled planning meetings. In addition to conferring on specific instructional design and outcomes, the psychologist offers the teacher his objective view of the classroom environment and how it could be altered to suit the student's needs—for example, minimizing or maximizing lectures, suggesting alternatives to written tests, or planning material to suit a variety of learning styles.

Acting as Agency Liaison

In the course of diagnostic testing and consultation, help for the student and his family outside the classroom is sometimes indicated—for example, the need for a medical or psychiatric evaluation; family support; or more confidential, individual psychotherapy. The school psychologist is the "crossing guard" for this process. As agency liaison, she operates as a "primary care" professional within the school who refers to community-based specialists, including counselors and social workers for the student and the family, pediatric neurologists and child psychiatrists for behavioral medicine concerns, and clinics that offer a combination of all support services. After referral has been made and therapeutic intervention initiated, the psychologist provides ongoing clinical information during regular phone or office contacts with treating physicians or therapists. In every respect, the school psychologist remains the primary facilitator between community mental health services and the school.

Participating as a Multidisciplinary Team Member

As a multidisciplinary team member, the psychologist is a participant in—and brings expertise in learning theory, behavior, personality development, and therapeutic interventions to—the group process of reviewing evaluation results and planning the IEP. The group is charged with devising instructional methods and classroom management techniques and often includes regular and specialized classroom teachers, speech–language pathologists, counselors, physical and occupational therapists, parents, and administrators. The psychologist's role often extends beyond the formal meetings to one-on-one meetings with various clinicians to compare test results and brainstorm possible interventions.

Acting as a Facilitator

During consultation, the psychologist often finds himself in the role of a facilitator. As such, he uses his knowledge of resources within the school to assist teachers and other professionals in their efficient use. This is a networking process, in which teachers are introduced to each other and strategies are compared and exchanged and teaching styles are matched to student learning styles. The psychologist's mobility and contacts within the school environment place him in a logical position to take this role.

Providing Supportive Counseling

The school psychologist's ability to provide counseling services is sometimes diminished by demands for testing, crisis management, and consultation. Many psychologists express frustration that they are often unable to serve in this function, especially since they recognize that counseling focuses on the fundamental, often unseen causes for a student's school problems. Ideally, counseling is provided for both individuals and groups of various sizes. Individual counseling is usually requested by a parent, teacher, or student; is often related to behavioral problems in the classroom; and sometimes extends into other areas of student life, for example, family and social relationship problems. Individual school-based counseling can include play therapy to help young children manage emotional issues without direct verbal mediation, or it can feature information about learning disabilities, so that older students can learn self-advocacy skills that will enable them to demand compensatory teaching strategies.

While counseling has the goal of establishing a therapeutic, supportive relationship with the student in order to develop the student's self-understanding and self-direction toward an improved quality of life, it is different from psychotherapy. The latter is more intensive and is best delivered in a private, agency-based setting. Small-group counseling obviously can make services available to larger numbers of students. Its primary benefit lies in its opportunity for students to learn that their problems, fears, and anxieties are shared by others, that they are not alone, and that they can learn from another's experience. Groups also provide an excellent setting for teaching positive social skills. Play groups, in which early elementary students are provided models and guidance in social pragmatics, are of particular value in this respect. Finally, the school psychologist can provide counseling to whole classes, discussing broad issues such as character development, social and moral dilemmas, values, and making productive decisions.

Engaging in Staff Development

Finally, the school psychologist serves as a valuable resource during staff development and education. Formal group presentations and informal consultations are provided to teachers on subjects as diverse as inclusion, learning diversity, disorders of regulation (attention-deficit/hyperactivity disorder, obsessive–compulsive disorder, Tourette's syndrome), the rising occurrence of autistic spectrum disorders, emotional disturbance, classroom management, and learning differences. Current information is gathered as part of the psychologist's ongoing professional development during seminars, research reviews, and membership in professional organizations (e.g., the National Association of School Psychologists).

Specific Tests and Diagnostic Procedures

As stated earlier, one of the primary functions of the school psychologist is assessing student potential and how it is realized in learning. As in all areas relating to human functioning, this a complex process and, by its nature, imperfect. The tools used in diagnostic measurement present a series of questions and tasks that are associated with concepts fundamental to human development and learning. These tools are imperfect as well, in no way encompassing the multifaceted nature of human functioning. They can provide only "snapshots" of the dynamic and ever changing process of learning and adjustment and the conditions under which this process is most efficiently realized. If that snapshot is taken under favorable circumstances—good examiner–examinee rapport, good examinee attention, high examinee motivation to demonstrate ability, reliable and valid test materials—the attending examiner can begin to understand the full-length "moving picture" from which the snapshot was derived. No test of intelligence provides an all-inclusive measure of the full range of intellectual functioning. However, scientific research into learning and behavior has provided us with a representation of what is considered typical intellectual development as it relates to learning, both in life and in school. For school-age children, the most commonly used instruments to compare a student's performance on a variety of tasks to that of their age mates are the Wechsler tests, the Stanford-Binet fourth edition, and the *Kaufman Assessment Battery for Children.*

The Wechsler tests include the *Wechsler Preschool and Primary Scale of Intelligence* (3rd ed.; WPPSI–3; Wechsler, 2002) for ages 3 to 7, the *Wechsler Intelligence Scale for Children* (4th ed.; WISC–4; Wechsler, 2004) for ages 6 to 16, and the *Wechsler Adult Intelligence Scale* (3rd ed.; WAIS–III; Wechsler, 1997). One of the most relevant features of the tests is the grouping of intellectual tasks into verbal and nonverbal domains, the former of which has obvious diagnostic significance for speech–language pathologists. These instruments render a verbal intelligence quotient, a nonverbal intelligence quotient, and a full-scale intelligence score. In the verbal area, skills related to general knowledge, abstract and concrete verbal reasoning, auditory memory, and attention are assessed in a question-and-answer format. In the nonverbal area, skills related to visual perceptual organization and visual motor integration and visual processing are assessed in a given series of tasks. Materials used in this assessment include puzzles, paper–pencil tasks, and picture cards.

The *Stanford-Binet Intelligence Scale* (5th ed.; SB–5; Roid, 2003) is an alternate, less frequently used instrument that provides a comparison of the subject's performance to age mates from 2 to 23 years of age. It is often used in assessing preschool children because of the early age at which normative comparisons can be made. The SB–5 seeks to estimate intellectual development with regard to general knowledge, crystallized abilities, fluid-analytical abilities, and memory. Crystallized ability refers to those cognitive skills necessary for acquiring and using information about verbal and quantitative concepts to solve problems. They are greatly influenced by schooling. Fluid-analytic ability refers to cognitive skills necessary in spontaneous problem solving that involve figural or other nonverbal stimuli. They are closely related to invention, strategy, and flexibility in novel situations. Memory ability is assessed in both short- and long-term aspects of visual, auditory, and tactile modalities.

The *Kaufman Assessment Battery for Children* (2nd ed.; K-ABC–II; Kaufman & Kaufman, 2004) assesses intelligence as it pertains to cognitive ability in processing auditory and visual stimuli across simultaneous and sequential paradigms. This test has been useful to school psychologists interested in a match between learning and instructional styles. Results are represented in mental processing composite scores. Separate scaled scores for verbal and nonverbal test performances are also obtained.

When these intelligence measures are administered, diagnostic hypotheses begin to emerge that must be verified with additional testing, using a variety of norm-referenced tests that are less concerned with estimating general intelligence and more concerned with patterns of strength and weakness that may underlie learning difficulties. The following are those most commonly used for that purpose by school psychologists:

- *Woodcock-Johnson Psycho-Educational Cognitive Battery* (3rd. ed.; WJPB–III/Cognitive; McGrew & Mather, 2001): a variety of primary and supplemental subtests designed to measure auditory and visual processing ability. The test also offers achievement subtests in core academic and content areas.
- *Peabody Picture Vocabulary Test* (3rd ed.; PPVT–III; Dunn & Dunn, 1997): primarily a test of single-word receptive language that allows the examinee to demonstrate acquired knowledge and concepts without verbal responses.
- *Bender Gestalt Test* (2nd ed.; Brannigan & Decker, 2003): designed to measure visual motor integration and perceptual organization in copying designs and shapes from a given stimulus—important when considering the possibility of nonverbal learning or motor expression disabilities. Many years of behavioral research have also allowed the use of this test as a projective indicator of personality and emotional adjustment.
- *Beery-Buktenica Test of Visual Motor Integration* (5th ed.; Beery, Buktenica, & Beery, 2004): similar to the *Bender*, it measures visual perceptual, motor, and visual motor integration in a more structured drawing format and is useful for preschool and early elementary students.
- *Visual–Aural Digit Span Test* (VADS; Koppitz, 1977): a test of visual and auditory and short-term sequential memory, requiring the subject to recite and write verbally a visually presented number series from memory. Although it is presently in dire need of updated norming, it remains useful in understanding the student's efficiency in learning and recalling auditory and visual symbol relationships for reading, spelling, and writing.

Individual achievement tests provide norm-referenced age and grade comparisons of anticipated core academic achievement. Although their importance in the array of various psychoeducational assessment tools is obvious, results are interpreted with caution. The match between test items at any particular grade or age level must have a positive correlation with the curriculum to which the examinee has been exposed. Where this relationship between the test and curriculum is limited, curriculum-based assessments are favored. Curriculum-based assessment, as the name implies, uses a variety of techniques to employ the actual classroom methods and instructional materials in placing a student at a level of mastery. When norm-referenced test materials are used, some of the most common instruments chosen are the following:

- *Woodcock-Johnson Psycho-Educational Achievement Battery* (3rd ed.; WJPB–III/Achievement; Woodcock, McGrew, & Mather, 2001): the achievement part of the WJPB, offering age and grade norm comparisons in all core academic and content areas, is of particular value in its evaluation of specific skills of written expression.

- *Woodcock Reading Mastery Tests* (Rev.; WRMT–R; Woodcock, 1998): evaluates an in-depth catalogue of reading skills.
- *Kaufman Test of Educational Achievement* (2nd ed.; K-TEA; Kaufman & Kaufman, 2004): compares core academic test performance to age- and grade-normed population, particularly popular because of its high content validity with typical school curricula.
- *Wechsler Individual Achievement Test* (2nd ed.; WIAT–II; Zimmerman, Steiner, & Pond, 2001): authored in concert with the WISC–III, it attends to all basic academic areas including written expression. It provides a composite standard score specifically for expressive language that correlates to the verbal portion of the WISC–III.
- *Test of Written Language* (3rd ed.; TOWL–3; Hammill & Larsen, 1996): a well-constructed measure of various aspects of written language, providing a scaled-score measurement in contrived and spontaneous writing tasks. While its normative group is not fully representative of early primary writing, it is sensitive to the ability of students fourth grade and above.
- *Key Math Diagnostic Arithmetic Test* (Rev.; KM–R; Connolly, 1998): offers an in-depth evaluation of math concepts, calculating ability, and application. With the exception of some of its calculation subtests, it is considered precise in assigning a student's performance accurately within a given age range.

A number of commonly used test instruments are concerned with the dynamics of personality development and emotional adjustment. They are termed *projective* measures because they attempt to safely evoke the subject's unconscious or preconscious nature, needs, anxieties, and conflicts as he negotiates various ambiguous materials and activities. While these projective activities have been subject to many years of scientific research, they remain subjective, and interpretation of their results requires much training and careful analysis. Psychologists must consider how neurological factors interact with developmental psychology, learned behavior, and unconscious experience (anxiety, defense mechanisms, etc.). Projective measures are often considered when behavioral concerns are expressed by teachers and parents in the process of referral, and no psychoeducational assessment is complete without at least one projective measure. Of the wide variety of projective tests, the following reflect those most commonly used by the school psychologist:

- The *Draw-A-Person* (DAP-IQ; Reynolds & Hickman, 2004) test requests that students simply draw male and female figures. The subject's approach to this task, final product, and verbal responses to inquiry are assessed for indicators of intellectual development, self-concept and self-esteem, emotional experience, and overall adjustment.

- The *Incomplete Sentence Blank* (ISB; Rotter, Lau, & Rafferty, 1992), similar to the more widely known word association exercise common in psychoanalysis, requires the examinee to complete a series of partial sentences with the first idea that comes to mind. Responses or lack of them sometimes reveal significant information related to the subject's view of self, family, school, and degree of conflicts presented.

- The *Rorschach Test* (Herausgegeben, Morgenthaler, Bash, & Nachduck, 1999) presents a series of inkblot cards that are designed to evoke unconscious personality aspects. Response to location, color, shading, and so forth are compared with well-researched personality dynamics to form hypotheses regarding the student's unconscious experience.

- The *Lowenfeld Mosaic Test* (Lowenfeld, 2004) is an especially useful measure with children. It offers the subject a variety of colored tiles and shapes with which to construct designs and pictures on a blank surface. Efficient material use, color forms, and interview responses are assessed in terms of well-researched associated psychodynamics.

Another format for assessing personality and emotional and behavior dynamics are behavior rating scales that provide scaled listings of behaviors associated with a number of disorders of maladjustment. They are considerably more objective in their design than the previously described more subjective projective measures; subjectivity does exist in their application, however. They are also less useful in gaining a comprehensive understanding of the etiology of the conditions they identify. They include the *Achenbach Child Behavior Rating Scales* (CBRS; Achenbach, 2003a), the *Achenbach Teacher Rating Form* (TRF; Achenbach, 2003b), the *Behavior Assessment System for Children* (2nd ed.; BASC–II; Reynolds & Kamphaus, 2004), and the *Conners' Rating Scale–Revised* (CRS–R; Conners, 1997). These scales have grown in popularity because they provide criteria for identifying children with attention deficits and other neurological disorders of regulation.

There are many subtests contained in the testing instruments described previously that deal directly with auditory and verbal processes. The findings generated by these subtests (see Appendix 12.A for sample assessment report) inexorably bind the school psychologist and the speech–language pathologist into a common diagnostic effort. The verbal sections of the Wechsler tests provide an illustration. Responses in this question-and-answer format can offer the clinician valuable data about the student's understanding of simple and complex questions and about her ability to use language accurately in verbal responses. Subtests requiring the student to establish a common theme for two given concepts reveal abstract reasoning ability necessary for verbal comprehension, independent application of knowledge, and categorical thinking as an aid to memory. Responses to questions about everyday situations provide a measure of social understanding and pragmatics. Rote repetition of number serials relates directly to auditory short-term sequential memory, an important skill in ordering sounds for speech production and learning to use orthographic symbols. Further auditory processing subtests are included in the *Woodcock-*

Johnson Psycho-Educational Battery (3rd ed.; McGrew & Mather, 2001). Here the student's responses in subtests measuring auditory closure, sound blending, auditory discrimination, and sentence memory are combined into a composite score for auditory processing. This type of subtest performance is of obvious value to the SLP evaluating a child for a central auditory processing deficit.

Conclusion: School Psychologist

It should be clear from the above that there are many commonalities between the interests and roles of a school psychologist and a speech–language pathologist. Assessment and intervention are equally important to both. The differences that exist between the two professions afford an opportunity to expand information and insights about the student both practitioners seek to serve. For that to occur, communication must be open, frank, and cordial. Regular meetings and sharing of resources are but two of the ways for cooperation to occur; the time spent can reap rich benefits.

PUBLIC SCHOOL LIBRARIAN: LINDA ROBINSON

Many people still picture a school librarian as a little old lady with her hair in a bun, telling students to be quiet in the library and inadvertently making it difficult for them to acquire the resources they need to be successful students. In actuality, today's school library media specialists are active participants in student-centered learning. Their role is to help students become independent, information literate, lifelong learners. Guided by the concepts in *Information: Power: Building Partnerships for Learning* (American Association of School Librarians, 1998), the current standard for school library media center stakeholders, school librarians are committed to using their collaborative, leadership, and technology skills in achieving an integral partnership in the learning community that supports all students.

The School Librarian and the Team Concept

Within the school community, the library media specialist should be part of the team that works with the speech–language pathologist and other specialists to meet the unique needs of children with communication disorders. The librarian is the expert in the area of book selection, research skills, and information literacy. This knowledge is a tremendous asset when the school media specialist works with the speech–language pathologist to provide resources for a child.

Determining and meeting the particular needs of students is an everyday task for the school librarian. Each student enters the library with unique research needs, as well as her own level of understanding and reading ability.

This daily challenge is what drives the good librarian to search for just the right piece of information or that special book to help a student succeed in the classroom. Unfortunately, the school library media specialist is usually not part of the IEP team and remains an overlooked resource. It is often assumed that students with special needs will automatically receive the assistance they need when they visit the library. Many times, however, students don't realize that help is available or find it difficult to approach adults and ask for assistance.

Therefore, as a speech–language pathologist, you should locate your school library media specialist and discuss the issues surrounding specific students. Keep him informed of developments or needs so he can help those students whenever they are in the library media center. Since many students with disabilities are mainstreamed, they often visit the library as part of an entire class without the speech–language pathologist present for consultation. So sharing information ahead of time can alert the librarian and help him guide the student more effectively. If you are in a school without a full-time librarian, consider making contact with your local public library to determine the support that might be available through that avenue.

Relevant Materials

Finding the best materials for a student is what it is all about. The school library media specialist is committed to providing unfettered access to library resources and services for all students (American Library Association [ALA], 1996). Students who struggle with basic communication skills are at a real disadvantage in the traditional school environment since that setting operates often based on the assumption that students are functioning at a standard reading level.

Students with communication difficulties may also have special reading and research needs. If students' reading abilities are significantly below their grade level, they may not enjoy reading. Finding a book that sparks interest and is a quick read is critical to engaging this type of student. Books specifically designed for the high-interest, low-level reader are available if you know where to look. This is where the librarian's broad knowledge of reading materials is critical and where access to other library collections becomes important. Visually impaired students might need access to either large-print materials or books on tape. Many libraries, especially public libraries, offer large-print materials for their older readers, and libraries with large commuter populations often offer books on tape or on CD. Your librarian can also investigate the availability of illustrated, adapted, or condensed versions of materials if those meet the needs of your students.

Sometimes helping a student engage in literature requires more than just providing materials. Your librarian can help "sell" a book or resource to your students. Book talks and storytelling opportunities are often enough to connect a struggling student with a great read. You can approach the school librarian about designing book talk opportunities specifically geared to students with speech, language, and hearing impairments. This can be an entertaining opportunity and may stimulate peer recommendations and discussions about different books that will entice your student to read.

Reading Power

How does a librarian know what book to suggest to a student with reading difficulties? Generally, experience and a wide exposure to children's literature help the school library media specialist select the right book. However, librarians have other tools at their disposal. One of those is the book's readability level, often calculated using the Degrees of Reading Power (DRP) developed by TASA Literacy (Gunning, 2003). Any book or other reading material can be evaluated to determine its text difficulty. Software is also available to help determine the DRP, and some book publishers include the DRP in their grade-level assignment of material.

DRP tests are also administered to students in Grades 1 through 12+ to determine individual reading performance. They attempt to establish how well students understand the meaning of text. Test results are reported on a readability scale, the same scale used to quantify reading materials. By correlating student DRP scores with book DRP reading levels, one can locate materials that are appropriate to a student's reading ability, saving time and decreasing student frustration. In addition to the DRP, a variety of other methods to determine readability are available. Software used by school districts includes the Star Reading Program from Advantage Learning Systems. This program uses in-context vocabulary questions and text passages to determine reading levels. The *Gates-MacGinitie Reading Tests* (GMRT) measure beginning reading skills, primary-level developmental reading skills, and continuing growth in reading competence.

No matter what method your school uses to determine student reading abilities, reading is more than just numbers. Book selection cannot exclusively rely on the DRP or other scores. Students often read because they are engaged in a book. Your school library media specialist is a good resource to suggest ways to blend quantitative measurements with student interests.

Technology Assistance

Technology has greatly augmented the level of library service. With the advent of the online card catalog, many libraries can access materials outside of their building. Online Public Access Catalogs (OPACs) provide search capabilities previously unavailable with the old print card catalog system. A school district whose card catalog is shared among all of its schools can thereby increase materials available to students—a student at the middle school would have easy access to materials at an elementary school, for example. The first step, however, is notifying the school librarians of the need to borrow materials from other libraries. The technology that permitted the development of the online card catalog facilitates this process enormously.

In addition, the resources at your local public library should not be overlooked. They often have significantly larger collections and offer books on subjects that may be of real interest to the nonreader. Consider asking your local government to establish weekly runs between the school and public library to simplify access between the two resources. Many towns already have mail or delivery runs that could be altered at little cost. This access can be a wonderful resource for families who do not have easy access to library materials.

If your students are unable to access the OPAC themselves because of their limitations, explore assistive technologies that will allow this to happen. Touch screens, audio devices, and young reader library software are only some of the devices available to supplement traditional access to library electronic resources. If your school library does not have access to funds to purchase these types of devices, remember to involve your school librarian in the next round of grant writing you undertake. Your willingness to partner in this effort could help provide these hardware resources to your students.

Student Self-Efficacy

According to Bandura (1997), children are extremely sensitive to their relative standing among peers: "Students publicly label, rank, and discuss with one another how smart their classmates are" (p. 22). This is important to remember when helping students locate materials that are obviously below the reading abilities of their peers. Minimizing where the materials have come from can be critical to student self-esteem. Books should not be labeled or placed on a special shelf that publicizes that they are below the "normal" reading level.

This can be difficult if a librarian also wants to make the materials easy to locate for teachers or other service providers. One of the advantages of the new computerized card catalogs is that materials can be cataloged using unique subject headings that allow one to search for resources without advertising their special support opportunities. Also, when requesting materials from other libraries, you can ask for a large selection of books, so students have a choice. If everyone else in the class can select materials from the entire library, a student with disabilities should not be provided with only two books to pick from.

Finding Resources

There are numerous places on the Internet to access information on books you might suggest for your students. Bookwire (http://www.bookwire.com/bookwire/reviews.htm) offers reviews from a number of great library resources including the periodicals *Library Journal, Hungry Mind Review,* and *Boston Book Review.*

The American Library Association has a feature called Booklist Editors' Choice that provides short reviews on a wide range of new books. It is available at http://www.ala.org/ala/booklist/editorschoice/2004abcd/Youth.htm. You can find your own favorite book review resource by selecting one of the numerous Web sites indexed on AcqWeb's Directory of Book Reviews at http://acqweb. library.vanderbilt.edu/bookrev.html. The Children's Literature Web Guide (http:// ucalgary.ca/~dkbrown) provides information specifically about literature for children and includes information on Newberry and Caldecott award-winning books.

The Internet also offers online versions of many texts. A great place to search for available titles is the Internet Public Library Online Texts Collection at http:// www.ipl.org/div/books/. This site provides access to thousands of titles. Works can be offered in many different formats, so you may need to search to locate the version that you need. A similar collection of resources can be found at the Literature Project's Web page, http://www.literatureproject.com. A focused site offering short story resources can be found at Classic Short Stories at http:// www.bnl/com/shorts.

The Internet allows you easy access to libraries in your district and across the world as well. Some great resources to get you started are the Internet Public Library at www.ipl.org, the Library of Congress (http://catalog.loc/gov), and the New York Public Library (http://www.nypl.org). If you want to see which libraries have an Internet presence, you can use the Libweb Directory of Libraries (http://lists.webjunction.org/libweb), the comprehensive list available on the St. Joseph County Public Library Web site (sjcpl.lib.in.us/homepage/ PublicLibraries/PublicLibraryServers.html) or at the Library Index Web site (http://www.libdex.com).

Conclusion: Public School Librarian

Your school library media specialists or public librarians can provide numerous resources to help your students be more successful in the classroom. Their commitment to collaboration, appropriate use of technology, and equitable access of information for all students should place them on the same team as the speech, language, and hearing specialist when advocating for student needs. Remember to seek out their support, advice, and input in addressing the literacy challenges your students must overcome. In order to build a community of learners that includes all students, we must provide a culture of support. Make your school library media specialist part of that culture.

SCHOOL OCCUPATIONAL AND PHYSICAL THERAPISTS: KAREN BROWNING AND KIM M. NEVINS

Speech–language pathologists are often seen as kindred spirits by occupational and physical therapists when it comes to practice in a school setting. All three services are viewed as "related services" under Part B of IDEA. All three professions have roots in the medical–diagnostic model of assessment and intervention. As practitioners in the school setting, we are frequently thrown together to work as collaborative team members to serve the same children.

History

The treatment of children within educational settings by physical therapists (PTs) and occupational therapists (OTs) has been a part of both professions for nearly as long as both professions have existed. A review of the early physical therapy literature shows articles from the 1930s pertaining to the treatment of "crippled children" who attended "special schools" (Batten, 1933; Mulcahey, 1936; Severs, 1938). At that time in history, these special schools represented the cutting edge in care for children with primarily physically disabling conditions. The schools and the children who attended were generally segregated from the community and educational settings in which children without disabilities were enrolled.

Traditionally trained in a medical model of service delivery, PTs and OTs who worked in special schools during the early segregated years tended to apply the medical model of service delivery to the special school setting (Severs, 1938). In fact, the schools themselves more often resembled medical or rehabilitation institutions than primary educational facilities. This theoretical approach focused on remediating the dysfunctional components of disabling conditions by removing children from their classrooms or other more routine environments for isolated treatment or rehabilitation. Therapists assumed that appropriate treatment meant maximizing function through direct "hands-on" intervention. The assessment and treatment methodologies of the time supported (a) neuromaturational and reflex hierarchical models of assessment and intervention; (b) assessment and measurement of disabling conditions through a developmental framework; and (c) child-centered service provision (McEwen & Sheldon, 1995).

It was not until the federal legislation of the 1970s, which provided that children with disabilities should have access to the public schools, that therapists began to treat children in those settings on a regular basis. As OTs and PTs began to provide services in the relatively foreign professional arena of the public schools, they found that their traditional service delivery models and practice patterns were often in conflict with the tenets of the Education for All Handicapped Children Act (P.L. 94-142; 1975). For example, the law stipulated that children should receive services in "the least restrictive environment." It was difficult for therapists to resolve how to provide services to children in the classroom or "less restricted" environment, when they had been taught that direct "hands-on" treatment in a "private" room was the best way to minimize dysfunction.

While therapists were struggling with this conflict of medical versus educational models, teachers and administrators (as reported in the education and related services literature) were struggling to find ways to integrate children with disabilities into general education environments. This included the provision of support services within the general classroom, instead of providing "pull-out" resource support or isolated episodic therapy in a separate room. Later, with the passage of the Individuals with Disabilities Education Act (IDEA; 1990), more refined interpretation of the least restrictive environment concept demanded that educators, therapists, and other specialists justify removing a student from his peers to provide intervention.

Along with this philosophical change in where to serve children with disabilities, the literature now addressed how to serve them. Research studies in the PT and OT literature began to support the idea that motor skill problems were best addressed within the context of daily activities and with the combined expertise of a variety of disciplines (Campbell, 1987; Rainforth & York, 1987, 1987). In addition, these studies reported the positive benefits of using collaborative practices among team members to ensure successful integration of students as well as to improve goal attainment. This collaborative teamwork has also been referred to as an integrated therapy approach or a type of transdisciplinary approach to teamwork (Giangreco, York, & Rainforth, 1989; Rainforth & York-Barr, 1997; Sternat, Messina, Nietupske, Lyon, & Brown, 1997). As research studies and outcomes were helping to redefine appropriate practice approaches, case law based on litigation was also having a major influence on "best practice." Best practices are those that represent the most current beliefs about how professionals should provide their range of services. They evolve over time, and best practices for occupational and physical therapists have undergone many changes since the federal legislation of the 1970s. For example, in 1982, the U.S. Supreme Court clarified an "appropriate" education as one based on an IEP that was reasonably calculated by the educational team to enable the student to receive meaningful educational benefit (*Board of Education v. Rowley*, 1982). The Rowley decision informed OT and PT therapists that although their intervention could not be trivial, it should be designed not to maximize potential, but to show educational benefit.

The practice of school-based treatment performed by OTs and PTs in the 1980s began to evolve to incorporate these changes, but not without resistance and conflict over treatment methodology and models of service provision (Campbell, 1987; Giangreco, 1986; Orelove & Sobsey, 1987, 1996). We have seen that best practice now supports working with children in classrooms and other natural environments (Bundy & Carter, 1991; McEwen & Sheldon, 1995). Best practice also supports teachers, therapists, speech–language pathologists, and other service providers collaborating to develop an integrated therapy approach, in which the IEP team members focus on prioritizing a child's educational needs. From those needs, the team then develops "discipline-free" goals, described as goals that teams develop without regard to individual disciplines. In essence, those goals represent a child's meaningful and relevant goals, not the OT, PT, or SLP goals (McEwen, 2000).

Other significant changes in practice patterns adopted by therapists in the 1990s were seen in assessment and therapeutic intervention models. As changes in contemporary theories of motor development and motor learning began to be accepted by therapists, they shifted from a model that uses a developmental sequence of tasks to one that focuses on functional task acquisition (Atwater, 1991; McEwen & Sheldon, 1995).

Despite these changes in best practice and nearly a century of PT and OT therapists serving children within educational settings, a sense of uncertainty concerning their appropriate roles and responsibilities on a day-to-day basis remains. Much of the confusion exists because of the ever shifting interpretation of federal legislation, as well as the unknown outcomes of ongoing litigation that may have an impact on future practice patterns. On the positive side, this uncertainty leads to some creative and exciting days (albeit sometimes frustrating and scary, as well) as we try to serve children as appropriately as possible in a challenging and rewarding environment.

Frequently Asked Questions

Despite the frequent interactions and similarities in background among PTs, OTs, and SLPs, speech–language pathologists (as well as many other school faculty members) often have questions about the roles that occupational and physical therapists play in the public school setting. Indeed, as occupational and physical therapists who work for a school district, much of our day is spent in answering basic questions about the nature of our responsibilities within this unique setting. So, when we were approached with the opportunity to write about our services, we saw it as a way to articulate answers to some of the most frequently asked questions from our fellow school team members.

We felt organizing this chapter in a question-and-answer format would allow readers to "jump" to the question that is most pertinent or critical to them now and read the material more completely at a later time.

Q *Who may provide occupational and physical therapy services in the school setting?*

The Individuals with Disabilities Education Act (1990) states that occupational and physical therapy services are to be provided by "qualified, trained practitioners." The only "qualified and trained" people are those who have a license to practice occupational or physical therapy. In occupational therapy, this includes occupational therapists and certified occupational therapy assistants (COTA). In physical therapy, the designation includes physical therapists and licensed physical therapy assistants (PTA). The COTA and PTA may provide occupational therapy and physical therapy under the direction of a qualified licensed OT or PT. The OT, PT, COTA, or PTA may direct other professionals or paraprofessionals to carry out integrated or supportive activities in the school setting following training by the PT or OT. It must be stressed, however, that these activities are not included in the number of minutes listed on a student's IEP under the heading of "Occupational or Physical Therapy Intervention." The use of personnel other than therapists for supporting children in the classroom is explained in greater detail later in this chapter.

Q *What is the role and expertise of occupational therapists in educational environments?*

Occupational therapists are licensed or certified health-care professionals who use purposeful activities, environmental modifications, and adapted methods and equipment to promote an individual's independent function in her life roles or occupations. As a related service, OT may be provided to promote improved movement and coordination, visual motor function, and organization and use of school materials to increase focus or attention on instruction or to improve interaction with peers. The role or occupation of a student is to learn and to demonstrate what she has learned. To participate as fully as possible in the educational process, a student must be able to participate in those activities that are a part of the daily school routine. Eating lunch, using the toilet, dressing in the locker room for physical education, playing on the playground, accessing a locker for books or a coat, accessing equipment and tools for industrial technology class, and using the computer in the computer lab are examples of activities in which an OT may be asked to assist a student.

Fundamental to the practice of OT is its focus on supporting students' self-initiated adaptive behaviors as they engage in purposeful activities within an ever changing environment. Consequently, school-based occupational therapists attempt to structure activities and to adapt the school environment within natural, goal-directed contexts in a manner designed to facilitate learning skills that will generalize to similar situations. Therapy and therapeutic intervention strategies are incorporated into students' daily activities and routines, allowing repeated opportunities to learn, practice, and develop skills in natural environments where they will be needed and are meaningful. Services delivered in this fashion take on increased relevance to the educational program. These services function as they are intended, to assist a child to benefit from his or her educational program by decreasing the effects of the handicapping condition on the student's ability to participate effectively in the educational process.

Occupational therapy interventions may address behavioral or sensorimotor problems, functional musculoskeletal limitations, perceptual problems, and the use of assistive or other technology. OTs recommend, construct, and teach others to maintain and use adaptive equipment for such activities as positioning, feeding, helping children write, and helping children use other school tools. Assistance is also provided with transition planning for those students who are moving from one grade level to the next or preparing to enter postschool community life.

Q *What is the role and expertise of physical therapists in educational environments?*

Physical therapists who work with the pediatric population are licensed health-care professionals who provide services to children with acute and chronic conditions or disabilities in order to promote improved performance and health by preventing, evaluating, and treating movement dysfunction. Movement problems may include limitations such as muscle weakness, paralysis, poor motor coordination, painful movement, lack of endurance, poor posture, soft tissue restriction, or joint instability (American Physical Therapy Association [APTA], 1992). In the public school setting, physical therapists use techniques that facilitate, correct, or adapt a child's functional performance in

- using muscle strength, motor control, mobility patterns, muscle coordination, and endurance needed for school performance;
- posture, balance, gait, and body awareness skills needed for school-related functional tasks;
- use of mobility devices such as walkers, crutches, and wheelchairs; and
- use of specialized positioning and other equipment that assists with access to the educational environment.

Similar to their occupational therapy colleagues, physical therapists attempt to structure their therapeutic interventions and activities in a way that will support the acquisition of skills within natural, goal-directed contexts and provide many opportunities for practice. Physical therapists who work in educational environments may provide services related to the functional use of the body for

- postural alignment and balance (e.g., to maintain sitting, standing, or upright mobility in the classroom as needed for educational activities);
- mobility around the school (e.g., wheelchair mobility, stair climbing, walking);
- the use of braces or prostheses;
- maintaining or improving general endurance for school participation;
- the use of adaptive equipment to support posture or movement for the school routine; and
- positioning needs required for independent school participation.

Q *How are the roles of the COTA and PTA different from those of the OT and PT?*

Both assistants work under the supervision of a licensed professional (OT or PT) in directing and monitoring the intervention plans the IEP team has developed. The level of supervision by the OT or PT is determined by factors such as the experience of the assistant, the stability of the child's condition or situation, and the assistant's familiarity with the type of intervention being provided. Neither COTAs nor PTAs may perform or interpret comprehensive initial evaluations or reevaluations on students who have been referred or develop a student's initial treatment plan. Assistants may perform some aspects of an evaluation, such as classroom observations, or undertake procedures they have been appropriately trained to execute. They may delegate tasks to other school professionals and paraprofessionals, but it is the supervising therapist who has ultimate responsibility. COTAs and PTAs should attend IEP meetings to report on progress and to be a part of any intervention activity revisions. For PTAs, the section on pediatrics in *Guide to Physical Therapy Practice* (APTA, 1997a) and *the Utilization of Physical Therapist Assistants in Various Pediatric Settings* (APTA, 1997b) provide useful information. The American Occupational Therapy Association (AOTA) has published *Standards of Practice for Occupational Therapy Services in the Schools* (1987) to assist school districts in implementing occupational therapy services.

Q *It seems that the OT and PT disciplines have overlapping areas of expertise. How are roles and responsibilities differentiated?*

It is true that occupational and physical therapists appear to have expertise in similar areas of performance, such as motor control, coordination, mobility, equipment use, and activities of daily living. Despite this appearance of duplication, each discipline brings its own perspective when assessing and providing intervention plans. It is the prerogative of the educational teams to determine who has the most appropriate level of expertise (within the established scope of their practice) to provide the required services. The "most appropriate" person may be the person with the best qualifications in terms of training and experience in treating a particular problem.

OTs and PTs also share areas of expertise with other professionals. For example, both the occupational therapist and the SLP may share expertise in evaluating and treating children with swallowing difficulties or oral motor control. Each discipline contributes information and important intervention strategies to support students with these difficulties. The OT and SLP may also share expertise in evaluating students for assistive technology—for example, for augmentative communication devices or devices that might assist in alternative communication. Once again, the OT and SLP have significant areas of specialized training that when combined will provide a more complete assessment of the child and contribute to better planning for the use and application of such devices.

In another example, physical therapists share similar knowledge with adapted physical education teachers in such areas as gross motor skill development and coordination. The PT and the adapted physical educator each bring a unique perspective to serving students. For instance, the adapted physical education teacher may have responsibilities in curriculum development, whereas the cooperating physical therapist has responsibilities in developing individual exercise programs to be used in the adapted physical education class. As noted above, knowledge about motor skill development does not lie solely in the domains of OT and PT. Many special education teachers (especially those in early childhood) have expertise in assessing a child's motor skills, as well as developing intervention strategies and making adaptations to the physical environment. When the special educator's level of expertise is not adequate to assess or intervene effectively in areas such as sensory integration problems or the use of assistive technology, consultation or direct services may be required from either an OT or PT. Another example of shared expertise is seen between elementary or secondary classroom teachers and OTs, who may each have knowledge about the skills of keyboarding, handwriting, and organization.

It should be noted that shared areas of expertise should not lead to duplication of services, nor should they lead to a substitution for the most appropriate service or service provider (California Department of Education, 1996).

Collaboration among classroom teachers, therapists, and other related service providers should always be emphasized.

Q *What are the educational backgrounds, qualifications, and supervision requirements of the OT, PT, COTA, and PTA?*

Each state's licensing or professional registration board regulates OT, PT, COTA, and PTA requirements for training and qualifications for licensure. Generally, therapists and assistants are regulated as health-care professionals; thus, their licensing and renewal processes may look different from those of teachers and other related service providers.

The specialized education that OTs, PTs, COTAs, and PTAs receive from approved and accredited educational programs in their respective areas provides the foundation of each practitioner's expertise. A person who does not hold the appropriate credentials (license, certificate, or registration) in accordance with his state's requirements may not refer to himself as a licensed or registered practitioner in any setting. In addition, unless a provider possesses the credentials, he may not state that he is providing physical or occupational therapy services. There is some confusion about this when paraprofessionals or teacher's aides are following through with suggestions or activities that therapists have provided to them. This will be addressed later.

The education and licensure requirements for OTs and COTAs are similar: The registered or licensed occupational therapist must graduate from an accredited educational program (or have met the equivalency educational requirements) and receive certification after passing a nationally recognized examination. Although their educational backgrounds are similar, OTs must complete a wider range of courses and the content of those courses reflects greater depth. Courses include specific biological and physical sciences; human development and behavior, including social, emotional, and physiological implications of illness and injury; clinical courses featuring the analysis and application of theory to practice; ethics; and supervised fieldwork experience.

Entry level for the professional occupational therapist is the bachelor's degree; however, many therapists enter the profession holding a master's degree. COTAs must have an associate degree and a certificate from a program sanctioned by their professional accrediting body. Licensure for both therapists is determined by specific state regulations. There is no national certification for an occupational therapist or a COTA to work within the school setting. Individual states may have requirements for continuing education to maintain a current license. Individual states may also have particular requirements for professional development for therapists who are working in the public school setting.

The education and licensure requirements for PTs include a minimum of a bachelor's or master's degree in physical therapy from an educational program approved and accredited by the Commission on Accreditation in Physical Therapy Education or the equivalency education requirements for eligibility to sit for the certification examination (APTA, 1997a). The coursework for PTAs differs in the length of training and the depth of covered material. The educational background of PTs and PTAs generally includes significant background in biological and physical sciences; human growth and development, including congenital developmental and acute and chronic disease processes; clinical therapy theory and practice; statistics and research methodology; and supervised clinical experience.

Licensure is required to practice as either a PT or a PTA, and eligibility requirements must be met as designated by the specific state's Physical Therapy Practice Act. Some states require varying hours of continuing education to maintain a license in good standing. As is the case with OTs, there is no specific qualifying exam that allows a PT or PTA to practice in a school setting. Many states, however, have developed guidelines for PT (and OT) practice in the public schools to assist with continuity of practice patterns within those states. In addition, the American Physical Therapy Association has published *Providing Physical Therapy Services Under Parts B and C of the Individuals with Disabilities Education Act* (2000) to assist therapists with negotiating this area of practice.

Q *Who provides supervision of PTs, OTs, COTAs, and PTAs in the school setting?*

Other experienced therapists, school principals, special education administrators, or other designated facility or district administrators may supervise PTs and OTs. PTs and OTs who are new to the public school setting should receive a complete orientation to this unique area of practice, as well as close mentoring or supervision by an experienced therapist in the district; the level of supervision should be determined by the therapist's past clinical and school-based practice and level of responsibility.

As implied in the answer to a preceding question on the role of COTAs and PTAs, the licensed PT or OT is responsible for evaluating the standard of work performed by the assistants, including the safety of the children being served. The supervisor should meet with the COTA or PTA on a frequent and regular basis to review the progress of children receiving intervention. Supervision of assistants should be performed according to the manuals provided by their respective professional organizations (AOTA, 1986; APTA, 1997b). Individual states may have established standards regarding how PTAs and COTAs are to be appropriately monitored. Supervision of COTAs and PTAs may range from on-site daily supervision to intermittent supervision, in which the PT or OT may not be on site every day.

Q *How may other personnel be used to support OT and PT services?*

OT and PT practitioners frequently collaborate with educational professionals, paraprofessionals, and other related service providers (including SLPs) to facilitate or enhance a child's performance within the context of the school environment. The literature pertaining to best practice in educational environments supports an integrated service delivery model (Effgen, 1994a; Rainforth, York, & McDonald, 1992). This model of service delivery assumes that specialists such as the OT and PT will need to instruct a variety of professionals and paraprofessionals regarding intervention strategies employed throughout a child's day. The use of intervention in this manner helps ensure that children will have opportunities to practice the skills they need in the context of the school environment. Teachers and paraprofessionals may assist children with activities or interventions that are within the scope of their education and experience, that they can carry out safely, and that are in accordance with state and federal laws and regulations (APTA, 1997a). If physical and occupational therapy personnel delegate activities or instruct school staff in the use of specialized equipment, they are responsible for the training and monitoring of those activities or equipment.

One misconception of this service delivery model is that collaborative integrated services can be used to decrease the amount of time required for OT or PT services. School districts may also misinterpret this model to use unqualified staff without adequate supervision or instruction (Effgen & Klepper, 1994). Under IDEA, neither of these scenarios is allowed.

Skilled tasks that require the use of ongoing and changing clinical judgments or hands-on skills, or necessitate on-site decisions in order to be safely administered should be undertaken only by licensed OT or PT personnel. Before delegating any services, the therapist should determine that the situation is safe and stable and that there are predictable outcomes and consequences (Watts, 1971). It is the OT or PT's responsibility to provide initial training and guidance, as well as to exercise ongoing, intensive supervision if necessary. As stated previously, if a COTA or PTA provides supervision of delegated tasks, the supervising OT or PT maintains ultimate responsibility for the treatment plan. Selection of which activities to teach other professionals and paraprofessionals in school-based practice must be a "professional decision based on the characteristics of the individual child, the specific activity, and the capabilities and interest of other individuals" (Effgen, 1994a).

Q *How do OTs and PTs evaluate and assess children in the public school-setting?*

From Chapter 3 on speech–language assessment, you know how incredibly complex the process of assessment can be. OTs and PTs ask themselves the same questions about the "hows and whys" of choosing tools that will determine the most complete and appropriate evaluation of each child referred to our services. It is our intent here not to provide detailed descriptions of every tool that we have at our disposal, but to describe briefly the current thinking in our professions in terms of best practice as it relates to assessment.

Like our SLP colleagues, OTs and PTs have a number of standardized assessment tools that assist with determining a child's skills in relation to his or her peers. These "discriminative" measures are useful in distinguishing between children who may have particular skills or characteristics (Kirshner & Guyatt, 1985). The areas of assessment range from general gross and fine motor skill development to instruments for specific motor skills such as handwriting or ambulating. In addition, there are assessment tools that focus on other areas of physical development or function, such as sensorimotor development and visual motor integration. It is important to note that the primary purpose of these discriminative tools is to determine whether a child varies from the norm. They are not designed to "diagnose" why a child has a difference, to predict a particular outcome, or to evaluate performance of functional skills over time. Examples of this type of assessment tool, familiar to our SLP colleagues, are the *Peabody Developmental Motor Scales* (2nd ed.; Folio & Fewell, 2000), the *Bruininks-Oseretsky Test of Motor Proficiency* (Bruininks, 1978), the *Sensory Profile* (Dunn, 1999), and the *Sensory Integration and Praxis Tests* (Ayres, 1989). Although it has been a common practice in the past, it is important to note that using failed items from discriminative tests is not supported by either the tenets of IDEA or the OT and PT literature. As mentioned previously, current best practice supports an IEP that reflects meaningful and functional goals in the context of the school environment. The only time that failed items on discriminative tests may be useful is when the child has a mild delay and the expectation is that they will make progress in a more typical sequence of development (McEwen, 2000).

Just as the SLP uses observations as a part of a complete evaluation, OTs and PTs rely on clinical observations that reflect our training and expertise, specifically in the areas of muscle strength and range; coordination; dexterity; posture and positioning; environmental factors; and general neurological assessment, including level of alertness and sensitivity to touch, sound, visual stimuli, and movement.

Clinical observations are an area where an SLP and either an OT or a PT can evaluate a student together to obtain a more complete and integrated picture of the child's skills or functional abilities. Examples include oral motor assessment or factors involved in assessing a student with cerebral palsy. Using their combined expertise, they are able to assess the effect of sitting posture on such areas as ability to use sign language or augmentative communication devices.

In evaluating a child with autism who may be nonverbal and highly distractible, the SLP and OT may work together to evaluate which type of sensory stimulus is most effective for attention and focus. As OTs and PTs assume greater roles in the acquisition and application of assistive technology, they may be able to assist the SLP in determining what communication system may be the least taxing and most efficient in terms of a child's motor skills.

In any assessment, after therapists have determined a student's strengths and deficits, they must discern how those factors affect a child's ability to perform within the school environment (Dunn, Brown, & McGuigan, 1994; IDEA, 1997, 2004; Royeen, 1992). As in speech pathology, observing a student as he interacts with elements in the school environment is described in our literature as an ecological approach to assessment and planning (Dunn et al., 1994; Rainforth & York-Barr, 1997; Royeen, 1992). In terms of OT and PT, an ecologically referenced assessment focuses on the pertinent sensory, motor, self-help, and social skills that the child or student will require to be successful in all present school environments (regular and special education classrooms, physical education class, cafeteria, playground, music and art rooms), as well as the skills the student will need in future school environments. Once the student's abilities and interests have been determined, the IEP team members develop a plan that prioritizes the skills required for success (Rainforth & York-Barr, 1997). This approach can also be used in planning for transitions and challenges as students advance from grade to grade.

Clearly, the ecological approach is as helpful in program planning for the OT and PT as it is for the SLP. It may not be useful in determining program eligibility, however. It is distinguished from other assessment approaches (e.g., the developmental approach) by the development of student goals prior to assessment. In other words, assessment takes place after the student's goals have been determined and is specifically referenced to those goals and the environments in which the student will achieve them (Kelly et al., 1991).

Two standardized instruments that assist OTs and PTs in an ecological assessment approach are the *Pediatric Evaluation of Disability Inventory* (PEDI; Haley, Coster, Ludlow, Haltiwanger, & Andrellos, 1992) and the *School Function Assessment* (SFA; Coster, Deeney, Haltiwanger, & Haley, 1998). Both the SFA and PEDI can be used to identify functional abilities and limitations in school-related activities, such as mobility, social interactions, self-care, and communication (both of these tools were developed to be used by a number of professionals, including the SLP). The SFA and the PEDI can be used for program planning, as well as to monitor and measure progress over time. As previously noted, a primary concern for therapists who are using an ecological approach is that individual states may require some other type of percentile ranking or discrepancy measure in order for a child to qualify for services under Part B or C of IDEA.

Q *Following evaluation, how does a child become eligible for OT or PT services?*

A child does not automatically become eligible for OT or PT because of a particular cutoff score on a specialized test or diagnosed physical or cognitive disability. Children generally become eligible for OT and PT only after they have met the criteria for one of the 13 diagnostic categories in special education (as determined by each state's plan for special education). In other words, for the majority of states, children have to qualify for special education first. They also have to be within the age range specified by the state (usually 3–21). Following the satisfaction of these criteria, the student may receive occupational or physical therapy if the educational team determines that therapy is required for the child to benefit from the child's individually designed education program (AOTA, 1998; APTA, 2000). To be even more specific, the educational goals for the child should be determined prior to deciding who is needed and what services are required to support the student appropriately (Hanft & Place, 1996). The IEP goals should ultimately drive the support services necessary for each student.

As mentioned in the preceding paragraph, a disability diagnosis does not mean that a child automatically qualifies for special education or related services. If a child's disabling condition does not adversely affect his educational performance, he does not require special education or related services. If he needs only OT or PT and does not satisfy the criteria for specialized instruction according to state standards, the child is not considered to have a disability under IDEA. There are exceptions in some states, where the standards dictate that the provision of OT or PT alone can be considered to be special education. Students who are diagnosed with a disability but do not qualify as being disabled under IDEA (i.e., don't meet their state's standards for one of the diagnostic categories) may qualify for services under Section 504 (Rehabilitation Act of 1973).

Q *What are the roles of the OT and PT in developing an IEP?*

Although best practice would dictate otherwise, we are aware that many PTs and OTs who work in the public school setting submit their own discipline-specific Present Level of Performance statements, as well as discipline-specific goals and benchmarks, prior to the IEP meeting. They may not even be present at the meeting. PTs and OTs are not required to be present at IEP meetings under IDEA, but they should be involved in the IEP process because they have knowledge and expertise that can assist in determining the most appropriate educational program for a child.

Another issue of concern in regard to OT and PT practices is developing meaningful and functional goals. As noted in the section on assessment, therapists in the past frequently used failed items on discriminative tests to develop goals and objectives. Although this was an easy way for therapists to write goals, those goals were not necessarily meaningful in the context of the school environment (Harris, 1981). Instead of writing functional goals such as maneuvering a wheelchair safely in the hallway, handling art supplies independently, getting to class in a timely manner, or eating independently during snack time, therapists wrote goals for skipping 20 feet, walking a 4-inch-wide balance beam, or stringing 10 beads in 60 seconds. Implied in the development of such goals is the idea that achievement requires isolated and episodic "therapy." Although each of these skills may be justified as meaningful to an individual child, OTs and PTs have to discern how the use of these skills can be translated to meaningful functions. Goals should address tasks that children will have many opportunities to practice as they go about a daily routine, such as climbing the steps to a classroom, operating the elevator from their wheelchair, or using a computer and word prediction software to complete a class assignment.

We suggest that the OT and PT should be involved prior to the IEP meeting. They should consult and collaborate with classroom teachers and other related service providers (as well as the student and family if appropriate) and serve as contributing members to the development of an integrated Present Level of Performance statement. In that statement, information describing a child's function should provide the reader with a realistic and holistic view of the child (Rainforth & York-Barr, 1997). Although each team member contributes a disciplinary perspective, the focus should be on the child and not on the individual disciplines that serve the child. Since IDEA intends that the student's educational plan be developed at the IEP meeting (where the goals are child centered and not discipline specific), it follows that OTs and PTs should not submit "OT or PT goals" prior to that meeting. If an OT or PT is not able to attend an IEP meeting, she has an obligation to the child and other team members to clearly communicate her assessment of the child's strengths and concerns, as well as ideas for possible goals, beforehand. She should also communicate whether her expertise will be required to achieve particular goals, either on a direct service or consultative basis.

Q *How is "benefit from special education" determined?*

This question has probably given therapists more headaches, caused more confusion, and led to more heated debate than any other single subject. In the past, some school districts have attempted to limit services provided by OTs and PTs to those activities that directly affected academic performance, while others limited services to those activities that simply assisted a child's free access to the educational environment (Effgen, 1994b). Case law that resulted from litigation (several cases went all the way to the Supreme Court) has helped to define "benefit." It should come as a relief to the educational team that special education can be anything that the team determines it to be. A philosophy has emerged that states that the greater purpose of education is to prepare children for independent living and self-sufficiency. It is critical that IEP teams embrace this concept. If the team decides that an OT or PT has the required expertise to help a child meet one or more of the IEP goals, services should be secured as needed in an appropriate and "educationally relevant" manner.

Q *What are the roles of the OT and PT in 504 plans?*

As discussed in Chapter 1, Section 504 of the Rehabilitation Act (1973) deals with discrimination against people with disabilities. It prohibits any state or local government or private organization that receives federal funds from discriminating against children or adults with disabilities solely on the basis of their disability; in essence, it protects the civil rights of those individuals against discrimination. A person with a disability is defined in Section 504 as one who (a) has a physical or mental impairment that substantially limits one or more major life activities, (b) has a record of having a physical or mental impairment that limits one or more life activities, or (c) does not have an impairment but is regarded as having an impairment. Section 504 defines major life activities as "functions such as caring for one's self, performing manual tasks, walking, seeing, hearing, speaking, breathing, learning, and working."

Like IDEA, Section 504 requires schools to provide children with disabilities with a free and appropriate public education. Like speech–language services, OT and PT are not specifically mentioned, but regular or special education and "related aids and services" designed to meet children's educational needs are included. Under Section 504, neither occupational nor physical therapy is considered to be a related service or special education, but the services must be made available to children to accommodate for a disability that affects one or more of their major life activities. For a child who is diagnosed with either a temporary or permanent physical disability but does not qualify for services under IDEA, the issue of PT and OT supporting access to the educational program or environment through accommodations clearly falls within their scope of practice.

For instance, a child who has paraplegia but functions independently for learning and communication in the general classroom may not qualify for services under IDEA. But because this child uses a wheelchair and may have difficulty getting to the playground, passing through the lunch line, or taking care of hygiene needs during the school day, a PT or OT could assist the general educators in developing a plan that allows the child access to the physical environment of the school. Using 504 plans to accommodate for difficulties with some other major life activities is not so clear. For example, if a child has poor handwriting but exhibits no other problems in the classroom and has no medical diagnosis that explains the etiology of the poor handwriting, would that student qualify for OT under a 504 plan because the teacher regards the child as having an impairment? If the answer is yes, to what extent may the OT provide services to accommodate the child's limitations? What are "reasonable" accommodations? If the answer is no, is the school in violation of a child's civil rights? Although there are documents to help guide the application of 504 plans, available through the Council of Administrators of Special Education, there is still confusion about the issue. Like issues raised under IDEA, litigation and case law may be the ultimate determinants of how Section 504 is applied within the public schools.

Q *What service delivery models do occupational and physical therapists use?*

Hanft and Place (1996) stated that the exclusive use of one model of service delivery is ineffective and violates the IDEA mandate for individualized services for children. Dunn (1991) noted that educationally services require therapists to consider multiple options to meet the divergent needs of children. Fortunately (or perhaps unfortunately) for OTs and PTs, as we're sure it is for our SLP colleagues, we are not lacking in models for service delivery or team interaction. We too have encountered and used terms such as *direct, indirect, monitoring, transdisciplinary, collaboration, consultation,* and *push-in* or *pull-out services.* This wide variety of models has created confusion. Depending on the source used to describe individual models, the different definitions often contain conflicting information (Effgen, 2000). Even the meaning and functional definition of the word *collaboration,* which continues to be one of the buzzwords from the 1980s and 1990s (Benard, 1989), continue to be debated.

We will take the risk of being accused of oversimplification by limiting our discussion to three service delivery models, as each relates to OT and PT practice in the schools: the direct model, the consultation model, and the integrated therapy model of team interaction. We apologize to our SLP readers in advance for any confusion or frustration that definitions from our literature may cause.

As noted in the historical narrative at the beginning of this section, the direct service model was the preferred model initially used by OTs and PTs who served children in educational environments. In this model, the OT or PT served as the primary service provider, and therapists developed their own discipline-specific goals that were typically delivered in a "hands on" or one-to-one interaction in an isolated and episodic manner (Dunn, 1991). Although this model is still employed today, applying it has evolved to reflect contemporary theories of motor skill acquisition. It is now suggested that when direct services are used, they be limited to situations where the emphasis is on the child's acquiring new motor skills or when specific techniques cannot be safely delegated to other IEP team members (Effgen, 2000). Once the skill or critical components of the skill have been acquired, the child should receive intervention that promotes frequent practice and integration into natural environments (McEwen, 2000).

Even when a direct service model is employed, best practice in OT and PT directs that there should be ongoing consultation with teachers, parents, and other team members (Hanft & Place, 1996). Consultation occurs when the therapist uses discipline-specific professional expertise to address the needs of another adult on the intervention team (AOTA, 1998). The OT or PT works together with other IEP team members to create appropriate intervention plans that use their combined knowledge. Dunn and Campbell (1991) state that "the therapist provides consultative services when he or she adjusts task demands to enable task performance, adapts environmental conditions to improve integration, alters materials to address specific strengths and needs, creates optimal postural conditions, establishes movement parameters within the educational environment and instructs the classroom personnel about specific methods that can improve learning" (p. 142).

In the consultative model, the OT or PT provides instruction and information to other team members who are the providers of skill or activities practice. Consultation may not be limited to child-specific concerns but may include subjects that affect school district programming, such as issues related to safety, architectural barriers, transportation, equipment, and documentation (Lindsey, O'Neal, Haas, & Tervey, 1980). As with the direct service model, consultation is rarely used in isolation but is typically provided using a variety of service delivery models such as the integrated therapy model (Hanft & Place, 1996).

The integrated therapy model has been defined as a model in which the therapist's contact is not limited to a specific child but includes the teacher, teacher's aide, and other team members including the child's family (Iowa Department of Education, 1996). Integrated therapy is based on an approach in which team interaction and collaboration promote achievement of functional goals within the context of the natural environment (McEwen & Sheldon, 1995). Because of this dynamic team interaction, the integrated therapy approach may include direct and consultative service delivery approaches.

Dunn (1991) describes the integrated model as consisting of four components, identified as peer integration, functional integration, practice integration, and comprehensive integration. *Peer integration* occurs when children with disabilities function in the classroom or in social situations with children who are not disabled. *Functional integration* is achieved when a child with a disability is able to use a new skill in the natural environment. This provides support for the rationale behind providing therapeutic intervention within the natural environment. *Practice integration* is achieved when professionals collaborate to serve a child's individual needs. *Comprehensive integration* is described as the combination of all the areas of integration.

Because OTs and PTs are instructing other team members in therapeutic strategies or delegating specific activities, a certain amount of role release is inherent in the integrated therapy model. Therapists should be familiar with their individual states' practice acts so they can determine how this delegation may occur. It should always be emphasized that delegation of tasks or activities is not the same as abdication of a therapist's obligation to provide appropriate training and supervision (McEwen, 2000).

As noted at the beginning of this section on service delivery models, therapists have an array of models to choose from when attempting to meet the needs of individual students. We have seen that there is often confusion and conflict in the use of terminology to describe different models. What is ultimately important in using whatever model is currently viewed as "best practice" is clearly describing to all team members how we are going to provide our services. This means that we may need to forego the terminology or vernacular of the OT and PT disciplines and use instead common language and terms that can be understood by all team members, especially families.

Q *What is the role of the OT or PT in acquiring and using assistive technology?*

Historically, a significant part of pediatric occupational and physical therapy practice has been the process of providing children with disabilities with environmental adaptations, devices, and specialized equipment to assist with improving function. Physical and occupational therapists are frequently involved in recommending and procuring equipment such as posture supports (seating systems and upright or prone standers), mobility devices (wheelchairs and walkers), and adapted aids for skills such as dressing, eating, and writing. Many professionals outside of our professions assume that assistive technology refers only to expensive devices that involve electronic parts, such as computers, power-assisted wheelchairs, or switches. OTs and PTs generally view any environmental adaptation or device that increases function, no matter how readily available or seemingly insignificant, as assistive technology. Simple devices like a pencil grip, left-handed scissors, or a piece of tape that keeps a student's paper from sliding off the desk are assistive technology in the same sense that custom seating, voice-activated computer software, alternative computer keyboards, and complex environmental control systems are. During the last two decades, many advances in the general and assistive technology sectors have led to the development of what is now a vast array of types of devices, materials, and designs available to therapists (Carlson & Ramsey, 2000). While we welcome more options and choices when searching for equipment that will best address a child's needs, the explosion of available resources has made it increasingly difficult to keep pace with the latest innovations and applications.

The 1997 and 2004 amendments of IDEA emphasize the expanding role of technology in the educational setting and strengthen the requirement that IEP teams carefully consider children's needs for assistive technology devices and services. In addition, they mandate public schools to "make available" assistive technology devices and service if children with disabilities require them as a part of their special education, part of related services, or a supplementary aid or service in the general education classroom. The identification, procurement, and application of assistive technology by a number of school personnel now assume a greater role in their already busy schedules.

It should be noted that although IDEA mandates that assistive technology be considered and provided in public schools when appropriate, therapists and other IEP team members must show that the technology is "necessary and reasonable" to the specific needs in the context of the setting. As with the term *educational benefit,* the phrase may be interpreted differently by teachers, therapists, parents, and administrators (Hammel & Niehues, 1998).

PTs and OTs, operating within an ecological or functional framework, generally attempt to consider the broad range of activities that children take part in during their daily school routine. In other words, therapists would not limit the application of technology to classroom performance in math and reading. They would assess the need for technology in essential functional skills required in the cafeteria, restroom, playground, school bus, and music room, as well. PTs and OTs work with teachers, speech pathologists, classroom paraprofessionals, and others to address the proper use of seating and positioning equipment that enables improved function. They would also address the environmental barriers across multiple areas of the school that might inhibit a child from participating effectively. The challenge for therapists and other team members is to make the appropriate connection between technology and an individual child's needs. The ultimate goal in providing assistive technology is that the technology serve as an equalizer, allowing the child's access to the same environments that students without disabilities have. The focus should remain on the child's needs and not on the seductive "bells and whistles" pictured in glossy catalogs. Most therapists agree that using technology that is "low tech," minimally intrusive into a child's daily life, and requiring low maintenance or monitoring (but still appropriately serving the child's needs) is preferable to high-tech, high-maintenance technology.

In addition, when evaluating a child for assistive technology, OTs and PTs should not limit their assessment to physical access but should address the social and communication aspects of the school day. For example, an OT and an SLP might collaborate to assess a student for an augmentative communication system, keeping in mind that the system will be used to socialize with friends in the hallway, participate in a group activity in a classroom, or deliver messages to the office. The OT may assist the SLP to ensure that the system can be used safely and efficiently across a number of areas in the school environment. If the OT and SLP combine their knowledge and expertise in this manner, technology can be used to address multiple IEP goals (Hammel & Niehues, 1998). Chapter 8 includes additional perspectives and describes a specific model used to choose AAC devices and adaptations.

Conclusion: School Occupational and Physical Therapists

The purpose of this chapter segment is to inform the speech–language pathologist about the roles, responsibilities, and best practice considerations of their occupational and physical therapist colleagues. The definition and implementation of best practice has evolved for OTs and PTs since the inception of the special education legislation of the 1970s. Current best practice dictates that a collaborative and integrated process be the means to prioritize and select the most educationally meaningful goals for the student. Each member's expertise should be included in the decision-making process, but the focus should be on choosing the most appropriate integrated goals, not on creating goals that represent team members' backgrounds. To do this, we have to work together in a truly collaborative manner.

CHAPTER CONCLUSION

In learning about the roles of the professionals described in this chapter, it should have become clear that speech–language pathologists have much to gain from truly collaborative interaction with these educational allies. The insights that colleagues from other backgrounds bring to the table can only enhance the services that we all provide. Understanding what we each offer a student can also help prevent fragmentation and encourage thinking of the needs of the whole child as goals are developed. If it is possible for you to observe a classroom or special education teacher, a school psychologist, an OT, a PT, or the school librarian as she goes about her day, embrace the opportunity. It will enrich your specialized training as an SLP.

STUDY QUESTIONS

1. What are the similarities among teachers, school psychologists, librarians, and occupational, physical, and speech–language therapists?
2. List four general questions SLPs should ask their school psychologist about his findings concerning a student they have in common.
3. Borrow six tests from your school psychologist and write a brief summary of them, indicating information from each that would prove useful to an SLP.
4. SLPs often describe a student's pragmatics—in what ways does a school psychologist address a child's social communication skills?
5. How are the roles of teachers and SLPs alike? different?
6. How do the roles of the classroom teacher differ from those of a special educator?
7. Ask a grade-level teacher to see a copy of the science (or social studies, math, or language arts) curriculum used in her grade. Discuss how specific

language deficits could keep a student from accessing this information within a typical classroom.

8. What are the similarities and differences in service delivery models of OTs and PTs compared with those of an SLP?

9. What are some of the differences between the roles of OTs, PTs and their respective assistants?

10. In recent years, how have assessment and evaluation changed for OTs and PTs who are in school-based practice, compared to the medical model used previously?

11. Given the new emphasis on literacy in speech–language pathology, cite the advantages of a speech–language pathologist's close working relationship with the school librarian.

12. What has been the impact of the computer on the role of the librarian?

13. Why should SLPs care about a student's reading level? How could this knowledge influence your intervention?

14. Using the curriculum from question 7, discuss with your school librarian books that he could recommend for a student on your caseload with a language-based learning disability, with a specific emphasis on vocabulary.

15. Cite the advantages of a team approach in developing IEP goals.

REFERENCES

Achenbach, T. (2003a). *The Achenbach child behavior rating scales checklist*. Itasca, IL: Riverside.

Achenbach, T. (2003b). *The Achenbach teacher rating form*. Itasca, IL: Riverside.

AcqWeb Directory of Book Reviews. (n.d.). Retrieved September 7, 2005, from the AcqWeb site: http://acqweb.library.vanderbilt.edu/bookrev.html.

American Association of School Librarians. (1998). *Information power: Building partnerships for learning*. Chicago: Author.

American Library Association. (1996). *ALA library bill of rights*. Retrieved September 2, 2005 from the American Library Association Web site: http://www.ala.org/ala/cif/statementsspots/statementsif/librarybillright.htm

American Library Association. (2004). *Booklist editors' choice*. Retrieved September 7, 2005 from the American Library Association Web site: http://www.ala.org/ala/booklist/editorschoice/2004abcd/Youth.htm.

American Occupational Therapy Association. (1986). *Guide for supervision of occupational therapy personnel*. Bethesda, MD: Author.

American Occupational Therapy Association. (1987). *Standards of practice for occupational therapy services in the schools*. Bethesda, MD: Author.

American Occupational Therapy Association. (1998). *Occupational therapy: Making a difference in school system practice*. Bethesda, MD: Author.

American Physical Therapy Association. (1990). *Physical therapy practice in educational environments*. Alexandria, VA: Author.

American Physical Therapy Association. (1992). *Accreditation handbook*. Alexandria, VA: Author.

American Physical Therapy Association. (1997a). *Guide to physical therapy practice*. Alexandria, VA: Author.

American Physical Therapy Association. (1997b). *Utilization of physical therapy assistants in various pediatric settings*. Alexandria, VA: Author.

American Physical Therapy Association. (2000). *Providing physical therapy services under parts B and C of the Individuals with Disabilities Education Act*. Alexandria, VA: Author.

Atwater, S. (1991). Should the normal developmental sequence be used as a theoretical model in pediatric physical therapy? In M. Lister (Ed.), *Contemporary management of motor control problems: Proceedings of the II step conference* (pp. 89–93). Alexandria, VA: Foundations for Physical Therapy.

Ayres, A. (1989). *Sensory Integration and Praxis Tests*. Los Angeles: Western Psychological Services.

Bandura, A. (1997). *Self-efficacy: The exercise of control*. New York: W.H. Freeman.

Batten, H. E. (1993). The industrial school for the crippled and deformed children. *Physical Therapy Review, 13,* 112–113.

Beery, K., Buktenica, N., & Beery, N. (2004). *Beery-Buktenica Test of Visual Motor Integration* (5th ed.). Austin, TX: PRO-ED.

Benard, B. (1989). Working together: Principles of effective collaboration. *Prevention Forum, 10*(1), 4–9.

Board of Education v. Rowley 458 U.S. 176, 203 (1982).

Bookwire. (n.d.). Retrieved September 7, 2005 from Bookwire Web site: http://www.bookwire.com/bookwire/reviews.htm

Brannigan, G., & Decker, S. (2003). *Bender-Gestalt Visual Motor Test* (2nd ed.). Itasca, IL: Riverside.

Bruininks, R. H. (1978). *Bruininks-Oseretsky Test of Motor Proficiency*. Circle Pines, MN: American Guidance Service.

Bundy, A. C., & Carter, R. A. (1991). *Conceptual model of practice for school system therapists*. Occupational and Physical Therapy Departments at the University of Illinois at Chicago, College of Associated Health Professions.

California Department of Education. (1996). *Guidelines for occupational therapy and physical therapy in California public schools*. Sacramento, CA: Author.

Campbell, P. H. (1987). The integrated programming team: An approach for coordinating professionals of various disciplines in programs for students with severe and multiple handicaps. *Journal of the Association for Persons with Severe Handicaps, 12,* 107–118.

Carlson, S. J., & Ramsey, C. (2000). Assistive technology. In S. K. Campbell (Ed.), *Physical therapy for children* (pp. 671–708). Philadelphia: W.B. Saunders.

Children's Literature Web Guide. (n.d.). Retrieved September 7, 2005 from the Children's Literature Web Guide Web site: http://ucalgary.ca/~dkbrown

Classic Short Stories. (n.d.). Retrieved September 7, 2005 from the Classic Short Stories Web site: http://www.bnl.com/shorts.

Conners, C. (1997). *Conners' Behavior Rating Scale* (Rev.). San Antonio, TX: Psychological Corp.

Connolly, A. (1998). *The Key Math Diagnostic Arithmetic Test* (Rev.). Circle Pines, MN: AGS.

Coster, W., Deeney, T., Haltiwanger, J., & Haley, S. (1998). *School Function Assessment*. San Antonio, TX: Psychological Corp.

Dunn, W. (1991). Integrated related services. In L. Meyer, C. Peck, & L. Brown (Eds.), *Critical issues in the lives of people with severe disabilities*. Baltimore: Brookes.

Dunn, W. (1999). *Sensory profile*. San Antonio, TX: Therapy Skill Builders.

Dunn, W., Brown, C., & McGuigan, A. (1994). The ecology of human performance: A framework for considering the impact of context. *American Journal of Occupational Therapy, 48,* 595–607.

Dunn, W., & Campbell, P. H. (1991). Designing pediatric service provision. In W. Dunn (Ed.), *Pediatric occupational therapy* (pp. 139–159). Thorofare, NJ: Slack.

Dunn, L., & Dunn, L. (1997). *Peabody Picture Vocabulary Test* (3rd ed.). Circle Pines, MN: AGS.

Education of All Handicapped Children Act. (1975). Public Law 94-142.

Effgen, S. K. (1994a). The educational setting. In S. K. Campbell (Ed.), *Physical therapy for children* (pp. 847–872). Philadelphia: W.B. Saunders.

Effgen, S. K. (1994b). Survey of physical therapy practice in educational settings. *Pediatric Physical Therapy, 6,* 15–21.

Effgen, S. K. (2000). The educational environment. In S. K. Campbell (Ed.), *Physical therapy for children* (pp. 910–933). Philadelphia: W.B. Saunders.

Ehren, B. (2000). Maintaining a therapeutic focus and sharing responsibility for student success: Keys to in-classroom speech–language services. *Language, Speech and Hearing Services in Schools, 31*(3), 219–229.

Folio, M., & Fewell, R. (2000). *Peabody Developmental Motor Scales* (2nd ed.). Austin, TX: PRO-ED.

Giangreco, M. F. (1986). Effects of integrated therapy: A pilot study. *Journal of Association of Persons with Severe Handicaps, 11,* 205–208.

Giangreco, M. F., York, J., & Rainforth, B. (1989). Providing related services to learners with severe handicaps in educational settings: Pursuing the least restrictive option. *Pediatric Physical Therapy, 1,* 55–63.

Gunning, T. T. (2003). The role of readability in today's classrooms. *Topics in Language Disorders, 23,* 175–189.

Haley, S. M., Coster, W. J., Ludlow, L. H., Haltiwanger, J. T., & Andrellos, P. (1992). *Pediatric evaluation of disability inventory.* Boston: New England Medical Center Hospital.

Hammel, J., & Niehues, A. (1998). Integrating general and assistive technology into school based practice: Process and information resources. In J. Case-Smith (Ed.), *Occupational therapy: Making a difference in school system practice* (pp. 1–54). Bethesda, MD: American Occupational Therapy Association.

Hammill, D., & Larsen, S. (1996). *Test of Written Language* (3rd ed.). Austin, TX: PRO-ED.

Hanft, B. E., & Place, P. A. (1996). *The consulting therapist.* San Antonio, TX: Therapy Skill Builders.

Harris, S. (1981). Effects of neurodevelopmental treatment on improving motor performance in Down syndrome. *Developmental Medicine and Child Neurology, 23,* 477.

Herausgegeben, W., Morgenthaler, V., Bash, K., & Nachduck, J. (1999). *The Rorschach Test.* Berne, Switzerland: Hogrefe and Huber Publishers.

Individuals with Disabilities Education Act. (1990). Public Law 101-476.

Individuals with Disabilities Education Act Amendments of 1991. (1991). Public Law 102-19.

Individuals with Disabilities Education Act Amendments of 1997. (1997). Public Law 105-17.

Individuals with Disabilities Education Improvement Act. (2004). Public Law 108-446.

Internet Public Library Online Texts Collection. (n.d.). Retrieved September 7, 2005 from Internet Public Library Web site: http://www.ipl.org/div/books/

Iowa Department of Education. (1996). *Iowa guidelines for educationally related physical services.* Des Moines, IA: Author.

Kaufman, A. (1994). *Intelligent testing with the WISC–III.* New York: Wiley.

Kaufman, A., & Kaufman, N. (1997). *Kaufman Test of Educational Achievement.* Circle Pines, MN: AGS.

Kaufman, A., & Kaufman, N. (2004). *Kaufman Test of Educational Achievement* (2nd ed.). Circle Pines, MN: AGS.

Kaufman, A., & Kaufman, N. (2004). *Kaufman Assessment Battery for Children* (2nd ed.). Circle Pines, MN: AGS.

Kelly, L. E., et al. (1991). *Achievement-based curriculum: Teaching manual*. Charlottesville: University of Virginia.

Kirshner, B., & Guyatt, G. H. (1985). A methodologic framework for assessing health indices. *Journal of Chronic Disease, 38,* 27–36.

Koppitz, E. (1977). *Visual-Aural Digit Span Test*. San Antonio, TX: Psychological Corp.

Library of Congress. (n.d.). Retrieved September 7, 2005 from the Library of Congress Web site: http://catalog.loc/gov

Library Index. (n.d.). Retrieved on September 7, 2005 from the Library Index (Libdex) Web site: http://www.libdex.com

Libweb Directory of Libraries. (n.d.). Retrieved September 7, 2005 from the Library on the Web site: http://lists.webjunction.org/libweb

Lindsey, D., O'Neal, J., Haas, J., & Tervey, S. M. (1980). Physical therapy services in North Carolina schools. *Clinical Management in Physical Therapy, 4,* 40–43.

Literature Project. (n.d.). Retrieved September 7, 2005 from The Literature Project's Web site: http://www.literatureproject.com

Lowenfeld, M. (2004). *Lowenfeld Mosaic Test*. Sussex, England: Sussex Academic Press.

McEwen, I. (Ed.). (2000). *Providing physical therapy services under parts B and C of the Individuals with Disabilities Education Act*. Alexandria, VA: American Physical Therapy Association.

McEwen, I. R., & Sheldon, M. L. (1995). Pediatric therapy in the 1990s: The demise of the educational versus medical dichotomy. *Occupational and Physical Therapy in Pediatrics. 15*(2), 33–45.

Mulcahey, A. L. (1936). Detroit schools for crippled children. *Physical Therapy, 16,* 63–64.

New York Public Library. (n.d.). Retrieved September 7, 2005 from the New York Public Library Web site: http://www.nypl.org

Orelove, F. P., & Sobsey, D. (1987). *Educating children with multiple disabilities*. Baltimore: Brookes.

Orelove, F. P., & Sobsey, D. (1996). Designing transdisciplinary services. In F. P. Orelove & D. Sobsey (Eds.), *Educating students with multiple disabilities: A transdisciplinary approach* (3rd ed., pp. 1–33). Baltimore: Brookes.

Rainforth, B., & York, J. (1987). Integrating related services in community instruction. *Journal of the Association of the Severely Handicapped, 12,* 190–198.

Rainforth, B., York, J., & McDonald, C. (1992). *Collaborative teams for students with severe disabilities*. Baltimore: Brookes.

Rainforth, B., & York-Barr, J. (1997). *Collaborative teams for students with severe disabilities* (2nd ed.). Baltimore: Brookes.

Rehabilitation Act of 1973. (1973). Pub. L. No. 93-112 Sec. 504, 87 Stat. 355.

Reynolds, C., & Hickman, J. (2004). *Draw-A-Person Intellectual Ability Test for Children, Adolescents and Adults*. Austin, TX: PRO-ED.

Reynolds, C., & Kamphaus, R. (2004). *Behavior Assessment System for Children* (2nd ed.). Circle Pines, MN: AGS.

Roid, G. (2003). *Stanford-Binet Intelligence Scale* (5th ed.). Itasca, IL: Riverside.

Rotter, J., Lau, M., & Rafferty, J. (1992). *Incomplete Sentence Blank Test*. San Antonio, TX: Psychological Corp.

Rowley v. Board of Education of Hendrick Hudson Central School District, 458 U.S. 176 (1982).

Royeen, C. B. (1992). Educationally related assessment and evaluation. In C. B. Royeen (Ed.), *Classroom applications for school-based practice: Lesson 1*. Rockville, MD: American Occupational Therapy Association.

Royeen, C. (1994). *School-based therapy … What's next?* Paper presented at Professional Education Programs, Kansas City, MO.

St. Joseph County Public Library. (n.d.). Retrieved September 7, 2005 from the St. Joseph's County Public Library Web site: sjcpl.lib.in.us/homepage/PublicLibraries/PublicLibrary Servers.html

Severs, J. W. (1938). Physical therapy in schools for crippled children. *Physical Therapy Review, 18,* 298–303.

Sternat, J., Messina, R., Nietupske, J., Lyon, S., & Brown, L. (1997). Occupational therapy and physical therapy services for severely handicapped students: Toward a naturalized public school delivery model. In E. Sontag (Ed.), *Educational programming for the severely and profoundly handicapped.* Reston, VA: Council for Exceptional Children.

Thomas, A., & Grimes, J. (1990). *Best practices in school psychology–II.* Washington, DC: National Association of School Psychologists.

Watts, N. T. (1971). Task analysis and division of responsibility in physical therapy. *Physical Therapy, 51,* 22–25.

Wechsler, D. (1997). *Wechsler Adult Intelligence Scale* (3rd ed.). San Antonio, TX: Psychological Corp.

Wechsler, D. (2002). *Wechsler Pre-School and Primary Scale of Intelligence* (Rev.). San Antonio, TX: Psychological Corp.

Wechsler, D. (2004). *Wechsler Intelligence Scale for Children* (4th ed., Integrated). San Antonio, TX: Psychological Corp.

Woodcock, R. (1998). *Woodcock Reading Mastery Test* (Rev.). Itasca, IL: Riverside.

Woodcock, R., McGrew, K., & Mather, N. (2001a). *Woodcock-Johnson Psychoeducational Battery* (3rd ed.). Itasca, IL: Riverside.

Woodcock, R., McGrew, K., & Mather, N. (2001b). *Woodcock-Johnson Test of Achievement* (3rd ed.). Itasca, IL: Riverside.

Zimmerman, I., Steiner, J., & Pond, R. (2001). *Wechsler Individual Achievement* (2nd ed.). San Antonio, TX: Psychological Corp.

Appendix 12.A

Psychological Assessment Report

GENERAL INFORMATION

Name:	Zachary Johnson	**Birth date:**	8/28/97
Age:	6-6	**School:**	Smallville School
Address:	24 Winget Road	**Grade:**	First
	Anywhere, Illinois	**Teacher:**	Mrs. Cato
Parents:	Susan & Samuel	**CSE status:**	Initial referral
	Johnson		
Testing dates:	2/14–2/21/04	**Examiner:**	Edward Grimly, MS, CAS

EVALUATION INSTRUMENTS AND PROCEDURES

Wechsler Intelligence Scale for Children–Third Edition (WISC–III)
Woodcock-Johnson Psycho-Educational Battery–Revised, Cognitive Battery
  (WJ–R/C)
Bender Gestalt Test
Peabody Picture Vocabulary Test–3rd Edition (PPVT–III)
Kaufman Test of Educational Achievement (K-TEA)
Key Math–Revised (KM–R)
Draw-A-Person (DAP)
Review of records
Classroom observation
Parent, child, teacher interviews

BACKGROUND AND OBSERVATIONS

Zachary was referred for an evaluation by his father due to concern about his reading achievement and readiness for second grade.

Zachary is a youngster of slightly below average weight and height who resides with his mother and older brother, age 11; he visits with his father regularly. Mrs. Johnson recalls a normal pregnancy, but Zachary's birth was complicated by anoxia. Developmental milestones are reported as attained within normal limits. Zachary's medical history is remarkable for recurrent ear infections until the age of 2½ and minor surgery in 3/2000 for removal of adenoids. Described as a warm and caring child with a good-natured disposition, Zachary enjoys a variety of activities such as video games, computer programs, sports, looking at books, and watching television. He occupies his time independently, yet plays well with others. His mother notes, however, that Zachary has problems expressing himself when he is frustrated and has difficulty following directions. She describes him as sometimes fearful, quite dependent, easily overwhelmed, and at times reluctant to leave the house. Home tutoring by his parents has been ongoing, and Mr. Johnson has noted that his son has had considerable difficulty learning basic phonic word attack skills.

During May 2002, Zachary took part in the school's kindergarten screening. He was described by the examiner as very quiet and cooperative during testing. At mid-year, his kindergarten teacher noted he had difficulty identifying letters and counting beyond 20. At the end of the year, he continued to exhibit below-average academic readiness, with specific weaknesses in printing his last name, reading simple sight words, naming letters, and printing numbers 11–20. His teacher also characterized him as a very caring and considerate child with good listening skills and work habits. His present teacher reports continuing basic skill weakness. She also states that he lacks confidence and often copies from others in completing his work. He is attentive during instruction but does not retain information. In recent weeks, she notes some improvement in most areas. School vision and hearing screenings have been within normal limits.

Psychological assessment took place from 2/14–2/21/04. Zachary arrived at all testing sessions appropriately dressed and groomed. He was quite timid, and his responses to general queries during conversation with the examiner were minimal. He responded, "I don't know" to many questions. He also complained about forgetting "what I want to say when someone says something." His responsiveness and understanding of a task were improved when he worked on visually oriented test items. Conversely, his responses to verbally oriented questions were minimal, and he appeared overwhelmed and frightened at times. His approach to construction designs and puzzles was slow yet very precise. His rather fearful, minimally responsive style of interaction with the examiner was far less in evidence during interactions with peers during the classroom observation. At these times, he initiated and participated spontaneously in conversations and open play activities.

Test Results

WISC–III (Age norms, 7–13 approximates the average range)

Verbal	Scaled Score	Performance	Scaled Score
Information	11	Picture Completion	14
Similarities	11	Coding	4
Arithmetic	9	Picture Arrangement	11
Vocabulary	10	Block Design	13
Comprehension	7	Object Assembly	18
(Digit Span)	(5)	(Symbol Search)	(11)
		(Mazes)	(14)

Verbal IQ	98	45%ile
Performance IQ	127	96%ile
Full Scale IQ	112	79%ile
Verbal Comprehension Index	99	47%ile
Perceptual Organization Index	124	95%ile

Freedom from Distractibility Index	84	14%ile
Processing Speed Index	114	82%ile

This test compares Zachary's performance to that of his age mates on various verbal and nonverbal intellectual tasks. While these results do not represent the full range of his intelligence, they provide information about his intellectual ability with respect to learning potential in school and life experiences. His high-average overall performance, composed of average verbal and superior nonverbal performances, is not considered an accurate measure of his true intelligence because of the considerable verbal–nonverbal difference. It is evident, however, that his greatest intellectual proficiencies lie in the visual–perceptual organization area. This agrees with test behavior observations of increased confidence and spontaneity in his approach to visually oriented areas.

In the verbal area, Zachary demonstrated average skill in understanding and answering orally presented questions about general facts, word definitions, math word problems, and common themes. This suggests adequately developed skills related to long-term memory, fund of knowledge, numerical and abstract verbal reasoning, and word knowledge. His answers to questions about common scenarios were low average. This task requires solutions to situational dilemmas; his performance suggests considerable weakness in the areas of social knowledge and practical judgment. When asked to immediately recall number serials, he demonstrated a most significant weakness in the area of short-term auditory sequential memory. This supports parent reports of his difficulty remembering directions, his teachers' reports of difficulty learning sound–symbol relationships, and his own description of easily forgetting what he intends to say.

In the nonverbal area, Zachary demonstrated a number of strengths that represent the best estimate of his true intelligence. His skill in finding missing picture parts, transcribing symbols, constructing designs and puzzles, and negotiating mazes ranged from high average to significantly above average. This suggests significant strengths in visual areas of attention, spatial reasoning, part–whole reasoning, motor planning, and psychomotor speed. His highly proficient performance in these areas indicates high aptitude in organizing and manipulating visual configurations and materials. The least advanced of his nonverbal performances was his average arrangement of pictures into logical sequences and timely matching of nonmeaningful symbols. These tasks involve social knowledge and planning, and visual processing speed, respectively. The former of these skills, when considered with the low-average practical reasoning observed in his verbal performance, further suggests limited social awareness. The latter of these skills suggests possible weakness in the speed with which he processes rote visual material.

WJ–R/C (Age norms, 25–80 percentile approximates the average range)

	SS	%ile		SS	%ile
Memory for names	110	75	Visual closure	109	73
Memory for sentences	47	0.1	Picture vocabulary	103	57
Visual matching	117	88	Analysis–synthesis	128	97
Incomplete words	82	12			

This test compares Zachary's skill development in various areas of visual and auditory processing to that of his age mates and sometimes provides diagnostic information about learning style and preferences. His performance indicates a marked difference between auditory and visual processing similar to that seen in the significant difference between his verbal and nonverbal WISC–III performances. When he was asked to recall named characters, quickly match numbers, identify partially obscured pictures by name, and solve visual puzzles, his performances were average to well above average. When he was asked to repeat sentences and recognize partially pronounced words, his performances were significantly below average. These results further highlight a considerable strength in visual learning in contrast to marked processing difficulty in the auditory verbal domain.

BENDER

Zachary achieved a developmental score of 6 on this measure of visual motor integration. This places his performance in the 7-0 to 7-5 age range, which corresponds to a percentile rank of 60; this is considered average for his age. His responses to inquiry were minimal, in keeping with previously described timidity. His performance suggests average skill in paper–pencil tasks and organization.

PPVT–III	SS	%ile	Age Equivalent
	111	77	8-02

This instrument compares Zachary's general knowledge and receptive language development to that of his age mates. His performance places his development in these areas in the high-average range and indicates very good acquisition and retention of general concepts gained through school and life experiences.

K-TEA (Grade norms, 25–80 percentile approximates the average range)

	Scaled Score	%ile Rank
Math applications	88	21
Reading decoding	81	10
Spelling	84	14
Reading comprehension	88	21
Math computation	75	05
Reading composite	83	13
Math composite	81	10
Battery composite	81	10

This test compares Zachary's academic achievement to that of his grade mates. His overall performance suggests a discrepancy from his potential as predicted by his intelligence test performance. His greatest relative skills were demonstrated when he was asked to apply math concepts to solve word problems and answer questions about self-read simple sentences with picture cues. When required to encode, decode, and work efficiently with letters or number sound symbols, he demonstrated his greatest weakness. Review of classroom curriculum suggests that the math computational weakness may be attributed to his lack of exposure, as his present program is highly focused on math concept development rather than math operations.

KM–R (25–80 percentile approximates the average range)

	Scaled Score	%ile Rank
Basic concepts		
Numeration	11	63
Geometry	13	84
Operations		
Addition	08	25
Subtraction	09	37
Application		
Measurement	15	95
Time & money	12	75
Estimation	09	37
Basic concepts area	105	63
Operations area	91	27
Applications area	108	70
Total test	**104**	**61**

This test provides a diagnostic inventory of Zachary's essential math skills as compared to those of his age mates. Despite slight computational weakness, which again is likely the result of lack of exposure, he demonstrated average skill in numerical reasoning, basic figural perception, and math applications.

DAP

These are projective activities that sometimes provide information about emotional experience, adjustment, and personality development. Considerable timidity, as observed in his general interactions with the examiner, was evident in the diminutive and restricted quality of his figure drawings. This is also apparent in the paucity of his responses to inquiry, which consisted of "I don't know" answers to most questions. Suggestions of limited independence and self-reliance are also noted.

It should be noted that several of the above describe instruments that were current at the time of this writing, have been updated. For example, the *Wechsler,* the *Stanford-Binet Intelligence Test,* and the *Woodcock-Johnson Psycho-Educational Battery* have recently been renormed and altered.[1] The fundamental nature of these instruments, however, remains the same. Wholly new tests are also to have been introduced since the time of this review. Publishers' Web pages should be consulted frequently to stay updated about new and revised test instruments.

SUMMARY

Zachary is a very enjoyable but shy youngster of superior intelligence, which is primarily evident in his performance of visual perceptual and motor integration tasks. His particular strength in visual part–whole reasoning suggests extremely well-developed visual understanding of construction and figural composition. His verbal intelligence, while generally average, appears to be relatively less well developed. While this result may in part be due to extreme timidity in direction question–answer testing formats, it is also likely to be related to auditory processing weakness. This was quite evident in Zachary's very limited ability to recall orally presented number series, repeat simple sentences, and make auditory closure in partially presented words. In the presence of superior general intelligence, this processing weakness is likely to be a primary learning inhibitor in his ongoing struggles in reading. Although his progress in math concepts appears adequate at this time, auditory processing weakness affecting efficient sound–symbol learning may also extend into this area. A relative weakness in his overall social awareness and practical judgment was noted in his test results. This may relate to his extreme timidity, especially in new and unfamiliar situations.

RECOMMENDATIONS

I. Zachary should be considered for special educational instruction in the area of reading. Suggested clinical teaching strategies are as follows:
   A. Instruction should favor visual and manipulative cues and formats whenever possible.

---

[1]The latest editions of these tests are listed in the references.

    B. Specific instruction in evaluating and responding to real-life situations could include activities such as
      1. playing Simon Says or other games requiring specific body movements;
      2. inventing missing parts and details to stories; completing unfinished stories;
      3. direct instruction of logical and illogical concepts;
      4. role-playing problem-solving situations and social situations;
      5. solving simple riddles; and
      6. searching for absurdities or words that do not belong.
    C. Specific instruction and activities to improve ability to retain, recall, and repeat auditorily presented information in correct sequence and detail could include
      1. repeating simple letter & number sequences of increasing difficulty;
      2. coloring or drawing activities with step-by-step directions;
      3. repeating increasingly difficult series of nonsense syllables;
      4. repeating sequences of 2 or more unrelated words;
      5. repeating a sequence of named objects and arranging pictures of the objects in same order;
      6. repeating words, letters, sounds, and number series in correct sequence after time intervals of 30 to 60 seconds; and
      7. repeating short poems and rhymes from memory.

II. While home instruction is an important support, care should be taken that Zachary also has ample noninstructional time away from school requirements. He needs plentiful opportunities to explore and discover himself through his choices for free-time activity. His participation in team sporting groups, scouts, day camp, and sleepovers should be facilitated. Home supportive instruction should be limited to reinforcement of previously learned material. Time allotted for such instruction should not be excessive.

III. Suggested classroom and instructional modifications are as follows:
    A. Provide Zachary with preteaching before requiring him to respond independently during class discussions and lessons.
    B. Provide him the opportunity to use his visual perceptual strengths to help students of lesser skill.

IV. Zachary should be referred for a speech–language screening to determine whether auditory processing difficulties have in any way affected his expressive ability.

(signed)

Edward M. Grimly, MS, CAS
School Psychologist, Smallville School

Chapter 13

◆ ◆

Epilogue

Eileen H. Gravani
and Jacqueline Meyer

he purpose of this edition mirrors editor Pamela O'Connell's final comments in the initial edition:

> The overall aim of this book has been to help prepare the novice school practitioner or the practitioner-in-training to function in today's schools. Effective performance in this setting depends on many things.... Each contributor has presented a part or parts of the complex and interlocking structure that houses school programs in speech, language, and hearing within the edifice of contemporary education.... Yet what is current is also subject to change ... (1997, p. 372)

It is with this acknowledgment of change that we close this second edition of the text. Each modification and expansion noted in this edition has moved school-based speech–language pathologists and audiologists in many directions. Some changes lead to paths that appear clear; others, however, seem quite capable of branching toward unforeseen destinations.

In fall 2004, a single issue of the *ASHA Leader* featured nine articles describing factors that, among others, will shape the future of speech–language pathology in the schools: salary supplements for school-based clinicians, the No Child Left Behind Law (NCLB), evidence-based practice, AAC, English-language learners, the 2004 revision and reauthorization of IDEA, the National Center for Speech Language Pathology in Schools, the role of SLPs in dealing with school bullies, and the "no-win" system of due process. With some additions, we have divided the subjects of the nine articles into three categories that are likely to bring about alterations in the role of SLPs in the schools: (a) new legislation or governmental actions, (b) technological developments, and (c) accelerated expansion into areas of current involvement.

The current and future reauthorizations of IDEA remain key, because the legislation will indicate what school districts and school-based SLPs must do to be in compliance with the law. The question that remains is what new roles will be required of us, and, as a corollary, what tasks and ways of completing them must be discarded. Within IDEA, the concept of highest-qualified provider is crucial to our profession (Snyder, 2004). This is also related to the controversy surrounding the role of individual states in defining who we are, in terms of both educational certification and professional licensure and the relationship of either to ASHA's Certificate of Clinical Competence. Definitions count in practical as well as philosophical terms because they will help determine the standard for third-party payment.

Presently, some states are providing salary supplements to all clinicians who hold ASHA CCCs because they recognize that those professionals represent assets to the school system (Boswell & Crowe, 2004). However, as stated in the U.S. Department of Education's *Executive Summary—Twenty-Fourth Annual Report to Congress on the Implementation of the Individuals with Disabilities Act,* "Having an adequate supply of school-based speech–language pathologists is as important as the quality of those available because shortages typically force administrators to hire less qualified individuals" (n.d., p. 3). If speech–pathology assistants, whose salaries cost districts less, are sanctioned by the law to provide a wide variety of services, schools may be more inclined to hire them, potentially affecting Medicaid reimbursement, as well as quality of service for our most challenged students. Considering the shortage of SLPs in many districts, the issue of highest-qualified provider can have far-reaching results.

It seems clear that changes in the No Child Left Behind segments of the Elementary and Secondary Education Act will also continue to affect speech–language pathologists in a number of ways. SLPs are struggling to develop new means to assess and provide intervention for children with speech and language deficits who must take state-mandated tests. In addition, referring to adolescent students, Conley and Hinchman state, "Many secondary teachers remain ill-equipped with strategies that could help them build bridges between adolescent, classroom and community" (2004, p. 47). Because of our training and experience in developing programs based on an individual's strengths and challenges, SLPs can also help teachers learn new ways to assist students who are failing the new high-stakes tests but do not qualify for an IEP. We can share our knowledge of different types of strategies with others who can apply them to any subject, adjust them for various grade levels, and tailor them to serve the needs of individual students. Although many teachers are aware of strategies, they may need help in adjusting their teaching of them to students who have limited language skills. During push-in intervention or an in-service presentation, we can model scaffolding techniques that are equally useful to other professionals. Ehren (2002) states the situation clearly: "High school faculty and administrators must be encouraged to act on the notion that problems encountered by low achievers are frequently language related. All students will not meet the high expectations of standards-based education without attention to the language underpinnings of the curriculum" (p. 70). Consulting on this level, however, means time away from students on caseloads and consequently will require consistent and long-term administrative support.

As school districts attempt to meet the requirements of IDEA and NCLB, they may feel pressured by the "rise in the current legal and regulatory climate ... [and the fact that] the days are gone when we could work things out without lawyers" (Boswell, 2004, p. 18). This has added new urgency to SLPs following correct procedures, developing goals on IEPs that can reasonably be met, and meticulously documenting results, even though P.L. 108-446 eliminates most benchmarks and short-term objectives from IEP requirements (IDEA, 2004). Compliance monitoring under IDEA (2004) specifically requires professionals to focus on student performance, not compliance with procedures, and the new revision and reauthorization also emphasizes the point that assessment measures must be technically sound (Council for Exceptional Children, 2004). Boswell quotes a statement from a director of special education that applies to us, as well: "Be very objective in what you write in all of your documentation. All of it can be admitted into evidence—right down to a casual remark on a sticky note" (Boswell, 2004, p. 18).

A closely related subject is the new emphasis on evidence-based practice, or as Justice and Fey (2004) put it, "emphasiz[ing] the systematic and deliberate integration of science and craft or alternatively, data and theory … in which consideration of the preponderance of evidence from scientific investigations is systematically integrated with clinical expertise and contextual factors" (p. 4). To accomplish this, SLPs must depend on a continuing stream of well-designed, relevant research by professionals in our field, "presented in forms that are readily accessible to and assimilable by busy practitioners with little time to separate the wheat from the chaff … [but] currently school-based SLPs who turn to the accumulated evidence on a particular treatment have no guidance on determining the adequacy of the evidence in quality and quantity" (2004, pp. 30, 31). The need is urgent, but it puts increasing pressure on the already limited number of faculty members in departments of speech pathology. Collaborative research between school-based SLPs and their university counterparts may be a partial solution.

One attempt to distribute information on current issues was the formation of the National Center for Speech Language Pathology in Schools, the result of collaboration between the University of Cincinnati and Miami University of Ohio. The Center is an example of one response to the 1997 reauthorization of IDEA mandate to establish an "educational planning process to promote meaningful access to training for school-based clinicians in subjects such as authentic assessment, curriculum-based intervention and collaborative IEP training" (Creaghead et al., 2004, p. 11). Although not directly related to legislation, the Center represents an acknowledgment that continuing education in our profession has moved from a recommendation to a requirement. Consequently, easy access to current, accurate, unbiased information for school-based speech–language pathologists will likely be explored in many new and exciting ways.

One of the ways the roles of school-based SLPs will most certainly continue to expand is in providing services to children who represent increasingly diverse backgrounds. Roseberry-McKibbin, O'Hanlon, and Brice (2004) report that since the 1990–1991 school year, the English-language learner (ELL) population in the schools has grown 105% while the general school population has grown only 12%. The authors posit that one of the implications of this growth will be the increasing "importance of improved service delivery to ELL students with communication disorders [and] … the need for more valid, reliable methods and materials for less biased assessment of ELL students" (p. 8). The authors conclude, "Our profession needs to continue to recruit and retain bilingual SLPs to provide services to our increasingly diverse public school population … educate SLPs regarding appropriate intervention … [and help them] understand the effects of bilingualism and second-language acquisition on … those ELL students referred for services" (p. 35).

Another rapidly expanding area of responsibility will be in the provision of services to children with language-based deficits as they struggle to gain acceptable skills in reading, writing, and spelling. The issues addressed in Chapter 7 represent only the beginning. A recent advertisement for software that determines which language-knowledge deficits underlie spelling errors is an indication of how quickly our profession is moving into literacy assessment practices that take advantage of our background in language development and disorders (Masterson, Apel, & Wasowicz, 2004). Massey and Heafner's (2004) article on reading comprehension in social studies, authored by a reading educator and a social studies teacher, describes strategies that speech–language pathologists could use as they develop and implement relevant IEP goals to address the underlying language deficits interfering with a student's reading comprehension. This source also represents the need for SLPs to gain information from sources other than those directly related to speech pathology, another daunting task.

McKinley's (2004) suggestions on how SLPs can respond to the problem of bullying is based on her assertion that "children with mental and physical disabilities are two to three times more likely to be targets of bullies … includ[ing] those with language and learning disabilities, fluency disorders, intelligibility problems, cognitive disabilities and autism spectrum disorders" (p. 16). The problem described in her article is one that is not contained within the traditional areas of phonology, syntax, morphology, and semantics. McKinley asserts that as part of the school community, SLPs must be part of the solution to the bullying problem, an indication of how many hats we will be expected to (and should) wear when we work in this particular setting.

Ehren's (2002) work with high school students makes the case that more SLPs can and should address the needs of students in Grades 9–12 who are presently underidentified and consequently underserved. A report by the National Assessment of Educational Progress (NAEP) reported by Ehren (2002) indicates that 23% of 12th graders had scores below a basic level in reading, and 60% of them were below a proficiency level. Similarly sobering percentages for writing, 22% and 78%, respectively, were reported. Ehren states that the "problem of adolescent literacy warrants serious and continuing attention" (p. 65). She argues that SLPs should consider identifying high school students with language-based learning disabilities as a justification for both direct and indirect services. With national concerns about workload and a shortage of SLPs in some areas, it remains to be seen how this need can be met in the future.

Finally, to technology. In the field of audiology, it seems likely that we will provide more speech and language services to students who have received cochlear implants (Chute & Nevins, 2003). The exponential overall growth of high-tech industries argues for improvements in hearing aids and other assistive devices. How these will affect classroom participation and overall learning of those students wearing and using them is another area we cannot plan for in detail. Similarly, improved AAC devices will necessitate adaptations of therapy. It is interesting to note, however, that experts in this area argue that we not become so enamored with new gadgets, no matter how glamorous, that we neglect simpler strategies: "For some potential users, the most ideal AAC systems are often low-tech solutions with a minimal price tag. The key … is identifying appropriate [ones] and pairing them with motivating classroom activities that are rich with communication prospects" (Downey, Daugherty, Helt, & Daugherty, 2004, p. 6).

A similar comparison can be made to the increasing role of technology in our everyday interaction with students during assessment and intervention. The explosion of Internet sites and computer software is almost overwhelming. The list of Web sites in the Appendix to the text contains only the tiniest fraction of what is available. Identifying the most efficacious resources and determining how, when, and whether to use them for a particular student will remain a real challenge. A further use of technology will be to gather new information in our field, as implied in the previous paragraphs. Conferences will continue to exist, but outlines of conference presentations, chat rooms, online courses, self-instruction modules, and other new uses of technology will surely change and expand. We will all have to adjust to new ways of thinking and to different, sometimes frustrating, rules. Judith Kuster (2004) writes a valuable column addressing Internet issues in the *ASHA Leader;* over the years, her columns and materials have come to represent a ready source of information for many SLPs. However, when the name of her home base—her university—changed, anyone attempting to link to her materials was met with the message "That server is not available." The balance of her column dealt with how to finesse a paperless paper trail, valuable information indeed.

In the "Introduction" to this text, we indicated that the field of school-based speech–language pathology is exciting, rewarding, and never dull, partly because our profession is now and always has been marked by change. Let us close with a quote from the first edition, from Marcel Proust:

> We don't receive wisdom; we must discover it for ourselves after a journey no one else can take for us or spare us.

We wish you well on your journey. We hope we have provided a few signposts along your way.

REFERENCES

Boswell, S. (2004, September 21). Due process: No-win system. *ASHA Leader, 9*(17), 18, 20.

Boswell, S., & Crowe, E. (2004, September 21). Delaware adds salary supplement for school-based clinicians. *ASHA Leader, 9*(17), 1, 37, 38.

Chute, P. M., & Nevins, M. E. (2003). Educational challenges for children with cochlear implants. *Topics in Language Disorders, 23*, 57–67.

Conley, M. W., & Hinchman, K. A. (2004). No Child Left Behind: What it means for U.S. adolescents and what we can do about it. *Journal of Adolescent and Adult Literacy, 48*(1), 42–50.

Council for Exceptional Children. (2004). *The new IDEA-CEC's summary of significant issues.* Retrieved January 30, 2004 from Council for Exceptional Children Web site: http://www.cec.sped.org/

Creaghead, N. A., Glaser, A., Prendeville, J., Secord, W. A., Wellman, L. L., & Williams, S. (2004, September 21). The national center for speech–language pathology in the schools. *ASHA Leader, 9*(17), 11, 12, 53.

Downey, D., Daugherty, P., Helt, S., & Daugherty, D. (2004, September 21). Integrating AAC into the classroom: Low-tech strategies. *ASHA Leader, 9*(17), 6, 7, 36.

Ehren, B. J. (2002). Speech–language pathologists contributing significantly to the academic success of high school students: A vision for professional growth. *Topics in Language Disorders, 22*(2), 60–80.

Individuals with Disabilities Education Improvement Act. (2004). Public Law 108-446.

Justice, L. M., & Fey, M. E. (2004, September 21). Evidence-based practice in schools: Integrating craft and theory with science and data. *ASHA Leader, 9*(17), 4, 5, 30–32.

Kuster, J. (2004, November 2). Dealing with change. *ASHA Leader, 9*(20), 18.

Massey, D. D., & Heafner, T. L. (2004). Promoting reading comprehension in social studies. *Journal of Adolescent and Adult Literacy, 48*(1), 26–40.

Masterson, J. J., Apel, K., & Wasowicz, J. (2004). Spelling Performance Evaluation for Language & Literacy [Computer software]. Evanston, IL: Learning by Design.

McKinley, N. (2004, September 21). Braving the bullies: What speech–language pathologists can do. *ASHA Leader, 9*(17), 16–17.

O'Connell, P. (Ed.). (1997). *Speech, language, and hearing programs in schools: A guide for students and practitioners.* Gaithersburg, MD: Aspen.

Roseberry-McKibbin, C., O'Hanlon, L., & Brice, A. (2004, September 21). Service delivery to English language learners in the public schools: A national survey. *ASHA Leader, 9*(17), 8, 34, 35.

Snyder, N. (2004, September 21). As schools open, Congress eyes IDEA reauthorization. *ASHA Leader, 9*(17), 2, 21.

U.S. Department of Education. (n.d.). *Executive summary—Twenty-fourth annual report to Congress on the implementation of the Individuals with Disabilities Act.* Retrieved July 30, 2005, from http://www.ed.gov/about/reports/annual/osep/2002/execsumm.html

◆ ◆

A Sampling of Web Sites for the School-Based Speech– Language Pathologist

Web sites are constantly changing. We have made an effort to choose sites that present practical, useful information and are likely to be in existence for the lifetime of this edition of the text. Inevitably, however, some will disappear and be replaced by exciting new ones. You are encouraged to share news of helpful sites with your colleagues as you discover them. All of the sites listed here were retrieved on August 28, 2005.

Search engines enable the school-based SLP to find Web sites that deal with every conceivable subject; use your favorite or one of these:

www.google.com	uses text-matching techniques to find pages to aid the search.
www.yahoo.com	provides a category-based Web directory.

An excellent continuing Web resource specific to speech pathology is Judith Kuster's column *Internet,* which regularly appears in the *ASHA Leader.* A list of her past columns with links to the full text of those that are still available can be found at either www.asha.org/about/publications/leader-online/archives/news.htm or www.mnsu.edu/comdis/kuster4/leader.html. For Kuster's Net Connections for Communication Disorders and Sciences, an Internet guide of links and original material on a variety of topics related to speech–language pathology, she suggests www.communicationdisorders.com. Her guide to therapy materials on the Internet can be found at www.mnsu.edu/dept/comdis/kuster2/sptherapy.html.

The following sampling of suggestions comes from one of Kuster's columns (January 20, 2003) featuring templates and generators available on the Internet. Templates allow users to adapt or customize an activity, e.g., flashcards; a generator can produce material online that can be printed out later. Kuster comments that both are "useful in developing individualized treatment materials" (p. 15). The entire column from which this information was selected is available at the Web site listed previously for past columns.

www.teachnet.com	provides several PowerPoint presentations that can be adapted to make materials that feature game show formats, e.g., *Jeopardy* or *Who Wants To Be a Millionaire.*
www.searsportrait.com/StoryBook/StoryBook_StoryIndex.asp?tag	can be used to create personalized stories and letters by entering answers to questions; results can be printed out.
www.puzzle-maker.com/CW	online crossword puzzle makers that can be used for word-finding problems, vocabulary work, or articulation practice.

www.digitalbookindex.com/	links to 1,200 free online versions of many classic children's books. Can be used in a parent–child literacy program. Other free online book sites are listed in Kuster's column in the *ASHA Leader* May 11, 2004.

Another place to look for information is organizations devoted to different disorders and special interests. All of the following sites have subdivisions that can be easily accessed, and many have links to other related sites. To find Web pages for organizations not listed here, type the name in the search box at google.com or yahoo.com.

www.asha.org	American Speech-Language-Hearing Association, a huge site that is a starting place for information. Its "Search for" window acts like a search engine within ASHA. Special Divisions number 1 (Language Learning and Education), 12 (Augmentative and Alternative Communication), 14 (Communication Disorders and Sciences in Culturally and Linguistically Diverse Populations), and 16 (School-Based Issues) are especially good for current material. Represents a good source of different types of continuing education.
www.interdys.org	International Dsylexia Association
www.reading.org/index.html	International Reading Association
www.nea.org/index.html	National Education Association
www.ala.org/Template.cfm? Section=proftools	American Library Association
www.ed.gov	U.S. Department of Education. This is another huge site but very helpful for all aspects of education.
www.autism-society.org	Autism Society of America
www.asperger.org	Asperger Association
www.biausa.org/	Brain Injury Association of America
www.nifl.gov/	National Institute of Literacy
www.isaac-online.org	International Society of Augmentative & Alternative Communication

Be sure to check your own state's department of education site. In addition to volumes of general information, statistical and otherwise, on educational matters, most such sites have helpful links to developing IEPs that meet both federal and specific state requirements. These sites can be found through Google or Yahoo. One example, from North Dakota: http://www.dpi.state.nd.us/speced/guide/iep/index.shtm

Listed below is a very small sampling of the many sites dealing with curriculum or grade-level activities from pre-K through Grade 12; many contain links to additional Web sites that feature related material. Some of the activities and lesson plans are directed at classroom teachers, but you can use them to familiarize yourself with curriculum or adapt them to meet your speech–language goals. Many sites provide speech–language therapy ideas directly, including sites that focus on reading or subcategories of language areas, e.g. vocabulary. Although some of these are commercial sites that sell materials, all of them contain activities, lesson plans, and so forth that can be downloaded without cost.

www.funbrain.com	educational activities by grade level and subject; games adaptable for speech–language goals; grammar games for beginners and more advanced students.
teacher.scholastic.com	many activities tied to their materials are common in school curricula.
teacher.scholastic.com/lessonplans/graphicorg/	a subsite of *Scholastic, Inc.* that features graphic organizers for teaching organizational schemas and strategies that can be downloaded.
www.mcrel.org/standards-benchmarks/(Mid Continent Research for Education and Learning)	general site with lesson plans and activities, plus standards for writing, reading, listening, and speaking.
www.edstandards.org/StSu/ELA.html	an index of sources of information about standards and curriculum frameworks taken from sites (national, state, local, and other). The sites can be accessed directly. This site has not been updated recently, but the list of sources is valuable.
www.wordcentral.com (Merriam-Webster)	an interactive site for building language, complete with daily buzzwords, spelling bee quizzes, student dictionaries, etc.
www.creativekidsathome.com/activities	craft ideas, recipes, science projects, with links to 100 other craft sites and specific links for parents and teachers; could be used in conjunction with literature or social studies.

www.lessonplanz.com	lists children's books with activities to go with them; how to use computers and technology in the classroom; sections on phonemic awareness, spelling and writing; how to use literacy centers; printable books for emergent readers; lesson plans by topic and grade including special education.
school.discovery.com/ lessonplans/	lesson plans written by teachers organized by subject, grade (K–12), or both. Many are science based; easily adjusted to speech–language goals.
www.lessonplanspage.com	lesson plans for Grades pre-K through high school, searchable by subject and grade level. Includes art, music, health, and computers; easily adjustable to speech–language goals; can sign up for a free lesson plans newsletter.
teachology.com/ webtools	good source of other Web sites; curriculum, lesson plans, Web site reviews, printable lesson plans and activities, scoring rubrics (e.g., for scoring paragraph writing, oral presentations, many others), thematic units; links for "teacher" subjects: behavior management, parent conferences, bulletin boards. See this site also under crossword puzzles.
www.ccc.commnet.edu/ grammar	an information treasure for all aspects of syntax at various grade levels.
http://www.eduref.org/ cgi-bin/lessons.cgi/ Language_Arts/Reading	educator's reference desk; a large site with resources for many subject areas, including language arts. One activity involves reading lesson plans to be used with specific, commonly used children's books.
www.nationalgeo graphic.com/kids/	games, activites, experiments, downloadable coloring books of animals, etc.; children's magazine. Good for social studies.
www.lessonplancentral.com	worksheets; links for children; Web quests. Clipart; lesson plans.
www.atozteacherstuff.com	teacher-created lesson plans, thematic units; source of online resources, downloadable teacher material.
www.reading.org/resources/ index.html	book lists for the classroom; parent resources, position statements regarding reading; lesson plans.

enchantedlearning.com/home.html	many printable activity sheets based on themes, plus geography, history, language, science, and writing materials for K–12.
www.abcteach.com	reading comprehension, math, writing, handwriting, colors, shapes, theme units tied to curriculum, plus information on student portfolios; 5,000 pages of free printable pages and worksheets.
www.funschool.com	games on computer to be used in a lab or classroom; adaptable to speech–language goals; printable interactive games by grade, pre K–6, e.g., a matching rhyme game with sound and colorful graphics.
www.nick.com/all_nick/tv_supersites/spongebob/main.jhtml	an example of one Web site to familiarize yourself with programs popular with children. Find sites featuring other characters by typing in the name of the character on Google or Yahoo.
newslink.org	links to worldwide newspapers and 4,000 U.S. online newspapers; helpful for social studies alternate sources.
www.onelook.com	a search engine for words and phrases, providing definitions for more than 5 million words; also a general dictionary clearinghouse site: can link to specific dictionary sites for sports words, technology words, etc.
www.quia.com/dir/speechandlanguagetherapy	activities for articulation and language, e.g., analogies, WH questions.
home.comcast.net/~speechguide/sample.html	therapy ideas for different areas, e.g., apraxia, articulation, augmentative communication, autism spectrum disorders, fluency, language pragmatics, and voice.
www.cyberbee.com	how to integrate the Internet into the classroom curriculum. Includes many projects and how to use the Web in class.
www.pbs.org/teachersource	lesson plans related to PBS programs; allows users to build a personal profile for future use.
www.apraxia-kids.org/resources/online.html	links for activities for students with articulation deficits, including home activities, a moving diagram of the articulators, a sign language dictionary, and a materials exchange.

www.education-world.com/	sample curriculum-oriented lesson plans; links to individual state standards; search engine for lesson plans by topic, e.g., idioms.
www.speakingofspeech.com	a site to exchange ideas, techniques, lesson plans, advice through e-mails with other school-based SLPs; supplies links to other sites; free items.

For current assessment information relating to specific instruments, contact the publisher online.

www.proedinc.com	PRO-ED, Inc.
www.linguisystems.com	LinguiSystems
www.PsychCorp.com (now harcourtassessment.com)	The Psychological Corporation
www.acadcom.com	Academic Communication Associates
www.thinkingpublications.com	Thinking Publications
www.agsnet.com	American Guidance Service

Index

About the Authors

Helen Arvidson

Helen Arvidson provides speech–language services at the Porter County Education Interlocal in Valparaiso, Indiana. Dr. Arvidson has presented at conferences on the topic of AAC. She is a co-editor of *Augmentative and Alternative Communication: New Directions in Research and Practice*. Dr. Arvidson is co-editing the Augmentative and Alternative Perspectives Series, which currently includes *The Efficacy of Augmentative and Alternative Communication: Toward Evidence-Based Practice* and *Literacy and Augmentative and Alternative Communication.*

Arlene Balestra-Marko

Arlene Balestra-Marco, AuD, is a licensed audiologist and a certified auditory verbal therapist. She founded *Hear 2 Learn,* which provides a variety of services to children with cochlear implants and to their parents and families. *Hear 2 Learn* serves many children with cochlear implants living in the central New York area.

Karen Browning

Karen Browning holds a BA in special education, an MS in curriculum and instruction, and certification in occupational therapy. She was a teacher of special education before the enactment of P.L. 94-142 and now serves as a school-based occupational therapist. She primarily serves adolescent students; her therapeutic focus is on providing appropriate transitions as students move from the elementary grades to secondary education to work sites. She recently contributed to the development of *Guidelines for School Based Occupational and Physical Therapists for the State of Missouri.*

Li-Rong Lilly Cheng

Li-Rong Lilly Cheng is a professor in the Department of Communication Disorders at San Diego State University. She has a wealth of experience working with bilingual children and adults. Dr. Cheng has made multiple presentations and published several books and numerous professional articles. She is an ASHA Fellow and has received the Multicultural Affairs Award from ASHA. She is on the editorial board of several major journals and has served on ASHA's Legislative Council.

Nanette Clapper

Nanette Clapper holds the Certificate of Clinical Competence in Speech Pathology and was a school-based speech–language pathologist for 10 years in a school serving children from kindergarten through Grade 12. She has published articles, including one on a program to integrate language therapy into the classroom setting. She has also worked in private practice, specializing in auditory processing disorders and apraxia. She has presented on these topics throughout New York State. Currently she is a speech pathologist–2 at the New York State Office of Mental Retardation and Developmental Disabilities.

Tracy Crouch

Tracy Crouch has a BA in speech therapy, a master's degree in speech pathology, and a Certificate of Clinical Competence in speech pathology. She provided early intervention services during the first years of her career before moving to the schools. She has worked as a school-based SLP in Grades K–4 for 13 years in central New York and is known in the area for her innovative therapy techniques. She is interested in autism spectrum disorders and has worked extensively with students with Asperger syndrome. She sees herself "as a teacher first" and is involved in all aspects of the educational system in her school.

Regina B. Grantham

Regina Grantham is chair of the Department of Speech Pathology and Audiology at the State University of New York at Cortland. She has been very active in ASHA, serving on its Legislative Council, ASHA-PAC, and a variety of committees. She has recently been named an ASHA Fellow. She was a member of the task force that developed the ASHA position statement on social dialects. She has presented and authored chapters on African American English and multicultural assessment and treatment. She has served on the New York State Licensure Board and has also presented and written on ethics in speech–language pathology and audiology.

Eileen H. Gravani

Eileen Gravani is an assistant professor in the Department of Speech Pathology and Audiology at the State University of New York at Cortland. She has worked in the public schools and now teaches in the areas of language development, phonetics, and phonology and teaching children with limited English proficiency; she also supervises speech pathology students during their student teaching placements. Currently, Dr. Gravani is working on a research project with Jacqueline Meyer on preliteracy intervention. Dr. Gravani has presented on this topic, as well as on methods to incorporate New York State learning standards into speech–language goals.

Nancy P. Huffman

Nancy P. Huffman is an audiologist and retired from the Board of Cooperative Educational Services No. 1, Monroe County, New York as Chair of Speech–Language and Audiology Services. She is an ASHA Fellow and has received the ASHA Outstanding Service Award and the Van Hattum Award from ASHA for her work in educational audiology. She has presented and written in this area and has co-authored (with Mary Ann O'Brien) a manual, *A Comparison of Federal Regulations as Regarding Provision of Related Services in Schools: IDEA, Section 504 of the Vocational Rehabilitation Act and the ADA.* She is the co-author with Susan Brannen, Joan Marttila, and Evelyn Williams of an issues brief submitted by ASHA to the Center for Personnel Studies in Special Education (COPSE) titled *Audiology Services in the School Issues Brief.* She continues to consult on topics relating to audiology both in New York State and nationally.

Donna McGhie-Richmond

Donna McGhie-Richmond, PhD, is a special educator with over 25 years experience. She has worked in clinical, academic, and research capacities in the field of augmentative and alternative communication (AAC) for 15 years. She has taught in the preservice and graduate education programs at the Ontario Institute for Studies in Education of the University of Toronto, Canada. She is currently an instructor in the Department of Educational Psychology at the University of Alberta, Canada. She has been involved in a variety of research and community development projects related to children, youth, and adults who have special learning needs and has presented locally and internationally.

Jacqueline Meyer

Jacqueline Meyer is lecturer Emerita in the Department of Speech Pathology and Audiology at the State University College at Cortland. She has worked extensively in the public schools, receiving grants and awards for innovative approaches to therapy. At the college level, she taught in the areas of assessment and intervention and providing speech–language services in the public schools. She is working in preliteracy research with Eileen Gravani. She has presented on that topic, as well as on innovative teaching and therapy programs and on incorporating the New York State learning standards into students' speech–language goals.

Jill Modafferi

Jill Modafferi holds a BS in elementary and special education and an MA in learning disabilities. She served as a special education teacher for 15 years in a variety of settings, including self-contained and resource rooms. For the past 12 years she has taught fifth grade. She has received a number of grants and served on too many committees to mention, including various curriculum committees, the school improvement team, and a committee to revamp report cards. Her particular area of professional interest is written language: "giving the kids the tools they need to write."

Kim M. Nevins

Kim Nevins holds a BS in physical therapy, an MS in adaptive physical education, and a PhD in educational counseling and psychology. Her research deals with best practice for school-based physical therapists. She has worked in critical care and pediatrics in the hospital setting. She was the coordinator of occupational therapy, physical therapy, and adaptive physical therapy for the Columbia Missouri Public School system. Currently, she is an assistant professor in the Department of Physical Therapy, School of Health Professions, University of Missouri, Columbia. Her primary area of interest is school-based practice and the appropriate use of physical therapy and occupational therapy services in schools. She recently contributed to the development of *Guidelines for School Based Occupational and Physical Therapists for the State of Missouri.*

Mary Ann O'Brien

Mary Ann O'Brien is a speech–language pathologist and is retired from the Board of Cooperative Educational Services No. 1, Monroe County, New York, as director of support services. She is a past president of the New York State Speech Language and Hearing Association. She served on the NYS Licensure Board and on the ASHA Task Force on IDEA Regulations. She testified before Congress on the reauthorization of IDEA. She is an ASHA Fellow. She has published a variety of articles and recently co-authored (with Nancy Huffman) a manual, *A Comparison of Federal Regulations as Regarding Provision of Related Services in Schools: IDEA, Section 504 of the Vocational Rehabilitation Act and the ADA.*

Luis Riquelme

Luis Riquelme is a lecturer in the Department of Communication Sciences and Disorders at Long Island University, Brooklyn Campus. He is the co-director of Riquelme & Santos, PC, a private practice in Brooklyn. He has been president of the New York State Speech-Language-Hearing Association and serves on state and national committees. He has presented locally and nationally on the topics of multiculturalism and bilingualism, dysphagia, report writing, and quality improvement for service delivery.

Linda Robinson

Linda Robinson is the coordinator of library and media services for Mansfield Connecticut Public Schools. She has worked in a variety of different libraries: academic, school, public and community, as well as special libraries. She has presented to a variety of audiences on technology and currently has a large grant from the State of Connecticut to assess how hand-held computers assist learning. She is enrolled in a doctoral program in adult learning in the School of Education, University of Connecticut.

Ralf W. Schlosser

Ralf W. Schlosser is an associate professor in the Department of Speech Pathology and Audiology at Northeastern University. He is frequently consulted on matters concerning augmentative and alternative communication (AAC) in the schools. He has presented and written a variety of articles on AAC and is co-author of *The Efficacy of Augmentative and Alternative Communication.* He is currently involved in research on the effect of synthetic speech output and visually displayed feedback on spelling in children with autism.

Joseph Sheedy

Joseph Sheedy has a BS in elementary education, an MS in special education, and a Certificate of Advanced Study in school psychology. He has worked as a school psychologist for 16 years in a K–8 school in central New York. He also sees children privately. His private practice reflects his area of particular professional interests, learning disabilities and emotional disturbances. In recent years, he has become increasingly interested in neuropsychology.